POCKET GUIDE TO
Psychiatric
Nursing

ELEVENTH EDITION

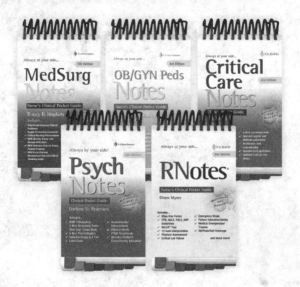

POCKET GUIDE TO
Psychiatric Nursing

ELEVENTH EDITION

Karyn I. Morgan, RN, MSN, APRN, CNS
Psychiatric Clinical Nurse Specialist
Professor of Instruction
University of Akron
Akron, Ohio

Mary C. Townsend, DSN, PMHCNS-BC
Clinical Specialist/Nurse Consultant
Adult Psychiatric Mental Health Nursing
Former Assistant Professor and
Coordinator, Mental Health Nursing
Kramer School of Nursing
Oklahoma City University
Oklahoma City, Oklahoma

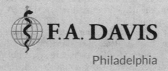

F.A. DAVIS
Philadelphia

F. A. Davis Company
1915 Arch Street
Philadelphia, PA 19103
www.fadavis.com

Printed in the United States of America

Last digit indicates print number: 10 9 8 7 6 5 4 3 2

Publisher, Nursing: Susan Rhyner
Senior Content Project Manager: Amy M. Romano
Design and Illustrations Manager: Carolyn O'Brien

As new scientific information becomes available through basic and clinical research, recommended treatments and drug therapies undergo changes. The author(s) and publisher have done everything possible to make this book accurate, up to date, and in accord with accepted standards at the time of publication. The author(s), editors, and publisher are not responsible for errors or omissions or for consequences from application of the book, and make no warranty, expressed or implied, in regard to the contents of the book. Any practice described in this book should be applied by the reader in accordance with professional standards of care used in regard to the unique circumstances that may apply in each situation. The reader is advised always to check product information (package inserts) for changes and new information regarding dose and contraindications before administering any drug. Caution is especially urged when using new or infrequently ordered drugs.

Library of Congress Cataloging-in-Publication Data

Names: Townsend, Mary C., 1941- author. | Morgan, Karyn I., author.
Title: Pocket guide to psychiatric nursing / Karyn I. Morgan,
  Mary C. Townsend.
Description: 11th edition. | Philadelphia : F.A. Davis, [2021] |
  Mary C. Townsend's name appears first in the previous edition. | Includes
  bibliographical references and index.
Identifiers: LCCN 2020026062 (print) | LCCN 2020026063 (ebook) |
  ISBN 9780803699953 (library binding) | ISBN 9781719643016 (ebook)
Subjects: MESH: Mental Disorders—nursing | Nursing Diagnosis | Patient
  Care Planning | Psychotropic Drugs—therapeutic use | Handbook
  Classification: LCC RC440 (print) | LCC RC440 (ebook) | NLM WY 49 |
  DDC 616.89/0231—dc23
LC record available at https://lccn.loc.gov/2020026062
LC ebook record available at https://lccn.loc.gov/2020026063

I dedicate this book to my mother Mary, my sister Cindy, and my Aunt Jane; the three most inspirational nurses and women in my life.

Karyn I. Morgan

To my husband, Jim, who encouraged and supported me throughout all my writing projects, and whose love continues to nurture and sustain me, even after 56 years.

To my daughters Kerry and Tina, my grandchildren Meghan, Matthew, and Catherine, and my sons-in-law Ryan and Jonathan. You are the joys of my life.

And finally, to the memory of my father and mother, Francis and Camalla Welsh, who reared my sister Francie and me without knowledge of psychology or developmental theories, but with the kind of unconditional love I have come to believe is so vital to the achievement and maintenance of emotional wellness.

Mary C. Townsend

Consultants

Maude H. Alston, RN, PhD
Assistant Professor of Nursing
University of North Carolina at Greensboro
Greensboro, North Carolina

Betty J. Carmack, RN, EdD
Assistant Professor
University of San Francisco
School of Nursing
San Francisco, California

Doris K. DeVincenzo, PhD
Professor
Pace University
Lienhard School of Nursing
Pleasantville, New York

Mary Jo Gorney-Fadiman, RN, PhD
Assistant Professor
San Jose State University
School of Nursing
San Jose, California

Mary E. Martucci, RN, PhD
Associate Professor and Chairman
Saint Mary's College
Notre Dame, Indiana

Sheridan V. McCabe, BA, BSN, MSN, PhD
Assistant Professor of Nursing
University of Virginia
School of Nursing
Charlottesville, Virginia

Elizabeth Anne Rankin, PhD
Psychotherapist and Consultant
University of Maryland
School of Nursing
Baltimore, Maryland

Judith M. Saunders, DNS, FAAN
Postdoctoral Research Fellow
University of Washington
School of Nursing
Seattle, Washington

Gail Stuart, RN, CS, PhD
Associate Professor
Medical University of South Carolina
College of Nursing
Charleston, South Carolina

Reviewers

Susan Atwood
Faculty
Antelope Valley College
Lancaster, California

Jaynee R. Boucher, MS, RN
St. Joseph's College of Nursing
Syracuse, New York

Sherry Campbell
Allegany College of Maryland
Cumberland, Maryland

Lorraine Chiappetta
Professor
Washtenaw Community College
Ann Arbor, Michigan

Ileen Craven
Instructor
Roxborough Memorial Hospital
Philadelphia, Pennsylvania

Marcy Echternacht
College of St. Mary
Omaha, Nebraska

Susan Feinstein
Instructor, Psychiatric Nursing
Cochran School of Nursing
Yonkers, New York

Mavonne Gansen
Northeast Iowa Community College
Peosta, Iowa

Diane Gardner
Assistant Professor
University of West Florida
Pensacola, Florida

Jo Anne C. Jackson, EdD, RN
Middle Georgia College
Cochran, Georgia

Elizabeth Kawecki
South University
Royal Palm Beach, Florida

Florence Keane, DNSc, MSN, BSN
Assistant Professor
Florida International University
Miami, Florida

Gayle Massie, MSN, RN
Professor
Shawnee State University
Portsmouth, Ohio

Mary McClay
Walla Walla University
Portland, Oregon

Judith Nolen
Clinical Assistant Professor
University of Arizona
Tucson, Arizona

Pamela Parlocha
California State University–East Bay
Hayward, California

Joyce Rittenhouse
Burlington County College
Pemberton, New Jersey

Phyllis Rowe, DNP, RN, ANP
Riverside Community College
Riverside, California

Georgia Seward
Baptist Health Schools–Little Rock
Little Rock, Arkansas

Anna Shanks
Shoreline Community College
Seattle, Washington

Rhonda Snow
Stillman College
Tuscaloosa, Alabama

Karen Tarnow, RN, PhD
Clinical Associate Professor
University of Kansas Medical Center
Kansas City, Kansas

Shirley Weiglein
South University
Tampa, Florida

Tammie Willis
Penn Valley Community College
Kansas City, Missouri

Acknowledgments

Special thanks and appreciation:

To Susan Rhyner, who provides ongoing wisdom and encouragement; to Amy Romano for her expertise, organizational skills, and availability and to Kathleen Scogna for all of her brilliant queries.

To the editorial and production staffs of the F. A. Davis Company, who are always willing to provide assistance when requested and whose consistent excellence in publishing is a special blessing.

To the gracious individuals who read and critiqued the original manuscript, providing valuable input into the final product.

And finally, a special acknowledgment to the nurses who staff the psychiatric units of the clinical agencies where nursing students go to learn about psychiatric nursing. To those of you who willingly share your knowledge and expertise with, and act as role models for, these nursing students: you are the heroes of our profession, and we hope this book provides a useful tool to support your efforts.

Karyn Morgan and Mary Townsend

Contents

UNIT THREE

SPECIAL TOPICS IN PSYCHIATRIC-MENTAL HEALTH NURSING

Introduction

■ *How to Use This Book*

This book is designed as a guide in the construction of care plans for various psychiatric clients. The concepts are presented in such a manner that they may be applied to various types of health-care settings: inpatient hospitalization, outpatient clinic, home health, partial hospitalization, and private practice, to name a few. Major divisions in the book are identified by psychiatric diagnostic categories as they appear in the *Diagnostic and Statistical Manual of Mental Disorders (DSM-5)* (American Psychiatric Association [APA], 2013). The nursing diagnoses used in this textbook are from the nomenclature of Taxonomy II that has been adopted by NANDA International (NANDA-I, 2018). The use of this format is not to imply that nursing diagnoses are based on, or flow from, medical diagnoses; it is meant only to enhance the usability of the book. It is valid, however, to state that certain nursing diagnoses are indeed common to individuals with specific psychiatric disorders.

In addition, nursing diagnoses presented with each psychiatric category are not intended to be all-inclusive. The diagnoses presented in this book are intended to be used as guidelines for construction of care plans that must be individualized for each patient on the basis of the nursing assessment. The interventions can also be used in areas in which interdisciplinary treatment plans take the place of the nursing care plan.

Each chapter in Unit Two begins with an overview of information related to the psychiatric diagnostic category, which may be useful to the nurse as background assessment data. This section includes:

1. **The Disorder:** A definition and common types or categories that have been identified.
2. **Predisposing Factors:** Information regarding theories of etiology, which the nurse may use in formulating the "related to" portion of the nursing diagnosis, as it applies to the patient.
3. **Symptomatology:** Subjective and objective data identifying behaviors common to the disorder. These behaviors, as they apply to the individual patient, may be pertinent to the "evidenced by" portion of the nursing diagnosis.

Information presented with each nursing diagnosis includes the following:

1. **Definition:** The approved NANDA definition from the Taxonomy II nomenclature (NANDA-I, 2018).
2. **Possible Etiologies ("related to"):** This section suggests possible causes for the problem identified. Those not listed by NANDA-I are identified by brackets [ ].
3. **Related/Risk Factors** are given for diagnoses for which the patient is at risk. *Note:* **Defining characteristics are replaced by "related/risk factors" for the "Risk for" diagnoses.**
4. **Defining Characteristics ("evidenced by"):** This section includes signs and symptoms that may be evident to indicate that the problem exists. Again, as with etiologies, those not identified by NANDA-I are noted by brackets [ ].
5. **Goals/Objectives:** These statements are made in patient behavioral objective terminology. They are measurable short- and long-term goals, to be used in evaluating the effectiveness of the nursing interventions in alleviating the identified problem. There may be more than one short-term goal, and they may be considered "stepping stones" to fulfillment of the long-term goal. For purposes of this book, "long-term," in most instances, is designated as "by time of discharge from treatment," whether the patient is in an inpatient or outpatient setting.
6. **Interventions with *Selected Rationales:*** Only those interventions that are appropriate to a particular nursing diagnosis within the context of the psychiatric setting are presented. Rationales for selected interventions are included to provide clarification beyond fundamental nursing knowledge and to assist in the selection of appropriate interventions for individual patients. Important interventions related to communication may be identified by a communication icon.
7. **Outcome Criteria:** These are behavioral changes that can be used as criteria to determine the extent to which the nursing diagnosis has been resolved.

To use this book in the preparation of psychiatric nursing care plans, find the section in the text applicable to the patient's psychiatric diagnosis. Review background data pertinent to the diagnosis, if needed. Complete a biopsychosocial history and assessment on the patient. Select and prioritize nursing diagnoses appropriate to the patient. Using the list of NANDA-I approved nursing diagnoses, be sure to include those that are patient-specific and not just those that have been identified as "common" to a particular psychiatric diagnosis. Select nursing interventions and outcome criteria appropriate to the patient for each nursing diagnosis identified. Include all of this information on the care plan, along with a date for evaluating the status of each problem. On the evaluation date, document success of the nursing interventions in achieving the goals of care, using the desired patient outcomes as criteria. Modify the plan as required.

Unit Three addresses patient populations with special psychiatric nursing needs. These include survivors of abuse or neglect, patients at risk for suicide, patients who are homeless, patients who are experiencing bereavement, and military families. Topics related to forensic nursing, psychiatric home nursing care, and complementary therapies are also included.

Unit Four, Psychotropic Medications, has been updated to include new medications that have been approved by the FDA since the last edition. This information should facilitate use of the book for nurses administering psychotropic medications and also for nurse practitioners with prescriptive authority. The major categories of psychotropic medications are differentiated by chemical class. Information is presented related to indications, actions, contraindications and precautions, interactions, route and dosage, and adverse reactions and side effects. Examples of medications in each chemical class are presented by generic and trade name, along with information about half-life, controlled substance schedules and available forms of the medication. Therapeutic plasma level ranges are provided, where appropriate. Nursing diagnoses related to each category, along with nursing interventions, and patient and family education are included in each chapter.

Another helpful feature of this text is the table in Appendix L, which lists some patient behaviors commonly observed in the psychiatric setting and the most appropriate nursing diagnosis for each. It is hoped that this information will broaden the understanding of the need to use a variety of nursing diagnoses in preparing the patient treatment plan.

This book helps to familiarize the nurse with the current NANDA-I approved nursing diagnoses and provides information useful to clinical reasoning and clinical judgment in the preparation of nursing care plans. It is expected that additional information will be required for each nursing diagnosis as the nurse individualizes care for psychiatric patients.

 INTERNET REFERENCES

- https://www.apna.org
- www.nanda.org
- www.ispn-psych.org

Index of *DSM-5* Psychiatric Diagnoses

THE FOUNDATION FOR PLANNING PSYCHIATRIC NURSING CARE

CHAPTER **1**

The Nursing Process in Psychiatric-Mental Health Nursing

Nursing has struggled for many years to achieve recognition as a profession. Out of this struggle has emerged an awareness of the need to do the following:

1. Define the boundaries of nursing (What is nursing?).
2. Identify a scientific method for delivering nursing care.

The American Nurses Association (ANA, no date) presents the following description:

> Beyond the time-honored reputation for compassion and dedication lies a highly specialized profession that is constantly evolving to address the needs of society. From ensuring the most accurate diagnoses to the ongoing education of the public about critical health issues, nurses are indispensable in safeguarding public health…. Through the critical thinking exemplified in the nursing process, nurses use their judgment to integrate objective data with subjective experience of a patient's biological, physical, and behavioral needs. This ensures that every patient, from city hospital to community health center, state prison to summer camp, receives the best possible care regardless of who they are, or where they may be.

The nursing process has been identified as nursing's scientific methodology for the delivery of nursing care. The curricula of most nursing schools include nursing process as a component of their conceptual frameworks. The National Council of State Boards of Nursing (NCSBN) has integrated the nursing process throughout the test plan for the National Council Licensure Examination for Registered Nurses (NCSBN, 2016). Questions that relate to nursing behaviors in a variety of patient situations are presented according to the steps of the nursing process:

1. **Assessment:** Establishing a database on a patient.
2. **Diagnosis:** Identifying the patient's health-care needs and selecting goals of care.
3. **Outcome Identification:** Establishing criteria for measuring achievement of desired outcomes.
4. **Planning:** Designing a strategy to achieve the goals established for patient care.
5. **Implementation:** Initiating and completing actions necessary to accomplish the goals.
6. **Evaluation:** Determining the extent to which the goals of care have been achieved.

By following these six steps, the nurse has a systematic framework for decision making and problem-solving in the delivery of nursing care. The nursing process is dynamic, not static. It is an ongoing process that continues for as long as the nurse and patient have interactions directed toward change in the patient's physical or behavioral responses. Figure 1–1 presents a schematic of the ongoing nursing process.

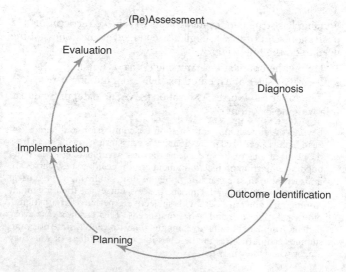

FIGURE 1–1 The ongoing nursing process.

Diagnosis is an integral part of the nursing process. In this step, the nurse identifies the human responses to actual or potential health problems. In some states, diagnosing is identified within the nurse practice act as a legal responsibility of the professional nurse. Nursing diagnosis provides the basis for prescribing the specific interventions for which the nurse is accountable.

As an inherent part of the nursing process, nursing diagnosis is included in the ANA Standards of Practice. These standards provide one broad basis for evaluating practice and reflect recognition of the person's rights when receiving nursing care (ANA, 2015).

■ CONCEPT MAPPING

Concept mapping is a diagrammatic teaching and learning strategy that allows students and faculty to visualize interrelationships between medical diagnoses, nursing diagnoses, assessment data, and treatments. Concept maps have been used in other professions, such as engineering and instructional design, to organize and visualize different aspects of a concept. When applied to nursing, the concept map is a strategy for planning, organizing, and visualizing nursing care. Basically, it is a diagram of patient problems and interventions. Compared to the commonly used column-format care plans, concept map care plans provide a more succinct picture of various factors as they influence nursing care. As nursing continues to explore ways to promote the Quality and Safety in Education for Nurses (QSEN) competency related to teamwork and collaboration, the concept map can be expanded to describe interdisciplinary relationships and their impact on nursing care. For example, medical interventions such as prescribing medication and social services interventions with regard to discharge planning will influence nursing care and may be visualized in the concept map. The concept map is a visual, adaptable, creative way to conceptualize nursing care and serves to enhance critical-thinking skills and clinical reasoning ability.

The nursing process is foundational to developing and using the concept map care plan, just as it is with all types of nursing care plans. Patient data are collected and analyzed, nursing diagnoses are formulated, outcome criteria are identified, nursing actions are planned and implemented, and the success of the interventions in meeting the outcome criteria is evaluated.

The concept map care plan may be presented in its entirety on one page, or the assessment data and nursing diagnoses may appear in diagram format on one page, with outcomes, interventions, and evaluation written on a second page. Additionally, the diagram may appear in circular format, with nursing diagnoses and interventions branching off the "patient" in the center of the diagram. Or, it may begin with the "patient" at the top of the diagram, with branches emanating in a linear fashion downward.

Since the concept map care plan is based on the components of the nursing process, it is assembled in a stepwise fashion, beginning with the patient and his or her reason for needing care, nursing diagnoses with subjective and objective clinical evidence for each, nursing interventions, and outcome criteria for evaluation.

Various colors may be used in the diagram to designate various components of the care plan. Lines are drawn to connect the various components to indicate any relationships that exist. For example, there may be a relationship between two nursing diagnoses (e.g., there may be a relationship between the nursing diagnoses of pain, anxiety, and disturbed sleep pattern). A line between these nursing diagnoses should be drawn to show the relationship.

Concept map care plans allow for a great deal of creativity on the part of the user, and they permit viewing the "whole picture" without generating a great deal of paperwork. Concept map care plans may also provide valuable guides for documentation of patient care.

An example of one format for a concept map care plan is presented in Figure 1–2.

The purpose of this book is to assist students and staff nurses as they endeavor to provide high-quality nursing care to their psychiatric patients. Following is an example of a nursing history and assessment tool that may be used to gather information about the patient during the assessment phase of the nursing process.

■ NURSING HISTORY AND ASSESSMENT TOOL

I. General Information

Patient name:_____ Allergies: _____

Room number:_____ Diet: _____

Doctor: _____ Height/weight: _____

Age: _____ Vital signs: TPR/BP _____

Sex: _____ Name and phone no. of
  significant other: _____

Race: _____

Dominant language:_____ City of residence: _____

Marital status: _____ Diagnosis (admitting
  & current): _____

Chief complaint:_____ _____

_____ _____

II. Conditions of Admission

Date: _____ Time: _____
Accompanied by: _____
Route of admission (wheelchair; ambulatory; cart): _____
Admitted from: _____

III. Precipitating Event

Describe the situation or events that precipitated this illness/hospitalization (patient's perception and family's or significant other's perception when available): _____
_____
_____

III. Predisposing Factors

A. Family History and Genetic Vulnerabilities

1. Family configuration (use genograms):
   Family of origin: _____ Present family: _____
   Family dynamics (describe significant relationships between family members):
   _____
   _____
   _____
   _____

2. Medical/psychiatric history:
   a. Patient:
   _____
   _____

   b. Family members:
   _____
   _____

3. Other family and/or genetic influences affecting present adaptation not addressed elsewhere in the assessment:
   _____

B. Past Experiences

1. Cultural and social history:
   a. Environmental factors (family living arrangements, type of neighborhood, special working conditions):
   _____
   _____
   _____

   b. Health beliefs and practices (personal responsibility for health; special self-care practices): _____
   _____
   _____

   c. Religious beliefs and practices: _____
   _____
   _____

    d. Educational background: _____

    _____

    e. Significant losses/changes (include dates): _____

    _____

    f. Peer/friendship relationships: _____

    _____

    g. Occupational history: _____

    _____

    h. Previous pattern of coping with stress: _____

    _____

    i. Other lifestyle factors contributing to present
       adaptation: _____

    _____

    _____

C. *Existing Conditions*
    1. Stage of development (Erikson):
       a. Theoretically: _____
       b. Behaviorally: _____
       c. Rationale: _____

    _____

    2. Patient perception of support systems: _____

    _____

    3. Patient perception of economic security: _____

    _____

    4. Avenues of productivity/contribution:
       a. Current job status: _____

    _____

       b. Role contributions and responsibility for others:

    _____

IV. Patient's Perception of the Stressor

The patient's understanding or description of stressor/illness and
expectations of hospitalization (include family/significant other's
perception as available): _____

_____

_____

_____

V. Adaptation Responses

A. Psychosocial

1. Anxiety level (circle level, and check the behaviors that apply):

    Mild   *Moderate*   *Severe*   *Panic*

    Calm _____ Friendly _____ Passive _____
    Alert _____ Perceives environment correctly _____
    Cooperative _____ Impaired attention _____
    "Jittery" _____ Unable to concentrate _____
    Hypervigilant _____ Tremors _____ Rapid speech _____
    Withdrawn _____ Confused _____
    Disoriented _____ Fearful _____ Hyperventilating _____
    Misinterpreting the environment _____
    Hallucinations   Yes   No
    (if yes, describe) _____
    _____
    Delusions   Yes   No
    (if yes, describe) _____
    _____
    Depersonalization _____ Obsessions _____
    Compulsions _____ Somatic complaints _____
    Excessive hyperactivity _____ Other _____
    Judgment: Intact _____ Impaired _____
    Associated behaviors: _____
    _____
    Insight: Intact _____ Impaired _____
    Associated patient statements: _____
    _____

2. Mood/affect (circle as many as apply):
    Happy   Sad   Dejected   Despondent
    Elated   Euphoric   Suspicious
    Apathetic (little emotional tone)   Angry/hostile

3. Patient's perception of self-esteem (circle one):
    Low   *Moderate*   *High*
    Things patient likes about self: _____
    _____
    Things patient would like to change about self: _____
    Nurse's objective assessment of self-esteem:
    _____
    Eye contact _____
    General appearance _____
    _____
    Personal hygiene _____
    Patient's interest in activities and interactions with others _____
    _____

4. Stage and manifestations of grief (circle one):
   *Denial   Anger   Bargaining   Depression
   Acceptance*
   Describe the patient's behaviors and communication
   that are associated with this stage of grieving in
   response to loss or change: _____
   _____
   _____

5. Thought processes (circle as many as apply):
Clear	Logical	Easy to follow	Relevant
Confused	Blocking	Delusional	Rapid flow of thoughts

   Thought retardation (slow thought   Suspicious
   processes)

6. Memory
Recent memory:	Loss	Intact
Remote memory:	Loss	Intact

   Other: _____
   _____

7. Communication patterns (circle as many as apply):
Clear	Coherent	Slurred speech	Incoherent

   Neologisms   Loose associations (disconnected
   thoughts)
   Flight of ideas (racing thoughts)
   Aphasic   Perseveration   Rumination
   Tangential   Loquaciousness
   speech
   Slow, impoverished speech
   Speech impediment (describe): _____
   Other: _____
   _____

8. Interaction patterns (describe the patient's pattern
   of interpersonal interactions with staff and peers on
   the unit; e.g., manipulative, withdrawn, isolated,
   verbally or physically hostile, argumentative, passive,
   assertive, aggressive, passive-aggressive, other):
   _____
   _____
   _____

9. Reality orientation (check those that apply):
   Oriented to: Time _____ Person _____
                   Place _____ Situation _____
10. Ideas of harm to self/others?   Yes   No
11. Nonsuicidal intent to self-injury?   Yes   No

12. Intent to die?   Yes   No
    If yes, consider plan; available means: _____
    _____
    _____
    _____

13. Previous history of ideation and/or attempts
    (describe): _____
    _____

14. Intensity of current ideation (if present): _____

15. Other risk factors: _____
    _____

16. Other warning signs: _____
    _____

B. *Physiological*

1. Psychosomatic manifestations (describe any somatic
   complaints that may be stress related): _____
   _____
   _____
   _____

2. Drug history and assessment:
   Use of prescribed drugs:

Name	*Dosage*	*Prescribed For*	*Results*

   Use of over-the-counter drugs (including herbal
   remedies):

Name	*Dosage*	*Used For*	*Results*

   Medication Side Effects:
   What symptoms is the patient experiencing that may
   be attributed to current medication usage?
   _____

   Use of street drugs or alcohol (include name of
   substance, how often used, when last used, effects
   produced): _____
   _____
   _____
   _____

3. Pertinent physical assessments:
   a. Respirations: Normal _____ Labored _____
      Rate _____ Rhythm _____
   b. Skin: Warm _____ Dry _____ Moist _____
      Cool _____ Clammy _____ Pink _____
      Cyanotic _____ Poor turgor _____ Edematous _____
      Evidence of: Rash _____ Bruising _____
      Needle tracks _____ Hirsutism _____ Loss of hair _____
      Other _____
   c. Musculoskeletal status: Weakness _____
      Tremors _____
      Degree of range of motion (describe limitations)
      _____
      _____
      Pain (describe) _____
      _____
      Skeletal deformities (describe) _____
      Coordination (describe limitations) _____
   d. Neurological status:
      History of (check all that apply):
      Seizures (describe method of control) _____
      _____
      Headaches (describe location and frequency) _____
      Fainting spells _____ Dizziness _____
      Tingling/numbness (describe location) _____
   e. Cardiovascular: B/P _____ Pulse _____
      History of (check all that apply):
      Hypertension _____ Palpitations _____
      Heart murmur _____ Chest pain _____
      Shortness of breath _____ Pain in legs _____
      Phlebitis _____ Ankle/leg edema _____
      Numbness/tingling in extremities _____
      Varicose veins _____
   f. Gastrointestinal:
      Usual diet pattern _____
      Food allergies _____
      Dentures? Upper _____ Lower _____
      Any problems with chewing or swallowing? _____
      Any recent change in weight? _____
      Any problems with:
      Indigestion/heartburn? _____
      Relieved by _____
      Nausea/vomiting? _____
      Relieved by _____
      History of ulcers? _____
      Usual bowel pattern _____
      Constipation? _____ Diarrhea? _____

Type of self-care assistance provided for either of the above problems _____

c. Genitourinary/Reproductive:
Usual voiding pattern _____
Urinary hesitancy? _____
Frequency? _____
Nocturia? _____ Pain/burning? _____
Incontinence? _____
Any genital lesions? _____
Discharge? _____ Odor? _____
History of sexually transmitted disease? _____
If yes, please explain: _____
_____

Any concerns about sexuality/sexual activity? _____
_____

Method of birth control used _____
Females:
Date of last menstrual cycle _____
Length of cycle _____
Problems associated with menstruation? _____
_____

Breasts: Pain/tenderness? _____
Swelling? _____ Discharge? _____
Lumps? _____ Dimpling? _____
Practice breast self-examination? _____
Frequency? _____
Males:
Penile discharge? _____
Prostate problems? _____

g. Eyes:

	Yes	No	Explain
Glasses?	____	____	_____
Contacts?	____	____	_____
Swelling?	____	____	_____
Discharge?	____	____	_____
Itching?	____	____	_____
Blurring?	____	____	_____
Double vision?	____	____	_____

h. Ears:

	Yes	No	Explain
Pain?	____	____	_____
Drainage?	____	____	_____
Difficulty hearing?	____	____	_____
Hearing aid?	____	____	_____
Tinnitus?	____	____	_____

i. Altered lab values and possible significance:
_____
_____

j. Activity/rest patterns:
Exercise (amount, type, frequency) _____
_____

Leisure time activities: _____
_____

Patterns of sleep: Number of hours per night ____
Use of sleep aids? _____
Pattern of awakening during the night? _____
Feel rested upon awakening? _____

k. Personal hygiene/activities of daily living:
Patterns of self-care: Independent _____
Requires assistance with: Mobility _____
                             Hygiene _____
                             Toileting _____
                             Feeding _____
                             Dressing _____
                             Other _____
Statement describing personal hygiene and
general appearance: _____
_____

l. Other pertinent physical assessments: _____
_____
_____

VII. Summary of Initial Psychosocial/Physical Assessment:

Knowledge Deficits Identified: _____
Nursing Diagnoses Indicated: _____

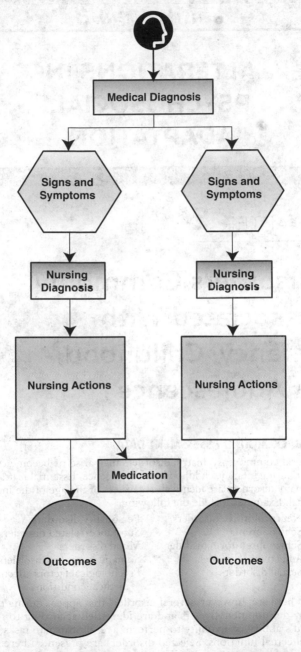

FIGURE 1–2 Example of a format for a concept map care plan.

ALTERATIONS IN PSYCHOSOCIAL ADAPTATION

CHAPTER **2**

Disorders Commonly Associated With Infancy, Childhood, or Adolescence

■ BACKGROUND ASSESSMENT DATA

Several common psychiatric disorders may arise or become evident during infancy, childhood, or adolescence. Essential features of many disorders are identical, regardless of the age of the individual. Examples include the following:

Neurocognitive disorders
Schizophrenia
Schizophreniform disorder
Adjustment disorder
Sexual disorders

Personality disorders
Substance-related disorders
Mood disorders
Somatic symptom disorders
Psychological factors affecting medical condition

There are, however, several disorders that appear during the early developmental years and are identified according to the child's ability or inability to perform age-appropriate tasks or intellectual functions. Selected disorders are presented here. It is essential that the nurse working with these patients understands normal behavior patterns characteristic of the infant, childhood, and adolescent years.

■ INTELLECTUAL DISABILITY (INTELLECTUAL DEVELOPMENTAL DISORDER)

Defined

The *Diagnostic and Statistical Manual of Mental Disorders, Fifth Edition* (*DSM-5*, American Psychiatric Association [APA], 2013) defines intellectual disability as a "disorder with onset during the developmental period that includes both intellectual and adaptive functioning deficits in conceptual, social, and practical domains" (p. 33). Onset of intellectual and adaptive deficits occurs during the developmental period. Level of severity (mild, moderate, severe, or profound) is based on adaptive functioning within the three domains.

Predisposing Factors

1. Physiological
   a. About 5% of cases of intellectual disability are caused by genetic factors, such as Tay-Sachs disease, phenylketonuria, and hyperglycinemia. Chromosomal disorders, such as Down syndrome and Klinefelter's syndrome, have also been implicated.
   b. Events that occur during the prenatal period (e.g., fetal malnutrition, viral and other infections, maternal ingestion of alcohol or other drugs, and uncontrolled diabetes) and perinatal period (e.g., birth trauma or premature separation of the placenta) can result in intellectual disability.
   c. Intellectual disability can occur as an outcome of childhood illnesses, such as encephalitis or meningitis, or be the result of poisoning or physical trauma in childhood.
2. Sociocultural Factors and Other Mental Disorders
   a. An estimated 15% to 20% of cases of intellectual disability may be attributed to deprivation of nurturance and social stimulation and to impoverished environments associated with poor prenatal and perinatal care and inadequate nutrition. Additionally, severe mental disorders, such as autism spectrum disorder, can result in intellectual disability.

Symptomatology (Subjective and Objective Data)

1. At the mild level (IQ in the range of 50 to 70), the individual can live independently but with some assistance. He or she is capable of work at the sixth-grade level and can learn a vocational skill. Social skills are possible, but the individual functions best in a structured, sheltered setting. Coordination may be slightly affected.

2. At the moderate level (IQ in the range of 35 to 49), the individual can perform some activities independently but requires supervision. Academic skill can be achieved to about the second-grade level. The individual may experience some limitation in speech communication and in interactions with others. Motor development may be limited to gross motor ability.
3. The severe level of intellectual disability (IQ in the range of 20 to 34) is characterized by the need for complete supervision. Systematic habit training may be accomplished, but the individual does not have the ability for academic or vocational training. Verbal skills are minimal, and psychomotor development is poor.
4. The individual with profound intellectual disability (IQ commonly less than 20) has no capacity for independent living. Constant aid and supervision are required. No ability exists for academic or vocational training. There is a lack of ability for speech development, socialization skills, and fine or gross motor movements. The individual requires constant supervision and care.

Common Nursing Diagnoses and Interventions for the Patient With Intellectual Disability

(Interventions are applicable to various health-care settings, such as inpatient and partial hospitalization, community outpatient clinic, home health, and private practice.)

■ RISK FOR INJURY

Definition: Susceptible to physical damage due to environmental conditions interacting with the individual's adaptive and defensive resources, which may compromise health (NANDA International [NANDA-I], 2018, p. 393)

Risk Factors ("related to")

Alteration in psychomotor functioning
[Aggressive behavior]
[Developmental immaturity]

Goals/Objectives
Short-/Long-term Goal
The patient will not experience injury.

Interventions

1. To ensure patient safety:
   a. Create a safe environment for the patient. Remove small items from the area where the patient will be ambulating and move sharp items out of his or her reach.

  b. Store items that the patient uses frequently within easy reach.
  c. Pad side rails and headboard for the patient who has a history of seizures.
  d. Prevent physical aggression and acting-out behaviors by learning to recognize signs that the patient is becoming agitated.

Outcome Criteria

1. Patient has experienced no physical harm.
2. Patient responds to attempts to inhibit agitated behavior.

■ SELF-CARE DEFICIT

Definition: Inability to independently perform task associated with [activities of daily living] (NANDA-I, 2018, pp. 243–246)

Possible Contributing Factors ("related to")

Musculoskeletal impairment
Cognitive impairment

Defining Characteristics ("evidenced by")

Inability to wash body
Inability to put on clothing
Inability to bring food from receptacle to the mouth
[Inability to toilet self without assistance]

Goals/Objectives

Short-term Goal

Patient will be able to participate in aspects of self-care.

Long-term Goal

Patient will have all self-care needs met.

Interventions With *Selected Rationales*

1. Identify aspects of self-care that may be within the patient's capabilities. Work on one aspect of self-care at a time. Provide simple, concrete explanations. *Because patients' capabilities vary so widely, it is important to know each patient individually and to ensure that no patient is set up to fail.*
2. Offer positive feedback for efforts at assisting with own self-care. *Positive reinforcement enhances self-esteem and encourages repetition of desirable behaviors.*
3. When one aspect of self-care has been mastered to the best of the patient's ability, move on to another. Encourage independence but intervene when the patient is unable to perform. *Patient comfort and safety are nursing priorities.*

Outcome Criteria

1. The patient assists with self-care activities to the best of his or her ability.
2. The patient's self-care needs are being met.

■ IMPAIRED VERBAL COMMUNICATION

Definition: Decreased, delayed, or absent ability to receive, process, transmit, and/or use a system of symbols [to communicate] (NANDA-I, 2018, p. 263)

Possible Contributing Factors ("related to")

Alteration in development

Defining Characteristics ("evidenced by")

Speaks or verbalizes with difficulty
Difficulty forming words or sentences
Difficulty expressing thought verbally
Inappropriate verbalization
Does not or cannot speak

Goals/Objectives

Short-term Goal

The patient will establish trust with caregiver and a means of communicating needs.

Long-term Goals

1. The patient's needs are being met through established means of communication.
2. If the patient cannot speak or communicate by other means, needs are met by caregiver's anticipation of the patient's needs.

Interventions With *Selected Rationales*

1. Maintain consistency of staff assignment over time. *This facilitates trust and the ability to understand the patient's actions and communication.*
2. Anticipate and fulfill the patient's needs until satisfactory communication patterns are established. Learn (from family, if possible) special words the patient uses that are different from the norm.
3. Identify nonverbal gestures or signals that the patient may use to convey needs if verbal communication is absent. Practice these communication skills repeatedly. *Some children with intellectual disability, particularly at the severe level, can learn only by systematic habit training.*

Outcome Criteria

1. Patient is able to communicate with consistent caregiver.
2. For patient who is unable to communicate: Patient's needs, as anticipated by caregiver, are being met.

■ IMPAIRED SOCIAL INTERACTION

Definition: Insufficient or excessive quantity or ineffective quality of social exchange (NANDA-I, 2018, p. 301)

Possible Contributing Factors ("related to")

[Speech deficiencies]
[Difficulty adhering to conventional social behavior (because of delayed maturational development)]

Defining Characteristics ("evidenced by")

Use of unsuccessful social interaction behaviors
Dysfunctional interaction with others
[Observed] discomfort in social situations

Goals/Objectives

Short-term Goal

Patient will attempt to interact with others in the presence of trusted caregiver.

Long-term Goal

Patient will be able to interact with others using behaviors that are socially acceptable and appropriate to developmental level.

Interventions With *Selected Rationales*

1. Remain with patient during initial interactions with others. *The presence of a trusted individual provides a feeling of security.*
2. Explain to other patients the meaning of some of the patient's nonverbal gestures and signals. *Others may be more accepting of the patient's differentness if they have a better understanding of his or her behavior.*
3. Use simple language to explain to patient which behaviors are acceptable and which are not. Establish a procedure for behavior modification that offers rewards for appropriate behaviors and renders an aversive reinforcement in response to the use of inappropriate behaviors. *Positive, negative, and aversive reinforcements can contribute to desired changes in behavior. The privileges and penalties are individually determined as caregiver learns the likes and dislikes of the patient.*

Outcome Criterion

The patient interacts with others in a socially appropriate manner.

■ AUTISM SPECTRUM DISORDER

Defined

Autism spectrum disorder (ASD) is characterized by a withdrawal of the child into the self and into a fantasy world of his or her own creation. Activities and interests are restricted and may be considered somewhat bizarre. The Autism and Developmental Disabilities Monitoring (ADDM) Network, a group of programs funded by the Centers for Disease Control and Prevention (CDC), estimates that 1 in 59 children in the United States are identified with ASD (CDC, 2019a). ASD includes a spectrum of symptoms based on level of severity. ASD occurs about 4 times more often in boys than in girls. Onset of the disorder occurs in early childhood, and, in most cases, it runs a chronic course, with symptoms persisting into adulthood.

Predisposing Factors

1. Physiological
   a. **Genetics:** Studies have shown that parents who have one child with ASD are at increased risk for having more than one child with the disorder. Other studies with both monozygotic and dizygotic twins have also provided evidence of a genetic involvement. Genetic studies have identified genes that are linked to both autism and schizophrenia, suggesting the two conditions are related (Gilman et al, 2012), but the same genetic variations appear to confer risk for some other neurodevelopmental disorders as well (Volkmar et al, 2017).
   b. **Neurological:** Abnormalities in brain structures or functions have been correlated with ASD. Total brain volume, the size of the amygdala, and the size of the striatum have all been identified as enlarged in about 9% to 16% of children younger than age 4 with ASD. Volkmar and associates (2017) report that the Infant Brain Imaging Study, a national study of developmental changes in at-risk infants, has repeatedly demonstrated abnormal organizational properties in white matter within the first year of life that accentuate over time. Certain developmental problems, such as postnatal neurological infections, congenital rubella, phenylketonuria, and fragile X syndrome, also have been implicated.
2. Environmental
   a. The *DSM-5* reports that "a variety of nonspecific risk factors, such as advanced parental age, low birth weight, or fetal exposure to valproate, may contribute to risk of ASD" (APA, 2013, p. 56). Volkmar and associates (2017) note that "despite multiple focused investigations, there is no evidence that vaccinations play a role in the environmental liability for ASD" (p. 3576).

Symptomatology (Subjective and Objective Data)

1. Failure to form interpersonal relationships, characterized by unresponsiveness to people, lack of eye contact and facial responsiveness, indifference or aversion to affection and physical contact. In early childhood, there is a failure to develop cooperative play and friendships.
2. Impairment in communication and imaginative activity. Language may be totally absent or characterized by immature grammatical structure, incorrect use of words, echolalia, or inability to use abstract terms. Accompanying nonverbal expressions may be inappropriate or absent.
3. Bizarre responses to the environment, characterized by resistance or extreme behavioral reactions to minor occurrences; abnormal, obsessive attachment to peculiar objects; ritualistic behaviors.
4. Extreme fascination for objects that move (e.g., fans, trains). Special interest in music, playing with water, buttons, or parts of the body.
5. Unreasonable insistence on following routines in precise detail (e.g., insisting that exactly the same route always be followed when shopping).
6. Marked distress over changes in trivial aspects of environment (e.g., when a vase is moved from its usual position).
7. Stereotyped body movements (e.g., hand flicking or clapping, rocking, or whole-body swaying).
8. Behaviors that are self-injurious, such as head banging or biting the hands or arms, may be evident.

Common Nursing Diagnoses and Interventions for the Patient With ASD

(Interventions are applicable to various health-care settings, such as inpatient and partial hospitalization, community outpatient clinic, home health, and private practice.)

■ RISK FOR SELF-MUTILATION

Definition: Susceptible to deliberate self-injurious behavior causing tissue damage with the intent of causing nonfatal injury to attain relief of tension (NANDA-I, 2018, p. 420)

Risk Factors ("related to")

[Neurological alterations]
[History of self-mutilative behaviors in response to increasing anxiety]
[Obvious indifference to environment or hysterical reactions to changes in the environment]
Inability to express tension verbally

Goals/Objectives

Short-term Goal

The patient will demonstrate alternative behavior (e.g., initiating interaction between self and nurse) in response to anxiety within specified time. (Length of time required for this objective will depend on severity and chronicity of the disorder.)

Long-term Goal

The patient will not harm self.

Interventions With *Selected Rationales*

1. Intervene to protect child when self-mutilative behaviors, such as head banging or other hysterical behaviors, become evident. *The nurse is responsible for ensuring patient safety.*
2. A helmet may be used to protect against head banging, hand mitts to prevent hair pulling, and appropriate padding to protect extremities from injury during hysterical movements.
3. Try to determine if self-mutilative behaviors occur in response to increasing anxiety, and if so, to what the anxiety may be attributed. *Mutilative behaviors may be averted if the cause can be determined.*
4. Work on one-to-one basis with child *to establish trust.*
5. Offer self to child during times of increasing anxiety, *in order to decrease need for self-mutilative behaviors and provide feelings of security.*

Outcome Criteria

1. Anxiety is maintained at a level at which the patient feels no need for self-mutilation.
2. When feeling anxious, the patient initiates interaction between self and nurse.

■ IMPAIRED SOCIAL INTERACTION

Definition: Insufficient or excessive quantity or ineffective quality of social exchange (NANDA-I, 2018, p. 301)

Possible Contributing Factors ("related to")

Self-concept disturbance
Absence of [available] significant others
[Unfulfilled tasks of trust versus mistrust]
[Neurological alterations]

Defining Characteristics ("evidenced by")

[Lack of responsiveness to, or interest in, people]
[Failure to cuddle]

[Lack of eye contact and facial responsiveness]
[Indifference or aversion to affection and physical contact]
[Failure to develop cooperative play and peer friendships]

Goals/Objectives

Short-term Goal

The patient will demonstrate trust in one caregiver (as evidenced by facial responsiveness and eye contact) within specified time (depending on severity and chronicity of disorder).

Long-term Goal

The patient will initiate social interactions (physical, verbal, nonverbal) with caregiver by time of discharge from treatment.

Interventions With *Selected Rationales*

1. Assign a limited number of caregivers to the child. Ensure that warmth, acceptance, and availability are conveyed. *Warmth, acceptance, and availability, along with consistency of staff assignment, enhance the establishment and maintenance of a trusting relationship.*
2. Provide child with familiar objects (favorite toys, blanket). *These items will offer security during times when the child feels distressed.* Go slowly. Do not force interactions. Begin with positive reinforcement for eye contact.
3. Gradually introduce touch, smiling, hugging. *The patient with ASD may feel threatened by an onslaught of stimuli to which he or she is unaccustomed.*
4. Support the patient with your presence as he or she endeavors to relate to others in the environment. *The presence of an individual with whom a trusting relationship has been established provides a feeling of security.*

Outcome Criteria

1. The patient initiates interactions between self and others.
2. The patient uses eye contact, facial responsiveness, and other nonverbal behaviors in interactions with others.
3. The patient does not withdraw from physical contact.

■ IMPAIRED VERBAL COMMUNICATION

Definition: Decreased, delayed, or absent ability to receive, process, transmit, and/or use a system of symbols [to communicate] (NANDA-I, 2018, p. 263)

Possible Contributing Factors ("related to")

[Inability to trust]
[Withdrawal into the self]
[Neurological alterations]

Defining Characteristics ("evidenced by")

Does not or cannot speak
[Immature grammatical structure]
[Echolalia]
[Pronoun reversal]
[Inability to name objects]
[Inability to use abstract terms]
[Absence of nonverbal expression (e.g., eye contact, facial responsiveness, gestures)]

Goals/Objectives

Short-term Goal

The patient will establish trust with one caregiver (as evidenced by facial responsiveness and eye contact) by specified time (depending on severity and chronicity of disorder).

Long-term Goal

The patient will establish a means of communicating needs and desires to others by time of discharge from treatment.

Interventions With *Selected Rationales*

1. Maintain consistency in assignment of caregivers. *Consistency facilitates trust and enhances the caregiver's ability to understand the child's attempts to communicate.*
2. Anticipate and fulfill the patient's needs until satisfactory communication patterns are established. *Anticipating needs helps to minimize frustration as the child is learning communication skills.*
3. Use the techniques of *consensual validation* and *seeking clarification* to decode communication patterns. (Examples: "I think you must have meant ..." or "Did you mean to say that ... ?" [see Appendix E].) *These techniques work to verify the accuracy of the message received or to clarify any hidden meanings within the message. Take caution not to "put words into the patient's mouth."*
4. Give positive reinforcement when eye contact is used to convey nonverbal expressions. *Positive reinforcement increases self-esteem and encourages repetition of the behavior.*

Outcome Criteria

1. The patient is able to communicate in a manner that is understood by others.
2. The patient's nonverbal messages are congruent with verbalizations.
3. The patient initiates verbal and nonverbal interaction with others.

■ DISTURBED PERSONAL IDENTITY

Definition: Inability to maintain an integrated and complete perception of self (NANDA-I, 2018, p. 269)

Possible Contributing Factors ("related to")

[Unfulfilled tasks of trust versus mistrust]
[Neurological alterations]
[Inadequate sensory stimulation]

Defining Characteristics ("evidenced by")

[Inability to separate own physiological and emotional needs from those of others]
[Increased levels of anxiety resulting from contact with others]
[Inability to differentiate own body boundaries from those of others]
[Repeating words he or she hears others say or mimicking movements of others]
Unable to distinguish between inner and outer stimuli

Goals/Objectives

Short-term Goal

The patient will name own body parts as separate and individual from those of others (within specified time, depending on severity and chronicity of disorder).

Long-term Goal

The patient will develop ego identity (evidenced by ability to recognize physical and emotional self as separate from others) by time of discharge from treatment.

Interventions With *Selected Rationales*

1. Function in a one-to-one relationship with the child. *Consistency of staff-patient interaction enhances the establishment of trust.*
2. Assist child to recognize separateness during self-care activities, such as dressing and feeding. *These activities increase child's awareness of self as separate from others.*
3. Point out and assist child in naming own body parts. *This activity may increase the child's awareness of self as separate from others.*
4. Gradually increase amount of physical contact, using touch to point out differences between the patient and nurse. Be cautious with touch until trust is established *because this gesture may be interpreted by the patient as threatening.*
5. Use mirrors and drawings or pictures of the child to reinforce the child's learning of body parts and boundaries.

Outcome Criteria

1. The patient is able to differentiate own body parts from those of others.
2. The patient communicates ability to separate self from environment by discontinuing use of echolalia (repeating words heard) and echopraxia (imitating movements seen).

■ DISRUPTIVE BEHAVIOR DISORDERS

Attention-Deficit/Hyperactivity Disorder

Defined

Attention-deficit/hyperactivity disorder (ADHD) is characterized by a "persistent pattern of inattention and/or hyperactivity-impulsivity that interferes with functioning or development" (APA, 2013, p. 61). The disorder often is not diagnosed until the child begins school because, prior to that time, childhood behavior is much more variable than that of older children. It is more common in boys (14.2%) than girls (6.4%), and the overall prevalence among school-aged children in the United States is 10.4% (CDC, 2019b). It is estimated that in 50% to 70% of the cases, ADHD persists into young adulthood and beyond, and unlike other psychiatric disorders that are typically episodic, the adult with ADHD has symptoms that are chronic and unrelenting (McGough, 2017). The *DSM-5* further categorizes the disorder according to current clinical presentation. These subtypes include a combined presentation (meeting the criteria for both inattention and hyperactivity/impulsivity), a predominantly inattentive presentation, and a predominantly hyperactive/impulsive presentation.

Predisposing Factors

1. Physiological
   a. **Genetics:** Twin and family studies showed that the heritability for ADHD exceeds 75% (McGough, 2017). Studies of genetic evidence for ADHD have found genetic variants and mutations such as copy number variants on a specific region of chromosome 16 (Acosta et al, 2016; Williams et al, 2010). The researchers also found that copy number variants overlap with chromosomal regions previously linked to ASD and schizophrenia.
   b. **Biochemical:** Several studies, using single photon emission computed tomography (SPECT), have now demonstrated increased dopamine transporter-binding densities in the striatal regions (McGough, 2017). Not surprisingly, researchers have also found a significant risk of new onset psychosis in ADHD patients taking amphetamines, almost double the risk than for those taking methylphenidate (Griffin & Harari, 2019).
   c. **Prenatal, Perinatal, and Postnatal:** Early risk factors for the development of ADHD include prenatal tobacco exposure, premature birth, and low birth weight (ADHD Institute,

2019). Froehlich and associates (2009) in a large U.S. study found that maternal cigarette smoking during pregnancy was significantly associated with childhood ADHD. Intrauterine exposure to toxic substances, including alcohol, can produce effects on behavior. Premature birth, fetal distress, precipitated or prolonged labor, and perinatal asphyxia have also been implicated. Postnatal factors include cerebral palsy, epilepsy, and other central nervous system abnormalities resulting from trauma, infections, or other neurological disorders.

2. Environmental Influences
   a. Disorganized or chaotic environments or a disruption in family equilibrium may predispose some individuals to ADHD. Galéra and colleagues (2011) identified several psychosocial influences associated with the development of ADHD, including nonintact family, young maternal age at birth of the target child, paternal history of antisocial behavior, and maternal depression.
   b. Studies continue to provide evidence of the adverse effects of elevated body levels of lead on cognitive and behavioral development in children (Froehlich et al, 2009; Rossignol & Frye, 2016).

Symptomatology (Subjective and Objective Data)

1. Difficulties in performing age-appropriate tasks.
2. Highly distractible.
3. Extremely limited attention span.
4. Shifts from one uncompleted activity to another.
5. Impulsivity, or deficit in inhibitory control, is common.
6. Difficulty forming satisfactory interpersonal relationships.
7. Disruptive and intrusive behaviors inhibit acceptable social interaction.
8. Difficulty complying with social norms.
9. Some children with ADHD are very aggressive or oppositional. Others exhibit more regressive and immature behaviors.
10. Low frustration tolerance and outbursts of temper are common.
11. Boundless energy, exhibiting excessive levels of activity, restlessness, and fidgeting.
12. Often described as "perpetual motion machines," continuously running, jumping, wiggling, or squirming.
13. They experience a greater than average number of accidents, from minor mishaps to more serious incidents that may lead to physical injury or the destruction of property.

Oppositional Defiant Disorder

Defined

Oppositional defiant disorder (ODD) is characterized by a pattern of angry mood and defiant behavior that occurs more frequently than is usually observed in individuals of comparable age and developmental level and interferes with social, occupational, or other important areas of functioning (APA, 2013). The disorder typically begins by 8 years of age and usually not later than early adolescence. The disorder is more prevalent in boys than in girls before puberty, but the rates are more closely equal after puberty. The symptoms of ODD are generally considered less severe than those of conduct disorder (CD) but ODD may progress to CD, and both ODD and CD confer greater risk for antisocial personality disorder in adulthood (Connor, 2017). The *DSM-5* identifies that ODD often precedes CD, especially in children with onset of CD prior to 10 years of age (APA, 2013).

Predisposing Factors

1. Physiological
   a. Refer to this section under Conduct Disorder.
2. Psychosocial
   a. **Theory of Family Dynamics:** It is thought that some parents interpret average or increased levels of developmental oppositionalism as hostility and a deliberate effort on the part of the child to be in control. If power and control are issues for parents or if they exercise authority for their own needs, a power struggle can be established between the parents and the child that sets the stage for the development of ODD.

Symptomatology (Subjective and Objective Data)

1. Characterized by passive-aggressive behaviors such as stubbornness, procrastination, disobedience, carelessness, negativism, testing of limits, resistance to directions, deliberately ignoring the communication of others, and unwillingness to compromise.
2. Other symptoms that may be evident are running away, school avoidance, school underachievement, temper tantrums, fighting, and argumentativeness.
3. In severe cases, there may be elective mutism, enuresis, encopresis, or eating and sleeping problems.
4. Blames others for mistakes and misbehavior.
5. Has poor peer relationships.

Conduct Disorder

Defined

The *DSM-5* describes the essential feature of this disorder as a "repetitive and persistent pattern of behavior in which the basic rights of others or major age-appropriate societal norms or rules are violated" (APA, 2013, p. 472). The behavior is more serious than the ordinary mischief and pranks of children and adolescents. The disorder is more common in boys than in girls, and the behaviors may continue into adulthood, often meeting the criteria for antisocial personality disorder. CD is divided into two subtypes based on the age at onset: childhood-onset type (onset of symptoms before age 10 years) and adolescent-onset type (absence of symptoms before age 10 years).

Predisposing Factors

1. Physiological
   a. **Birth Temperament:** The term *temperament* refers to personality traits that become evident very early in life and may be present at birth. Evidence suggests a genetic component in temperament and an association between temperament and behavioral problems later in life.
   b. **Genetics:** Family, twin, and adoptive studies have revealed a significantly higher number of conduct disorders among those who have family members with the disorder.
2. Psychosocial
   a. **Peer Relationships:** Social groups have a significant impact on a child's development. Peers play an essential role in the socialization of interpersonal competence, and skills acquired in this manner affect the child's long-term adjustment. "Considerable research indicates that the deviant peer group provides training in criminal and delinquent behavior including substance abuse" (Bernstein, 2018). In addition to evidence that engaging in risk-taking behaviors can yield reinforcement (acceptance within a peer group), Bernstein notes that "studies of neural processing show that risk-taking may be associated with reward-related brain activation."
   b. **Theory of Family Dynamics:** The following factors related to family dynamics have been implicated as contributors in the predisposition to CD (Bernstein, 2018; Mayo Clinic, 2019; Sadock et al, 2015):
      * Parental rejection
      * Inconsistent management with harsh discipline
      * Early institutional living
      * Frequent shifting of parental figures
      * Large family size
      * Absent father
      * Parents with antisocial personality disorder and/or alcohol dependence
      * Marital conflict and divorce
      * Inadequate communication patterns
      * Parental permissiveness

Symptomatology (Subjective and Objective Data)

1. Uses physical aggression in the violation of the rights of others.
2. The behavior pattern manifests itself in virtually all areas of the child's life (home, school, with peers, and in the community).
3. Stealing, fighting, lying, and truancy are common problems.
4. There is an absence of feelings of guilt or remorse.
5. The use of tobacco, liquor, or nonprescribed drugs, as well as the participation in sexual activities, occurs earlier than the peer group's expected age.
6. Projection is a common defense mechanism.

7. Low self-esteem is manifested by a "tough guy" image. Often threatens and intimidates others.
8. Characteristics include poor frustration tolerance, irritability, and frequent temper outbursts.
9. Symptoms of anxiety and depression are not uncommon.
10. Level of academic achievement may be low in relation to age and IQ.
11. Manifestations associated with ADHD (e.g., attention difficulties, impulsiveness, and hyperactivity) are very common in children with CD.

Common Nursing Diagnoses and Interventions for Patients With Disruptive Behavior Disorders

(Interventions are applicable to various health-care settings, such as inpatient and partial hospitalization, community outpatient clinic, home health, and private practice.)

■ RISK FOR SELF-DIRECTED OR OTHER-DIRECTED VIOLENCE

Definition: Susceptible to behaviors in which an individual demonstrates that he or she can be physically, emotionally, and/or sexually harmful [either to self or to others] (NANDA-I, 2018, pp. 416–417)

Risk Factors ("related to")

[Unsatisfactory parent-child relationship]
[Neurological alteration related to premature birth, fetal distress, precipitated or prolonged labor]
[Dysfunctional family system]
[Disorganized or chaotic environments]
[Child abuse or neglect]
[Birth temperament]
Negative body language (e.g., rigid posture, clenching of fists and jaw, hyperactivity, pacing, breathlessness, threatening stances)
[History or threats of violence toward self or others or of destruction to the property of others]
Impulsivity
[History of] cruelty to animals
Suicidal ideation, plan, [available means]

Goals/Objectives

Short-term Goals

1. The patient will seek out staff at any time if thoughts of harming self or others should occur.
2. The patient will not harm self or others.

Long-term Goal
The patient will not harm self or others.

Interventions With *Selected Rationales*

1. Observe the patient's behavior frequently. Do this through routine activities and interactions to avoid appearing watchful and suspicious. *Patients at high risk for violence require close observation to prevent harm to self or others.*
2. Observe for suicidal behaviors: Verbal statements, such as "I'm going to kill myself" or "Very soon my mother won't have to worry herself about me any longer," or nonverbal behaviors, such as giving away cherished items or mood swings. *Most patients who attempt suicide have communicated their intent, either verbally or nonverbally.*
3. Determine suicidal intent and available means. Ask, "Do you plan to kill yourself?" and "How do you plan to do it?" *Direct, closed-ended questions are appropriate in this instance. The patient who has a usable plan is at higher risk than one who does not.*
4. Conduct a thorough assessment of risk factors and warning signs for suicide, including history of ideation and attempts, and engage the patient in collaborating to identify a safety plan.
5. Help the patient to recognize when anger occurs and to accept those feelings as his or her own. Have the patient keep an "anger notebook," in which a record of anger experienced on a 24-hour basis is kept. Information regarding source of anger, behavioral response, and the patient's perception of the situation should also be noted. Discuss entries with the patient, suggesting alternative behavioral responses for those identified as maladaptive.
6. Act as a role model for appropriate expression of angry feelings, and give positive reinforcement to the patient for attempting to conform. *It is vital that the patient express angry feelings, because suicide and other self-destructive behaviors are often viewed as a result of anger turned inward on the self.*
7. Remove all dangerous objects from the patient's environment. *The patient's physical safety is a nursing priority.*
8. Try to redirect violent behavior with physical outlets for the patient's anxiety (e.g., physical exercise, jogging, volleyball). *Anxiety and tension can be relieved safely and with benefit to the patient in this manner.*
9. Be available to stay with the patient as anxiety level and tensions begin to rise. *The presence of a trusted individual provides a feeling of security.*
10. Staff should maintain and convey a calm attitude to the patient. Anxiety is contagious and can be communicated from staff to the patient and vice versa. *A calm attitude conveys a sense of control and a feeling of security to the patient.*

11. Have sufficient staff available to indicate a show of strength to the patient if it becomes necessary. *This conveys to the patient an evidence of control over the situation and provides some physical security for staff.*

12. Administer tranquilizing medications as ordered by physician, or obtain an order if necessary. Monitor medication for effectiveness and for adverse side effects. *Short-term use of antianxiety medications (e.g., chlordiazepoxide, alprazolam, lorazepam) provides relief from the immobilizing effects of anxiety and facilitates patient's cooperation with therapy.*

13. Mechanical restraints, holding the patient, or isolation room may be required if less restrictive interventions are unsuccessful. *It is the patient's right to expect the use of the least restrictive means needed to ensure safety of the patient and others.*

Outcome Criteria

1. Anxiety is maintained at a level at which the patient feels no need for aggression.
2. The patient seeks out staff to discuss true feelings.
3. The patient recognizes, verbalizes, and accepts possible consequences of own maladaptive behaviors.
4. The patient does not harm self or others.

■ DEFENSIVE COPING

Definition: Repeated projection of falsely positive self-evaluation based on a self-protective pattern that defends against underlying perceived threats to positive self-regard (NANDA-I, 2018, p. 326)

Possible Contributing Factors ("related to")

[Low self-esteem]
[Negative role models]
[Lack of positive feedback]
[Repeated negative feedback, resulting in feelings of diminished self-worth]
[Unsatisfactory parent-child relationship]
[Disorganized or chaotic environments]
[Child abuse or neglect]
[Dysfunctional family system]
[Neurological alteration related to premature birth, fetal distress, precipitated or prolonged labor]

Defining Characteristics ("evidenced by")

Denial of obvious problems or weaknesses
Projection of blame or responsibility
Rationalization of failures

Hypersensitivity to criticism
Grandiosity
Superior attitude toward others
Difficulty establishing or maintaining relationships
Hostile laughter or ridicule of others
Difficulty in perception of reality testing
Lack of follow-through or participation in treatment or therapy

Goals/Objectives

Short-term Goal

The patient will verbalize personal responsibility for difficulties experienced in interpersonal relationships.

Long-term Goal

The patient will demonstrate ability to interact with others without becoming defensive, rationalizing behaviors, or expressing grandiose ideas.

Interventions With *Selected Rationales*

1. Recognize and support basic ego strengths. *Focusing on positive aspects of the personality may help to improve self-concept.*
2. Encourage the patient to recognize and verbalize feelings of inadequacy and need for acceptance from others and to recognize how these feelings provoke defensive behaviors, such as blaming others for own behaviors. *Recognition of the problem is the first step in the change process toward resolution.*
3. Provide immediate, matter-of-fact, nonthreatening feedback for unacceptable behaviors. *The patient may not realize how these behaviors are being perceived by others. Providing this information in a nonthreatening manner may help to eliminate these undesirable behaviors.*

> 🍏 **CLINICAL PEARL** Say to the patient, "When you say those things to people, they don't like it, and they don't want to be around you. Try to think how you would feel if someone said those things to you."

4. Help the patient identify situations that provoke defensiveness, and practice through role-play more appropriate responses. *Role-playing provides confidence to deal with difficult situations when they actually occur.*
5. Provide immediate positive feedback for acceptable behaviors. *Positive feedback enhances self-esteem and encourages repetition of desirable behaviors.*
6. Help the patient set realistic, concrete goals and determine appropriate actions to meet those goals. *Success increases self-esteem.*
7. With the patient, evaluate the effectiveness of the new behaviors and discuss any modifications for improvement. *Because of*

limited problem-solving ability, assistance may be required to reassess and develop new strategies in the event that some new coping methods prove ineffective.

Outcome Criteria

1. The patient verbalizes and accepts responsibility for own behavior.
2. The patient verbalizes correlation between feelings of inadequacy and the need to defend the ego through rationalization and grandiosity.
3. The patient does not ridicule or criticize others.
4. The patient interacts with others in group situations without taking a defensive stance.

■ IMPAIRED SOCIAL INTERACTION

Definition: Insufficient or excessive quantity or ineffective quality of social exchange (NANDA-I, 2018, p. 301)

Possible Contributing Factors ("related to")

Self-concept disturbance
[Neurological alterations related to premature birth, fetal distress, precipitated or prolonged labor]
[Dysfunctional family system]
[Disorganized or chaotic environments]
[Child abuse or neglect]
[Unsatisfactory parent-child relationship]
[Negative role models]

Defining Characteristics ("evidenced by")

[Verbalized or observed] discomfort in social situations
[Verbalized or observed] inability to receive or communicate a satisfying sense of belonging, caring, interest, or shared history
[Observed] use of unsuccessful social interaction behaviors
Dysfunctional interaction with others
[Behavior unacceptable for appropriate age by dominant cultural group]

Goals/Objectives

Short-term Goal

The patient will interact in age-appropriate manner with nurse in one-to-one relationship within 1 week.

Long-term Goal

By time of discharge from treatment, the patient will be able to interact with staff and peers using age-appropriate, acceptable behaviors.

Interventions With *Selected Rationales*

1. Develop trusting relationship with the patient. Be honest; keep all promises; convey acceptance of the person, separate from unacceptable behaviors ("It is not *you*, but *your behavior*, that is unacceptable.") *Acceptance of the patient increases his or her feelings of self-worth.*
2. Offer to remain with the patient during initial interactions with others. *Presence of a trusted individual provides a feeling of security.*
3. Provide constructive criticism and positive reinforcement for the patient's efforts. *Positive feedback enhances self-esteem and encourages repetition of desirable behaviors.*
4. Confront the patient and withdraw attention when interactions with others are manipulative or exploitative. *Attention to the unacceptable behavior may reinforce it.*
5. Act as a role model for the patient through appropriate interactions with other patients and staff members.
6. Provide group situations for the patient. *It is through these group interactions that the patient will learn socially acceptable behavior, with positive and negative feedback from his or her peers.*

Outcome Criteria

1. The patient seeks out staff member for social as well as therapeutic interaction.
2. The patient has formed and satisfactorily maintained one interpersonal relationship with another patient.
3. The patient willingly and appropriately participates in group activities.
4. The patient verbalizes reasons for past inability to form close interpersonal relationships.

■ INEFFECTIVE COPING

Definition: A pattern of invalid appraisal of stressors, with cognitive and/or behavioral efforts, that fails to manage demands related to well-being (NANDA-I, 2018, p. 327)

Possible Contributing Factors ("related to")

Situational crisis
Maturational crisis
[Inadequate support systems]
[Inadequate coping strategies]
[Negative role models]
[Neurological alteration related to premature birth, fetal distress, precipitated or prolonged labor]
[Low self-esteem]

[Dysfunctional family system]
[Disorganized or chaotic environments]
[Child abuse or neglect]

Defining Characteristics ("evidenced by")

Inability to meet [age-appropriate] role expectations
Inadequate problem-solving
Poor concentration
Risk taking
[Manipulation of others in the environment for purposes of fulfilling own desires]
[Verbal hostility toward staff and peers]
[Hyperactivity, evidenced by excessive motor activity, easily distracted, short attention span]
[Unable to delay gratification]
[Oppositional and defiant responses to adult requests or rules]

Goals/Objectives

Short-term Goal

Within 1 week, the patient will demonstrate ability and willingness to follow rules of the treatment setting.

Long-term Goal

By discharge from treatment, the patient will develop and utilize age-appropriate, socially acceptable coping skills.

Interventions With *Selected Rationales*

1. If the patient is hyperactive, make environment safe for continuous large muscle movement. Rearrange furniture and other objects to prevent injury. *Patient physical safety is a nursing priority.*
2. Provide large motor activities in which the patient may participate. Nurse may join in some of these activities *to facilitate relationship development. Tension is released safely and with benefit to the patient through physical activities.*
3. Provide frequent, nutritious snacks that the patient may "eat on the run" *to ensure adequate calories to offset the patient's excessive use of energy.*

> **CLINICAL PEARL** Set limits on manipulative behavior. Say, "I will not tolerate manipulative behaviors and communication." Take caution not to reinforce manipulative behaviors by providing desired attention but be willing to explore other alternatives for communicating needs and desires.

4. Identify for the patient the consequences of manipulative behavior (e.g., "If you decide to shout obscenities when you are told you are not allowed to stay up after 9 p.m., you will not be

permitted to join the group tomorrow for the movie"). All staff must follow through and be consistent. *The patient may try to play one staff member against another, so consistency is vital if intervention is to be successful. Aversive reinforcement may work to decrease unacceptable behaviors. Verbalizing that the patient is responsible for "deciding" communicates that he or she has the opportunity to make choices.*

5. Do not debate, argue, rationalize, or bargain with the patient. *Ignoring these attempts may work to decrease manipulative behaviors.*
6. Caution should be taken to avoid reinforcing manipulative behaviors by providing desired attention. *Attention provides positive reinforcement and encourages repetition of the undesirable behavior.*
7. Confront the patient's use of manipulative behaviors and explore their damaging effects on interpersonal relationships. *Manipulative patients often deny responsibility for their behaviors.*
8. Encourage discussion of angry feelings. Help the patient identify the true object of the hostility. *Dealing with the feelings honestly and directly will discourage displacement of the anger onto others.*
9. Explore with the patient alternative ways of handling frustration that would be most suited to his or her lifestyle. Provide support and positive feedback to the patient as new coping strategies are tried. *Positive feedback encourages use of the acceptable behaviors.*

Outcome Criteria

1. The patient is able to delay gratification without resorting to manipulation of others.
2. The patient is able to express anger in a socially acceptable manner.
3. Patient is able to verbalize alternative, socially acceptable, and lifestyle-appropriate coping skills he or she plans to use in response to frustration.

■ LOW SELF-ESTEEM

Definition: Negative evaluation and/or feelings about one's own capabilities (NANDA-I, 2018, pp. 272, 274)

Possible Contributing Factors ("related to")

[Negative role models]
Lack of approval
Repeated negative reinforcement
[Unsatisfactory parent-child relationship]
[Disorganized or chaotic environments]
[Child abuse or neglect]
[Dysfunctional family system]

Defining Characteristics ("evidenced by")

Lack of eye contact
Exaggerates negative feedback about self
Expressions of shame or guilt
Evaluation of self as unable to deal with events
Rejects positive feedback about self
Hesitant to try new things or situations
[Denial of problems obvious to others]
[Projection of blame or responsibility for problems]
[Rationalization of personal failures]
[Hypersensitivity to criticism]
[Grandiosity]

Goals/Objectives

Short-term Goal

The patient will independently direct own care and activities of daily living within 1 week.

Long-term Goal

By time of discharge from treatment, the patient will exhibit increased feelings of self-worth as evidenced by verbal expression of positive aspects about self, past accomplishments, and future prospects.

Interventions With *Selected Rationales*

1. Ensure that goals are realistic. It is important for the patient to achieve something, so plan for activities in which the possibility for success is likely. *Success enhances self-esteem.*
2. Convey unconditional positive regard for the patient. *Communication of your acceptance of him or her as a worthwhile human being increases self-esteem.*
3. Spend time with the patient, both on a one-to-one basis and in group activities. *This conveys to the patient that you feel he or she is worth your time.*
4. Assist the patient in identifying positive aspects of self and in developing plans for changing the characteristics he or she views as negative.
5. Help the patient decrease use of denial as a defense mechanism. Give positive reinforcement for problem identification and development of more adaptive coping behaviors. *Positive reinforcement enhances self-esteem and increases the patient's use of acceptable behaviors.*
6. Encourage and support the patient in confronting the fear of failure by having the patient attend therapy activities and undertake new tasks. Offer recognition of successful endeavors and positive reinforcement for attempts made. *Recognition and positive reinforcement enhance self-esteem.*

Outcome Criteria

1. The patient verbalizes positive perception of self.
2. The patient participates in new activities without exhibiting extreme fear of failure.

■ ANXIETY (Moderate to Severe)

Definition: Vague, uneasy feeling of discomfort or dread accompanied by an autonomic response (the source often nonspecific or unknown to the individual); a feeling of apprehension caused by anticipation of danger. It is an alerting signal that warns of impending danger and enables the individual to take measures to deal with threat (NANDA-I, 2018, p. 324)

Possible Contributing Factors ("related to")

Situational and maturational crises
Threat to self-concept [perceived or real]
Threat of death
Unmet needs
[Fear of failure]
[Dysfunctional family system]
[Unsatisfactory parent-child relationship]
[Innately, easily agitated temperament since birth]

Defining Characteristics ("evidenced by")

Overexcited
Fearful
Feelings of inadequacy
Fear of unspecified consequences
Restlessness
Insomnia
Poor eye contact
Focus on self
[Continuous attention-seeking behaviors]
Difficulty concentrating
Impaired attention
Increased respiration and pulse

Goals/Objectives

Short-term Goals

1. Within 1 week, the patient will be able to verbalize behaviors that become evident as anxiety starts to rise.
2. Within 1 week, the patient will be able to verbalize strategies to interrupt escalation of anxiety.

Long-term Goal

By time of discharge from treatment, the patient will be able to maintain anxiety below the moderate level as evidenced by absence of disabling behaviors in response to stress.

Interventions With *Selected Rationales*

1. Establish a trusting relationship with the patient. Be honest, consistent in responses, and available. Show genuine positive regard. *Honesty, availability, and acceptance promote trust in the nurse-patient relationship.*
2. Provide activities geared toward reduction of tension and decreasing anxiety (walking or jogging, volleyball, musical exercises, housekeeping chores, group games). *Tension and anxiety are released safely and with benefit to the patient through physical activities.*
3. Encourage the patient to identify true feelings and to acknowledge ownership of those feelings. *Anxious patients often deny a relationship between emotional problems and their anxiety. Use of the defense mechanisms of projection and displacement is exaggerated.*
4. The nurse must maintain an atmosphere of calmness; *anxiety is easily transmitted from one person to another.*
5. Offer support during times of elevated anxiety. Reassure the patient of physical and psychological safety. *Patient safety is a nursing priority.*
6. Use of touch is comforting to some patients. However, the nurse must be cautious with its use, *because anxiety may foster suspicion in some individuals who might misinterpret touch as aggression.*
7. As anxiety diminishes, assist the patient to recognize specific events that preceded its onset. Work on alternative responses to future occurrences. *A plan of action provides the patient with a feeling of security for handling a difficult situation more successfully should it recur.*
8. Help the patient recognize signs of escalating anxiety, and explore ways the patient may intervene before behaviors become disabling.
9. Administer tranquilizing medication, as ordered. Assess for effectiveness, and instruct the patient regarding possible adverse side effects. *Short-term use of antianxiety medications (e.g., lorazepam, chlordiazepoxide, alprazolam) provides relief from the immobilizing effects of anxiety and facilitates the patient's cooperation with therapy.*

Outcome Criteria

1. The patient is able to verbalize behaviors that become evident when anxiety starts to rise and takes appropriate action to interrupt progression of the condition.
2. The patient is able to maintain anxiety at a manageable level.

■ TOURETTE'S DISORDER

Defined

Tourette's disorder is characterized by the presence of multiple motor tics and one or more vocal tics, which may appear simultaneously or at different periods during the illness (APA, 2013). Onset of the disorder can be as early as 2 years, but it occurs most commonly during childhood (around age 6 to 7 years). Tourette's disorder is more common in boys than in girls. Although the disorder can be lifelong, the symptoms usually diminish during adolescence and adulthood and, in some cases, disappear altogether by early adulthood.

Predisposing Factors

1. Physiological
   a. **Genetics:** Family studies have shown that Tourette's disorder is more common in relatives of individuals with the disorder than in the general population. It may be transmitted in an autosomal pattern intermediate between dominant and recessive (Sadock et al, 2015). Although evidence supports that this is an inherited disorder, recent studies suggest that the pattern of inheritance is complex, probably involving several genes influenced by environmental factors (National Institutes of Health [NIH], 2019).
   b. **Brain Alterations:** Altered levels of neurotransmitters and dysfunction in the area of the basal ganglia have been implicated in the etiology of Tourette's disorder.
   c. **Biochemical:** Abnormalities in levels of dopamine, choline, N-acetylaspartate, creatine, myoinositol, and norepinephrine have all been demonstrated in neuroimaging studies.
2. Environmental
   a. The genetic predisposition to Tourette's disorder may be reinforced by certain factors in the environment, such as complications of pregnancy (e.g., severe nausea and vomiting or excessive stress), low birth weight, head trauma, carbon monoxide poisoning, and encephalitis.

Symptomatology (Subjective and Objective Data)

Signs and symptoms of Tourette's disorder are as follows (APA, 2013; NIH, 2019):

1. The disorder may begin with a single motor tic, such as eye blinking, neck jerking, shoulder shrugging, facial grimacing, or coughing.
2. Complex motor tics may follow and include touching, squatting, hopping, skipping, deep knee bends, retracing steps, and twirling when walking.
3. Vocal tics include various words or sounds such as clicks, grunts, yelps, barks, sniffs, snorts, coughs, and, in rare instances, a complex vocal tic involving uttering obscenities.

4. Vocal tics may include repeating certain words or phrases out of context, repeating one's own sounds or words (palilalia), or repeating what others say (echolalia).
5. The movements and vocalizations are experienced as compulsive and irresistible, but they can be suppressed for varying lengths of time.
6. Tics are exacerbated by stress and attenuated during periods in which the individual becomes totally absorbed by an activity.
7. Tics are markedly diminished during sleep.
8. Many children with tics manifest difficulty with reading, writing, and arithmetic (NIH, 2019). This may also be influenced by common comorbidities such as ADHD.

Common Nursing Diagnoses and Interventions for the Patient With Tourette's Disorder

(Interventions are applicable to various health-care settings, such as inpatient and partial hospitalization, community outpatient clinic, home health, and private practice.)

■ RISK FOR SELF-DIRECTED OR OTHER-DIRECTED VIOLENCE

Definition: Susceptible to behaviors in which an individual demonstrates that he or she can be physically, emotionally, and/or sexually harmful [either to self or to others] (NANDA-I, 2018, pp. 416–417)

Risk Factors ("related to")

[Low tolerance for frustration]
[Abnormalities in brain neurotransmitters]
Threatening body language (e.g., rigid posture, clenching of fists and jaw, hyperactivity, pacing, breathlessness, and threatening stances)
[History or threats of violence toward self or others or of destruction to the property of others]
Impulsivity
Suicidal ideation, plan, [available means]

Goals/Objectives

Short-term Goals
1. The patient will seek out staff or support person at any time if thoughts of harming self or others should occur.
2. The patient will not harm self or others.

Long-term Goal
The patient will not harm self or others.

Interventions With *Selected Rationales*

1. Observe the patient's behavior frequently through routine activities and interactions. Become aware of behaviors that indicate a rise in agitation. *Stress commonly increases tic behaviors. Recognition of behaviors that precede the onset of aggression may provide the opportunity to intervene before violence occurs.*

2. Monitor for self-destructive behavior and impulses. A staff member may need to stay with the patient to prevent self-mutilation. *Patient safety is a nursing priority.*

3. Provide hand coverings and other restraints that prevent the patient from self-mutilative behaviors. *Provides immediate external controls against self-aggressive behaviors.*

4. Redirect violent behavior with physical outlets for frustration. *Excess energy is released through physical activities and a feeling of relaxation is induced.*

5. Administer medication as ordered by the physician (when the tics are mild, medication may not be necessary). Several medications have been used to treat Tourette's disorder. The most common ones include the following:

   a. **Haloperidol (Haldol):** Haloperidol has been the drug of choice for Tourette's disorder. Children on this medication must be monitored for adverse effects associated with most antipsychotic medications (see Chapter 26). Because of the potential for adverse effects, haloperidol should be reserved for children with severe symptoms or with symptoms that interfere with their ability to function. Usual dosage for children 3 to 12 years of age is 0.05 to 0.075 mg/kg/day given in two to three divided doses.

   b. **Pimozide (Orap):** The response rate and side effect profile of pimozide are similar to haloperidol. It is used in the management of severe motor or vocal tics that have failed to respond to more conventional treatment. It is not recommended for children younger than age 12 years. Dosage is initiated at 0.05 mg/kg at bedtime; dosage may be increased every third day to a maximum of 0.2 mg/kg, not to exceed 10 mg/day.

   c. **Clonidine (Catapres):** Clonidine is an antihypertensive medication, the efficacy of which in the treatment of Tourette's disorder has been mixed. Some physicians use it as a drug of first choice because of its relative safety and few side effects. Recommended dosage is 150 to 200 mcg/day.

   d. **Atypical Antipsychotics:** Atypical antipsychotics are less likely to cause extrapyramidal side effects than the older antipsychotics (e.g., haloperidol and pimozide). Risperidone, olanzapine, and ziprasidone have demonstrated effectiveness in decreasing tic symptoms of Tourette's disorder.

    e. **Topiramate:** Recent studies have found that some individuals with Tourette's disorder respond to this antiseizure medication (Mayo Clinic, 2019).

    f. **Botulinum:** When injected into an affected muscle, this treatment may relieve a simple or vocal tic (Mayo Clinic, 2019).

6. Support and reinforce patient efforts related to CBIT (Comprehensive behavioral Intervention for tics) when this strategy is part of the overall treatment plan.

Outcome Criteria

1. Anxiety is maintained at a level at which the patient feels no need for aggression.
2. The patient seeks out staff or support person for expression of true feelings.
3. The patient has not harmed self or others.

■ IMPAIRED SOCIAL INTERACTION

Definition: Insufficient or excessive quantity or ineffective quality of social exchange (NANDA-I, 2018, p. 301)

Possible Contributing Factors ("related to")

Self-concept disturbance
[Low tolerance for frustration]
[Impulsiveness]
[Oppositional behavior]
[Aggressive behavior]

Defining Characteristics ("evidenced by")

[Verbalized or observed] discomfort in social situations
[Verbalized or observed inability] to receive or communicate a satisfying sense of belonging, caring, interest, or shared history
[Observed] use of unsuccessful social interaction behaviors
Dysfunctional interaction with others

Goals/Objectives

Short-term Goal

The patient will develop a one-to-one relationship with a nurse or support person within 1 week.

Long-term Goal

The patient will be able to interact with staff and peers using age-appropriate, acceptable behaviors.

Interventions With *Selected Rationales*

1. Develop a trusting relationship with the patient. Convey acceptance of the person separate from the unacceptable behavior. *Unconditional acceptance increases feelings of self-worth.*
2. Discuss with the patient which behaviors are and are not acceptable. Describe in matter-of-fact manner the consequences of unacceptable behavior. Follow through. *Aversive reinforcement can alter undesirable behaviors.*
3. Provide group situations for the patient. *Appropriate social behavior is often learned from the positive and negative feedback of peers.*
4. Act as a role model for the patient through appropriate interactions with others. *Role modeling of a respected individual is one of the strongest forms of learning.*

Outcome Criteria

1. The patient seeks out staff or support person for social as well as for therapeutic interaction.
2. The patient verbalizes reasons for past inability to form close interpersonal relationships.
3. The patient interacts with others using age-appropriate, acceptable behaviors.

■ LOW SELF-ESTEEM

Definition: Negative evaluation and/or feelings about one's own capabilities (NANDA-I, 2018, pp. 272, 274)

Possible Contributing Factors ("related to")

[Embarrassment associated with tic behaviors]

Defining Characteristics ("evidenced by")

Lack of eye contact
Self-negating verbalizations
[Expressions] of shame or guilt
Hesitant to try new things or situations

Goals/Objectives

Short-term Goal

The patient will verbalize positive aspects about self not associated with tic behaviors.

Long-term Goal

The patient will exhibit increased feeling of self-worth as evidenced by verbal expression of positive aspects about self, past accomplishments, and future prospects.

Interventions With *Selected Rationales*

1. Convey unconditional acceptance and positive regard. *Communication of the patient as worthwhile human being may increase self-esteem.*
2. If the patient chooses to suppress tics in the presence of others, provide a specified "tic time" during which the patient "vents" tics, feelings, and behaviors (alone or with staff). *Allows for release of tics and assists in sense of control and management of symptoms.*
3. Ensure that the patient has regular one-to-one time with staff or support person. *One-to-one time gives the nurse the opportunity to provide the patient with information about the illness and healthy ways to manage it. Exploring feelings about the illness helps the patient incorporate the illness into a healthy sense of self.*

Outcome Criteria

1. The patient verbalizes positive perception of self.
2. The patient willingly participates in new activities and situations.

■ SEPARATION ANXIETY DISORDER

Defined

The APA defines separation anxiety disorder as "excessive fear or anxiety concerning separation from home or attachment figures" (2013, p. 191). Onset may occur any time before age 18 years but is most commonly diagnosed around age 5 or 6, when the child goes to school. The disorder is more common in girls than in boys. Most children grow out of it, but in some instances, the symptoms can persist into adulthood.

Predisposing Factors

1. Physiological
   a. **Genetics:** The results of studies indicate that a greater number of children with relatives who manifest anxiety problems develop anxiety disorders themselves than do children with no such family patterns.
   b. **Temperament:** Studies have shown that differences in temperamental characteristics at birth may be correlated to the acquisition of fear and anxiety disorders in childhood. This may denote an inherited vulnerability or predisposition toward developing these disorders.
2. Psychosocial
   a. **Stressful Life Events:** Studies indicate that children who are predisposed to anxiety disorders may be affected significantly by stressful life events.
   b. **Family Influences:** Several theories exist that relate the development of separation anxiety to the following dynamics within the family:
      • Overattachment to the mother (primary caregiver)
      • Separation conflicts between parent and child

- Enmeshment of members within a family
- Overprotection of the child by the parents
- Transfer of parents' fears and anxieties to the children through role modeling

Symptomatology (Subjective and Objective Data)

Symptoms of separation anxiety disorder include the following:

1. In most cases, the child has difficulty separating from the mother, although occasionally the separation reluctance is directed toward the father, siblings, or other significant individual to whom the child is attached.
2. Anticipation of separation may result in tantrums, crying, screaming, complaints of physical problems, and clinging behaviors.
3. Reluctance or refusal to attend school is especially common in adolescence.
4. Younger children may "shadow" or follow around the person from whom they are afraid to be separated.
5. During middle childhood or adolescence, they may refuse to sleep away from home (e.g., at a friend's house or at camp).
6. Worrying is common and relates to the possibility of harm coming to self or to the attachment figure. Younger children may have nightmares to this effect.
7. Specific phobias may be present.
8. Depressed mood is frequently present and often precedes the onset of the anxiety symptoms, which commonly occur following a major stressor.

Common Nursing Diagnoses and Interventions for the Patient With Separation Anxiety Disorder

(Interventions are applicable to various health-care settings, such as inpatient and partial hospitalization, community outpatient clinic, home health, and private practice.)

■ ANXIETY (Severe)

Definition: Vague uneasy feeling of discomfort or dread accompanied by an autonomic response (the source is often nonspecific or unknown to the individual); a feeling of apprehension caused by anticipation of danger. It is an alerting signal that warns of impending danger and enables the individual to take measures to deal with threat (NANDA-I, 2018, p. 324).

Possible Contributing Factors ("related to")

Heredity
[Birth temperament]
[Overattachment to parent]
[Negative role modeling]

Defining Characteristics ("evidenced by")

[Excessive distress when separated from attachment figure]
[Fear or anticipation of separation from attachment figure]
[Fear of being alone or without attachment figure]
[Reluctance or refusal to go to school or anywhere else without attachment figure]
[Nightmares about being separated from attachment figure]
[Somatic symptoms occurring as a result of fear of separation]

Goals/Objectives

Short-term Goal

The patient will discuss fears of separation with trusted individual.

Long-term Goal

The patient will maintain anxiety at no higher than moderate level in the face of events that formerly have precipitated panic.

Interventions With *Selected Rationales*

1. Establish an atmosphere of calmness, trust, and genuine positive regard. *Trust and unconditional acceptance are necessary for satisfactory nurse-patient relationship. Calmness is important because anxiety is easily transmitted from one person to another.*
2. Assure patient of his or her safety and security. *Symptoms of panic anxiety are very frightening.*
3. Explore the child's or adolescent's fears of separating from the parents. Explore with the parents possible fears they may have of separation from the child. *Some parents may have an underlying fear of separation from the child, of which they are unaware and which they are unconsciously transferring to the child.*
4. Help parents and child initiate realistic goals (e.g., child to stay with sitter for 2 hours with minimal anxiety or child to stay at friend's house without parents until 9 p.m. without experiencing panic anxiety). *Parents may be so frustrated with the child's clinging and demanding behaviors that assistance with problem-solving may be required.*
5. Give and encourage parents to give positive reinforcement for desired behaviors. *Positive reinforcement encourages repetition of desirable behaviors.*

Outcome Criteria

1. The patient and parents are able to discuss their fears regarding separation.
2. The patient experiences no somatic symptoms from fear of separation.
3. The patient maintains anxiety at moderate level when separation occurs or is anticipated.

■ INEFFECTIVE COPING

Definition: A pattern of invalid appraisal of stressors, with cognitive and/or behavioral efforts, that fails to manage demands related to well-being (NANDA-I, 2018, p. 327)

Possible Contributing Factors ("related to")

[Unresolved separation conflicts]
[Inadequate coping skills]

Defining Characteristics ("evidenced by")

[Somatic complaints in response to occurrence or anticipation of separation from attachment figure]

Goals/Objectives

Short-term Goal

The patient will verbalize correlation of somatic symptoms to fear of separation.

Long-term Goal

The patient will demonstrate use of more adaptive coping strategies (than physical symptoms) in response to stressful situations.

Interventions With *Selected Rationales*

1. Encourage child or adolescent to discuss specific situations in life that produce the most distress and describe his or her response to these situations. Include parents in the discussion. *The patient and family may be unaware of the correlation between stressful situations and the exacerbation of physical symptoms.*
2. Help the child or adolescent who is perfectionistic to recognize that self-expectations may be unrealistic. Connect times of unmet self-expectations to the exacerbation of physical symptoms. *Recognition of maladaptive patterns is the first step in the change process.*
3. Encourage parents and child to identify more adaptive coping strategies that the child could use in the face of anxiety that feels overwhelming. Practice through role-play. *Practice facilitates the use of the desired behavior when the individual is actually faced with the stressful situation.*

Outcome Criteria

1. The patient and family verbalize the correlation between separation anxiety and somatic symptoms.
2. The patient verbalizes the correlation between unmet self-expectations and somatic symptoms.
3. The patient responds to stressful situations without exhibiting physical symptoms.

■ IMPAIRED SOCIAL INTERACTION

Definition: Insufficient or excessive quantity or ineffective quality of social exchange (NANDA-I, 2018, p. 301)

Possible Contributing Factors ("related to")

[Reluctance to be away from attachment figure]

Defining Characteristics ("evidenced by")

[Symptoms of severe anxiety]
[Verbalized or observed] discomfort in social situations
[Verbalized or observed] inability to receive or communicate a satisfying sense of belonging, caring, interest, or shared history
[Observed] use of unsuccessful social interaction behaviors
Dysfunctional interaction with others

Goals/Objectives

Short-term Goal

The patient will spend time with staff or other support person (without presence of attachment figure) without excessive anxiety.

Long-term Goal

The patient will be able to spend time with others (without presence of attachment figure) without excessive anxiety.

Interventions With *Selected Rationales*

1. Develop a trusting relationship with the patient. *This is the first step in helping the patient learn to interact with others.*
2. Attend groups with the child, and support efforts to interact with others. Give positive feedback. *Presence of a trusted individual provides security during times of distress. Positive feedback encourages repetition.*
3. Convey to the child the acceptability of his or her not participating in group in the beginning. Gradually encourage small contributions until the patient is able to participate more fully. *Small successes will gradually increase self-confidence and decrease self-consciousness, so that the patient will feel less anxious in the group situation.*
4. Help the patient set small personal goals (e.g., "Today I will speak to one person I don't know"). *Simple, realistic goals provide opportunities for success that increase self-confidence and may encourage the patient to attempt more difficult objectives in the future.*

Outcome Criteria

1. The patient spends time with others using acceptable, age-appropriate behaviors.
2. The patient is able to interact with others away from the attachment figure without excessive anxiety.

@ INTERNET REFERENCES

Additional information about ADHD may be located at the following Web sites:

- www.chadd.org
- https://www.nimh.nih.gov/health/topics/attention-deficit-hyperactivity-disorder-adhd/index.shtml

Additional information about ASD may be located at the following Web sites:

- www.autism-society.org
- https://www.nimh.nih.gov/health/topics/autism-spectrum-disorders-pervasive-developmental-disorders/index.shtml

Additional information about medications to treat ADHD and Tourette's disorder may be located at the following Web sites:

- www.drugs.com
- www.nlm.nih.gov/medlineplus/druginformation.html

Movie Connections

Bill (Intellectual disability) • *Bill, On His Own* (Intellectual disability) • *Sling Blade* (Intellectual disability) • *Forrest Gump* (Intellectual disability) • *Rain Man* (ASD) • *Mercury Rising* (ASD) • *Niagara, Niagara* (Tourette's disorder) • *Phoebe in Wonderland* (Tourette's disorder) • *Toughlove* (Conduct disorder)

CHAPTER 3

Neurocognitive Disorders

■ BACKGROUND ASSESSMENT DATA

Delirium

Defined

The American Psychiatric Association (APA, 2013) *Diagnostic and Statistical Manual of Mental Disorders, Fifth Edition (DSM-5)* defines *delirium* as a disturbance in attention and awareness and a change in cognition that develop rapidly over a short period of time (usually hours to a few days). Duration is usually brief (e.g., 1 week; rarely more than 1 month), and the disorder subsides completely on recovery from the underlying determinant. If the underlying condition persists, the delirium may gradually progress to stupor, coma, seizures, or death (APA, 2013).

Etiology

The *DSM-5* differentiates among the disorders of delirium by their etiology, although they share a common symptom presentation. Categories of delirium include the following:

1. **Substance Intoxication Delirium:** Delirium symptoms can occur in response to taking high doses of cannabis, cocaine, hallucinogens, alcohol, anxiolytics, or narcotics.
2. **Substance Withdrawal Delirium:** Reduction or termination of long-term, high-dose use of certain substances, such as alcohol, sedatives, hypnotics, or anxiolytics, can result in withdrawal delirium symptoms.
3. **Medication-Induced Delirium:** The symptoms of delirium can occur as a side effect of a medication taken as prescribed. Medications that have been known to precipitate delirium include anticholinergics, antihypertensives, corticosteroids, anticonvulsants, cardiac glycosides, analgesics, anesthetics, antineoplastic agents, antiparkinson drugs, H_2-receptor antagonists (e.g., cimetidine), and others.
4. **Delirium Due to Another Medical Condition:** Certain medical conditions, such as systemic infections, metabolic disorders, fluid and electrolyte imbalances, liver or kidney disease, thiamine deficiency, postoperative states, hypertensive

encephalopathy, postictal states, and sequelae of head trauma can cause the symptoms of delirium.

5. **Delirium Due to Multiple Etiologies:** Symptoms of delirium may be related to more than one medical condition or to the combined effects of another medical condition and substance use or medication side effects. Current evidence suggests that delirium is usually the result of many factors rather than one (Fabian & Solai, 2017).

Symptomatology (Subjective and Objective Data)

The following symptoms have been identified with the syndrome of delirium:

1. Alteration in awareness (reduced orientation to the environment).
2. Extreme distractibility with difficulty focusing attention.
3. Disorientation to time and place.
4. Impaired reasoning ability and goal-directed behavior.
5. Disturbance in the sleep-wake cycle.
6. Emotional instability as manifested by fear, anxiety, depression, irritability, anger, euphoria, or apathy.
7. Misperceptions of the environment, including illusions and hallucinations.
8. Autonomic manifestations, such as tachycardia, sweating, flushed face, dilated pupils, and elevated blood pressure.
9. Incoherent speech.
10. Impairment of recent memory.

Neurocognitive Disorder

Defined

Neurocognitive disorder (NCD) is defined by the *DSM-5* as "evidence of significant cognitive decline from a previous level of performance in one or more cognitive domains (complex attention, executive function, learning and memory, language, perceptual-motor, or social cognition)" (APA, 2013, p. 602). The disorder is identified as *Major NCD* or *Mild NCD* according to the degree of impairment. The symptoms usually have a slow, insidious onset and are chronic, progressive, and irreversible.

Predisposing Factors to NCD

Following are major etiological categories for the syndrome of NCD:

1. **NCD Due to Alzheimer's Disease:** The exact cause of Alzheimer's disease is unknown, but several theories have been proposed, such as reduction in brain acetylcholine, the formation of plaques and tangles, serious head trauma, inflammation, and genetic factors. Pathological changes in the brain include atrophy, enlarged ventricles, and the presence of numerous neurofibrillary plaques and tangles. Definitive diagnosis is by biopsy or autopsy examination of brain tissue, although refinement of diagnostic

criteria and discriminating diagnostic instruments such as amyloid PET scans now enable clinicians to identify the disease at a high rate of accuracy. Current research is focusing on identifying early biomarkers that might be useful in preventing the illness or the minimizing the extent of progressive brain damage.

2. **Vascular NCD:** This type of NCD is caused by significant cerebrovascular disease. The patient suffers the equivalent of small strokes caused by arterial hypertension or cerebral emboli or thrombi, which destroy many areas of the brain. The onset of symptoms is more abrupt than in Alzheimer's disease and runs a highly variable course, progressing in steps rather than as a gradual deterioration.

3. **Frontotemporal NCD:** Symptoms from frontotemporal NCD occur as a result of shrinking of the frontal and temporal anterior lobes of the brain. The cause is unknown, but a genetic factor appears to be involved. Symptoms may include behavioral and personality changes, speech and language problems, or both. Apathy, a decline in social cognition, and compulsive/ritualistic behaviors are common. The disease progresses steadily and often rapidly, ranging from less than 2 years in some individuals to more than 10 years in others.

4. **NCD With Lewy Bodies:** Clinically, Lewy body NCD is fairly similar to Alzheimer's disease; however, it tends to progress more rapidly, and there is an earlier appearance of visual hallucinations and parkinsonian features. This disorder is distinctive by the presence of Lewy bodies—eosinophilic inclusion bodies—seen in the cerebral cortex and brainstem. Acetylcholinesterase (ACh) concentrations are reduced in the brains of people with Lewy body NCD, and as such, cholinesterase inhibitors are likely to be more effective for this population than for those with Alzheimer's dementia (Crystal, 2018).

5. **NCD Due to Traumatic Brain Injury:** *DSM-5* criteria states that this disorder "is caused by an impact to the head or other mechanisms of rapid movement or displacement of the brain within the skull, with one or more of the following: loss of consciousness, posttraumatic amnesia, disorientation and confusion, or neurological signs (e.g., positive neuroimaging demonstrating injury, a new onset of seizures or a marked worsening of a preexisting seizure disorder, visual field cuts, anosmia, hemiparesis)" (APA, 2013, p. 624). Depending on the severity of the injury, the symptoms may eventually subside or may become permanent.

6. **NCD Due to HIV Infection:** The immune dysfunction associated with HIV disease can lead to brain infections by other organisms. HIV also appears to cause NCD directly.

7. **NCD Due to Prion Disease:** This disorder is identified by its insidious onset, rapid progression, and manifestations of motor features of prion disease, such as myoclonus or ataxia, or biomarker evidence (APA, 2013). The clinical presentation

is typical of the syndrome of mild or major NCD, along with involuntary movements, muscle rigidity, and ataxia. The clinical course is extremely rapid, with progression from diagnosis to death in less than 2 years.

8. **NCD Due to Parkinson's Disease:** Parkinson's disease is caused by a loss of nerve cells in the substantia nigra of the basal ganglia. NCD is observed in as many as 75% of patients with Parkinson's disease (APA, 2013). The symptoms of NCD associated with Parkinson's disease often closely resemble those of Alzheimer's disease.

9. **NCD Due to Huntington's Disease:** This disease is transmitted as a Mendelian dominant gene, and damage occurs in the areas of the basal ganglia and the cerebral cortex. The onset of symptoms (i.e., involuntary twitching of the limbs or facial muscles, mild cognitive changes, depression, and apathy) usually occurs between age 30 and 50 years. The patient usually declines into a profound state of cognitive impairment and **ataxia** (muscular incoordination). The average duration of the disease is 10 to 20 years depending on the severity of symptoms. As the disease progresses, the weakened individual usually dies secondary to pneumonia, heart failure, choking, or other complications (Huntington's Disease Society of America [HDSA], 2019). About 10% of the cases occur in children and adolescents, and the progression is typically more rapid than it is in adult-onset Huntington's disease.

10. **NCD Due to Another Medical Condition:** A number of other general medical conditions can cause NCD. Some of these include hypothyroidism, hyperparathyroidism, pituitary insufficiency, uremia, encephalitis, brain tumor, pernicious anemia, thiamine deficiency, pellagra, uncontrolled epilepsy, cardiopulmonary insufficiency, fluid and electrolyte imbalances, central nervous system and systemic infections, systemic lupus erythematosus, and multiple sclerosis (APA, 2013).

11. **Substance/Medication-Induced NCD:** NCD can occur as the result of substance reactions, overuse, or abuse. Symptoms are consistent with major or mild NCD and persist beyond the usual duration of intoxication and acute withdrawal (APA, 2013). Substances that have been associated with the development of NCDs include alcohol, sedatives, hypnotics, anxiolytics, and inhalants. Drugs that cause anticholinergic side effects and toxins such as lead and mercury have also been implicated.

Symptomatology (Subjective and Objective Data)

Symptoms that have been identified with the syndrome of NCD include:

1. Memory impairment (impaired ability to learn new information or to recall previously learned information).

2. Impairment in abstract thinking, judgment, and impulse control.
3. Impairment in language ability, such as difficulty naming objects. In some instances, the individual may not speak at all (aphasia).
4. Personality changes.
5. Impaired ability to perform motor activities despite intact motor abilities (apraxia).
6. Disorientation.
7. Wandering.
8. Delusions (particularly delusions of persecution).

Common Nursing Diagnoses and Interventions for Delirium and NCD

(Interventions are applicable to various health-care settings, such as inpatient and partial hospitalization, community outpatient clinic, home health, and private practice.)

■ RISK FOR PHYSICAL TRAUMA

Definition: Susceptible to physical injury of sudden onset and severity which require immediate attention (NANDA International [NANDA-I], 2018, p. 401)

Risk Factors ("related to")

[Chronic alteration in structure or function of brain tissue, secondary to the aging process, multiple infarcts, HIV disease, head trauma, chronic substance abuse, or progressively dysfunctional physical condition resulting in the following symptoms:
    Disorientation; confusion
    Weakness
    Muscular incoordination
    [Seizures]
    Memory impairment
    Poor vision
    [Extreme psychomotor agitation observed in the late stages of delirium]
[Frequent shuffling of feet and stumbling]
[Falls, caused by muscular incoordination or seizures]
[Bumping into furniture]
[Exposing self to frigid conditions with insufficient protective clothing]
[Cutting self when using sharp instruments]
[History of attempting to light burner or oven and leaving gas on in house]
[Smoking and leaving burning cigarettes in various places; smoking in bed; falling asleep sitting on couch or chair with lighted cigarette in hand]
[Purposeless, thrashing movements; hyperactivity that is out of touch with the environment]

Goals/Objectives

Short-term Goals

1. The patient will call for assistance when ambulating or carrying out other activities.
2. The patient will not experience physical injury.

Long-term Goal

The patient will not experience physical injury.

Interventions With *Selected Rationales*

1. Assess the patient's level of disorientation and confusion to determine specific requirements for safety. *Knowledge of the patient's level of functioning is necessary to formulate appropriate plan of care.*
2. Institute appropriate safety measures, such as the following:
   a. Place furniture in the room in an arrangement that best accommodates the patient's disabilities.
   b. Observe patient behaviors frequently; assign staff on one-to-one basis if condition warrants; accompany and assist the patient when ambulating; use wheelchair for transporting long distances.
   c. Store items that the patient uses frequently within easy access.
   d. Remove potentially harmful articles from the patient's room: cigarettes, matches, lighters, and sharp objects.
   e. Supervise the patient when engaged in any activities that may increase risk of personal injury.
   f. Pad side rails and headboard of the patient with seizure disorder. Institute seizure precautions as described in procedure manual of individual institution.
   g. If the patient is prone to wander, provide an area within which wandering can be carried out safely.
3. Frequently orient the patient to reality and surroundings. *Disorientation may endanger patient safety if he or she unknowingly wanders away from safe environment.*
4. Use tranquilizing medications and soft restraints, as prescribed by physician, for the patient's protection during periods of excessive hyperactivity and assess patient carefully for evidence of adverse reaction to these medications. *Use restraints judiciously and only as a last resort, because they can increase agitation. They may be required, however, to provide for patient safety. Black box warnings for antipsychotic medication in elderly with dementia note that there is increased risk for death secondary to cardiovascular events.*
5. Teach prospective caregivers methods that have been successful in preventing patient injury. *These caregivers will be responsible for the patient's safety after discharge from the hospital. Sharing successful interventions may be helpful.*

Outcome Criteria

1. The patient is able to accomplish daily activities within the environment without experiencing injury.
2. Prospective caregivers are able to verbalize means of providing safe environment for the patient.

■ RISK FOR SELF-DIRECTED OR OTHER-DIRECTED VIOLENCE

Definition: Susceptible to behaviors in which an individual demonstrates that he or she can be physically, emotionally, and/or sexually harmful [either to self or to others] (NANDA-I, 2018, pp. 416–417)

Risk Factors ("related to")

[Chronic alteration in structure or function of brain tissue, secondary to the aging process, multiple infarcts, HIV disease, head trauma, chronic substance abuse, or progressively dysfunctional physical condition resulting in the following symptoms:
  Delusional thinking
  Suspiciousness of others
  Hallucinations
  Illusions
  Disorientation or confusion
  Impairment of impulse control
[Inaccurate perception of the environment]
Negative body language—rigid posture, clenching of fists and jaw, hyperactivity, pacing, breathlessness, and threatening stances.
Suicidal ideation, plan, available means
Cognitive impairment
[Depressed mood]

Goals/Objectives

Short-term Goals

1. The patient will maintain agitation at manageable level so as not to become violent.
2. The patient will not harm self or others.

Long-term Goal

The patient will not harm self or others.

Interventions With *Selected Rationales*

1. Assess the patient's level of anxiety and behaviors that indicate the anxiety is increasing. *Recognizing these behaviors, the nurse may be able to intervene before violence occurs.*

2. Assess the patient's level of orientation. *The patient's level of orientation may be variable, so ongoing assessment is important in protecting patient safety. This assessment is also valuable in differentiating pseudodementia (depression) in the older adult; patients with pseudodementia typically have more prominent symptoms of depression and more insight into their symptoms, and they improve with treatment for depression* (APA, 2013; Sadock et al, 2015).

3. Maintain low level of stimuli in the patient's environment (low lighting, few people, simple decor, low noise level). *Anxiety increases in a highly stimulating environment.*

4. Remove all potentially dangerous objects from the patient's environment. *In a disoriented, confused state, the patient may use these objects to harm self or others.*

5. Have sufficient staff available to execute a physical confrontation, if necessary. *Assistance may be required from others to provide for physical safety of the patient or primary nurse or both.*

6. Maintain a calm manner with the patient. Attempt to prevent frightening the patient unnecessarily. Provide continual reassurance and support. *Anxiety is contagious and can be transferred to the patient.*

7. Reorient to surroundings as needed. *Patient safety is jeopardized during periods of disorientation.*

8. Use tranquilizing medications and soft restraints, as prescribed by physician. Use restraints judiciously and only as a last resort for the protection of patient at imminent risk for harm to self or others. *Risk for confusion and falls is increased with use of sedating medications. Black box warnings for antipsychotic medication in elderly with dementia note that there is increased risk for death secondary to cardiovascular events.*

9. Sit with the patient and provide one-to-one observation if assessed to be actively suicidal. *Patient safety is a nursing priority, and one-to-one observation may be necessary to prevent a suicidal attempt.*

10. Teach relaxation exercises *to intervene in times of increasing anxiety.*

11. Incorporate person-centered activities, exercise, and social interaction. *This program, called "Well-Being and Health for People With Dementia (WHELD)," is a nonpharmacological, psychosocial intervention that focuses on tailored person-centered activities, exercise, and social interaction and has demonstrated benefits for decreasing agitation, decreasing use of antipsychotic medication, and improving quality of life for patients with dementia in long-term care settings* (Ballard et al, 2018).

12. Teach prospective caregivers to recognize patient behaviors that indicate anxiety is increasing and ways to intervene before violence occurs.

Outcome Criteria

1. Prospective caregivers are able to verbalize behaviors that indicate an increasing anxiety level and ways they may assist the patient to manage the anxiety before violence occurs.

2. With assistance from caregivers, the patient is able to control impulse to perform acts of violence against self or others.

■ CHRONIC CONFUSION

Definition: Irreversible, progressive, insidious, and long-term alteration of intellect, behavior, and personality, manifested by impairment in cognitive functions (memory, speech, language, decision-making, and executive function), and dependency in execution of daily activities (NANDA-I, 2018, p. 256)

Possible Contributing Factors ("related to")

[Alteration in structure/function of brain tissue, secondary to the following conditions:
  Vascular disease
  Hypertension
  Cerebral hypoxia
  Long-term abuse of mood- or behavior-altering substances
  Exposure to environmental toxins
  Various other physical disorders that predispose to cerebral abnormalities (see Predisposing Factors)]

Defining Characteristics ("evidenced by")

Altered interpretation
Altered personality
Altered response to stimuli
Clinical evidence of organic impairment
Impaired long-term memory
Impaired short-term memory
Impaired socialization
Long-standing cognitive impairment
No change in level of consciousness
Progressive cognitive impairment

Goals/Objectives

Short-term Goal

The patient will accept explanations of inaccurate interpretations within the environment.

Long-term Goal

With assistance from caregiver, the patient will be able to interrupt nonreality-based thinking.

Interventions With *Selected Rationales*

1. Frequently orient the patient to reality and surroundings. Allow the patient to have familiar objects around him or her. Use other items, such as clock, calendar, and daily schedules, to assist in maintaining reality orientation. *Patient safety is jeopardized during*

periods of disorientation. Maintaining reality orientation enhances cognitive function (Alzheimer's Australia, 2017) and may enhance the patient's sense of self-worth and personal dignity.

2. Teach prospective caregivers how to orient the patient to time, person, place, and circumstances as required. *These caregivers will be responsible for patient safety after discharge from the hospital. Sharing successful interventions may be helpful.*

3. Give positive feedback and validation when thinking and behavior are appropriate or when the patient verbalizes that certain ideas expressed are not based in reality. *Positive feedback increases self-esteem and enhances desire to repeat appropriate behaviors.*

4. Use simple explanations and face-to-face interaction when communicating with the patient. Do not shout message into the patient's ear. *Speaking slowly and in a face-to-face position is most effective when communicating with an elderly individual experiencing a hearing loss. Visual cues facilitate understanding. Shouting causes distortion of high-pitched sounds and in some instances creates a feeling of discomfort for the patient.*

5. Express reasonable doubt if the patient relays suspicious beliefs in response to delusional thinking. Discuss with the patient the potential personal negative effects of continued suspiciousness of others. Reinforce accurate perception of people and situations. *Expressions of doubt by a trusted individual may foster similar uncertainties about the delusion on the part of the patient.*

6. Do not focus on discussing false ideas. Instead talk to the patient about real people and real events. Validate the patient's feelings. *Reality orientation and validation increases the patient's sense of self-worth and personal dignity.*

7. Close observation of the patient's behavior is indicated if delusional thinking reveals an intention for violence. *Patient safety is a nursing priority.*

CLINICAL PEARL **Medications for Alzheimer's disease.** Cholinesterase inhibitors are used for mild to moderate cognitive impairment in patients with Alzheimer's disease. Examples include *donepezil (Aricept), rivastigmine (Exelon),* and *galantamine (Razadyne).* (Higher-dose donepezil has also been approved for moderate to severe Alzheimer's disease.) Common side effects include dizziness, headache, and gastrointestinal upset. *Memantine (Namenda),* an N-methyl-D-aspartate receptor antagonist, is used for treatment of moderate to severe cognitive impairment in patients with Alzheimer's disease. Common side effects of memantine include dizziness, headache, and constipation. These medications do not stop or reverse the disease process but may slow down the progression of the decline in functionality.

Outcome Criteria

1. With assistance from caregiver, the patient is able to distinguish between reality-based and nonreality-based thinking.

2. Prospective caregivers are able to verbalize ways in which to orient the patient to reality as needed.

■ SELF-CARE DEFICIT

Definition: Inability to independently perform tasks associated with [activities of daily living (ADLs)] (NANDA-I, 2018, pp. 243–246)

Possible Contributing Factors ("related to")
Cognitive impairment

Defining Characteristics ("evidenced by")
Inability to wash body
Inability to put on clothing
Inability to bring food from receptacle to the mouth
[Inability to toilet self without assistance]

Goals/Objectives
Short-term Goal
The patient will participate in ADLs with assistance from caregiver.
Long-term Goal
The patient will accomplish ADLs to the best of his or her ability.
   Unfulfilled needs will be met by caregiver.

Interventions With *Selected Rationales*
1. Provide a simple, structured environment *to minimize confusion:*
   a. Identify self-care deficits and provide assistance as required.
   b. Allow plenty of time for the patient to perform tasks.
   c. Provide guidance and support for independent actions by talking the patient through the task one step at a time.
   d. Provide a structured schedule of activities that does not change from day to day.
   e. Ensure that ADLs follow home routine as closely as possible.
   f. Provide for consistency in assignment of daily caregivers.
2. In planning for discharge:
   a. Perform ongoing assessment of the patient's ability to fulfill nutritional needs, ensure personal safety, follow medication regimen, and communicate need for assistance with those activities that he or she cannot accomplish independently. *Patient safety and security are nursing priorities.*
   b. Assess prospective caregivers' ability to anticipate and fulfill the patient's unmet needs. Provide information to assist caregivers with this responsibility. Ensure that caregivers are aware of available community support systems from which they can seek assistance when required.

This will facilitate transition to discharge from treatment center.

c. National support organizations can provide information:

National Parkinson Foundation
www.parkinson.org
1-800-4PD-INFO (1-800-473-4636)

Alzheimer's Association
www.alz.org
1-800-272-3900

Outcome Criteria

1. The patient willingly participates in ADLs.
2. The patient accomplishes ADLs to the best of his or her ability.
3. The patient's unfulfilled needs are met by caregivers.

■ DISTURBED SENSORY PERCEPTION (Specify)

Definition: Change in the amount or patterning of incoming stimuli [either internally or externally initiated] accompanied by a diminished, exaggerated, distorted, or impaired response to such stimuli (Note: This diagnosis has been retired by NANDA-I but is retained in this text because of its appropriateness in describing these specific behaviors.)

Possible Contributing Factors ("related to")

[Alteration in structure/function of brain tissue, secondary to the following conditions:
   Advanced age
   Vascular disease
   Hypertension
   Cerebral hypoxia
   Abuse of mood- or behavior-altering substances
   Exposure to environmental toxins
   Various other physical disorders that predispose to cerebral abnormalities (see Predisposing Factors)]

Defining Characteristics ("evidenced by")

Poor concentration
Sensory distortions
Hallucinations
[Disorientation to time, place, person, or circumstances]
[Inappropriate responses]
[Talking and laughing to self]
[Suspiciousness]

Goals/Objectives

Short-term Goal

With assistance from caregiver, the patient will maintain orientation to time, place, person, and circumstances for specified period of time.

Long-term Goal

The patient will demonstrate accurate perception of the environment by responding appropriately to stimuli indigenous to the surroundings.

Interventions With *Selected Rationales*

1. Decrease the amount of stimuli in the patient's environment (e.g., low noise level, few people, simple decor). *This decreases the possibility of the patient's forming inaccurate sensory perceptions.*
2. Do not reinforce the hallucination. Let the patient know that you do not share the perception. Maintain reality through re-orientation and focus on real situations and people. *Reality orientation enhances cognitive function and the patient's sense of personal dignity.*
3. Provide reassurance of safety if the patient responds with fear to inaccurate sensory perception. *Patient safety and security are nursing priorities.*
4. Correct the patient's description of inaccurate perception, and describe the situation as it exists in reality. *Explanation of and participation in real situations and real activities interferes with the ability to respond to hallucinations.*
5. Allow for care to be given by same personnel on a regular basis, if possible, *to provide a feeling of security and stability in the patient's environment.*
6. Teach prospective caregivers how to recognize signs and symptoms of the patient's inaccurate sensory perceptions. Explain techniques they may use to restore reality to the situation.

Outcome Criteria

1. With assistance from caregiver, the patient is able to recognize when perceptions within the environment are inaccurate.
2. Prospective caregivers are able to verbalize ways in which to correct inaccurate perceptions and restore reality to the situation.

■ CHRONIC LOW SELF-ESTEEM

Definition: Negative evaluation and/or feelings about one's own capabilities, lasting at least three months (NANDA-I, 2018, p. 272)

Possible Contributing Factors ("related to")

[Loss of independent functioning]
[Loss of capacity for remembering]
[Loss of capability for effective verbal communication]

Defining Characteristics ("evidenced by")

[Withdraws into social isolation]
Lack of eye contact
[Excessive crying alternating with expressions of anger]
[Refusal to participate in therapies]
[Refusal to participate in own self-care activities]
[Becomes increasingly dependent on others to perform ADLs]
Expressions of shame or guilt

Goals/Objectives

Short-term Goal

The patient will voluntarily spend time with staff and peers in day-room activities (time dimension to be individually determined).

Long-term Goal

The patient will exhibit increased feelings of self-worth as evidenced by voluntary participation in own self-care and interaction with others (time dimension to be individually determined).

Interventions With *Selected Rationales*

1. Encourage the patient to express honest feelings in relation to loss of prior level of functioning. Acknowledge pain of loss. Support the patient through process of grieving. *The patient may be fixed in anger stage of grieving process, which is turned inward on the self, resulting in diminished self-esteem.*
2. Devise methods for assisting the patient with memory deficit. *These aids may assist the patient to function more independently, thereby increasing self-esteem.* Examples follow:
   a. Name sign on door identifying the patient's room
   b. Identifying sign on outside of dining room door
   c. Identifying sign on outside of restroom door
   d. Large clock, with oversized numbers and hands, appropriately placed
   e. Large calendar, indicating one day at a time, with month, day, and year identified in bold print
   f. Printed, structured daily schedule, with one copy for the patient and one posted on unit wall
   g. "News board" on unit wall on which current national and local events may be posted
3. Encourage the patient's attempts to communicate. If verbalizations are not understandable, express to the patient what you think he or she intended to say. It may be necessary to reorient

the patient frequently or use validation therapy as a person-centered strategy to preserve self-esteem. *The ability to communicate effectively with others may enhance self-esteem.*

4. Encourage reminiscence and discussion of life review. Also discuss present-day events. Sharing picture albums, if possible, is especially good. *Reminiscence and life review help the patient resume progression through the grief process associated with disappointing life events and increase self-esteem as successes are reviewed.*

5. Encourage participation in group activities. Caregiver may need to accompany the patient at first, until he or she feels secure that the group members will be accepting, regardless of limitations in verbal communication. *Positive feedback from group members will increase self-esteem.*

6. Offer support and empathy when the patient expresses embarrassment at inability to remember people, events, and places. Focus on accomplishments *to promote positive self-esteem.*

7. Encourage the patient to be as independent as possible in self-care activities. Provide written schedule of tasks to be performed. Intervene in areas in which the patient requires assistance. *The ability to perform independently preserves self-esteem.*

Outcome Criteria

1. The patient initiates own self-care according to written schedule and willingly accepts assistance as needed.
2. The patient interacts with others in group activities, maintaining anxiety at minimal level in response to difficulties with verbal communication.

■ CAREGIVER ROLE STRAIN

Definition: Difficulty in fulfilling care responsibilities, expectations and/or behaviors for family or significant others (NANDA-I, 2018, p. 278)

Possible Contributing Factors ("related to")

Severity of the care receiver's illness
Chronicity of the care receiver's illness
[Lack of respite and recreation for the caregiver]
Caregiver's competing role commitments
Inadequate physical environment for providing care
Family or caregiver isolation
Complexity and amount of caregiving activities

Defining Characteristics ("evidenced by")

Apprehension about possible institutionalization of care receiver
Apprehension about future regarding care receiver's health and
caregiver's ability to provide care

Difficulty performing and/or completing required tasks

Apprehension about care receiver's care if caregiver unable to provide care

Goals/Objectives

Short-term Goal

Caregivers will verbalize understanding of ways to facilitate the caregiver role.

Long-term Goal

Caregivers will demonstrate effective problem-solving skills and develop adaptive coping mechanisms to regain equilibrium.

Interventions With *Selected Rationales*

1. Assess caregivers' ability to anticipate and fulfill the patient's unmet needs. Provide information to assist caregivers with this responsibility. *Caregivers may be unaware of what the patient will realistically be able to accomplish. They may be unaware of the progressive nature of the illness.*
2. Ensure that caregivers are aware of available community support systems from which they can seek assistance when required. Examples include adult day-care centers, housekeeping and homemaker services, respite-care services, and a local chapter of the Alzheimer's Association. This organization sponsors a nationwide 24-hour hotline to provide information and link families who need assistance with nearby chapters and affiliates. The hotline number is 1-800-272-3900. *Caregivers require relief from the pressures and strain of providing 24-hour care for their loved one. Studies show that elder abuse arises out of caregiving situations that place overwhelming stress on caregivers.*
3. Encourage caregivers to express feelings, particularly anger. *Release of these emotions can serve to prevent psychopathology, such as depression or psychophysiological disorders, from occurring.*
4. Encourage participation in support groups composed of members with similar life situations. *Hearing others who are experiencing the same problems discuss ways in which they have coped may help caregiver adopt more adaptive strategies. Individuals who are experiencing similar life situations provide empathy and support for each other.*

Outcome Criteria

1. Caregivers are able to problem-solve effectively regarding care of the elderly patient.
2. Caregivers demonstrate adaptive coping strategies for dealing with stress of caregiver role.
3. Caregivers express feelings openly.
4. Caregivers express desire to join support group of other caregivers.

@ INTERNET REFERENCES

Additional information about Alzheimer's disease may be located at the following Web sites:

- www.alz.org
- https://www.nia.nih.gov
- https://www.ninds.nih.gov/Disorders/All-Disorders/Alzheimers-Disease-Information-Page

Information on caregiving can be located at the following Web site:

- www.aarp.org/home-family/caregiving

Additional information about medications to treat Alzheimer's disease may be located at the following Web sites:

- https://medlineplus.gov/druginformation.html
- https://www.drugs.com/condition/alzheimer-s-disease.html

Movie Connections

The Notebook (Alzheimer's disease) • *Away From Her* (Alzheimer's disease) • *Iris* (Alzheimer's disease) • *Still Alice* (Early onset Alzheimer's disease)

CHAPTER 4

Substance-Related and Addictive Disorders

■ BACKGROUND ASSESSMENT DATA

The substance-related disorders are composed of two groups: substance use disorders (addiction) and substance-induced disorders (intoxication and withdrawal). Other disorders that may be substance-induced (delirium, neurocognitive disorder, psychotic disorders, bipolar disorders, depressive disorders, anxiety disorders, obsessive-compulsive and related disorders, and sexual dysfunctions) are included in the chapters with which they share symptomatology (e.g., substance-induced anxiety disorder is included in Chapter 8; substance-induced sexual dysfunction is included in Chapter 12). Also included in this chapter is a discussion of gambling disorder, a nonsubstance addiction disorder.

■ SUBSTANCE USE DISORDERS
Substance Addiction
Defined

The American Society of Addiction Medicine (ASAM) defines addiction as "a treatable, chronic medical disease involving complex interactions among brain circuits, genetics, the environment, and an individual's life experiences. People with addiction use substances or engage in behaviors that become compulsive and often continue despite harmful consequences" (ASAM, 2019).

The *Diagnostic and Statistical Manual of Mental Disorders, Fifth Edition (DSM-5)* (American Psychiatric Association [APA], 2013) lists diagnostic criteria for addiction to specific substances, including alcohol, cannabis, hallucinogens, inhalants, opioids, stimulants, tobacco, sedatives, hypnotics, and anxiolytics. Individuals are considered to have a substance use disorder when use of the substance interferes with their ability to fulfill role obligations, such as at work, school, or home. Often the individual would like to cut down or control use of the substance but attempts fail, and use of the substance continues to increase. There is an intense craving for the substance, and an excessive amount of time is spent trying to procure more of the substance or recover from the effects of its use. Use of the substance causes problems with interpersonal relationships, and the individual may become socially isolated. Individuals with substance use disorders often participate in hazardous activities when they are impaired by the substance and continue to use the substance despite knowing that its use is contributing to a physical or psychological problem. Addiction is evident when tolerance develops and the amount required to achieve the desired effect continues to increase. A syndrome of symptoms, characteristic of the specific substance, occurs when the individual with the addiction attempts to discontinue use of the substance.

■ SUBSTANCE-INDUCED DISORDERS

Substance Intoxication

Defined

Substance intoxication is a state of disturbance in cognition, perception, behavior, level of consciousness, judgment, and other functions that is directly attributable to the effects of a psychoactive drug. Manifestations include a physical and mental state of exhilaration and emotional frenzy or lethargy and stupor. The mood alteration and behavior changes can be attributed to the physiological effects of the substance on the central nervous system (CNS).

Substance Withdrawal

Defined

Substance withdrawal is a syndrome of symptoms that occur upon abrupt reduction or discontinuation of a substance that has been used regularly over a prolonged period of time. The substance-specific syndrome includes clinically significant physical signs and symptoms as well as psychological changes such as disturbances in thinking, feeling, and behavior. The effects are of sufficient significance to interfere with usual role performance and, in some cases, can be life threatening.

■ CLASSIFICATION OF SUBSTANCES

Alcohol

Although alcohol is a CNS depressant, it is considered separately because of the complex effects and widespread nature of its use. Low to moderate consumption produces a feeling of well-being and reduced inhibitions. At higher concentrations, both motor and intellectual functioning are impaired; mood becomes very labile; and behaviors characteristic of depression, euphoria, and aggression are exhibited. Historically, alcohol was used to treat a variety of conditions, including pain, but currently the only medical use for alcohol (with the exception of its inclusion in a number of pharmacological concentrates) is as an antidote for methanol consumption.

Examples: Beer, wine, bourbon, scotch, gin, vodka, rum, tequila, liqueurs

Common substances containing alcohol and used by some dependent individuals to satisfy their need include liquid cough medications, liquid cold preparations, mouthwashes, isopropyl rubbing alcohol, nail polish removers, colognes, and aftershave and preshave preparations.

Opioids

Opioids have a medical use as analgesics, antitussives, and antidiarrheals. They produce the effects of analgesia and euphoria by stimulating the opiate receptors in the brain, thereby mimicking the naturally occurring endorphins. Currently being abused in epidemic proportions in the United States, opiates have been implicated in alarming numbers of drug-related deaths, especially when mixed with fentanyl or an even more potent version, carfentanyl. The U.S. Food and Drug Administration (FDA, 2016) began requiring black-box warnings, its strongest warning label, for opioid analgesics, opioid cough products, and benzodiazepines based on evidence that the combination of opioids and benzodiazepines carries a particularly high risk for excessive sleepiness, respiratory depression, coma, and death.

Examples: Opioids of natural origin (opium, morphine, codeine), kratom (a plant indigenous to Southeast Asia that has opiate-like effects), opioid derivatives (heroin, hydromorphone, hydrocodone, oxycodone), synthetic opiate-like drugs (meperidine, methadone, pentazocine, fentanyl, sufentanil, and tramadol).

Common Street Names: Horse, junk, H (heroin); black stuff, poppy, big O (opium); M, white stuff, Miss Emma (morphine); dollies (methadone); terp (terpin hydrate or cough syrup with codeine); oxy, O.C. (oxycodone); vike (hydrocodone); doctors (meperidine); Apache, China girl, goodfella (fentanyl); U47700 (synthetic opiate)

■ CNS DEPRESSANTS

CNS depressants have a medical use as antianxiety agents, sedatives, hypnotics, anticonvulsants, and anesthetics. They depress the action of the CNS, resulting in an overall calming, relaxing effect on the individual. At higher dosages they can induce sleep.

Examples: Benzodiazepines, barbiturates, nonbarbiturate hypnotics (e.g., chloral hydrate, eszopiclone, ramelteon, zaleplon, zolpidem), meprobamate, club drugs (e.g., flunitrazepam, gamma-hydroxybutyrate [GHB])

Common Street Names: Peter, Mickey (chloral hydrate); green and whites, roaches (Librium); blues (Valium, 10 mg); yellows (Valium, 5 mg); candy, tranks (other benzodiazepines); red birds, red devils (secobarbital); downers (barbiturates; tranquilizers); rophies, roofies, forget-me pill, R2 (flunitrazepam [Rohypnol]); G, liquid X, grievous bodily harm, easy lay (GHB)

CNS Stimulants

CNS stimulants have a medical use in the management of hyperactivity disorders, narcolepsy, and weight control. They stimulate the action of the CNS, resulting in increased alertness, excitation, euphoria, increased pulse rate and blood pressure, insomnia, and loss of appetite. One research study found that their effectiveness in the treatment of hyperactivity disorders was based on the activation of dopamine D4 receptors in the basal ganglia and thalamus, which depress, rather than enhance, motor activity (Erlij et al, 2012).

Examples: Amphetamines (e.g., dextroamphetamine, methamphetamine, 3,4-methylene-dioxyamphetamine [MDMA]), nonamphetamine stimulants (e.g., phendimetrazine, benzphetamine, methylphenidate, dexmethylphenidate, modafinil), synthetic stimulants (e.g., mephedrone, methylone, ethylone, dibutylone), cocaine, caffeine, tobacco (Note: MDMA, mephedrone, and methylone are cross-listed with the hallucinogens.)

Common Street Names: Dexies, pep pills, black beauties, pick me ups, pickups, uppers, amps, speed (amphetamines); coke, snow, gold dust, girl (cocaine); crack, kryptonite, cookies, strong, rock (hydrochloride cocaine); speedball (mixture of heroin and cocaine); Adam, ecstasy, XTC (MDMA); bath salts (mephedrone, methylone); flakka, gravel (synthetic stimulant alpha-PVP cathinone)

Hallucinogens

Hallucinogens act as sympathomimetic agents, producing effects resembling those resulting from stimulation of the sympathetic nervous system (e.g., excitation, increased energy, distortion of the senses). Therapeutic medical uses for lysergic acid diethylamide (LSD) have been proposed in the treatment of chronic alcoholism and in the reduction of intractable pain, such as terminal malignant disease and phantom limb sensations. In 2018 the FDA approved the use of psilocybin for clinical trials to explore its benefits in treatment-resistant depression.

Examples: Naturally occurring hallucinogens (e.g., mescaline, psilocybin, ololiuqui), synthetic compounds (e.g., LSD, 2,5-dimethoxy-4-methylamphetamine [DOM], phencyclidine [PCP], ketamine, 3,4-methylenedioxyamphetamine [MDMA], mephedrone, methylone)

Common Street Names: Cactus, mesc (mescaline); magic mushroom, shrooms (psilocybin); heavenly blue, pearly gates (ololiuqui); acid, cube, California sunshine (LSD); serenity, tranquility, peace; STP (DOM); angel dust (PCP); vitamin K (ketamine); XTC, ecstasy, Adam (MDMA); mephedrone, methylone (bath salts) (Note: MDMA, mephedrone, and methylone are cross-listed with the CNS stimulants.)

Cannabinoids

Cannabinoids depress higher centers in the brain and consequently release lower centers from inhibitory influence. They produce an anxiety-free state of relaxation characterized by a feeling of extreme well-being. Large doses of the drug can produce hallucinations. Marijuana has been used therapeutically in the relief of nausea and vomiting associated with antineoplastic chemotherapy and in the relief of chronic pain. Two medications that have components of the marijuana plant or related synthetic compounds are currently FDA approved. Dronabinol, a synthetic compound in the medication Marinol, is approved for nausea and vomiting associated with cancer treatment and for severe weight loss associated with AIDS. Nabilone, a chemical similar to THC and found in the medication Cesamet, is a similar FDA-approved drug. A third medication, Sativex, is an oromucosal spray containing THC and cannabidiol. It can be prescribed in the United States only with a special exemption from the FDA for use in select patients (Sadock et al, 2015). In 2018, the first cannabis-based drug (Epidiolex) became FDA-approved for the treatment of epilepsy. Several states have legalized marijuana for medical uses, recreational uses, or both. Synthetic cannabinoids are identified as a group of new psychoactive substances more powerful than the cannabinoids in marijuana, more unpredictable in their effects, and possibly life-threatening (National Institute on Drug Abuse, 2018).

Examples: Marijuana, hashish

Common Street Names: Joints, reefers, pot, grass, Mary Jane (marijuana); hash, bhang, ganja (hashish); K2, spice, joker, black mamba, kush, kronic (synthetic cannabinoids)

Inhalants

Inhalant disorders are induced by inhaling the aliphatic and aromatic hydrocarbons found in substances such as fuels, solvents, adhesives, aerosol propellants, and paint thinners. Inhalants are absorbed through the lungs and reach the CNS very rapidly. Inhalants generally act as a CNS depressant. The effects are relatively brief, lasting from several minutes to a few hours, depending on the specific substance and amount consumed.

Examples: Gasoline, varnish remover, lighter fluid, airplane glue, rubber cement, cleaning fluid, spray paint, shoe conditioner, typewriter correction fluid

A profile summary of these psychoactive substances is presented in Table 4–1.

■ PREDISPOSING FACTORS ASSOCIATED WITH SUBSTANCE-RELATED DISORDERS

1. Physiological
   a. **Genetics:** A genetic link may be involved in the development of substance-related disorders. This is especially evident with alcoholism, less so with other substances. Children of alcoholics are four times more likely than other children to become alcoholics (American Academy of Child and Adolescent Psychiatry, 2019). Studies with monozygotic and dizygotic twins have also supported the genetic hypothesis.

TABLE 4-1 Psychoactive Substances: A Profile Summary

Class of Drugs	Symptoms of Use	Therapeutic Uses	Symptoms of Overdose	Trade Names	Common Names
CNS Depressants					
Alcohol	Relaxation, loss of inhibitions, lack of concentration, drowsiness, slurred speech, sleep	Antidote for methanol consumption; ingredient in many pharmacological concentrates	Nausea, vomiting; shallow respirations; cold, clammy skin; weak, rapid pulse; coma; possible death	Ethyl alcohol, beer, gin, rum, vodka, bourbon, whiskey, liqueurs, wine, brandy, sherry, champagne	Booze, alcohol, liquor, drinks, cocktails, highballs, nightcaps, moonshine, white lightning, firewater
Other (barbiturates and nonbarbiturates)	Same as alcohol	Relief from anxiety and insomnia; as anticonvulsants and anesthetics	Anxiety, fever, agitation, hallucinations, disorientation, tremors, delirium, convulsions, possible death	Seconal, Amytal, Nembutal Valium Librium Noctec Miltown	Red birds, yellow birds, blue birds Blues/yellows Green & whites Mickeys Downers
CNS Stimulants					
Amphetamines and related drugs	Hyperactivity, agitation, euphoria, insomnia, loss of appetite	Management of narcolepsy, hyperkinesia, and weight control	Cardiac arrhythmias, headache, convulsions, hypertension, rapid heart rate, coma, possible death	Dexedrine, Didrex, Tenuate, Bontril, Ritalin, Focalin, Meridia, Provigil	Uppers, pep pills, wakeups, bennies, eye-openers, speed, black beauties, sweet A's, pick me ups, pick ups, kryptonite, amps, cookies, strong

Cocaine	Euphoria, hyperactivity, restlessness, talkativeness, increased pulse, dilated pupils, rhinitis	Hallucinations, convulsions, pulmonary edema, respiratory failure, coma, cardiac arrest, possible death	Cocaine hydrochloride	Coke, flake, snow, dust, happy dust, gold dust, girl, Cecil, C, toot, blow, crack
Synthetic stimulants	Agitation, insomnia, irritability, dizziness, decreased ability to think clearly, increased heart rate, chest pains	Paranoia, delusions, seizures, panic attacks, nausea, vomiting, heart attack, stroke, hallucinations, aggressive behavior	Mephedrone, MDPV (3,4-methylene-dioxypyrovalerone) 4-methylmeth-cathinone (mephedrone, 4-MMC)* Methylone* Ethylone Dibutylone Alpha-PVP	Bath salts, bliss, vanilla sky, ivory wave, purple wave, flakka, gravel

(Continued)

TABLE 4-1 Psychoactive Substances: A Profile Summary—cont'd

Class of Drugs	Symptoms of Use	Therapeutic Uses	Symptoms of Overdose	Trade Names	Common Names
Opioids	Euphoria, lethargy, drowsiness, lack of motivation, constricted pupils	As analgesics; antidiarrheals, and antitussives; methadone in substitution therapy; heroin has no therapeutic use	Shallow breathing, slowed pulse, clammy skin, pulmonary edema, respiratory arrest, convulsions, coma, possible death	Heroin	Snow, stuff, H, harry, horse
				Morphine	M, morph, Miss Emma
				Codeine	Schoolboy
				Dilaudid	Lords
				Demerol	Doctors
				Dolophine	Dollies
				Percodan	Perkies
				Talwin	Ts
				Opium	Big O, black stuff
				Carfentanyl	Kratom (opiate-like plant)
				Sufentanil	U47700 (synthetic opioid)
Hallucinogens	Visual hallucinations, disorientation, confusion, paranoid delusions, euphoria, anxiety, panic, increased pulse	LSD has been proposed in the treatment of chronic alcoholism, and in the reduction of intractable pain	Agitation, extreme hyperactivity, violence, hallucinations, psychosis, convulsions, possible death	LSD	Acid, cube, big D
				PCP	Angel dust, hog, peace pill
				Mescaline	Mesc
				DMT	Businessman's trip
				STP, DOM	Serenity and peace
				MDMA	Ecstasy, XTC

	Effects	Therapeutic Use	Adverse Effects	Source	Street Names
		Psilocybin is currently being tested in clinical trials for treatment-resistant depression		Ketamine MDPV	Special K, vitamin K, kit kat Bath salts
Cannabinoids	Relaxation, talkativeness, lowered inhibitions, euphoria, mood swings	Marijuana has been used for relief of nausea and vomiting associated with antineoplastic chemotherapy and to reduce eye pressure in glaucoma Treatment of epilepsy (Epidiolex)	Fatigue, paranoia, delusions, hallucinations, possible psychosis	Cannabis Hashish	Marijuana, pot, grass, joint, Mary Jane, MJ Hash, rope, Sweet Lucy Synthetic cannabinoids: K2, Kush, Joker, Black mamba, Spice, Kronic

b. **Biochemical:** Neurotransmitters that have been strongly linked to substance abuse include opioid, catecholamine (especially dopamine), glutamate (especially those binding to N-methyl-D-aspartate [NMDA]), and gamma-aminobutyric acid (GABA) systems (Sadock, Sadock, & Ruiz, 2015). Once activated, the neuronal pathways that sense pleasure and reward are believed responsible for pleasurable sensations associated with the substance, as well as creating a "memory" that triggers a desire for repeated use of the substance. These pathways are referred to as the *brain-reward circuitry*. Over time, the brain tries to compensate for this excessive activation by lowering levels of these neurotransmitters, and the result is that an individual begins to feel sick when he or she stops or attempts to curtail use of substance. At this point, the substance user needs to continue use of the substance simply to feel less sick.

2. Psychosocial
   a. **Psychodynamic Theory:** The psychodynamic approach to the etiology of substance abuse focuses on a punitive superego and fixation at the oral stage of psychosexual development which manifests as using alcohol to control panic, opioids to diminish anger, or amphetamines to counter depression (Sadock, Sadock, & Ruiz, 2015).
   b. **Social Learning Theory:** The effects of modeling, imitation, and identification on behavior can be observed from early childhood onward. In relation to drug consumption, the family appears to be an important influence. Various studies have shown that children and adolescents are more likely to use substances if they have parents who provide a model for substance use. Peers often exert a great deal of influence in the life of the child or adolescent who is being encouraged to use substances for the first time. Modeling may continue to be a factor in the use of substances once the individual enters the workforce. This is particularly true in the work setting that provides plenty of leisure time with coworkers and in which drinking is valued and is used to express group cohesiveness.

■ COMMON PATTERNS OF USE IN SUBSTANCE-RELATED DISORDERS

Symptomatology (Subjective and Objective Data)

Alcohol Use Disorder

1. Begins with social drinking that provides feeling of relaxation and well-being, which soon requires increasing amounts of alcohol to produce the same effects.
2. Drinks in secret; hides bottles of alcohol; drinks first thing in the morning (to "steady my nerves") and at any other opportunity that arises during the day.

3. As the disease progresses, the individual may drink in binges. During a binge, drinking continues until the individual is too intoxicated or too sick to consume any more. Behavior borders on the psychotic, with the individual wavering in and out of reality.
4. Begins to have blackouts. Periods of amnesia occur (in the absence of intoxication or loss of consciousness) during which the individual is unable to remember periods of time or events that have occurred.
5. Experiences multisystem physiological impairments from chronic use that include (but are not limited to) the following:
   a. **Peripheral Neuropathy:** Numbness, tingling, pain in extremities (caused by thiamine deficiency).
   b. **Wernicke-Korsakoff Syndrome:** Mental confusion, agitation, diplopia (caused by thiamine deficiency). Without immediate thiamine replacement, rapid deterioration to coma and death will occur.
   c. **Alcoholic Cardiomyopathy:** Enlargement of the heart caused by an accumulation of excess lipids in myocardial cells. Symptoms of tachycardia, dyspnea, and arrhythmias may be evident.
   d. **Esophagitis:** Inflammation of and pain in the esophagus.
   e. **Esophageal Varices:** Distended veins in the esophagus, with risk of rupture and subsequent hemorrhage.
   f. **Gastritis:** Inflammation of lining of stomach caused by irritation from the alcohol, resulting in pain, nausea, vomiting, and possibility of bleeding because of erosion of blood vessels.
   g. **Pancreatitis:** Inflammation of the pancreas, resulting in pain, nausea and vomiting, and abdominal distention. With progressive destruction to the gland, symptoms of diabetes mellitus could occur.
   h. **Alcoholic Hepatitis:** Inflammation of the liver, resulting in enlargement, jaundice, right upper-quadrant pain, and fever.
   i. **Cirrhosis of the Liver:** Fibrous and degenerative changes occurring in response to chronic accumulation of large amounts of fatty acids in the liver. In cirrhosis, symptoms of alcoholic hepatitis progress to include the following:
      • **Portal Hypertension:** Elevation of blood pressure through the portal circulation resulting from defective blood flow through the cirrhotic liver.
      • **Ascites:** An accumulation of serous fluid in the peritoneal cavity.
      • **Hepatic Encephalopathy:** Liver disorder caused by inability of the liver to convert ammonia to urea (the body's natural method of discarding excess ammonia); as serum ammonia levels rise, confusion occurs, accompanied by restlessness, slurred speech, fever, and without intervention, an eventual progression to coma and death.

Alcohol Intoxication

1. Symptoms of alcohol intoxication include disinhibition of sexual or aggressive impulses, mood lability, impaired judgment, impaired social or occupational functioning, slurred speech, incoordination, unsteady gait, nystagmus, and flushed face.
2. Physical and behavioral impairment based on blood alcohol concentrations differ according to gender, body size, physical condition, and level of tolerance.
3. The legal definition of intoxication in the United States is a blood alcohol concentration of 80 mg ethanol per deciliter of blood (mg/dL), which is also measured as 0.08 g/dL.
4. Nontolerant individuals with blood alcohol concentrations greater than 300 mg/dL are at risk for respiratory failure, coma, and death (Sadock et al, 2015).

Alcohol Withdrawal

1. Occurs within 4 to 12 hours of cessation of or reduction in heavy and prolonged alcohol use.
2. Symptoms include coarse tremor of hands, tongue, or eyelids; nausea or vomiting; malaise or weakness; tachycardia; sweating; elevated blood pressure; anxiety; depressed mood or irritability; transient hallucinations or illusions; headache; seizures; and insomnia.
3. Without aggressive intervention, the individual may progress to *alcohol withdrawal delirium* on the second or third day following cessation of or reduction in prolonged, heavy alcohol use. Symptoms include those described under the syndrome of delirium (see Chapter 3).

Amphetamine (or Amphetamine-type) Use Disorder

1. The use of amphetamines is often initiated for their appetite-suppressant effect in an attempt to lose or control weight.
2. Amphetamines are also taken for the initial feeling of well-being and confidence.
3. They are typically taken orally, intravenously, or by nasal inhalation.
4. Chronic daily (or almost daily) use usually results in an increase in dosage over time to produce the desired effect.
5. Episodic use often takes the form of binges, followed by an intense and unpleasant "crash" in which the individual experiences anxiety, irritability, and feelings of fatigue and depression with increased risk for suicide.
6. Continued use appears to be related to a craving for the substance rather than to prevention or alleviation of withdrawal symptoms.

Amphetamine (or Amphetamine-type) Intoxication

1. Amphetamine intoxication usually begins with a "high" feeling, followed by the development of symptoms of affective blunting;

changes in sociability; hypervigilance; interpersonal sensitivity; anxiety, tension, or anger; stereotyped behaviors; and impaired judgment.

2. Physical signs and symptoms that occur with amphetamine intoxication include tachycardia or bradycardia, pupillary dilation, elevated or lowered blood pressure, perspiration or chills, nausea or vomiting, weight loss, psychomotor retardation or agitation, muscular weakness, respiratory depression, chest pain or cardiac arrhythmias, confusion, seizures, dyskinesias, dystonia, or coma (APA, 2013).

Amphetamine (or Amphetamine-type) Withdrawal

1. Amphetamine withdrawal symptoms occur after cessation of (or reduction in) amphetamine (or a related substance) use that has been heavy and prolonged.

2. Symptoms of amphetamine withdrawal develop within a few hours to several days and include fatigue and depression with risk for suicide; vivid, unpleasant dreams; insomnia or hypersomnia; psychotic symptoms; increased appetite; headache; profuse sweating; and muscle cramps.

Cannabis Use Disorder

1. Cannabis preparations are almost always smoked but may also be taken orally.

2. It is commonly but incorrectly regarded to be a substance without potential for addiction. Synthetic cannabinoids are particularly associated with increased risk for addiction.

3. Tolerance to the substance may result in increased frequency of its use.

4. Abuse is evidenced by participation in hazardous activities when motor coordination is impaired from cannabis use.

Cannabis Intoxication

1. Cannabis intoxication is characterized by impaired motor coordination, euphoria, anxiety, sensation of slowed time, impaired judgment, and social withdrawal that develop during or shortly after cannabis use.

2. Physical symptoms of cannabis intoxication include conjunctival injection (redness), increased appetite, dry mouth, and tachycardia (APA, 2013).

3. The impairment of motor skills lasts for 8 to 12 hours.

Cannabis Withdrawal

1. The *DSM-5* (APA, 2013) describes a syndrome of symptoms that occur upon cessation of cannabis use that has been heavy and prolonged. Symptoms occur within a week following cessation of use and may include any of the following: irritability, anger, or aggression; nervousness or anxiety; sleep difficulty

(e.g., insomnia, disturbing dreams); decreased appetite or weight loss; restlessness; depressed mood.
2. Physical symptoms of cannabis withdrawal may include abdominal pain, tremors, sweating, fever, chills, or headache.

Cocaine Use Disorder

1. Various forms are smoked, inhaled, injected, or taken orally.
2. Chronic daily (or almost daily) use usually results in an increase in dosage over time to produce the desired effect.
3. Episodic use often takes the form of binges, followed by an intense and unpleasant crash in which the individual experiences anxiety, irritability, and feelings of fatigue and depression.
4. The drug user often abuses or is dependent on a CNS depressant to relieve the residual effects of cocaine.
5. Regular, prolonged use of cocaine leads to tolerance of the substance and subsequent use of increasing doses.
6. Continued use appears to be related to a craving for the substance rather than to prevention or alleviation of withdrawal symptoms.

Cocaine Intoxication

1. Symptoms of cocaine intoxication develop during or shortly after use of cocaine.
2. Symptoms of cocaine intoxication include euphoria, fighting, grandiosity, hypervigilance, psychomotor agitation, and impaired judgment.
3. Physical symptoms of cocaine intoxication include tachycardia, elevated blood pressure, papillary dilation, perspiration or chills, nausea or vomiting, chest pain, cardiac arrhythmias, hallucinations, seizures, and delirium.

Cocaine Withdrawal

1. Symptoms of withdrawal occur after cessation of or reduction in cocaine use that has been heavy and prolonged.
2. Symptoms of cocaine withdrawal include depression, anxiety, irritability, fatigue, insomnia or hypersomnia, psychomotor agitation, paranoid or suicidal ideation, apathy, and social withdrawal.

Hallucinogen Use Disorder

1. Hallucinogenic substances are taken orally.
2. The cognitive and perceptual impairment may last for up to 12 hours, so use is generally episodic because the individual must organize time during the daily schedule for its use.
3. Frequent use results in tolerance to the effects of the substance.
4. Addiction is rare, and most people are able to resume their previous lifestyle, following a period of hallucinogen use, without much difficulty.
5. Flashbacks may occur following cessation of hallucinogen use. These episodes consist of visual or auditory misperceptions

usually lasting only a few seconds but sometimes lasting up to several hours.

6. Hallucinogens are highly unpredictable in the effects they may induce each time they are used.

Hallucinogen Intoxication

1. Symptoms of intoxication develop during or shortly after hallucinogen use.
2. Symptoms include marked anxiety or depression, ideas of reference, fear of losing one's mind, paranoid ideation, and impaired judgment.
3. Other symptoms include subjective intensification of perceptions, depersonalization, derealization, illusions, hallucinations, and synesthesia.
4. Most hallucinogens have sympathomimetic effects, including tachycardia, hypertension, hyperthermia, sweating, pupillary dilation, and tremors (Delgado, Traub, & Grayzel, 2017).

Inhalant Use Disorder

1. Effects are induced by inhaling the vapors of volatile substances through the nose or mouth.
2. Examples of substances include glue, gasoline, paint, paint thinners, various cleaning chemicals, and typewriter correction fluid.
3. Use of inhalants often begins in childhood, and considerable family dysfunction is characteristic.
4. Use may be daily or episodic, and chronic use may continue into adulthood.
5. Tolerance has been reported among individuals with heavy use, but a withdrawal syndrome from these substances has not been well documented.

Inhalant Intoxication

1. Symptoms of intoxication develop during or shortly after use of or exposure to volatile inhalants.
2. Symptoms of inhalant intoxication include euphoria, excitation, disinhibition, belligerence, impaired judgment, and impaired social or occupational functioning.
3. Physical symptoms of inhalant intoxication include dizziness, ataxia, nystagmus, blurred vision, slurred speech, hypoactive reflexes, psychomotor retardation, lethargy, generalized muscular weakness, stupor, or coma (at higher doses) (APA, 2013).

Tobacco Use Disorder (Nicotine)

1. The effects of tobacco (nicotine) are induced through inhaling the smoke of cigarettes, cigars, or pipe tobacco, and orally through the use of snuff or chewing tobacco. The popular practice of "vaping" (inhaling vaporized smoke) exposes the user to potentially high doses of nicotine and other chemicals

and has been associated with significant, potentially fatal respiratory illness.
2. Continued use results in a craving for the substance.
3. Tobacco is commonly used to relieve or to avoid withdrawal symptoms that occur when the individual has been in a situation in which use is restricted.
4. Multiple medical problems are associated with prolonged tobacco use, including heart disease, stroke, asthma, COPD, emphysema, and lung cancer.

Tobacco (Nicotine) Withdrawal

1. Symptoms of withdrawal develop within 24 hours after abrupt cessation of (or reduction in) prolonged tobacco use.
2. Symptoms of tobacco (nicotine) withdrawal include dysphoric or depressed mood, insomnia, irritability, frustration, anger, anxiety, difficulty concentrating, restlessness, decreased heart rate, and increased appetite (APA, 2013).

Opioid Use Disorder

1. Various forms are taken orally, intravenously, by nasal inhalation, and by smoking.
2. Dependence occurs after recreational use of the substance "on the street" or after prescribed use of the substance for relief of pain or cough.
3. Chronic use leads to remarkably high levels of tolerance.
4. Once addiction is established, substance procurement often comes to dominate the person's life.
5. Cessation or decreased consumption results in a craving for the substance and produces a specific syndrome of withdrawal.

Opioid Intoxication

1. Symptoms of intoxication develop during or shortly after opioid use.
2. Symptoms of opioid intoxication include euphoria (initially) followed by apathy, dysphoria, psychomotor agitation or retardation, impaired judgment, and impaired social or occupational functioning.
3. Physical symptoms of opioid intoxication include pupillary constriction (or dilation due to anoxia from severe overdose), drowsiness, slurred speech, and impairment in attention or memory (APA, 2013).
4. Severe opioid intoxication can lead to respiratory depression, coma, and death.

Opioid Withdrawal

1. Symptoms of opioid withdrawal occur after cessation of (or reduction in) heavy and prolonged opioid use.
2. Symptoms of opioid withdrawal include dysphoric mood, nausea or vomiting, muscle aches, lacrimation or rhinorrhea,

pupillary dilation, piloerection, sweating, diarrhea, yawning, fever, and insomnia (APA, 2013).

3. Withdrawal symptoms are consistent with the half-life of the drug that is used. Withdrawal from the ultra-short-acting drugs such as meperidine begins quickly (within minutes to hours). With longer-acting drugs such as methadone, withdrawal begins within 1 to 3 days and may last for as long as 3 weeks.

Phencyclidine Use Disorder

1. PCP is taken orally, intravenously, or by smoking or inhaling.
2. Use can be on a chronic daily basis but more often is taken episodically in binges that can last several days.
3. Physical addiction does not occur with PCP; however, psychological addiction, characterized by craving for the drug, has been reported in chronic users, as has the development of tolerance.
4. Tolerance apparently develops quickly with frequent use.

Phencyclidine Intoxication

1. Symptoms of intoxication develop during or shortly after PCP use.
2. Symptoms of PCP intoxication include belligerence, assaultiveness, impulsiveness, unpredictability, psychomotor agitation, and impaired judgment.
3. Physical symptoms occur within an hour or less of PCP use and include vertical or horizontal nystagmus, hypertension, tachycardia, numbness or diminished responsiveness to pain, ataxia, muscle rigidity, and seizures.

Sedative, Hypnotic, or Anxiolytic Use Disorder

1. These substances are primarily taken orally.
2. Dependence can occur following recreational use of the substance "on the street" or after prescribed use of the substance for relief of anxiety or insomnia.
3. Chronic use leads to remarkably high levels of tolerance.
4. Once dependence develops, there is evidence of strong substance-seeking behaviors (obtaining prescriptions from several physicians or resorting to illegal sources to maintain adequate supplies of the substance).
5. Abrupt cessation of these substances can result in life-threatening withdrawal symptoms.

Sedative, Hypnotic, or Anxiolytic Intoxication

1. Symptoms of intoxication develop during or shortly after intake of sedatives, hypnotics, or anxiolytics.
2. Symptoms of intoxication include inappropriate sexual or aggressive behavior, mood lability, impaired judgment, and impaired social or occupational functioning.

3. Physical symptoms of sedative, hypnotic, or anxiolytic intoxication include slurred speech, incoordination, unsteady gait, nystagmus, impairment in attention or memory, stupor, or coma.

Sedative, Hypnotic, or Anxiolytic Withdrawal

1. Withdrawal symptoms occur after cessation of (or reduction in) heavy and prolonged use of sedatives, hypnotics, or anxiolytics.

2. Symptoms of withdrawal occur within several hours to a few days after abrupt cessation or reduction in use of the drug (depending on the half-life of the drug).

3. Symptoms of withdrawal include autonomic hyperactivity (e.g., sweating or pulse rate greater than 100); increased hand tremor; insomnia; nausea or vomiting; transient visual, tactile, or auditory hallucinations or illusions; psychomotor agitation; anxiety; or grand mal seizures.

A summary of symptoms associated with the syndromes of intoxication and withdrawal is presented in Table 4–2.

■ NONSUBSTANCE-RELATED DISORDERS
Gambling Disorder

This disorder is defined by the *DSM-5* as persistent and recurrent problematic gambling behavior leading to clinically significant impairment or distress (APA, 2013). The preoccupation with and impulse to gamble often intensifies when the individual is under stress. Many impulsive gamblers describe a physical sensation of restlessness and anticipation that can only be relieved by placing a bet. Often, the individual exhibits characteristics associated with narcissism and grandiosity and has difficulties with intimacy, empathy, and trust.

As the need to gamble increases, the individual is forced to obtain money by any means available. This may include borrowing money from illegal sources or pawning personal items (or items that belong to others). As gambling debts accrue or out of a need to continue gambling, the individual may desperately resort to forgery, theft, or even embezzlement. Family relationships are disrupted, and impairment in occupational functioning may occur because of absences from work in order to gamble.

Gambling behavior usually begins in adolescence; however, compulsive behaviors rarely occur before young adulthood. The disorder generally runs a chronic course, with periods of waxing and waning, largely dependent on periods of psychosocial stress. Prevalence estimates for problem gambling range from 3% to 5%, with about 1% meeting the criteria for a gambling disorder (Sadock et al, 2015). This condition is more common among men than women.

TABLE 4–2 Summary of Symptoms Associated With the Syndromes of Intoxication and Withdrawal

Class of Drugs	Intoxication	Withdrawal	Comments
Alcohol	Aggressiveness, impaired judgment, impaired attention, irritability, euphoria, depression, emotional lability, slurred speech, incoordination, unsteady gait, nystagmus, flushed face	Tremors, nausea/vomiting, malaise, weakness, tachycardia, sweating, elevated blood pressure, anxiety, depressed mood, irritability, hallucinations, headache, insomnia, seizures	Alcohol withdrawal begins within 4–6 hr after last drink. May progress to delirium tremens on second or third day. Use of Librium or Serax is common for substitution therapy.
Amphetamines and related substances	Fighting, grandiosity, hypervigilance, psychomotor agitation, impaired judgment, tachycardia, pupillary dilation, elevated blood pressure, perspiration or chills, nausea and vomiting	Anxiety, depressed mood, irritability, craving for the substance, fatigue, insomnia or hypersomnia, psychomotor agitation, paranoid and suicidal ideation	Withdrawal symptoms usually peak within 2–4 days, although depression and irritability may persist for months. Antidepressants may be used.
Caffeine	Restlessness, nervousness, excitement, insomnia, flushed face, diuresis, gastrointestinal complaints, muscle twitching, rambling flow of thought and speech, cardiac arrhythmia, periods of inexhaustibility, psychomotor agitation	Headache	Caffeine is contained in coffee, tea, colas, cocoa, chocolate, some over-the-counter analgesics, "cold" preparations, and stimulants.

(Continued)

TABLE 4-2 Summary of Symptoms Associated With the Syndromes of Intoxication and Withdrawal—cont'd

Class of Drugs	Intoxication	Withdrawal	Comments
Cannabis	Euphoria, anxiety, suspiciousness, sensation of slowed time, impaired judgment, social withdrawal, tachycardia, conjunctival redness, increased appetite, hallucinations	Restlessness, irritability, insomnia, loss of appetite	Intoxication occurs immediately and lasts about 3 hr. Oral ingestion is more slowly absorbed and has longer-lasting effects.
Cocaine	Euphoria, fighting, grandiosity, hypervigilance, psychomotor agitation, impaired judgment, tachycardia, elevated blood pressure, pupillary dilation, perspiration or chills, nausea/vomiting, hallucinations, delirium	Depression, anxiety, irritability, fatigue, insomnia or hypersomnia, psychomotor agitation, paranoid or suicidal ideation, apathy, social withdrawal	Large doses of the drug can result in convulsions or death from cardiac arrhythmias or respiratory paralysis.
Inhalants	Belligerence, assaultiveness, apathy, impaired judgment, dizziness, nystagmus, slurred speech, unsteady gait, lethargy, depressed reflexes, tremor, blurred vision, stupor or coma, euphoria, irritation around eyes, throat, and nose		Intoxication occurs within 5 min of inhalation. Symptoms last 60–90 min. Large doses can result in death from CNS depression or cardiac arrhythmia.

Tobacco (nicotine)		Craving for the drug, irritability, anger, frustration, anxiety, difficulty concentrating, restlessness, decreased heart rate, increased appetite, weight gain, tremor, headaches, insomnia	Symptoms of withdrawal begin within 24 hr of last drug use and decrease in intensity over days, weeks, or sometimes longer.
Opioids	Euphoria, lethargy, somnolence, apathy, dysphoria, impaired judgment, pupillary constriction, drowsiness, slurred speech, constipation, nausea, decreased respiratory rate and blood pressure	Craving for the drug, nausea/vomiting, muscle aches, lacrimation or rhinorrhea, pupillary dilation, piloerection or sweating, diarrhea, yawning, fever, insomnia	Withdrawal symptoms appear within 6–8 hr after last dose, reach a peak in the second or third day, and subside in 5–10 days. Times are shorter with meperidine and longer with methadone.
Phencyclidine and related substances	Belligerence, assaultiveness, impulsiveness, psychomotor agitation, impaired judgment, nystagmus, increased heart rate and blood pressure, diminished pain response, ataxia, dysarthria, muscle rigidity, seizures, hyperacusis, delirium		Delirium can occur within 24 hr after use of phencyclidine, or may occur up to a week following recovery from an overdose of the drug.
Sedatives, hypnotics, and anxiolytics	Disinhibition of sexual or aggressive impulses, mood lability, impaired judgment, slurred speech, incoordination, unsteady gait, impairment in attention or memory, disorientation, confusion	Nausea/vomiting, malaise, weakness, tachycardia, sweating, anxiety, irritability, orthostatic hypotension, tremor, insomnia, seizures	Withdrawal may progress to delirium, usually within 1 wk of last use. Long-acting barbiturates or benzodiazepines may be used in withdrawal substitution therapy.

Predisposing Factors Associated With Gambling Disorder

1. Biological
   a. **Genetics:** Familial and twin studies show an increased prevalence of pathological gambling in family members of individuals diagnosed with the disorder.
   b. **Physiological:** Studies of dopamine receptor systems have implicated this neurotransmitter in the development of addictive personality traits, including pathological gambling (Weiss & Pontone, 2014). Support for this association comes from studies that demonstrated a correlation between the development of pathological gambling behaviors after individuals were treated with dopamine receptor agonist drugs (Moore, Glenmullen, & Mattison, 2014).

      Biochemical theories suggest that, ironically, both winning and losing (perhaps related to the excitement of taking a risk) may stimulate the reward and pleasure centers of the brain. This response could contribute to persistent and repeated desire to gamble even when one is not winning.
2. Psychological
   a. Sadock and associates (2015) report that the following may be predisposing factors to the development of pathological gambling: "loss of a parent by death, separation, divorce, or desertion before the child is 15 years of age; inappropriate parental discipline (absence, inconsistency, or harshness); exposure to and availability of gambling activities for the adolescent; a family emphasis on material and financial symbols; and a lack of family emphasis on saving, planning, and budgeting" (p. 691).

Common Nursing Diagnoses and Interventions for Patients With Substance-Related and Addictive Disorders

(Interventions are applicable to various health-care settings, such as inpatient and partial hospitalization, community outpatient clinic, home health, and private practice.)

■ RISK FOR INJURY

Definition: Susceptible to physical damage due to [internal or external] environmental conditions interacting with the individual's adaptive and defensive resources, which may compromise health (NANDA International [NANDA-I], 2018, p. 393)

Risk Factors ("related to")

[Substance intoxication]
[Substance withdrawal]

[Disorientation]
[Seizures]
[Hallucinations]
[Psychomotor agitation]
[Unstable vital signs]
[Delirium]
[Flashbacks]
[Panic level of anxiety]

Goals/Objectives

Short-term Goal
The patient's condition will stabilize within 72 hours.

Long-term Goal
The patient will not experience physical injury.

Interventions With *Selected Rationales*

1. Assess the patient's level of disorientation to determine specific requirements for safety. *Knowledge of the patient's level of functioning is necessary to formulate appropriate plan of care.*
2. Obtain a drug history, if possible, to determine the following:
   a. Type of substance(s) used.
   b. Time of last ingestion and amount consumed.
   c. Length and frequency of consumption.
   d. Amount consumed on a daily basis.
3. Obtain urine sample for laboratory analysis of substance content. *Subjective history is often not accurate. Knowledge regarding substance ingestion is important for accurate assessment of patient condition.*
4. Place the patient in quiet, private room. *Excessive stimuli increase patient agitation.*
5. Institute necessary safety precautions (*patient safety is a nursing priority*):
   a. Observe patient behaviors frequently; assign staff on one-to-one basis if condition is warranted; accompany and assist patient when ambulating; use wheelchair for transporting long distances.
   b. Be sure that side rails are up when patient is in bed.
   c. Pad headboard and side rails of bed with thick towels to protect patient in case of seizure.
   d. Use mechanical restraints as necessary to protect patient if excessive hyperactivity accompanies the disorientation (e.g., as may occur in stimulant intoxication).

6. Ensure that smoking materials and other potentially harmful objects are stored away from the patient's access. *Patient may harm self or others in disoriented, confused state.*

7. Frequently orient the patient to reality and surroundings. *Disorientation may endanger patient safety if he or she unknowingly wanders away from safe environment.*

8. Monitor the patient's vital signs every 15 minutes initially and less frequently as acute symptoms subside. *Vital signs provide the most reliable information about the patient's condition and need for medication during acute intoxication and detoxification period.*

9. Follow medication regimen, as ordered by physician.* Common medical intervention for substance intoxication with the following substances includes:

    a. **Alcohol:** Alcohol intoxication and particularly alcohol poisoning require primarily supportive care including careful monitoring, assessment for breathing or choking problems, oxygen therapy, vitamins, and fluids to prevent dehydration (Mayo Clinic, 2019).

    b. **Narcotics**: Opioid antagonists such as naloxone (Narcan) may be administered through IV, intramuscular, subcutaneous, or intranasal routes to reverse CNS and respiratory depression associated with opioid overdose.

    c. **Stimulants:** Treatment of stimulant intoxication usually begins with minor tranquilizers such as chlordiazepoxide (Librium) and progresses to major tranquilizers such as haloperidol (Haldol). Antipsychotics should be administered with caution because of their propensity to lower seizure threshold. Repeated seizures are treated with intravenous diazepam.

    d. **Hallucinogens and Cannabinoids:** Substitution therapy is not required with these drugs. When adverse reactions such as anxiety or panic occur, benzodiazepines (e.g., diazepam or chlordiazepoxide) may be prescribed to prevent harm to the patient or others. Psychotic reactions may be treated with antipsychotic medications.

Outcome Criteria

1. Patient is no longer exhibiting any signs or symptoms of substance intoxication or withdrawal.

2. Patient shows no evidence of physical injury obtained during substance intoxication or withdrawal.

---

*See the next diagnosis for interventions specific to acute substance withdrawal syndrome.

■ ACUTE SUBSTANCE WITHDRAWAL SYNDROME

Definition: Serious multifactorial sequelae following abrupt cessation of an addictive compound. (NANDA-I, 2018, p. 351)

Possible Contributing Factors ("related to")

Sudden cessation of an addictive substance
Dependence on alcohol or other addictive substance
Heavy use of an addictive substance over time
Malnutrition

Defining Characteristics ("evidenced by")

Acute confusion
Anxiety
Disturbed sleep pattern
Nausea
Risk for electrolyte imbalance
Risk for injury

Goals/Objectives

Short-term Goal

Patient's condition will stabilize within 72 hours.

Long-term Goal

Patient will remain free of negative sequelae associated with acute substance withdrawal.

Interventions With *Selected Rationales*

1. Assess the patient's level for early symptoms of withdrawal and for level of disorientation to determine specific requirements for safety. *Knowledge of the patient's level of functioning is necessary to formulate appropriate plan of care.*
2. Institute necessary safety precautions *(patient safety is a nursing priority)*:
   a. Observe patient behaviors frequently; assign staff on one-to-one basis if condition is warranted; accompany and assist patient when ambulating; use wheelchair for transporting long distances.
   b. Be sure that side rails are up when the patient is in bed.
   c. Pad headboard and side rails of bed with thick towels to protect the patient in case of seizure.
3. Monitor the patient's vital signs every 15 minutes initially and less frequently as acute symptoms subside. *Vital signs provide the*

most reliable information about patient condition and need for med-ication during acute detoxification period.

4. Follow medication regimen, as ordered by physician. Common medical intervention for detoxification from the following sub-stances includes:

a. **Alcohol:** Benzodiazepines are the most widely used group of drugs for substitution therapy in alcohol withdrawal. They are administered in decreasing doses until withdrawal is complete. Commonly used agents include chlordiazepoxide (Librium), oxazepam (Serax), diazepam (Valium), and alpra-zolam (Xanax). In patients with liver disease, accumulation of the longer-acting agents, such as chlordiazepoxide, may be problematic, and the use of shorter-acting benzodi-azepines, such as oxazepam, is more appropriate. Some physicians may order anticonvulsant medication to be used prophylactically; however, this is not a universal in-tervention. Multivitamin therapy in combination with daily thiamine (either orally or by injection) is common protocol.

b. **Narcotics:** Opioid antagonists such as naloxone (Narcan) may be administered through IV, intramuscular, subcuta-neous, or intranasal routes to reverse CNS and respiratory depression associated with opioid overdose. Another opioid antagonist, naltrexone (ReVia, Vivitrol) may be adminis-tered via oral or intramuscular routes as part of an overall treatment program for management of alcohol and opioid dependence. Naltrexone blocks the opioid effects, but patient should be educated that there is risk for serious consequences, including death, if he or she takes higher doses of opioids to try to overcome naltrexone's antagonist effects. Patient should be assessed for the last time he or she used opioids or alcohol. Alcohol should be avoided during treatment with naltrexone; concurrent use increases the risk of liver damage. Patients must be free of opioids for 7 to 10 days before naltrexone therapy is initiated. One recent study, though, demonstrated effective results by rapid detoxification using buprenorphine for 1 day followed by low doses of naltrexone for the next 7 days followed by long-acting, injectable naltrexone (Sullivan et al, 2017). This alternative is attractive because the need to maintain abstinence from opioids for 7 to 10 days before initiating naltrexone treatment was associated with a higher risk for relapse and lack of follow-through with the treatment program. Otherwise, withdrawal is managed with rest and nutritional therapy, and substitution therapy may be instituted to decrease withdrawal symptoms using methadone (Dolophine) or buprenorphine (Subutex). Clonidine (Catapres) also has been used to suppress opiate withdrawal symptoms. As monotherapy, it is not as effective as substitution with methadone (an opioid agonist), but it is nonaddicting and serves effectively as a bridge that enables the patient to stay opiate-free long enough to facilitate termination of methadone maintenance.

c. **Depressants:** Substitution therapy may be instituted to decrease withdrawal symptoms using a long-acting barbiturate, such as phenobarbital (Luminal). The dosage required to suppress withdrawal symptoms is administered. When stabilization has been achieved, the dose is gradually decreased by 30 mg/day until withdrawal is complete. Long-acting benzodiazepines are commonly used for substitution therapy when the abused substance is a nonbarbiturate CNS depressant.

d. **Stimulants:** Withdrawal treatment is usually aimed at reducing drug craving and managing severe depression. The patient is placed in a quiet atmosphere and allowed to sleep and eat as much as is needed or desired. Suicide precautions may need to be instituted. Antidepressant therapy may be helpful in treating symptoms of depression. Desipramine has demonstrated efficacy not only in treating depression associated with cocaine withdrawal and abstinence but also in reducing cravings for the drug (American Addiction Centers, 2017).

e. **Hallucinogens and Cannabinoids**: Substitution therapy is not required with these drugs. When adverse reactions, such as anxiety or panic, occur, benzodiazepines (e.g., diazepam or chlordiazepoxide) may be prescribed to prevent harm to the patient or others. Psychotic reactions may be treated with antipsychotic medications.

■ DENIAL

Definition: Conscious or unconscious attempt to disavow the knowledge or meaning of an event to reduce anxiety/fear, leading to the detriment of health [or other aspects of the individual's life] (NANDA-I, 2018, p. 336)

Possible Contributing Factors ("related to")

[Weak, underdeveloped ego]
[Underlying fears and anxieties]
[Low self-esteem]
[Fixation in early level of development]

Defining Characteristics ("evidenced by")

[Denies substance-related or other addictions]

[Denies that substance use or gambling creates problems in his or her life]

[Continues to use substance or gamble, knowing it contributes to impairment in functioning, exacerbation of physical symptoms, or disruption on interpersonal relationships]

[Uses substance(s) in physically hazardous situations]

[Use of rationalization and projection to explain maladaptive behaviors]

Unable to admit impact of [the disorder] on life pattern

Goals/Objectives

Short-term Goal

Patient will divert attention away from external issues and focus on behavioral outcomes associated with substance-related or addictive disorder.

Long-term Goal

Patient will verbalize acceptance of responsibility for own behavior and acknowledge association between substance use or gambling and personal problems.

Interventions With *Selected Rationales*

1. Begin by working to develop a trusting nurse-patient relationship. Be honest. Keep all promises. *Trust is the basis of a therapeutic relationship.*
2. Convey an attitude of acceptance to the patient. Ensure that he or she understands, "It is not *you* but your *behavior* that is contributing to negative consequences and difficulty functioning." *An attitude of acceptance promotes feelings of dignity and self-worth.*
3. Incorporate motivational interviewing techniques to assess the patient's motivation to change. *Motivational interviewing is a patient-centered approach that incorporates open-ended questions, reflection, and a host of other therapeutic communication techniques that may reduce defensive responses by accepting the patient and initiating intervention with respect for where patient is in the process of recognizing the need for change.*
4. Provide information to correct misconceptions about the substance use or gambling behavior. Patient may rationalize his or her behavior with statements such as, "I'm not addicted. I can stop drinking (or gambling) any time I want," or "I only smoke pot to relax before class. So what? I know lots of people who do. Besides, you can't get hooked on pot."

Many myths abound regarding addictions. Factual information presented in a matter-of-fact, nonjudgmental way explaining what behaviors constitute substance-related and addictive disorders may help the patient focus on his or her own behaviors as an illness that requires help.

5. Identify recent maladaptive behaviors or situations that have occurred in the patient's life, and discuss how use of substances or gambling behavior may have been a contributing factor. *The first step in decreasing use of denial is for patient to see the relationship between substance use (or gambling) and personal problems.*

6. Use confrontation with caring. Do not allow patient to fantasize about his or her lifestyle. *Confrontation interferes with patient's ability to use denial; a caring attitude preserves self-esteem and avoids putting the patient on the defensive.*

🐟 **CLINICAL PEARL** It is important to speak objectively and nonjudgmentally to a person in denial. Examples: "It is my understanding that the last time you drank alcohol (gambled), you . . ." or "The lab report shows that your blood alcohol level was .25 when you were involved in that automobile accident" or "Your family is being evicted from their home because you lost the rent money when you bet on the horses."

---

7. Explore the use of rationalization or projection as the patient attempts to make excuses for or blame his or her behavior on other people or situations. *Rationalization and projection prolong the stage of denial that problems exist in the patient's life because of substance use or gambling.*

8. Encourage participation in group activities. *Peer feedback is often more accepted than feedback from authority figures. Peer pressure can be a strong factor as well as the association with individuals who are experiencing or who have experienced similar problems.*

9. Offer immediate positive recognition of patient's expressions of insight gained regarding illness and acceptance of responsibility for own behavior. *Positive reinforcement enhances self-esteem and encourages repetition of desirable behaviors.*

Outcome Criteria

1. Patient verbalizes understanding of the relationship between personal problems and the use of substances or gambling behaviors.

2. Patient verbalizes acceptance of responsibility for own behavior.

3. Patient verbalizes understanding of substance (or gambling) addiction as an illness requiring ongoing support and treatment.

■ INEFFECTIVE COPING

Definition: A pattern of invalid appraisal of stressors, with cognitive and/or behavioral efforts, that fails to manage demands related to well-being (NANDA-I, 2018, p. 327)

Possible Contributing Factors ("related to")

[Inadequate support systems]
[Inadequate coping skills]
[Underdeveloped ego]
[Possible hereditary factor]
[Dysfunctional family system]
[Negative role modeling]
[Personal vulnerability]

Defining Characteristics ("evidenced by")

[Low self-esteem]
[Chronic anxiety]
[Chronic depression]
Inability to meet role expectations
[Alteration in societal participation]
Inability to meet basic needs
[Inappropriate use of defense mechanisms]
Substance abuse
[Pathological gambling behaviors]
[Low frustration tolerance]
[Need for immediate gratification]
[Manipulative behavior]

Goals/Objectives

Short-term Goal

Patient will express true feelings associated with gambling or the use of substances as a method of coping with stress.

Long-term Goal

Patient will be able to verbalize adaptive coping mechanisms to use, instead of gambling or substance abuse, in response to stress.

Interventions With *Selected Rationales*

1. Establish trusting relationship with patient (be honest, keep appointments, be available to spend time). *The therapeutic nurse-patient relationship is built on trust.*
2. Set limits on manipulative behavior. Be sure the patient knows what is acceptable, what is not, and the consequences

for violating the limits set. Ensure that all staff maintains consistency with this intervention. *Patient is unable to establish own limits, so limits must be set for him or her. Unless administration of consequences for violation of limits is consistent, manipulative behavior will not be eliminated.*

3. Encourage patient to verbalize feelings, fears, and anxieties. Answer any questions he or she may have regarding the disorder. *Verbalization of feelings in a nonthreatening environment may help patient come to terms with long-unresolved issues.*

4. Explain the effects of substance abuse on the body. Emphasize that prognosis is closely related to abstinence. *Many patients lack knowledge regarding the deleterious effects of substance abuse on the body.*

5. Explore with patient the options available to assist with stressful situations rather than resorting to gambling or use of substances (e.g., contacting various members of Alcoholics Anonymous, Narcotics Anonymous, or Gamblers Anonymous; physical exercise; relaxation techniques; or meditation). *Patient may have persistently resorted to addictive behaviors and thus may possess little or no knowledge of adaptive responses to stress.*

6. Provide positive reinforcement for evidence of gratification delayed appropriately. *Positive reinforcement enhances self-esteem and encourages patient to repeat acceptable behaviors.*

7. Encourage patient to be as independent as possible in own self-care. Provide positive feedback for independent decision-making and effective use of problem-solving skills.

Outcome Criteria

1. Patient is able to verbalize adaptive coping strategies as alternatives to use of addictive behaviors in response to stress.
2. Patient is able to verbalize the names of support people from whom he or she may seek help when the desire to gamble or use substances is intense.

IMBALANCED NUTRITION: LESS THAN BODY REQUIREMENTS

Definition: Intake of nutrients insufficient to meet metabolic needs (NANDA-I, 2018, p. 157)

Possible Contributing Factors ("related to")

[Drinking alcohol instead of eating nourishing food]
[Eating only "junk food"]
[Eating nothing (or very little) while on a "binge"]

[No money for food (having spent what is available on substances)]
[Problems with malabsorption caused by chronic alcohol abuse]

Defining Characteristics ("evidenced by")

Loss of weight
Pale conjunctiva and mucous membranes
Poor muscle tone
[Poor skin turgor]
[Edema of extremities]
[Electrolyte imbalances]
[Cheilosis (cracks at corners of mouth)]
[Scaly dermatitis]
[Weakness]
[Neuropathies]
[Anemia]
[Ascites]

Goals/Objectives

Short-term Goals

1. Patient will gain 2 lb during next 7 days.
2. Patient's electrolytes will be restored to normal within 1 week.

Long-term Goal

Patient will exhibit no signs or symptoms of malnutrition by discharge. (This is not a realistic goal for a chronic alcoholic in the end stages of the disease. For such a patient, it is more appropriate to establish short-term goals as realistic step objectives to use in the evaluation of care given.)

Interventions With *Selected Rationales*

1. In collaboration with dietitian, determine number of calories required to provide adequate nutrition and realistic (according to body structure and height) weight gain.
2. Strict documentation of intake, output, and calorie count. *This information is necessary to make an accurate nutritional assessment and maintain patient safety.*
3. Weigh daily. *Weight loss or gain is important assessment information.*
4. Determine patient's likes and dislikes, and collaborate with dietitian to provide favorite foods. *Patient is more likely to eat foods that he or she particularly enjoys.*
5. Offer the patient small, frequent feedings, including a bedtime snack, if unable to tolerate three larger meals. *Large amounts of food may be objectionable, or even intolerable, to the patient.*
6. Administer vitamin and mineral supplements, as ordered by physician, *to improve nutritional state.*
7. If appropriate, ask family members or significant others to bring in special foods that patient particularly enjoys.

8. Monitor laboratory work, and report significant changes to physician.
9. Explain the importance of adequate nutrition. *Patient may have inadequate or inaccurate knowledge regarding the contribution of good nutrition to overall wellness.*

Outcome Criteria

1. Patient has achieved and maintained at least 90% of normal body weight.
2. Patient's vital signs, blood pressure, and laboratory serum studies are within normal limits.
3. Patient is able to verbalize importance of adequate nutrition.

■ CHRONIC LOW SELF-ESTEEM

Definition: Negative self-evaluation and/or feelings about one's own capabilities, lasting at least three months (NANDA-I, 2018, p. 272)

Possible Contributing Factors ("related to")

[Retarded ego development]
[Dysfunctional family system]
[Lack of positive feedback]
[Perceived failures]

Defining Characteristics ("evidenced by")

[Difficulty accepting positive reinforcement]
[Failure to take responsibility for self-care]
[Self-destructive behavior (substance use or pathological gambling)]
Lack of eye contact
Shame
[Withdraws into social isolation]
[Highly critical and judgmental of self and others]
[Sense of worthlessness]
[Fear of failure]
[Unable to recognize own accomplishments]
[Setting up self for failure by establishing unrealistic goals]
[Unsatisfactory interpersonal relationships]
[Negative or pessimistic outlook]
[Denial of problems obvious to others]
[Projection of blame or responsibility for problems]
[Rationalizing personal failures]
[Hypersensitivity to slight criticism]
[Grandiosity]

Goals/Objectives

Short-term Goal

Patient will accept responsibility for and verbalize the connection between substance use or gambling behaviors and negative consequences.

Long-term Goal

By time of discharge, patient will exhibit increased feelings of self-worth as evidenced by verbal expression of positive aspects about self, past accomplishments, and future prospects.

Interventions With *Selected Rationales*

1. Be accepting of patient and his or her negativism. *An attitude of acceptance enhances feelings of self-worth.*
2. Spend time with patient *to convey acceptance and contribute toward feelings of self-worth.*
3. Help patient to recognize and focus on strengths and accomplishments. Discuss past (real or perceived) negative consequences related to substance use or gambling, but minimize amount of attention devoted to them beyond patient's need to accept responsibility for them. *Patient must accept responsibility for own behavior before change in behavior can occur. Minimizing attention to past failures may help to eliminate negative ruminations and increase patient's sense of self-worth.*
4. Encourage participation in group activities *from which patient may receive positive feedback and support from peers.*
5. Help patient identify areas he or she would like to change about self and assist with problem-solving toward this effort. *Low self-worth may interfere with patient's perception of own problem-solving ability. Assistance may be required.*
6. Ensure that patient is not becoming increasingly dependent and that he or she is accepting responsibility for own behaviors. *Patient must be able to function independently if he or she is to be successful within the less-structured community environment.*
7. Ensure that therapy groups offer patient simple methods of achievement. Offer recognition and positive feedback for actual accomplishments. *Successes and recognition increase self-esteem.*
8. Provide instruction in assertiveness techniques: the ability to recognize the difference among passive, assertive, and aggressive behaviors and the importance of respecting the human rights of others while protecting one's own basic human rights. *Self-esteem is enhanced by the ability to interact with others in an assertive manner.*
9. Teach effective communication techniques, such as the use of "I" messages and placing emphasis on ways to avoid making judgmental statements.

Outcome Criteria

1. Patient is able to verbalize positive aspects about self.
2. Patient is able to communicate assertively with others.
3. Patient expresses an optimistic outlook for the future.

■ DEFICIENT KNOWLEDGE (About Effects of Substance Use on the Body)

Definition: Absence of cognitive information related to [the effects of substance abuse on the body and its interference with achievement and maintenance of optimal wellness], or its acquisition (NANDA-I, 2018, p. 259)

Possible Contributing Factors ("related to")

Lack of interest in learning
[Low self-esteem]
[Denial of need for information]
[Denial of risks involved with substance abuse]
Unfamiliarity with information resources

Defining Characteristics ("evidenced by")

[Abuse of substances]
[Statement of lack of knowledge]
[Statement of misconception]
[Request for information]
Verbalization of the problem

Goals/Objectives

Short-term Goal

Patient will be able to verbalize effects of [substance used] on the body following implementation of teaching plan.

Long-term Goal

Patient will verbalize the importance of abstaining from use of [substance] to maintain optimal wellness.

Interventions With *Selected Rationales*

1. Assess patient's level of knowledge regarding effects of [substance] on body. *Baseline assessment of knowledge is required to develop appropriate teaching plan for patient.*
2. Assess patient's level of anxiety and readiness to learn. *Learning does not take place beyond moderate level of anxiety.*
3. Determine method of learning most appropriate for patient (e.g., discussion, question and answer, use of audio or visual

aids, oral or written method). *Level of education and development are important considerations as to methodology selected.*

4. Develop teaching plan, including measurable objectives for the learner. *Measurable objectives provide criteria on which to base evaluation of the teaching experience.*
5. Include significant others, if possible. *Lifestyle changes often affect all family members.*
6. Implement teaching plan at a time that facilitates and in a place that is conducive to optimal learning (e.g., in the evening when family members visit; in an empty, quiet classroom or group therapy room). *Learning is enhanced by an environment with few distractions.*
7. Begin with simple concepts and progress to the more complex. *Retention is increased if introductory material presented is easy to understand.*
8. Include information on physical effects of [substance]: substance's capacity for physiological and psychological addiction, its effects on family functioning, its effects on a fetus (and the importance of contraceptive use until abstinence has been achieved), and the importance of regular participation in an appropriate treatment program.
9. Provide activities for patient and significant others in which to participate actively during the learning exercise. *Active participation increases retention.*
10. Ask patient and significant others to demonstrate knowledge gained by verbalizing information presented. *Verbalization of knowledge gained is a measurable method of evaluating the teaching experience.*
11. Provide positive feedback for participation as well as for accurate demonstration of knowledge acquired. *Positive feedback enhances self-esteem and encourages repetition of desired behaviors.*
12. Evaluate teaching plan. Identify strengths and weaknesses as well as any changes that may enhance the effectiveness of the plan.

Outcome Criteria

1. Patient is able to verbalize effects of [substance] on the body.
2. Patient verbalizes understanding of risks involved in use of [substance].
3. Patient is able to verbalize community resources for obtaining knowledge and support with substance-related problems.

■ DYSFUNCTIONAL FAMILY PROCESSES

Definition: Family functioning which fails to support the well-being of its members (NANDA-I, 2018, p. 290)

Possible Contributing Factors ("related to")

Substance abuse
Genetic predisposition [to addictions]
Lack of problem-solving skills
Inadequate coping skills
Family history of substance abuse
Biochemical influences
Addictive personality
[Pathological gambling]

Defining Characteristics ("evidenced by")

Anxiety, anger/suppressed rage; shame and embarrassment
Emotional isolation/loneliness; vulnerability; repressed emotions
Disturbed family dynamics; closed communication systems, in-
effective spousal communication and marital problems
Altered role function/disruption of family roles
Manipulation; dependency; blaming/criticizing; rationalization/
denial of problems
Enabling to maintain [addiction]; refusal to get help/inability to
accept and receive help appropriately

Goals/Objectives

Short-term Goals

1. Family members will participate in individual family programs
and support groups.
2. Family members will identify ineffective coping behaviors and
consequences.
3. Family will initiate and plan for necessary lifestyle changes.

Long-term Goal

Family members will take action to change self-destructive behaviors and alter behaviors that contribute to patient's addiction.

Interventions With *Selected Rationales*

1. Review family history; explore roles of family members, circumstances involving the addictive behavior, strengths, areas of growth.
This information determines areas for focus and potential for change.
2. Explore how family members have coped with the patient's
addiction (e.g., denial, repression, rationalization, hurt, loneliness, projection). *Persons who enable also suffer from the same
feelings as the patient and use ineffective methods for dealing
with the situation, necessitating help in learning new and effective
coping skills.*
3. Determine understanding of current situation and previous
methods of coping with life's problems. *Provides information
on which to base present plan of care.*

4. Assess current level of functioning of family members. *Affects individual's ability to cope with the situation.*

5. Determine extent of enabling behaviors being evidenced by family members; explore with each individual and patient. *Enabling is doing for the patient what he or she needs to do for self (rescuing). People want to be helpful and do not want to feel powerless to help their loved one to stop substance use or gambling and change the behavior that is so destructive. However, the addicted person often relies on others to cover up own inability to cope with daily responsibilities.*

6. Provide information about enabling behavior and addictive disease characteristics for both the user and nonuser. *Awareness and knowledge of behaviors (e.g., avoiding and shielding, taking over responsibilities, rationalizing, and subserving) provide opportunity for individuals to begin the process of change.*

7. Identify and discuss sabotage behaviors of family members. *Even though family member(s) may verbalize a desire for the individual to become addiction free, the reality of interactive dynamics is that they may unconsciously not want the individual to recover, as this would affect the family members' own role in the relationship. Additionally, they may receive sympathy or attention from others (secondary gain).*

8. Encourage participation in therapeutic writing, such as journaling (narrative), guided or focused. *Serves as a release for feelings (e.g., anger, grief, stress); helps move individual(s) forward in the treatment process.*

9. Provide factual information to patient and family about the effects of addictive behaviors on the family and what to expect after discharge. *Many people are unaware of the nature of addiction. If patient is using legally obtained drugs, he or she may believe this does not constitute abuse.*

10. Encourage family members to be aware of their own feelings, to look at the situation with perspective and objectivity. They can ask themselves: "Am I being conned? Am I acting out of fear, shame, guilt, or anger? Do I have a need to control?" *When the enabling family members become aware of their own actions that perpetuate the patient's problems, they need to decide to change themselves. If they change, the patient can then face the consequences of their own actions and may choose to get well.*

11. Provide support for enabling family members. *For change to occur, families need support as much as the person who has the problem with the addiction.*

12. Assist the patient's partner to become aware that the patient's behavior is not the partner's responsibility. *Partners need to learn that the patient's gambling or use of substances may or may not change despite partner's involvement in treatment.*

13. Help a recovering (formerly addicted) partner who is enabling to distinguish between destructive aspects of own behavior and genuine motivation to aid the patient. *Enabling behavior can be a recovering individual's attempts at personal survival.*

14. Note how the partner relates to the treatment team and staff. *Determines enabling style. A parallel exists between how partner relates to patient and to staff based on the partner's feelings about self and situation.*

15. Explore conflicting feelings the enabling partner may have about treatment (e.g., feelings similar to those of the person with the addiction [blend of anger, guilt, fear, exhaustion, embarrassment, loneliness, distrust, grief, and possibly relief]). *This is useful in establishing the need for therapy for the partner. This individual's own identity may have been lost—he or she may fear self-disclosure to staff and may have difficulty giving up the dependent relationship.*

16. Involve family in discharge referral plans. *Addiction is a family illness. Because the family has been so involved in dealing with the addictive behavior, family members need help adjusting to the new behavior of sobriety/abstinence. Incidence of recovery is almost doubled when the family is treated along with the patient.*

17. Encourage involvement with self-help associations, such as 12-step programs for patients, partners, and children, and professional family therapy. *Puts patient and family in direct contact with support systems necessary for continued sobriety/abstinence and assists with problem resolution.*

Outcome Criteria

1. Family verbalizes understanding of dynamics of enabling behaviors.
2. Family members demonstrate patterns of effective communication.
3. Family members regularly participate in self-help support programs.
4. Family members demonstrate behaviors required to change destructive patterns of behavior that contribute to and enable dysfunctional family process.

@ INTERNET REFERENCES

Additional information on addictions may be located at the following Web sites:

- https://www.samhsa.gov/
- https://www.well.com/user/woa
- www.addictions.com

Additional information on self-help organizations may be located at the following Web sites:
- https://ca.org (Cocaine Anonymous)
- www.aa.org (Alcoholics Anonymous)
- https://www.na.org (Narcotics Anonymous)
- www.al-anon.org
- www.gamblersanonymous.org/ga

Additional information about medications for treatment of alcohol and drug addiction may be located at the following Web sites:
- www.medicinenet.com/medications/article.htm
- https://medlineplus.gov
- https://www.drugs.com/condition/alcoholism.html

Movie Connections

Affliction (Alcoholism) • *Days of Wine and Roses* (Alcoholism) • *I'll Cry Tomorrow* (Alcoholism) • *When a Man Loves a Woman* (Alcoholism) • *Clean and Sober* (Addiction—cocaine) • *28 Days* (Alcoholism) • *Lady Sings the Blues* (Addiction—heroin) • *I'm Dancing as Fast as I Can* (Addiction—sedatives) • *The Rose* (Polysubstance addiction) • *The Gambler* (Gambling disorder) • *Requiem for a Dream* (Multisubstance addiction)

CHAPTER 5

Schizophrenia Spectrum and Other Psychotic Disorders

■ BACKGROUND ASSESSMENT DATA

The syndrome of symptoms associated with schizophrenia spectrum and other psychotic disorders may include alterations in content and organization of thoughts, perception of sensory input, affect or emotional tone, sense of identity, volition, psychomotor behavior, communication, and relationship skills. Cognitive deficits may affect memory, speed of processing thoughts, vigilance/attention, reasoning and problem-solving skills, and social cognition.

The *Diagnostic and Statistical Manual of Mental Disorders, Fifth Edition (DSM-5)* (American Psychiatric Association [APA], 2013) identifies a spectrum of psychotic disorders that are organized to reflect gradient of psychopathology from least to most severe. Degree of severity is determined by the level, number, and duration of psychotic signs and symptoms.

Several of the disorders may carry the additional specification of *With Catatonic Features.* Catatonia refers to a significant motor disturbance that may range from stupor (no motor activity) to excessive motor activity and agitation. The disorders to which this specifier may be applied include brief psychotic disorder, schizophreniform disorder, schizophrenia, schizoaffective disorder, and substance-induced psychotic disorder. It may also be applied to neurodevelopmental disorder, major depressive disorder, bipolar disorders I and II, and other mental disorders (APA, 2013).

The *DSM-5* initiates the spectrum of disorders with schizotypal personality disorder. For purposes of this textbook, this disorder is presented in Chapter 15, *Personality Disorders.*

Categories

Delusional Disorder

Delusional disorder is characterized by the presence of delusions that have been experienced by the individual for at least 1 month (APA, 2013). Hallucinatory activity is not prominent, and behavior is not bizarre. Delusional disorders are specified by subtypes based on the predominant delusional theme. The delusions, however, may be specified as having bizarre content if the thought is "clearly implausible, not understandable and not derived from ordinary life experiences" (APA, 2013, p. 91). Subtypes of delusional disorders include the following:

1. **Erotomanic Type:** Delusions that another person of higher status is in love with him or her
2. **Grandiose Type:** Delusions of inflated worth, power, knowledge, special identity, or special relationship to a deity or famous person.
3. **Jealous Type:** Delusions that one's sexual partner is unfaithful.
4. **Persecutory Type:** Delusions that one is being malevolently treated in some way.
5. **Somatic Type:** Delusions that the person has some physical defect, disorder, or disease.
6. **Mixed Type:** Prominent delusions but no single predominant theme.

Brief Psychotic Disorder

This disorder is identified by the sudden onset of psychotic symptoms that may or may not be preceded by a severe psychosocial stressor. These symptoms last at least 1 day but less than 1 month, and there is an eventual full return to the premorbid level of functioning (APA, 2013). The individual experiences emotional turmoil or overwhelming perplexity or confusion. Evidence of impaired reality testing may include incoherent speech, delusions, hallucinations, bizarre behavior, and disorientation. Individuals with preexisting personality disorders (most commonly histrionic, narcissistic, paranoid, schizotypal, and borderline personality disorders) appear to be susceptible to this disorder (Sadock, Sadock, & Ruiz, 2015). Catatonic features may also be associated with this disorder.

Schizophreniform Disorder

The essential features of schizophreniform disorder are identical to those of schizophrenia, with the exception that the duration is at least 1 month but less than 6 months. The diagnosis is termed *provisional* if a diagnosis must be made prior to recovery.

Schizophrenia

Characteristic symptoms of schizophrenia include dysfunctions in perception, inferential thinking, language, memory, and executive functions. Deterioration is evident in social, occupational, and interpersonal relationships. Symptoms of schizophrenia are commonly described as positive or negative. Positive symptoms reflect an alteration in or distortion of normal mental functions (e.g., delusions, hallucinations), whereas negative symptoms reflect a diminution or loss of normal functions (e.g., apathy, anhedonia, avolition, alogia, asociality). Most patients exhibit a mixture of both types of symptoms. Signs of the disturbance have been continuous for at least 6 months.

Schizoaffective Disorder

Schizoaffective disorder refers to behaviors characteristic of schizophrenia concurrent with an episode of a major mood disturbance, such as depression or mania and the presence of hallucinations and/or delusions for at least 2 weeks in the absence of a major mood episode over the lifetime of the illness (APA, 2013). However, prominent mood disorder symptoms must be evident for a majority of the time.

Substance/Medication-Induced Psychotic Disorder

The prominent hallucinations and delusions associated with this disorder are found to be directly attributable to substance intoxication or withdrawal or after exposure to a medication or toxin. This diagnosis is made when the symptoms are more excessive and more severe than those usually associated with the intoxication or withdrawal syndrome (APA, 2013). The medical history, physical examination, or laboratory findings provide evidence that the appearance of the symptoms occurred in association with a substance intoxication or withdrawal or exposure to a medication or toxin. Substances that are believed to induce psychotic disorders are presented in Table 5–1. Catatonic features may also be associated with this disorder.

Psychotic Disorder Due to Another Medical Condition

The essential features of this disorder are prominent hallucinations and delusions that can be directly attributed to another medical condition (APA, 2013). The diagnosis is not made if the symptoms occur during the course of a delirium. A number of medical conditions that can cause psychotic symptoms are presented in Table 5–1.

Catatonia Associated With Another Mental Disorder (Catatonia Specifier)

The characteristics of catatonia are identified by symptoms such as stupor; waxy flexibility; mutism; negativism; posturing; stereotypical, repetitive movements; agitation; grimacing; echolalia (mimicking another's speech); and echopraxia (mimicking another's movements) (APA, 2013). As previously stated, catatonia may be associated with brief psychotic disorder, schizophreniform disorder, schizophrenia, schizoaffective disorder, substance-induced psychotic disorder, neurocognitive disorder, depressive disorder, bipolar disorder, and other mental disorders such as post-traumatic stress disorder.

Catatonic Disorder Due to Another Medical Condition

Catatonic disorder is identified by the symptoms described in the previous section. This diagnosis is made when the symptomatology

TABLE 5–1	Substances and Medical Conditions That May Precipitate Psychotic Symptoms	
Substances	**Medical Conditions**	

Substances	Medical Conditions
Drugs of Abuse	Acute intermittent porphyria
Alcohol	Cerebrovascular disease
Amphetamines and related substances	Central nervous system (CNS)
Cannabis	infections
Cocaine	CNS trauma
Hallucinogens	Deafness
Inhalants	Fluid or electrolyte imbalances
Opioids	Hepatic disease
Phencyclidine and related substances	Herpes encephalitis
Sedatives, hypnotics, and anxiolytics	Huntington's disease
	Hypoadrenocorticism
Medications	Hypo- or hyperparathyroidism
Anesthetics and analgesics	Hypo- or hyperthyroidism
Anticholinergic agents	Metabolic conditions (e.g.,
Anticonvulsants	hypoxia; hypercarbia;
Antidepressant medication	hypoglycemia)
Antihistamines	Migraine headache
Antihypertensive agents	Neoplasms
Cardiovascular medications	Neurosyphilis
Antimicrobial medications	Normal pressure hydrocephalus
Antineoplastic medications	Renal disease
Antiparkinsonian agents	Systemic lupus erythematosus
Corticosteroids	Temporal lobe epilepsy
Disulfiram	Vitamin deficiency (e.g., B_{12})
Gastrointestinal medications	Wilson's disease
Muscle relaxants	
NSAIDs	
Toxins	
Anticholinesterase	
Organophosphate insecticides	
Nerve gases	
Carbon dioxide	
Carbon monoxide	
Volatile substances (e.g., fuel, paint, gasoline, toluene)	

Sources: American Psychiatric Association. (2013). *Diagnostic and statistical manual of mental disorders* (5th ed.). Washington, DC: American Psychiatric Publishing; Black, D.W., & Andreasen, N.C. (2014). *Introductory textbook of psychiatry* (6th ed.). Washington, DC: American Psychiatric Publishing; Freudenreich, O. (2010). Differential diagnosis of psychotic symptoms: Medical "mimics." *Psychiatric Times, 27*(12), 52–61; Sadock, B.J., Sadock, V.A., & Ruiz, P. (2015). *Synopsis of psychiatry: Behavioral sciences/clinical psychiatry* (11th ed.). Philadelphia, PA: Lippincott Williams & Wilkins.

is evidenced from medical history, physical examination, or laboratory findings to be directly attributable to the physiological consequences of another medical condition (APA, 2013). Some of the medical conditions associated with catatonia include metabolic disorders, encephalitis, nonconvulsive status epilepticus, subdural hematoma, neuroleptic malignant syndrome and several other drug toxicities, systemic lupus erythematosus, astrocytoma, carotid disease, manganese toxicity, meningioma, neurosyphilis, neurosarcoidosis, prion disease, and tuberculosis (Brasic, 2016).

Predisposing Factors

1. Physiological
   a. **Genetics:** Studies show that relatives of individuals with schizophrenia have a much higher probability of developing the disease than does the general population. Whereas the lifetime risk for developing schizophrenia is about 1% in most population studies, the risk for monozygotic twins is 50 times that of the general population (Sadock et al, 2015). Because in about one-half of the cases only one of a pair of identical twins develops schizophrenia, genetic makeup cannot be solely responsible for causing this disease. Os and Reininghaus (2017) suggest that additive and interacting combinations of genes, environmental factors, and the moderation of gene expression through interaction with environmental factors are probably all influential.
   b. **Histological Changes:** Sadock and colleagues (2015) report that epidemiological data indicate a high incidence of schizophrenia after prenatal exposure to influenza. The effect of autoimmune antibodies in the brain is being studied within the field of psychoneuroimmunology, and evidence suggests that these antibodies may be responsible for the development of at least some cases of schizophrenia following infection from a neurotoxic virus (particularly prenatal exposure to Toxoplasma gondii) (Matheson, Shepherd, & Carr, 2014). The role of cytokines in inflammation and the specific effects of these chemicals in the brain are still being explored through ongoing research.
   c. **Biochemical:** This theory suggests that schizophrenia (or schizophrenia-like symptoms) may be caused by an excess of dopamine-dependent neuronal activity in the brain. This excess activity may be related to increased production or release of the substance at nerve terminals, increased receptor sensitivity, too many dopamine receptors, or a combination of these mechanisms (Sadock et al, 2015). Various other biochemicals have also been implicated in the predisposition to schizophrenia. Abnormalities in the neurotransmitters norepinephrine, serotonin, acetylcholine, glutamate, and

gamma-aminobutyric acid and in the neuroregulators, such as prostaglandins and endorphins, have been suggested.

   d. **Anatomical Abnormalities:** With the use of neuroimaging technologies, structural brain abnormalities have been observed in individuals with schizophrenia. Ventricular enlargement is the most consistent finding; however, sulci enlargement and cerebellar atrophy are also reported. Reduction in the volume of the hippocampus observed in neuroimaging studies may signal risk for transition to a first psychotic episode (Harrisberger et al, 2016). Magnetic resonance imaging has revealed reduced symmetry in lobes of the brain and reductions in size of structures within the limbic system in patients with schizophrenia. Diffusion tensor imaging studies have identified widespread white matter abnormalities in schizophrenia (Viher et al, 2016). These abnormalities in white matter microstructure appear to be primarily associated with negative symptoms and psychomotor behavior abnormalities.

2. Environmental
   a. **Sociocultural:** Many studies have attempted to link schizophrenia to social class. Epidemiological statistics have shown that more individuals from lower socioeconomic classes experience symptoms associated with schizophrenia than do those from higher socioeconomic groups (Os & Reininghaus, 2017). These studies consistently find that lack of material resources (including housing and access to healthcare) and fragmented social relationships increase the risk for schizophrenia, whereas social cohesion and ethnic density (the concentration of a given ethnic group in a particular area) are protective.

   An alternative view is that of the *downward drift hypothesis*. This hypothesis suggests that, because of the characteristic symptoms of the disorder, individuals with schizophrenia have difficulty maintaining gainful employment and "drift down" to a lower socioeconomic level (or fail to rise out of a lower socioeconomic group). Proponents of this notion view poor social conditions as a consequence rather than a cause of schizophrenia.

   b. **Stressful Life Events:** Studies have been conducted in an effort to determine whether psychotic episodes may be precipitated by stressful life events. There is no scientific evidence to indicate that stress causes schizophrenia. It is very probable, however, that stress may contribute to the severity and course of the illness. It is known that extreme stress can precipitate psychotic episodes. Stress may indeed precipitate symptoms in an individual who possesses a genetic vulnerability to schizophrenia. Stressful life events may be associated with exacerbation of schizophrenic symptoms and increased rates of relapse.

c. **Cannabis and Genetic Vulnerability:** Studies of genetic vulnerability for schizophrenia have linked certain genes (COMT and ATK1) to increased risk for psychosis, particularly for adolescents with this genetic vulnerability who use cannabinoids (Radhakrishnan, Wilkinson, & D'Souza, 2014). Both cannabis and synthetic cannabinoids can induce schizophrenia-like symptoms. In individuals with a preexisting psychosis, cannabinoids can exacerbate symptoms. More important, the increased risk for psychotic disorders such as schizophrenia when combined with cannabis use suggests the influence of lifestyle factors in the expression of genes and points to the possibility of multiple factors playing a role in the causality of this illness.

Symptomatology–Positive Symptoms (Subjective/Objective Data)

Disturbances in Thought Content

1. **Delusions:** Delusions are fixed, false beliefs that are inconsistent with the person's intelligence or cultural background. The individual continues to have the belief in spite of obvious proof that it is false or irrational. Delusions are subdivided according to their content. Some of the more common ones are listed here.

   • **Delusion of Persecution:** The individual feels threatened and believes that others intend harm or persecution toward him or her in some way (e.g., "The FBI has bugged my room and intends to kill me," "I can't take a shower in this bathroom; the nurses have put a camera in there so that they can watch everything I do").

   • **Delusion of Grandeur:** The individual has an exaggerated feeling of importance, power, knowledge, or identity (e.g., "I am Jesus Christ").

   • **Delusion of Reference:** All events within the environment are referred by the psychotic person to him- or herself (e.g., "Someone is trying to get a message to me through the articles in this magazine [or newspaper or TV program]; I must break the code so that I can receive the message"). *Ideas* of reference are less rigid than delusions of reference. An example of an idea of reference is irrationally assuming that, when in the presence of others, one is the object of their discussion or ridicule.

   • **Delusion of Control or Influence:** The individual believes certain objects or persons have control over his or her behavior (e.g., "The dentist put a filling in my tooth; I now receive transmissions through the filling that control what I think and do") or the person believes that his or her thoughts or behaviors have control over specific situations or people (e.g., the mother who believes that if she scolds her son in any way, he will die). This type of delusion is similar to magical thinking, which is common in children (e.g., "The sky is raining because I'm sad").

- **Somatic Delusion:** The individual has a false idea about the functioning of his or her body (e.g., "I'm 70 years old and I will be the oldest person ever to give birth. The doctor says I'm not pregnant, but I know I am").
- **Nihilistic Delusion:** The individual has a false idea that the self, a part of the self, others, or the world is nonexistent (e.g., "The world no longer exists," "I have no heart").

2. **Paranoia:** Individuals with paranoia have extreme suspiciousness of others and of their actions or perceived intentions (e.g., "I won't eat this food. I know it has been poisoned").

Disturbances in Thought Processes Manifested in Speech

1. **Loose Association:** Thinking is characterized by speech in which ideas shift from one unrelated subject to another. Typically, the individual with loose association is unaware that the topics are disconnected. When the condition is severe, speech may be incoherent (e.g., "We wanted to take the bus, but the airport took all the traffic. No one needs a ticket to heaven. We have it all in our pockets").

2. **Neologisms:** Neologisms are newly invented words that are meaningless to others but have symbolic meaning to the individual (e.g., "She wanted to give me a ride in her new uniphorum").

3. **Clang Associations:** Choice of words is governed by sounds. Clang associations often take the form of rhyming (e.g., "It is very cold. I am cold and bold. The gold has been sold").

4. **Word Salad:** A word salad is a group of words that are put together randomly without any logical connection (e.g., "Most forward action grows life double plays circle uniform").

5. **Circumstantiality:** With circumstantiality, the individual delays in reaching the point of a communication because of unnecessary and tedious details. The point or goal is usually met but only with numerous interruptions by the interviewer to keep the person on track of the topic being discussed.

6. **Tangentiality:** Tangentiality differs from circumstantiality in that the person never really gets to the point of the communication. Unrelated topics are introduced, and the focus of the original discussion is lost.

7. **Echolalia:** The patient with schizophrenia may repeat words that he or she hears, which is called *echolalia*. This is an attempt to identify with the person speaking (e.g., the nurse says, "John, it's time for lunch." The patient may respond, "It's time for lunch, it's time for lunch," or sometimes, "Lunch, lunch, lunch, lunch").

8. **Perseveration:** The individual who exhibits perseveration persistently repeats the same word or idea in response to different questions.

Disturbances in Perception

1. **Hallucinations:** Hallucinations, or false sensory perceptions not associated with real external stimuli, may involve any of the five senses. Types of hallucinations include the following:
   - **Auditory:** Auditory hallucinations are false perceptions of sound. Most commonly they are of voices, but the individual may report clicks, rushing noises, music, and other noises. Command hallucinations may place the individual or others in a potentially dangerous situation. "Voices" that issue commands for violence to self or others may or may not be heeded by the psychotic person. Auditory hallucinations are the most common type in psychiatric disorders.
   - **Visual:** These are false visual perceptions. They may consist of formed images, such as of people, or of unformed images, such as flashes of light.
   - **Tactile:** Tactile hallucinations are false perceptions of the sense of touch, often of something on or under the skin. One specific tactile hallucination is formication, the sensation that something is crawling on or under the skin.
   - **Gustatory:** This type is a false perception of taste. Most commonly, gustatory hallucinations are described as unpleasant tastes.
   - **Olfactory:** Olfactory hallucinations are false perceptions of the sense of smell.
2. **Illusions:** Illusions are misperceptions or misinterpretations of real external stimuli.
3. **Echopraxia:** The patient who exhibits echopraxia may purposelessly imitate movements made by others. The mechanisms underlying echopraxia in schizophrenia are not well understood, but current evidence suggests that it may involve a disturbance in mirror neuron activity in the presence of social cognition impairments and self-monitoring deficits, culminating in imitative psychomotor behavior (Urvakhsh et al, 2014).

Symptomatology–Negative Symptoms (Subjective/Objective Data)

Disturbances in Affect

Affect describes the behavior associated with an individual's feeling state or emotional tone.

1. **Inappropriate Affect:** Affect is inappropriate when the individual's emotional tone is incongruent with the circumstances

(e.g., a young woman who laughs when told of the death of her mother).

2. **Bland or Flat Affect:** Affect is described as bland when the emotional tone is very weak. The individual with flat affect appears to be void of emotional tone (or overt expression of feelings).

3. **Apathy:** The patient with schizophrenia often demonstrates an indifference to or disinterest in the environment. The bland or flat affect is a manifestation of the emotional apathy.

Avolition

Impaired volition has to do with the inability to initiate goal-directed activity. In the individual with schizophrenia, this may take the form of inadequate interest, lack of motivation, neglect of activities of daily living (ADLs) including personal hygiene and appearance, or inability to choose a logical course of action in a given situation. Impairment in social functioning may be reflected in social isolation, emotional detachment, and lack of regard for social convention.

Lack of Interest or Skills in Interpersonal Interaction

Some patients with acute schizophrenia cling to others and intrude on the personal space of others, exhibiting behaviors that are not socially and culturally acceptable. Others may exhibit ambivalence in social relationships. Still others may withdraw from relationships altogether (asociality).

Lack of Insight

Some individuals lack awareness of having any illness or disorder even when symptoms appear obvious to others. The term for this state is *anosognosia*. The *DSM-5* identifies this symptom as the "most common predictor of nonadherence to treatment, and it predicts higher relapse rates, increased number of involuntary treatments, poorer psychosocial functioning, aggression, and poorer course of illness" (APA, 2013, p. 101).

Anergia

Anergia is a deficiency of energy. The individual with schizophrenia may lack sufficient energy to carry out ADLs or to interact with others.

Anhedonia

Anhedonia is the inability to experience pleasure. This is a particularly distressing symptom that compels some patients to attempt suicide.

Lack of Abstract Thinking Ability

Concrete thinking, or literal interpretations of the environment, represents a regression to an earlier level of cognitive development.

Abstract thinking becomes impaired in some individuals with schizophrenia. For example, the patient with schizophrenia may have great difficulty describing the abstract meaning of sayings such as "I'm climbing the walls" or "It's raining cats and dogs."

Associated Features
Waxy Flexibility
Waxy flexibility describes a condition in which the patient with schizophrenia allows body parts to be placed in bizarre or uncomfortable positions. This symptom is associated with catatonia. Once placed in position, the arm, leg, or head remains in that position for long periods, regardless of how uncomfortable it is for the patient. For example, the nurse may position the patient's arm in an outward position to take a blood pressure measurement. When the cuff is removed, the patient maintains the arm in the position in which it was placed to take the reading.

Posturing
This symptom is manifested by the voluntary assumption of inappropriate or bizarre postures.

Pacing and Rocking
Pacing back and forth and body rocking (a slow, rhythmic, backward-and-forward swaying of the trunk from the hips, usually while sitting) are common psychomotor behaviors of the patient with schizophrenia.

Regression
Regression is the retreat to an earlier level of development. This primary defense mechanism of schizophrenia may be a dysfunctional attempt to reduce anxiety. It provides the basis for many of the behaviors associated with schizophrenia.

Eye Movement Abnormalities
People with schizophrenia demonstrate difficulty tracking slow-moving objects: their eyes tend to fall behind the object and then attempt to catch up using rapid, jerking eye movements. In addition, instruction to gaze at an unmoving object is difficult for people with schizophrenia. Researchers (Benson et al, 2012) identify that simple eye movement tests can identify people with schizophrenia with 98% accuracy.

Common Nursing Diagnoses and Interventions for Individuals With Schizophrenia and other Psychotic Disorders
(Interventions are applicable to various health-care settings, such as inpatient and partial hospitalization, community outpatient clinic, home health, and private practice.)

■ RISK FOR SELF-DIRECTED OR OTHER-DIRECTED VIOLENCE

Definition: Susceptible to behaviors in which an individual demonstrates that he or she can be physically, emotionally, and/or sexually harmful [either to self or to others] (NANDA International [NANDA-I], 2018, pp. 416–417)

Risk Factors ("related to")

[Lack of trust (suspiciousness of others)]
[Panic level of anxiety]
[Negative role modeling]
[Rage reactions]
[Command hallucinations]
[Delusional thinking]
Negative body language—rigid posture, clenching of fists and jaw, hyperactivity, pacing, breathlessness, and threatening stances
[History or threats of violence toward self or others or of destruction to the property of others]
Impulsivity
Suicidal ideation, plan, available means
[Perception of the environment as threatening]
[Receiving auditory or visual commands of a threatening nature]

Goals/Objectives

Short-term Goals

1. Within [a specified time], the patient will recognize signs of increasing anxiety and agitation and report to staff (or other care provider) for assistance with intervention.
2. The patient will not harm self or others.

Long-term Goal

The patient will not harm self or others.

Interventions With *Selected Rationales*

1. Maintain low level of stimuli in patient's environment (low lighting, few people, simple decor, low noise level). *Anxiety level rises in a stimulating environment. A suspicious, agitated patient may perceive individuals as threatening.*
2. Observe patient's behavior frequently (every 15 minutes). Do this when carrying out routine activities *so as to avoid creating suspiciousness in the individual. Close observation is necessary so that intervention can occur if required to ensure patient (and others') safety.*
3. Remove all dangerous objects from patient's environment *so that in his or her agitated, confused state patient may not use them to harm self or others.*

4. Try to redirect the violent behavior with physical outlets for the patient's anxiety (e.g., physical exercise). *Physical exercise is a safe and effective way of relieving pent-up tension.*
5. Staff should maintain and convey a calm attitude toward patient. *Anxiety is contagious and can be transmitted from staff to patient.*
6. Have sufficient staff available to indicate a show of strength to patient if it becomes necessary. *This shows patient evidence of control over the situation and provides some physical security for staff.*
7. Administer tranquilizing medications as ordered by physician. Monitor medication for its effectiveness and for any adverse side effects. *The avenue of the "least restrictive alternative" must be selected when planning interventions for a psychiatric patient.*

   If patient is not calmed by "talking down" or by medication, use of mechanical restraints may be necessary. Restraints should be used only as a last resort, after all other interventions have been unsuccessful, and the patient is clearly at risk of harm to self or others. Be sure to have sufficient staff available to assist. Follow protocol established by the institution. Assess patient at least every 15 minutes to ensure that circulation to extremities is not compromised (check temperature, color, pulses); to assist the patient with needs related to nutrition, hydration, and elimination; and to position patient so that comfort is facilitated and aspiration is prevented. Continuous one-to-one monitoring may be necessary for the patient who is highly agitated or for whom there is a high risk of self- or accidental injury. *Patient safety is a nursing priority.*
8. As agitation decreases, assess patient's readiness for restraint removal or reduction. Remove one restraint at a time while assessing patient's response. *This minimizes risk of injury to patient and staff.*
9. Interact with the patient to better understand thought content, thought processes, and perceptions with particular attention to any content that might suggest risk for violence toward self or others. *Patient expression of suicidal or homicidal ideas or of command hallucinations that instruct patient to harm self or others increases the risk for violence and signals the need for additional safety precautions.*

Outcome Criteria

1. Anxiety is maintained at a level at which patient feels no need for aggression.
2. Patient demonstrates trust of others in his or her environment.
3. Patient maintains reality orientation.
4. Patient causes no harm to self or others.

■ SOCIAL ISOLATION

Definition: Aloneness experienced by the individual and perceived as imposed by others and as a negative or threatening state (NANDA-I, 2018, p. 455)

Possible Contributing Factors ("related to")

[Lack of trust]
[Panic level of anxiety]
[Regression to earlier level of development]
[Delusional thinking]
[Past experiences of difficulty in interactions with others]
[Repressed fears]
Unaccepted social behavior
Alterations in mental status

Defining Characteristics ("evidenced by")

[Staying alone in room]
Uncommunicative, withdrawn, no eye contact
Sad, dull affect
[Lying on bed in fetal position with back to door]
[Inappropriate or immature interests and activities for developmental age or stage]
Preoccupation with own thoughts; repetitive, meaningless actions
[Approaching staff for interaction, then refusing to respond to staff's acknowledgment]
Expression of feelings of rejection or of aloneness imposed by others

Goals/Objectives

Short-term Goal

The patient will willingly attend therapy activities accompanied by trusted staff member within 1 week.

Long-term Goal

The patient will voluntarily spend time with other patients and staff members in group activities.

Interventions With *Selected Rationales*

1. Convey an accepting attitude by making brief, frequent contacts and demonstrate willingness to listen. *An accepting attitude increases feelings of self-worth and facilitates trust.*
2. Show unconditional positive regard. *This conveys your belief in the patient as a worthwhile human being.*
3. Be with the patient to offer support during group activities that may be frightening or difficult for him or her. Offering

feedback about appropriate behavior in social situations promotes social skills and increases patient comfort in social situations. *The presence of a trusted individual provides emotional security for the patient.*

4. Be honest and keep all promises. *Honesty and dependability promote a trusting relationship.*

5. Orient patient to time, person, and place, as necessary.

6. Be cautious with touch. Allow patient extra space and an avenue for exit if he or she becomes too anxious. *A suspicious patient may perceive touch as a threatening gesture.*

7. Administer tranquilizing medications as ordered by physician. Monitor for effectiveness and for adverse side effects. *Antipsychotic medications help to reduce psychotic symptoms in some individuals, thereby facilitating interactions with others.*

8. Discuss with patient the signs of increasing anxiety and techniques to interrupt the response (e.g., relaxation exercises, thought stopping). *Maladaptive behaviors such as withdrawal and suspiciousness are manifested during times of increased anxiety.*

9. Give recognition and positive reinforcement for patient's voluntary interactions with others. *Positive reinforcement enhances self-esteem and encourages repetition of acceptable behaviors.*

Outcome Criteria

1. Patient demonstrates willingness and desire to socialize with others.

2. Patient voluntarily attends group activities.

3. Patient approaches others in appropriate manner for one-to-one interaction.

■ INEFFECTIVE COPING

Definition: A pattern of invalid appraisal of stressors, with cognitive and/or behavioral efforts, that fails to manage demands related to well-being (NANDA-I, 2018, p. 327)

Possible Contributing Factors ("related to")

Insufficient support system
[Inability to trust]
[Panic level of anxiety]
[Personal vulnerability]
[Low self-esteem]
[Inadequate support systems]
[Negative role model]
[Repressed fears]
[Possible hereditary factor]
[Dysfunctional family system]

Defining Characteristics ("evidenced by")

[Suspiciousness of others, resulting in:
- Alteration in societal participation
- Inability to meet basic needs
- Inappropriate use of defense mechanisms]

Goals/Objectives

Short-term Goal

The patient will develop trust in at least one staff member within 1 week.

Long-term Goal

The patient will demonstrate use of more adaptive coping skills as evidenced by appropriateness of interactions and willingness to participate in the therapeutic community.

Interventions With *Selected Rationales*

1. Encourage same staff to work with patient as much as possible *in order to promote development of trusting relationship.*
2. Avoid physical contact. *Patients with suspicious ideation may perceive touch as a threatening gesture.*
3. Avoid laughing, whispering, or talking quietly where patient can see but cannot hear what is being said. *Patients with suspicious ideation often believe others are discussing them, and secretive behaviors reinforce the paranoid feelings.*
4. Be honest and keep all promises. *Honesty and dependability promote a trusting relationship.*
5. A creative approach may have to be used to encourage food intake (e.g., canned food and own can opener or family-style meals). *Patients with suspicious ideation may believe they are being poisoned and refuse to eat food from the individually prepared tray.*
6. Mouth checks may be necessary following medication administration *to verify whether patient is swallowing the tablets or capsules. Suspicious patients may believe they are being poisoned with their medication and attempt to discard the pills.*
7. Activities should never include anything competitive. Activities that encourage a one-to-one relationship with the nurse or therapist are best. *Competitive activities are very threatening to suspicious patients.*
8. Encourage patient to verbalize true feelings. The nurse should avoid becoming defensive when angry feelings are directed at him or her. *Verbalization of feelings in a nonthreatening environment may help patient come to terms with long-unresolved issues.*
9. An assertive, matter-of-fact, yet genuine approach is least threatening and most therapeutic. *A person with suspicious ideation may misinterpret an attitude that seems overly friendly or overly cheerful.*
10. Empower the patient to be involved in decisions around his or her care to the best of their ability. *This approach establishes the*

foundation for patient-centered care and promotes a recovery-based focus.

Outcome Criteria

1. Patient is able to appraise situations realistically and refrain from projecting own feelings onto the environment.
2. Patient is able to recognize and clarify possible misinterpretations of the behaviors and verbalizations of others.
3. Patient eats food from tray and takes medications without evidence of mistrust.
4. Patient appropriately interacts and cooperates with staff and peers in therapeutic community setting.

■ DISTURBED SENSORY PERCEPTION: AUDITORY/VISUAL

Definition: Change in the amount or patterning of incoming stimuli [either internally or externally initiated] accompanied by a diminished, exaggerated, distorted, or impaired response to such stimuli (Note: This diagnosis has been retired by NANDA-I but is retained in this text because of its appropriateness in describing these specific behaviors.)

Possible Contributing Factors ("related to")

[Panic level of anxiety]
[Withdrawal into the self]
[Stress sufficiently severe to threaten an already weak ego]

Defining Characteristics ("evidenced by")

[Talking and laughing to self]
[Listening pose (tilting head to one side as if listening)]
[Stops talking in middle of sentence to listen]
[Rapid mood swings]
[Disordered thought sequencing]
[Inappropriate responses]
Disorientation
Poor concentration
Sensory distortions

Goals/Objectives

Short-term Goal

The patient will discuss content of hallucinations with nurse or therapist within 1 week.

Long-term Goal

The patient will be able to define and test reality, eliminating the occurrence of hallucinations. (This goal may not be realistic for the individual with chronic illness who has experienced auditory hallucinations for many years.) A more realistic goal may be: The patient will verbalize understanding that the sensory disturbances are a result of his or her illness and demonstrate ways to interrupt hallucinations.

Interventions With *Selected Rationales*

1. Observe patient for signs of hallucinations (listening pose, laughing or talking to self, stopping in midsentence). *Early intervention may prevent aggressive responses to command hallucinations.*

2. Avoid touching the patient or ask for permission before doing so. *Patient may perceive touch as threatening and respond in an aggressive manner.*

3. An attitude of acceptance encourages the patient to share the content of the hallucination with you. Ask, "What do you hear the voices saying to you?" *This is important in order to prevent possible injury to the patient or others from command hallucinations.*

4. Do not reinforce the hallucination. When referring to the hallucination, use impersonal words such as "the voices" or "the image you see" instead of descriptive words that support the hallucination, such as "the aliens" or "the starship." *Words that reiterate patient's description validate that the hallucination is real.*

> **CLINICAL PEARL** Let the patient who is "hearing voices" know that you do not share the perception. Say, "Even though I realize that the voices are real to you, I do not hear any voices speaking." The nurse must be honest with the patient so that he or she may realize that the hallucinations are not real.

5. Help the patient to understand the connection between increased anxiety and the presence of hallucinations. *If patient can learn to interrupt escalating anxiety, hallucinations may be prevented.*

6. Try to distract the patient from the hallucination. For some patients, auditory hallucinations persist after the acute psychotic episode has subsided. Listening to the radio or watching television helps distract some patients from attention to the voices. Others have benefited from an intervention called *voice dismissal*. With this technique, the patient is taught to say loudly, "Go away!" or "Leave me alone!" thereby exerting some conscious control over the behavior. *Involvement in activities, particularly intellectual activities or listening to music, is beneficial in distracting from and minimizing anxiety and associated perceptual disturbances.*

Outcome Criteria

1. Patient is able to recognize that hallucinations occur at times of extreme anxiety.

2. Patient is able to recognize signs of increasing anxiety and employ techniques to interrupt the response.

■ DISTURBED THOUGHT PROCESSES

Definition: Disruption in cognitive operations and activities (Note: This diagnosis has been retired by NANDA-I but is retained in this text because of its appropriateness in describing these specific behaviors.)

Possible Contributing Factors ("related to")

[Inability to trust]
[Panic level of anxiety]
[Repressed fears]
[Stress sufficiently severe to threaten an already weak ego]
[Possible hereditary factor]

Defining Characteristics ("evidenced by")

[Delusional thinking (false ideas)]
[Inability to concentrate]
Hypervigilance
[Altered attention span]—distractibility
Inaccurate interpretation of the environment
[Impaired ability to make decisions, problem-solve, reason, abstract or conceptualize, calculate]
[Inappropriate social behavior (reflecting inaccurate thinking)]
Inappropriate [nonreality-based] thinking

Goals/Objectives

Short-term Goal

[By specified time deemed appropriate], the patient will recognize and verbalize that false ideas occur at times of increased anxiety.

Long-term Goal

Depending on chronicity of disease process, choose the most realistic long-term goal for the patient:
1. By time of discharge from treatment, the patient's verbalizations will reflect reality-based thinking with no evidence of delusional ideation.
2. By time of discharge from treatment, the patient will be able to differentiate between delusional thinking and reality.

Interventions With *Selected Rationales*

1. Convey your acceptance of patient's need for the false belief, but indicate that you do not share the belief. *It is important to communicate to the patient that you do not view the idea as real.*
2. Do not argue or deny the belief. *Arguing with the patient or denying the belief serves no useful purpose, because delusional ideas are not eliminated by this approach, and the development of a trusting relationship may be impeded.*

> 🧠 **CLINICAL PEARL** Use *reasonable doubt* as a therapeutic technique: "I understand that you believe this is true, but I personally find it hard to accept."

3. Help the patient try to connect the false beliefs to times of increased anxiety. Discuss techniques that could be used to control anxiety (e.g., deep breathing exercises, other relaxation exercises, thought-stopping techniques). *If the patient can learn to interrupt escalating anxiety, delusional thinking may be prevented.*

4. Reinforce and focus on reality. Discourage long ruminations about the irrational thinking. Talk about real events and real people. *Discussions that focus on the false ideas are purposeless and useless and may even aggravate the psychosis.*

5. Assist and support patient in his or her attempt to verbalize feelings of anxiety, fear, or insecurity. *Verbalization of feelings in a nonthreatening environment may help patient come to terms with long-unresolved issues.*

6. Use a passive communication style whenever appropriate with patients who are extremely suspicious. For example, rather than telling the patient what he or she must do (e.g., "You need to go to group now"), using a passive approach empowers patient to decide (e.g., "Group will be starting in 15 minutes, and you are welcome to attend"). *A passive communication approach allows the patient to make choices whenever possible and may decrease the sense of threat or mistrust.*

Outcome Criteria

1. Verbalizations reflect thinking processes oriented in reality.
2. Patient is able to maintain ADLs to his or her maximal ability.
3. Patient is able to refrain from responding to delusional thoughts, should they occur.

■ IMPAIRED VERBAL COMMUNICATION

Definition: Decreased, delayed, or absent ability to receive, process, transmit, and use a system of symbols [to communicate] (NANDA-I, 2018, p. 263)

Possible Contributing Factors ("related to")

Altered perceptions
[Inability to trust]
[Panic level of anxiety]
[Regression to earlier level of development]
[Withdrawal into the self]
[Disordered, unrealistic thinking]

Defining Characteristics ("evidenced by")

[Loose association of ideas]
[Use of words that are symbolic to the individual (neologisms)]
[Use of words in a meaningless, disconnected manner (word salad)]
[Use of words that rhyme in a nonsensical fashion (clang association)]
[Repetition of words that are heard (echolalia)]
[Does not speak (mutism)]
[Verbalizations reflect concrete thinking (inability to think in abstract terms)]
[Poor eye contact (either no eye contact or continuous staring into the other person's eyes)]

Goals/Objectives

Short-term Goal

The patient will demonstrate ability to remain on one topic, using appropriate, intermittent eye contact for 5 minutes with nurse or therapist.

Long-term Goal

By time of discharge from treatment, the patient will demonstrate ability to carry on a verbal communication in a socially acceptable manner with health-care providers and peers.

Interventions With *Selected Rationales*

1. Maintain consistency of staff assignment as much as possible. In a nonthreatening manner, explain to the patient how his or her behavior and verbalizations are viewed by and may alienate others. *Consistency of staff assignment helps to facilitate trust and the ability to understand patient's actions and communication.*

> **CLINICAL PEARL** Attempt to decode incomprehensible communication patterns. Seek validation and clarification by stating, "Is it that you mean . . .?" or "I don't understand what you mean by that. Would you please explain it to me?" These techniques reveal to the patient how he or she is being perceived by others, and the responsibility for not understanding is accepted by the nurse.

2. Anticipate and fulfill the patient's needs until functional communication has been established. *Patient safety and comfort are nursing priorities.*
3. Orient the patient to reality as required. Call the patient by name. Validate those aspects of communication that help differentiate between what is real and not real. *These techniques may facilitate restoration of functional communication patterns in the patient.*

> 🔹 **CLINICAL PEARL** If the patient is unable or unwilling to speak (mutism), using the technique of verbalizing the implied is therapeutic. (Example: "That must have been very difficult for you when your mother left. You must have felt very alone.") This approach conveys empathy, facilitates trust, and eventually may encourage the patient to discuss painful issues.

4. Abstract phrases and clichés must be avoided, and explanations must be provided at the patient's level of comprehension. *Because concrete thinking prevails, misinterpretations are more likely to occur.*

Outcome Criteria

1. Patient is able to communicate in a manner that is understood by others.
2. Patient's nonverbal messages are congruent with verbalizations.
3. Patient is able to recognize that disorganized thinking and impaired verbal communication occur at times of increased anxiety and intervene to interrupt the process.

■ SELF-CARE DEFICIT (Identify Specific Area)

Definition: Inability to perform or complete [activities of daily livings] (NANDA-I, 2018, pp. 243–246)

Possible Contributing Factors ("related to")

[Withdrawal into the self]
[Regression to an earlier level of development]
[Panic level of anxiety]
Perceptual or cognitive impairment
[Inability to trust]

Defining Characteristics ("evidenced by")

Impaired ability to self-feed a complete meal
Inability [or refusal] to wash body
[Impaired ability or lack of interest in selecting appropriate clothing to wear, dressing, grooming, or maintaining appearance at a satisfactory level]
[Inability or unwillingness to carry out toileting procedures without assistance]

Goals/Objectives

Short-term Goal

The patient will verbalize a desire to perform ADLs by end of 1 week.

Long-term Goal

By time of discharge from treatment, the patient will be able to perform ADLs in an independent manner and demonstrate a willingness to do so.

Interventions With *Selected Rationales*

1. Encourage patient to perform normal ADLs to his or her level of ability. *Successful performance of independent activities enhances self-esteem.*
2. Encourage independence, but intervene when patient is unable to perform. *Patient comfort and safety are nursing priorities.*
3. Offer recognition and positive reinforcement for independent accomplishments (e.g., "Mrs. J., I see you have put on a clean dress and combed your hair"). *Positive reinforcement enhances self-esteem and encourages repetition of desirable behaviors.*

> **CLINICAL PEARL** Show the patient, on a concrete level, how to perform activities with which he or she is having difficulty. For example, if the patient is not eating, place a spoon in his or her hand, scoop some food into it, and say, "Now, eat a bite of mashed potatoes (or other food)." Speak plainly and clearly in words that cannot be misinterpreted.

4. Keep strict records of food and fluid intake. *This information is necessary to acquire an accurate nutritional assessment.*
5. Offer nutritious snacks and fluids between meals. *Patient may be unable to tolerate large amounts of food at mealtimes and may therefore require additional nourishment at other times during the day to receive adequate nutrition.*
6. If patient is not eating because of suspiciousness and fears of being poisoned, provide canned foods and allow patient to open them; or, if possible, suggest that food be served family-style *so that patient may see everyone eating from the same servings.*
7. If patient is soiling self, establish routine schedule for toileting needs. Assist patient to bathroom on hourly or bihourly schedule, as need is determined, until he or she is able to fulfill this need without assistance.

Outcome Criteria

1. Patient feeds self without assistance.
2. Patient selects appropriate clothing, dresses, and grooms self daily without assistance.
3. Patient maintains optimal level of personal hygiene by bathing daily and carrying out essential toileting procedures without assistance.

■ INSOMNIA

Definition: A disruption in amount and quality of sleep that impairs functioning (NANDA-I, 2018, p. 213)

Possible Contributing Factors ("related to")

[Panic level of anxiety]
[Repressed fears]
[Hallucinations]
[Delusional thinking]

Defining Characteristics ("evidenced by")

[Difficulty falling asleep]
[Awakening very early in the morning]
[Pacing; other signs of increasing irritability caused by lack of sleep]
[Frequent yawning, nodding off to sleep]

Goals/Objectives

Short-term Goal

Within first week of treatment, the patient will fall asleep within 30 minutes of retiring and sleep 5 hours without awakening, with use of sedative if needed.

Long-term Goal

By time of discharge from treatment, the patient will be able to fall asleep within 30 minutes of retiring and sleep 6 to 8 hours without a sleeping aid.

Interventions With *Selected Rationales*

1. Keep strict records of sleeping patterns. *Accurate baseline data are important in planning care to assist patient with this problem.*
2. Discourage sleep during the day *to promote more restful sleep at night.*
3. Administer antipsychotic medication at bedtime *so patient does not become drowsy during the day.*
4. Assist with measures that promote sleep, such as warm, non-stimulating drinks; light snacks; warm baths; and back rubs.
5. Performing relaxation exercises to soft music may be helpful prior to sleep.
6. Limit intake of caffeinated drinks such as tea, coffee, and colas. *Caffeine is a central nervous system stimulant and may interfere with the patient's achievement of rest and sleep.*

Outcome Criteria

1. Patient is able to fall asleep within 30 minutes after retiring.
2. Patient sleeps at least 6 consecutive hours without waking.
3. Patient does not require a sedative to fall asleep.

 INTERNET REFERENCES

Additional information about schizophrenia may be located at the following Web sites:

- www.schizophrenia.com
- https://www.nimh.nih.gov
- https://www.nami.org
- http://mentalhealth.com
- https://www.bbrfoundation.org

Additional information about medications to treat schizophrenia may be located at the following Web sites:

- www.medicinenet.com/medications/article.htm
- https://www.drugs.com
- https://medlineplus.gov

 Movie Connections

I Never Promised You a Rose Garden (Schizophrenia)
• *A Beautiful Mind* (Schizophrenia) • *The Fisher King* (Schizophrenia)
• *Bennie & Joon* (Schizophrenia) • *Out of Darkness* (Schizophrenia)
• *Conspiracy Theory* (Delusional disorder) • *The Fan* (Delusional disorder)
• *The Soloist* (Schizophrenia) and *Of Two Minds* (Schizophrenia)

CHAPTER 6

Depressive Disorders

■ BACKGROUND ASSESSMENT DATA

Depression is defined as an alteration in mood that is expressed by feelings of sadness, despair, and pessimism. There is a loss of interest in usual activities, and somatic symptoms may be evident. Changes in appetite and sleep patterns are common. Depression is one of the most frequently diagnosed psychiatric illnesses. It is so common in our society as to sometimes be called "the common cold of psychiatric disorders."

■ TYPES OF DEPRESSIVE DISORDERS

Disruptive Mood Dysregulation Disorder

Disruptive mood dysregulation disorder (DMDD) is a new diagnostic category in the *Diagnostic and Statistical Manual of Mental Disorders, Fifth Edition (DSM-5)* (American Psychiatric Association [APA], 2013), which describes a syndrome of persistent mood-related symptoms specifically in children. Onset of the disorder occurs before age 10 years, but the diagnosis is not applied to children younger than 6 years.

DMDD is characterized by chronic, severe, and persistent irritability. Clinical manifestations include frequent, developmentally inappropriate temper outbursts and persistently angry mood that is present between the severe temper outbursts. The behavior has been present for 12 or more months and occurs in more than one setting.

Major Depressive Disorder

Major depressive disorder (MDD) is described as a disturbance of mood involving depression or loss of interest or pleasure in usual activities and pastimes. There is evidence of interference in social and occupational functioning for at least 2 weeks. There is no history of manic behavior, and the symptoms cannot be attributed to use of substances or another medical condition. The diagnosis of MDD is specified according to whether it is a *single episode* (the individual's first encounter with a major depressive episode) or *recurrent* (the individual has a history of previous major depressive episodes). The diagnosis will also identify the degree of severity of symptoms (mild, moderate, or severe) and whether the disorder is in partial or full remission. Additionally, the following specifiers may be used to further describe the depressive episode:

1. **With Anxious Distress:** Feelings of restlessness, anxiety, and worry accompany the depressed mood.
2. **With Mixed Features:** The depression is accompanied by intermittent symptoms of mania or hypomania.
3. **With Melancholic Features:** The depressed mood is characterized by profound despondency and despair. There is an absence of the ability to experience pleasure and an expression of feelings of excessive or inappropriate guilt. Psychomotor agitation or retardation and anorexia or weight loss are evident.
4. **With Atypical Features:** This specifier indicates the individual has the ability for cheerful mood when presented with positive events. There may be increased appetite or weight gain and hypersomnia. Additional symptoms include long-standing sensitivity to interpersonal rejection and heavy, leaden feelings in the arms or legs.
5. **With Psychotic Features:** Depressive symptoms include the presence of delusions and/or hallucinations.
6. **With Catatonia:** Depressive symptoms are accompanied by additional symptoms associated with catatonia (e.g., stupor, waxy flexibility, mutism, posturing).
7. **With Peripartum Onset:** This specifier is used when symptoms of MDD occur during pregnancy or in the 4 weeks following delivery.
8. **With Seasonal Pattern:** This diagnosis indicates the presence of depressive episodes that occur at characteristic times of the year. Commonly, the episodes occur during the fall or winter months and remit in the spring. Less commonly, there may be recurrent summer depressive episodes (APA, 2013).

Persistent Depressive Disorder (Dysthymia)

Persistent depressive disorder is a mood disturbance with characteristics similar to, if somewhat milder than, those ascribed to MDD. There is no evidence of psychotic symptoms. The essential feature of the disorder is "a depressed mood that occurs for most of the day, for more days than not, for at least 2 years, or at least 1 year in children and adolescents" (APA, 2013, p. 169). Intermittent symptoms of MDD may or may not occur with this disorder. The same diagnostic specifiers described for MDD may also apply to persistent depressive disorder.

Premenstrual Dysphoric Disorder

The essential features of premenstrual dysphoric disorder include markedly depressed mood, excessive anxiety, mood swings, and decreased interest in activities during the week prior to menses, improving shortly after the onset of menstruation and becoming minimal or absent in the week postmenses (APA, 2013) (see Chapter 16).

Substance/Medication-Induced Depressive Disorder

The depressed mood associated with this disorder is considered to be the direct result of the physiological effects of a substance (e.g., a drug of abuse, a medication, or toxin exposure) and causes clinically significant distress or impairment in social, occupational, or other important areas of functioning.

Depressive Disorder Due to Another Medical Condition

This disorder is characterized by symptoms associated with a major depressive episode that are the direct physiological consequence of another medical condition (APA, 2013). The depression causes clinically significant distress or impairment in social, occupational, or other important areas of functioning.

■ PREDISPOSING FACTORS TO DEPRESSIVE DISORDER

1. Physiological
   a. **Genetics:** Numerous studies have been conducted that support the involvement of heredity in depressive illness. First-degree relatives of individuals with MDD have a two- to fourfold higher risk for the disorder than that of the general population (APA, 2013).
   b. **Biochemical:** Biochemical theory implicates the biogenic amines norepinephrine, dopamine, and serotonin. The levels of these chemicals are believed to be deficient in individuals with depressive illness. Glutamate receptors are also theorized to be influential in depression. One hypothesis is that down regulation of excess glutamate has antidepressant effects.
   c. **Neuroendocrine Disturbances:** Elevated levels of serum cortisol and increased levels of thyroid-stimulating hormone (triggered by low levels of thyroid hormones such as T_3 and T_4) have been associated with depressed mood in some individuals.
   d. **Substance Intoxication and Withdrawal:** Depressed mood may be associated with intoxication or withdrawal from substances such as alcohol, amphetamines, cocaine, hallucinogens, opioids, phencyclidine-like substances, sedatives, hypnotics, or anxiolytics. All of these substances increase the risk for suicide. Alcohol intoxication increases the risk for suicide associated not only with its depressant effects over time but also with its effect of decreasing inhibitions and impairing judgment. Amphetamine withdrawal carries a high risk for suicide related to the marked depression that accompanies "crashing."
   e. **Medication Side Effects:** A number of drugs can produce a depressive syndrome as a side effect. Common ones include

anxiolytics, antipsychotics, and sedative-hypnotics. Antihypertensive medications such as propranolol and reserpine have been known to produce depressive symptoms. Others include steroids, hormones, antineoplastics, analgesics, and antiulcer medications.

f. **Other Physiological Conditions:** Depressive symptoms may occur in the presence of electrolyte disturbances, hormonal disturbances, nutritional deficiencies, and with certain physical disorders, such as cerebrovascular accident, systemic lupus erythematosus, hepatitis, and diabetes mellitus.

2. Psychosocial

a. **Psychoanalytical Theory:** Freud observed that melancholia occurs after the loss of a loved object, either actually by death or emotionally by rejection, or the loss of some other abstraction of value to the individual. Freud indicated that in patients with melancholia, the depressed person's rage is internally directed because of identification with the lost object (Sadock, Sadock, & Ruiz, 2015).

b. **Cognitive Theory:** Beck and colleagues (1979) proposed that depressive illness occurs as a result of impaired cognition. Disturbed thought processes foster a negative evaluation of self by the individual. The perceptions are of inadequacy and worthlessness. Outlook for the future is one of pessimism and hopelessness.

c. **Learning Theory:** The learning theory (Seligman, 1974) proposes that a learned belief that there is a lack of control over his or her life situation predisposes an individual to depressive illness. Following numerous failures (either perceived or real), the individual develops a learned sense of helplessness and inability to succeed at any endeavor, which may culminate in clinical depression.

d. **Object Loss Theory:** The theory of object loss suggests that depressive illness occurs as a result of having been abandoned by, or otherwise separated from, a significant other during the first 6 months of life. Because during this period the mother represents the child's main source of security, she is the "object." The response occurs not only with a physical loss. This absence of attachment, which may be either physical or emotional, leads to feelings of helplessness and despair that contribute to lifelong patterns of depression in response to loss.

■ SYMPTOMATOLOGY (SUBJECTIVE AND OBJECTIVE DATA)

1. Typically, the affect of a depressed person is one of sadness, dejection, helplessness, and hopelessness. The outlook is gloomy and pessimistic. A feeling of worthlessness prevails. In

some cases, patients verbalize or demonstrate signs of marked depression (such as suicidal ideation) but their affect does not reveal their emotional state. This is referred to as *masked depression*.

2. Thoughts are slowed and concentration is difficult. Obsessive ideas and rumination of negative thoughts are common. In severe depression, psychotic features such as hallucinations and delusions may be evident, reflecting misinterpretations of the environment.

3. Physically, there is evidence of weakness and fatigue—very little energy to carry on activities of daily living (ADLs). The individual may express an exaggerated concern over bodily functioning, seemingly experiencing heightened sensitivity to somatic sensations.

4. Some individuals may be inclined toward excessive eating and drinking, whereas others may experience anorexia and weight loss. In response to a general slowdown of the body, digestion is often sluggish, constipation is common, and urinary retention is possible.

5. Sleep disturbances, either insomnia or hypersomnia, are common.

6. Individuals with severe depression often complain of feeling worse in the morning, with some improvement as the day progresses.

7. A general slowdown of motor activity commonly accompanies depression (called *psychomotor retardation*). At the severe level, energy is depleted, movements are lethargic, and performance of daily activities is extremely difficult. Regression is common, evidenced by withdrawal into the self and retreat to the fetal position. Conversely, severely depressed persons may manifest psychomotor activity through symptoms of agitation. These are constant, rapid, purposeless movements, out of touch with the environment.

8. Verbalizations are limited. When depressed persons do speak, the content may be either ruminations regarding their own life regrets or, in psychotic patients, a reflection of their delusional thinking.

9. Social participation is diminished. The depressed patient has an inclination toward egocentrism and narcissism—an intense focus on the self. This discourages others from pursuing a relationship with the individual, which increases his or her feelings of worthlessness and penchant for isolation.

Common Nursing Diagnoses and Interventions for Depression

(Interventions are applicable to various health-care settings, such as inpatient and partial hospitalization, community outpatient clinic, home health, and private practice.)

■ RISK FOR SUICIDE

Definition: Susceptible to self-inflicted, life-threatening injury (NANDA International [NANDA-I], 2018, p. 422)

Risk Factors ("related to")

[Depressed mood]
[Males over 65 years of age, adolescents]
Grief; hopelessness; social isolation
[Alienation from others; real or perceived]
[Purposelessness]
[Feeling trapped]
History of prior suicide attempt
Widowed or divorced
Chronic or terminal illness
Psychiatric illness or substance abuse
Threats of killing self
States desire to die
[Has a suicide plan and means to carry it out]
[Giving away possessions]

Goals/Objectives

Short-term Goals

1. The patient will seek out staff when feeling urge to harm self.
2. The patient will collaborate with a trusted staff member to identify a safety plan.
3. The patient will remain free of harm to self.

Long-term Goal

The patient will engage in his or her established plan to maintain personal safety.

Interventions With *Selected Rationales*

1. Create a safe environment for the patient. Remove all potentially harmful objects from patient's access (sharp objects, straps, belts, ties, glass items). Supervise closely during meals and medication administration. Perform room searches as deemed necessary. *Patient safety is a nursing priority.*
2. Conduct thorough, collaborative, and ongoing assessment of risk factors and warnings signs for suicide in the context of a therapeutic relationship with the patient. *Conveying an attitude of acceptance and willingness to collaborate with patients in maintaining their safety increases the potential for open and honest discussion of their thoughts and feelings. Suicide risk is variable over time, so regular assessment is warranted to protect patient safety.*

> **CLINICAL PEARL** Ask the patient directly, "Have you thought about killing yourself?" or "Have you thought about harming yourself in any way?" "If so, what do you plan to do? Do you have the means to carry out this plan?" "How strong would you say is your intention to die?" The risk of suicide is greatly increased if the patient has developed a plan, has intentions to die, and particularly if means exist for the patient to execute the plan.

3. Encourage the patient to seek out a staff member or support person if thoughts of suicide emerge or become more intense. *Suicidal patients are often very ambivalent about their feelings. Discussion of feelings with a trusted individual may provide assistance before the patient experiences a crisis situation.*

4. Maintain close observation. Depending on the level of suicide precautions, provide one-to-one contact, constant visual observation, or 15-minute checks (at irregular intervals). Place in room close to nurse's station; do not assign to private room. Accompany to off-unit activities if attendance is indicated. May need to accompany to bathroom. *Close observation is necessary to ensure that patient does not harm self in any way. Remaining alert for suicidal and escape attempts facilitates ability to prevent or interrupt harmful behavior.*

5. Maintain special care in administration of medications (e.g., assure that patient has swallowed pills). *Prevents patient from saving up to overdose or discarding and not taking. Antidepressant medication, as well as other medications, can be lethal in overdose.*

6. Make rounds at frequent, *irregular* intervals (especially at night, toward early morning, at change of shift, or during other predictably busy times for staff). *Prevents staff surveillance from becoming predictable. Awareness of patient's location is important, especially when staff is busy, unavailable, or less observable.*

7. Encourage verbalizations of honest feelings. Through exploration and discussion, help patient to identify symbols of hope in his or her life.

8. Encourage patient to express angry feelings within appropriate limits. Provide safe method of hostility release. Help patient to identify true source of anger and to work on adaptive coping skills for use outside the treatment setting. *Depression and suicidal behaviors may be viewed as anger turned inward on the self. If this anger can be verbalized in a nonthreatening environment, the patient may be able to eventually resolve these feelings.*

9. Identify community resources and other support systems that patient may use to maintain his or her plan for ongoing safety. *Having a concrete plan for seeking assistance during a crisis may discourage or prevent self-destructive behaviors.*

10. Orient patient to reality, as required. Point out sensory misperceptions or misinterpretations of the environment. Take care not to belittle patient's fears or indicate disapproval of verbal expressions.

11. Most important, spend time with the patient. *This provides a feeling of safety and security while also conveying the message, "I want to spend time with you because I think you are a worthwhile person."*

Outcome Criteria

1. The patient verbalizes no thoughts of suicide.
2. The patient commits no acts of self-harm.
3. The patient is able to verbalize names of resources outside the hospital from whom he or she may request help if feeling suicidal.

■ COMPLICATED GRIEVING

Definition: A disorder that occurs after the death of a significant other [or any other loss of significance to the individual], in which the experience of distress accompanying bereavement fails to follow normative expectations and manifests in functional impairment (NANDA-I, 2018, p. 340)

Possible Contributing Factors ("related to")

Unresolved anger
Lack of social support
[Real or perceived loss of any entity of value to the individual]
[Bereavement overload (cumulative grief from multiple unresolved losses)]
[Thwarted grieving response to a loss]
[Absence of anticipatory grieving]
[Feelings of guilt generated by ambivalent relationship with the lost entity]

Defining Characteristics ("evidenced by")

[Idealization of the lost entity]
[Denial of loss]
[Excessive anger, expressed inappropriately]
[Obsessions with past experiences]
[Ruminations of guilt feelings, excessive and exaggerated out of proportion to the situation]
[Developmental regression]
[Difficulty in expressing loss]
[Prolonged difficulty coping following a loss]
[Reliving of past experiences with little or no reduction of intensity of the grief]
[Prolonged interference with life functioning, with onset or exacerbation of somatic or psychosomatic responses]
[Labile affect]
[Alterations in eating habits, sleep patterns, dream patterns, activity level, libido]

Goals/Objectives

Short-term Goals

1. The patient will express anger regarding the loss.
2. The patient will verbalize behaviors associated with normal grieving.

Long-term Goal

The patient will be able to recognize his or her position in the grief process while progressing at own pace toward resolution.

Interventions With *Selected Rationales*

1. Determine the stage of grief in which the patient is fixed. Identify behaviors associated with this stage. *Accurate baseline assessment data are necessary to effectively plan care for the grieving patient.*
2. Develop trusting relationship. Show empathy, concern, and unconditional positive regard. Be honest and keep all promises. *Trust is the basis for a therapeutic relationship.*
3. Convey an accepting attitude, and encourage open expression of feelings. *An accepting attitude conveys to the patient that you believe he or she is a worthwhile person. Trust is enhanced.*
4. Encourage the patient to express anger. Do not become defensive if the initial expression of anger is displaced on the nurse or therapist. Help the patient to explore angry feelings so that they may be directed toward the intended person or situation. *Verbalization of feelings in a nonthreatening environment may help the patient come to terms with unresolved issues.*
5. Help the patient to discharge pent-up anger through participation in large motor activities (e.g., brisk walks, jogging, physical exercises, volleyball, exercise bike). *Physical exercise provides a safe and effective method for discharging pent-up tension.*
6. Teach the normal stages of grief and behaviors associated with each stage. Help patient to understand that feelings such as guilt and anger toward the lost entity are appropriate and acceptable during the grief process and should be expressed rather than held inside. *Knowledge of acceptability of the feelings associated with normal grieving may help to relieve some of the guilt that these responses generate.*
7. Encourage the patient to review relationship with the lost entity. With support and sensitivity, point out the reality of the situation in areas where misrepresentations are expressed. *The patient must give up an idealized perception and be able to accept both positive and negative aspects about the lost entity before the grief process is complete.*
8. Communicate to the patient that crying is acceptable. The use of touch may be therapeutic and appropriate. Assessment of cultural influences and history of trauma influence the clinical judgment about whether to use this intervention.

9. Assist the patient in problem-solving as he or she attempts to determine methods for more adaptive coping with the experienced loss. Provide positive feedback for strategies identified and decisions made. *Positive feedback increases self-esteem and encourages repetition of desirable behaviors.*

10. Encourage the patient to reach out for spiritual support during this time in whatever form is desirable to him or her. Assess spiritual needs of patient and assist as necessary in the fulfillment of those needs.

11. Encourage the patient to attend a support group of individuals who are experiencing life situations similar to his or her own. Help the patient to locate a group of this type.

Outcome Criteria

1. The patient is able to verbalize normal stages of the grief process and behaviors associated with each stage.

2. The patient is able to identify own position within the grief process and express honest feelings related to the lost entity.

3. The patient is no longer manifesting exaggerated emotions and behaviors related to complicated grieving and is able to carry out ADLs independently.

■ LOW SELF-ESTEEM (Situational)

Definition: Development of a negative perception of self-worth in response to a current situation (NANDA-I, 2018, p. 274)

Possible Contributing Factors ("related to")

Alteration in social role
Impaired functioning [may be social, financial, physical, psychological]
[Lack of positive feedback]
[Feelings of abandonment by significant other]
[Numerous failures (learned helplessness)]
[Underdeveloped ego and punitive superego]
[Impaired cognition fostering negative view of self]

Defining Characteristics ("evidenced by")

[Difficulty accepting positive reinforcement]
[Withdrawal into social isolation]
[Being highly critical and judgmental of self and others]
[Expressions of worthlessness]
[Fear of failure]
[Inability to recognize own accomplishments]
[Setting up self for failure by establishing unrealistic goals]
[Unsatisfactory interpersonal relationships]

[Negative, pessimistic outlook]
[Hypersensitive to slight or criticism]
[Grandiosity]

Goals/Objectives

Short-term Goals

1. Within reasonable time period, the patient will discuss fear of failure with nurse.
2. Within reasonable time period, the patient will verbalize things he or she likes about self.

Long-term Goals

1. By time of discharge from treatment, the patient will exhibit increased feelings of self-worth as evidenced by verbal expression of positive aspects of self, past accomplishments, and future prospects.
2. By time of discharge from treatment, the patient will exhibit increased feelings of self-worth by setting realistic goals and trying to reach them, thereby demonstrating a decrease in fear of failure.

Interventions With *Selected Rationales*

1. Be accepting of the patient and his or her negativism. Identify negative thinking as a symptom of depression rather than a trait. *An attitude of acceptance enhances feelings of self-worth. Identifying negative thinking as a symptom rather than a personality or character trait promotes the concept that negative thinking can be lessened in the course of treatment.*
2. Spend time with the patient *to convey acceptance and contribute toward feelings of self-worth.*
3. Help the patient to recognize and focus on strengths and accomplishments. Minimize attention given to past (real or perceived) failures. *Lack of attention may help to eliminate negative ruminations.*
4. Encourage participation in group activities *from which the patient may receive positive feedback and support from peers.*
5. Help the patient identify areas he or she would like to change about self, and assist with problem-solving toward this effort. *Low self-worth may interfere with the patient's perception of his or her own problem-solving ability. Assistance may be required.*
6. Assess the patient to ensure he or she is not becoming increasingly dependent and is accepting responsibility for own behaviors. *The patient must be able to function independently if he or she is to be successful within the less-structured community environment.*
7. Provide group activities that offer the patient simple methods of achievement. Offer recognition and positive feedback for actual accomplishments. *Successes and recognition increase self-esteem.*
8. Teach assertiveness techniques: the ability to recognize the differences among passive, assertive, and aggressive behaviors, and

the importance of respecting the human rights of others while protecting one's own basic human rights. *Self-esteem is enhanced by the ability to interact with others in an assertive manner.*

9. Teach effective communication techniques, such as the use of "I" messages. I-statements can be used to take ownership for one's feelings rather than saying they are caused by the other person (e.g., "I feel angry when you criticize me in front of other people, and I would prefer that you stop doing that"). You-statements put the other individual on the defensive (e.g., "You are a jerk for criticizing me in front of other people!").

10. Assist patient in performing aspects of self-care when required. Offer positive feedback for tasks performed independently. *Positive feedback enhances self-esteem and encourages repetition of desirable behaviors.*

Outcome Criteria

1. The patient is able to verbalize positive aspects about self.
2. The patient is able to communicate assertively with others.
3. The patient expresses some optimism and hope for the future.
4. The patient sets realistic goals for self and demonstrates willingness to attempt to reach them.

■ SOCIAL ISOLATION/IMPAIRED SOCIAL INTERACTION

Definition: Social isolation is the condition of aloneness experienced by the individual and perceived as imposed by others and as a negative or threatened state (NANDA-I, 2018, p. 455); impaired social interaction is an insufficient or excessive quantity or ineffective quality of social exchange (p. 301)

Possible Contributing Factors ("related to")

[Developmental regression]
[Egocentric behaviors (which offend others and discourage relationships)]
Disturbed thought processes [delusional thinking]
[Fear of rejection or failure of the interaction]
[Impaired cognition fostering negative view of self]
[Unresolved grief]
Absence of significant others

Defining Characteristics ("evidenced by")

Sad, dull affect
Being uncommunicative, withdrawn; lacking eye contact
Preoccupation with own thoughts; performance of repetitive, meaningless actions
Seeking to be alone

[Assuming fetal position]
Expression of feelings of aloneness or rejection
Discomfort in social situations
Dysfunctional interaction with others

Goals/Objectives

Short-term Goal

The patient will develop trusting relationship with nurse or counselor within time period to be individually determined.

Long-term Goals

1. The patient will voluntarily spend time with other patients and nurse or therapist in group activities by time of discharge from treatment.
2. The patient will refrain from using egocentric behaviors that offend others and discourage relationships by time of discharge from treatment.

Interventions With *Selected Rationales*

1. Spend time with the patient. This may mean just sitting in silence for a while. *Your presence may help improve the patient's perception of self as a worthwhile person.*
2. Develop a therapeutic nurse-patient relationship through frequent, brief contacts and an accepting attitude. Show unconditional positive regard. Encourage the patient to discuss his or her thoughts and feelings. *Your presence, acceptance, and conveyance of positive regard enhance the patient's feelings of self-worth. Conveying an attitude of interest in discussing the patient's thoughts and feelings may reduce his or her sense of isolation from others.*
3. After the patient feels comfortable in a one-to-one relationship, encourage attendance in group activities. May need to attend with the patient the first few times to offer support. Accept the patient's decision to remove self from group situation if anxiety becomes too great. *The presence of a trusted individual provides emotional security for the patient.*
4. Verbally acknowledge the patient's absence from any group activities. *Knowledge that his or her absence was noticed may reinforce the patient's feelings of self-worth.*
5. Teach assertiveness techniques. Interactions with others may be discouraged by the patient's use of passive or aggressive behaviors. *Knowledge of the use of assertive techniques could improve the patient's relationships with others.*
6. Provide direct feedback about the patient's interactions with others. Do this in a nonjudgmental manner. Help the patient learn how to respond more appropriately in interactions with others. Teach the patient skills that may be used to approach others in a more socially acceptable manner. Practice these skills through role-play. *The patient may not realize how he or she is being perceived*

by others. Direct feedback from a trusted individual may help to alter these behaviors in a positive manner. Having practiced these skills in role-play facilitates their use in real situations.

7. The depressed patient must have structure in his or her life because of the impairment in decision-making and problem-solving ability. Devise a plan of therapeutic activities and provide the patient with a written time schedule. Use an active (directive) communication approach when the patient is profoundly depressed and having difficulty making decisions (e.g., "It's time to go to group" rather than "Would you like to go to group today?"). *Remember:* The patient who is clinically depressed typically feels worse (less energy, more depressed) early in the day, so later in the day is a better time for the severely depressed individual to participate in activities. *It is important to plan activities at a time when the patient has more energy and is more likely to gain from the experience.*

8. Provide positive reinforcement for patient's voluntary interactions with others. *Positive reinforcement enhances self-esteem and encourages repetition of desirable behaviors.*

Outcome Criteria

1. The patient demonstrates willingness and desire to socialize with others.
2. The patient voluntarily attends group activities.
3. The patient approaches others in appropriate manner for one-to-one interaction.

■ POWERLESSNESS

Definition: The lived experience of lack of control over a situation, including a perception that one's actions do not significantly affect an outcome (NANDA-I, 2018, p. 343)

Possible Contributing Factors ("related to")

[Lifestyle of helplessness]
[Health-care] environment
[Complicated grieving process]
[Lack of positive feedback]
[Consistent negative feedback]

Defining Characteristics ("evidenced by")

Reports lack of control [e.g., over self-care, situation, outcome]
Nonparticipation in care
Reports doubt regarding role performance
[Reluctance to express true feelings]
[Apathy]

Dependence on others
[Passivity]

Goals/Objectives

Short-term Goal

The patient will participate in decision making regarding own care within 5 days.

Long-term Goal

The patient will be able to effectively solve problems in ways to take control of his or her life situation by time of discharge from treatment, thereby decreasing feelings of powerlessness.

Interventions With *Selected Rationales*

1. Encourage the patient to take as much responsibility as possible for own self-care practices (examples follow). *Providing the patient with choices will increase his or her feelings of control.*
   a. Include the patient in setting the goals of care he or she wishes to achieve.
   b. Allow the patient to establish own schedule for self-care activities.
   c. Provide the patient with privacy as need is determined.
   d. Provide positive feedback for decisions made. Respect the patient's right to make those decisions independently, and refrain from attempting to influence him or her toward those that may seem more logical.
2. Help the patient set realistic goals. *Unrealistic goals set the patient up for failure and reinforce feelings of powerlessness.*
3. Help the patient identify areas of his or her life situation that can be controlled. *Patient's emotional condition interferes with his or her ability to solve problems. Assistance is required to perceive the benefits and consequences of available alternatives accurately.*
4. Help patient identify areas of life situation that are not within his or her ability to control. Encourage verbalization of feelings related to this inability *in an effort to deal with unresolved issues and accept what cannot be changed.*
5. Identify ways in which patient can achieve. Encourage participation in these activities, and provide positive reinforcement for participation, as well as for achievement. *Positive reinforcement enhances self-esteem and encourages repetition of desirable behaviors.*

Outcome Criteria

1. Patient verbalizes choices made in a plan to maintain control over his or her life situation.
2. Patient verbalizes honest feelings about life situations over which he or she has no control.

3. Patient is able to verbalize system for problem-solving as required for adequate role performance.

■ DISTURBED THOUGHT PROCESSES

Definition: Disruption in cognitive operations and activities (Note: This diagnosis has been retired by NANDA-I but is retained in this text because of its appropriateness in describing these specific behaviors.)

Possible Contributing Factors ("related to")

[Withdrawal into the self]
[Underdeveloped ego; punitive superego]
[Impaired cognition fostering negative perception of self and the environment]

Defining Characteristics ("evidenced by")

[Inaccurate interpretation of environment]
[Delusional thinking]
[Altered attention span—distractibility]
[Egocentricity]
[Impaired ability to make decisions, problem-solve, reason]
[Negative ruminations]

Goals/Objectives

Short-term Goal

The patient will recognize and verbalize when interpretations of the environment are inaccurate within 1 week.

Long-term Goal

By time of discharge from treatment, the patient's verbalizations will reflect reality-based thinking with no evidence of delusional or distorted ideation.

Interventions With *Selected Rationales*

1. Convey your acceptance of the patient's need for the false belief, while letting him or her know that you do not share the delusion. *A positive response would convey to the patient that you accept the delusion as reality.*
2. Do not argue or deny the belief. Use *reasonable doubt* as a therapeutic technique: "I understand that you believe this is true, but I personally find it hard to accept." *Arguing with the patient or denying the belief serves no useful purpose because delusional ideas are not eliminated by this approach, and the development of a trusting relationship may be impeded.*

3. Use the techniques of *consensual validation* and *seeking clarification* when communication reflects alteration in thinking (e.g., "Is it that you mean . . . ?" or "I don't understand what you mean by that. Would you please explain?"). *These techniques reveal to the patient how he or she is being perceived by others, while the responsibility for not understanding is accepted by the nurse.*

4. Reinforce and focus on reality. Talk about real events and real people. Use real situations and events to divert the patient away from long, purposeless, repetitive verbalizations of false ideas.

5. Give positive reinforcement as the patient is able to differentiate between reality-based and nonreality-based thinking. *Positive reinforcement enhances self-esteem and encourages repetition of desirable behaviors.*

6. Teach patient to intervene, using thought-stopping techniques, when irrational or negative thoughts prevail. Thought stopping involves using the command "Stop!" or a loud noise (such as hand clapping) to interrupt unwanted thoughts. *This noise or command distracts the individual from the undesirable thinking that often precedes undesirable emotions or behaviors.*

7. Use touch cautiously, particularly if thoughts reveal ideas of persecution. *Patients who are suspicious may perceive touch as threatening and may respond with aggression.*

Outcome Criteria

1. The patient's thinking processes reflect accurate interpretation of the environment.

2. The patient is able to recognize negative or irrational thoughts and intervene to "stop" their progression.

■ IMBALANCED NUTRITION, LESS THAN BODY REQUIREMENTS

Definition: Intake of nutrients insufficient to meet metabolic needs (NANDA-I, 2018, p. 157)

Possible Contributing Factors ("related to")

Inability to ingest food because of:
    [Depressed mood]
    [Loss of appetite]
    [Energy level too low to meet own nutritional needs]
    [Regression to lower level of development]
    [Ideas of self-destruction]

Defining Characteristics ("evidenced by")

Loss of weight
Lack of interest in food

Pale mucous membranes
Poor muscle tone
[Amenorrhea]
[Poor skin turgor]
[Edema of extremities]
[Electrolyte imbalances]
[Weakness]
[Constipation]
[Anemia]

Goals/Objectives

Short-term Goal

The patient will gain 2 lb per week for the next 3 weeks.

Long-term Goal

The patient will exhibit no signs or symptoms of malnutrition by time of discharge from treatment (e.g., electrolytes and blood counts will be within normal limits; a steady weight gain will be demonstrated; constipation will be corrected; the patient will exhibit increased energy in participation in activities).

Interventions With *Selected Rationales*

1. In collaboration with dietitian, determine number of calories required to provide adequate nutrition and realistic (according to body structure and height) weight gain.
2. To prevent constipation, ensure that diet includes foods high in fiber content. Encourage increase in fluid consumption and physical exercise to promote normal bowel functioning. *Depressed patients are particularly vulnerable to constipation because of psychomotor retardation. Constipation is also a common side effect of many antidepressant medications.*
3. Keep strict documentation of intake, output, and calorie count. *This information is necessary to make an accurate nutritional assessment and maintain patient safety.*
4. Weigh patient daily. *Weight loss or gain is important assessment information.*
5. Determine patient's likes and dislikes and collaborate with dietitian to provide favorite foods. *Patient is more likely to eat foods that he or she particularly enjoys.*
6. Offer the patient small, frequent feedings, including a bedtime snack if he or she is unable to tolerate three larger meals. *Large amounts of food may be objectionable, or even intolerable, to the patient. Providing individualized care based on the patient's level of functioning supports maintaining adequate nutrition.*
7. Administer vitamin and mineral supplements and stool softeners or bulk extenders, as ordered by physician.

8. If appropriate, ask family members or significant others to bring in special foods that patient particularly enjoys.
9. Stay with the patient during meals *to assist as needed and to offer support and encouragement.*
10. Monitor laboratory values, and report significant changes to physician. *Laboratory values provide objective data regarding nutritional status.*
11. Explain the importance of adequate nutrition and fluid intake. *Patient may have inadequate or inaccurate knowledge regarding the contribution of good nutrition to overall wellness.*

Outcome Criteria

1. Patient has shown a slow, progressive weight gain during hospitalization.
2. Vital signs, blood pressure, and laboratory serum studies are within normal limits.
3. Patient is able to verbalize importance of adequate nutrition and fluid intake.

■ DISTURBED SLEEP PATTERN

Definition: Time-limited awakenings due to [internal or] external factors (NANDA-I, 2018, p. 216)

Possible Contributing Factors ("related to")

[Depression]
[Repressed fears]
[Feelings of hopelessness]
[Anxiety]
[Hallucinations]
[Delusional thinking]

Defining Characteristics ("evidenced by")

[Verbal complaints of difficulty falling asleep]
[Awakening earlier or later than desired]
[Interrupted sleep]
Reports not feeling well rested
[Awakening very early in the morning and being unable to go back to sleep]
[Excessive yawning and desire to nap during the day]
[Hypersomnia; using sleep as an escape]

Goals/Objectives

Short-term Goal
The patient will be able to sleep 4 to 6 hours within 5 days.

Long-term Goal

The patient will be able to fall asleep within 30 minutes of retiring and obtain 6 to 8 hours of uninterrupted sleep each night by time of discharge from treatment.

Interventions With *Selected Rationales*

1. Keep strict records of sleeping patterns. *Accurate baseline data are important in planning care to assist patient with this problem.*
2. Discourage sleep during the day *to promote more restful sleep at night.*
3. Antidepressant medications that are sedating may be administered at bedtime *so patient does not become drowsy during the day.*
4. Assist with measures that may promote sleep, such as warm, nonstimulating drinks, light snacks, warm baths, and back rubs.
5. Performing relaxation exercises to soft music may be helpful prior to sleep.
6. Limit intake of caffeinated drinks, such as tea, coffee, and colas. *Caffeine is a central nervous system stimulant that may interfere with the patient's achievement of rest and sleep.*
7. Administer sedative medications, as ordered, *to assist patient to achieve sleep until normal sleep pattern is restored.*
8. Some depressed patients may use excessive sleep as an escape. For the patient experiencing hypersomnia, set limits on time spent in room. Plan stimulating diversionary activities on a structured, daily schedule. Explore fears and feelings that sleep is helping to suppress.

Outcome Criteria

1. The patient is sleeping 6 to 8 hours per night without medication.
2. The patient is able to fall asleep within 30 minutes of retiring.
3. The patient is dealing with fears and feelings rather than escaping from them through excessive sleep.

@ INTERNET REFERENCES

Additional information about depressive disorders, including psychosocial and pharmacological treatment of these disorders, may be located at the following Web sites:

- www.dbsalliance.org
- www.mentalhealth.com
- www.mental-health-matters.com
- https://www.mentalhelp.net
- https://medlineplus.gov

- https://www.nami.org
- www.medicinenet.com/medications/article.htm
- https://www.drugs.com

Movie Connections

Prozac Nation (Depression) • *The Butcher Boy* (Depression)
• *Night, Mother* (Depression) • *The Prince of Tides* (Depression/Suicide)
• *The Perks of Being a Wallflower* (Depression) • *The Beaver* (Depression)
• *I'm Here Too* (Depression)

CHAPTER 7

Bipolar and Related Disorders

■ BACKGROUND ASSESSMENT DATA

Bipolar disorders are manifested by cycles of mania and depression. Mania is an alteration in mood that is expressed by feelings of elation, inflated self-esteem, grandiosity, hyperactivity, agitation, and accelerated thinking and speaking. A somewhat milder degree of this clinical symptom picture is called *hypomania*. Bipolar disorder affects about 4.4% of American adults and 82.9% of those cases are considered severe (National Institute of Mental Health, 2017). The average age of onset for bipolar disorder is around 18 years of age, and following the first manic episode, the disorder tends to be recurrent.

Types of Bipolar and Related Disorders

Bipolar I Disorder

Bipolar I disorder is the diagnosis given to an individual who is experiencing or has a history of one or more manic episodes. The patient may also have experienced episodes of depression. This diagnosis is further specified by the current or most recent behavioral episode experienced. For example, the specifier might be *single manic episode* (to describe individuals having a first episode of mania) or *current* (or most recent) *manic episode, hypomanic, mixed,* or *depressed* (to describe individuals who have had recurrent mood episodes). Psychotic or catatonic features and level of severity of symptoms may also be specified.

Bipolar II Disorder

Bipolar II disorder is characterized by recurrent bouts of major depression with the episodic occurrence of hypomania. The individual who is assigned this diagnosis may present with symptoms (or history) of depression or hypomania. The patient has never experienced a full manic episode. The diagnosis may specify whether the current or most recent episode is hypomanic, depressed, or with mixed features. If the current syndrome is a major depressive episode, psychotic or catatonic features may be noted.

Cyclothymic Disorder

The essential feature of cyclothymic disorder is a chronic mood disturbance with a duration of at least 2 years (at least 1 year in children and adolescents), involving numerous periods with hypomanic symptoms that do not meet the criteria for a hypomanic episode (i.e., too few hypomanic symptoms or not persistent for at least 4 consecutive days) and numerous periods of depressed mood of insufficient severity or duration to meet the criteria for major depressive episode (American Psychiatric Association [APA], 2013). The individual is never without the symptoms for more than 2 months.

Substance/Medication-Induced Bipolar Disorder

The disturbance of mood associated with this disorder is considered to be the direct result of physiological effects of a substance (e.g., ingestion of or withdrawal from a drug of abuse or a medication). The mood disturbance may involve elevated, expansive, or irritable mood, with inflated self-esteem, decreased need for sleep, and distractibility. The disorder causes clinically significant distress or impairment in social, occupational, or other important areas of functioning.

Bipolar Disorder Due to Another Medical Condition

This disorder is characterized by an abnormally and persistently elevated, expansive, or irritable mood and excessive activity or energy that is judged to be the result of direct physiological consequence of another medical condition (APA, 2013). The mood disturbance causes clinically significant distress or impairment in social, occupational, or other important areas of functioning.

■ PREDISPOSING FACTORS TO BIPOLAR DISORDER

1. Biological
   a. **Genetics:** Twin and family studies suggest that genes explain about 75% of risk for bipolar disorder (Kelsoe and Greenwood, 2017). If one parent has bipolar disorder, the risk that a child will have the disorder is around 25% (Sadock, Sadock, & Ruiz, 2015). If both parents have the disorder, the risk is two to three times as great. Increasing evidence continues to support the role of genetics in the predisposition to bipolar disorder. However, since genetic predisposition does not explain 100% of the risk, environmental and other nonheritable factors must be infuential, too.
   b. **Biochemical:** Just as there is an indication of lowered levels of norepinephrine and dopamine during an episode of depression, the opposite appears to be true of an individual experiencing a manic episode. Thus, the behavioral responses of elation and euphoria may be caused by an excess of these biogenic amines in the brain. It has also been suggested that manic individuals have increased intracellular

sodium and calcium. These electrolyte imbalances may be related to abnormalities in cellular membrane function in bipolar disorder.

2. Physiological
   a. **Neuroanatomical:** Right-sided lesions in the limbic system, temporobasal areas, basal ganglia, and thalamus have been shown to induce secondary mania. Magnetic resonance imaging studies have revealed enlarged third ventricles and subcortical white matter and periventricular hyperintensities in patients with bipolar disorder (Sadock et al, 2015).
   b. **Medication Side Effects:** Certain medications used to treat somatic illnesses have been known to trigger a manic response. The most common of these are the steroids frequently used to treat chronic illnesses such as multiple sclerosis and systemic lupus erythematosus. Some patients whose first episode of mania occurred during steroid therapy have reported spontaneous recurrence of manic symptoms years later. Amphetamines, antidepressants, and high doses of anticonvulsants and narcotics also have the potential for initiating a manic episode.
   c. **Substance Intoxication and Withdrawal:** Mood disturbances may be associated with intoxication from substances such as alcohol, amphetamines, cocaine, hallucinogens, inhalants, opioids, phencyclidine, sedatives, hypnotics, and anxiolytics. Symptoms can occur with withdrawal from substances such as alcohol, amphetamines, cocaine, sedatives, hypnotics, and anxiolytics.

■ SYMPTOMATOLOGY (SUBJECTIVE AND OBJECTIVE DATA)

(**NOTE:** The symptoms and treatment of bipolar depression are comparable to those of major depression that are addressed in Chapter 6. This chapter focuses on the symptoms and treatment of bipolar mania.)

1. The affect of an individual experiencing a manic episode is one of elation and euphoria—a continuous "high." However, the affect is very labile and may change quickly to hostility (particularly in response to attempts at limit setting) or to sadness, ruminating about past failures.
2. Alterations in thought processes and communication patterns are manifested by the following:
   a. **Flight of Ideas:** There is a continuous, rapid shift from one topic to another.
   b. **Loquaciousness:** The pressure of the speech is so forceful and strong that it is difficult to interrupt maladaptive thought processes.

   c. **Delusions of Grandeur:** The individual believes he or she is all-important, all-powerful, with feelings of greatness and magnificence.

   d. **Delusions of Persecution:** The individual believes someone or something desires to harm or violate him or her in some way.

3. Motor activity is constant. The individual is literally moving at all times.

4. Dress is often inappropriate: bright colors that do not match, clothing inappropriate for age or stature, excessive makeup and jewelry.

5. The individual has a meager appetite despite excessive activity level. He or she is unable or unwilling to stop moving in order to eat.

6. Sleep patterns are disturbed. The individual becomes oblivious to feelings of fatigue, and rest and sleep are abandoned for days or weeks.

7. Spending sprees are common. The individual spends large amounts of money, often beyond their available resources on numerous items, which are not needed.

8. Usual inhibitions are discarded in favor of sexual and behavioral indiscretions.

9. Manipulative behavior and limit testing are common in the attempt to fulfill personal desires. Verbal or physical hostility may follow failure in these attempts.

10. Projection is a major defense mechanism. The individual refuses to accept responsibility for the negative consequences of personal behavior.

11. There is an inability to concentrate because of a limited attention span. The individual is easily distracted by even the slightest stimulus in the environment.

12. Alterations in sensory perception may occur, and the individual may experience hallucinations.

13. As agitation increases, symptoms intensify. Unless the individual is placed in a protective environment, death can occur from exhaustion or injury.

Common Nursing Diagnoses and Interventions for Mania

(Interventions are applicable to various health-care settings, such as inpatient and partial hospitalization, community outpatient clinic, home health, and private practice.)

■ RISK FOR INJURY

Definition: Susceptible to physical damage due to environmental conditions interacting with the individual's adaptive and defensive resources, which may compromise health (NANDA International [NANDA-I], 2018, p. 393)

Risk Factors ("related to")

Biochemical dysfunction
Psychological (affective orientation)
[Extreme hyperactivity]
[Destructive behaviors]
[Anger directed at the environment]
[Hitting head (hand, arm, foot, etc.) against wall when angry]
[Temper tantrums—becomes destructive of inanimate objects]
[Increased agitation and lack of control over purposeless, potentially injurious movements]

Goals/Objectives

Short-term Goal

The patient will no longer exhibit potentially injurious level of activity after 24 hours with administration of tranquilizing medication.

Long-term Goal

The patient will experience no physical injury.

Interventions With *Selected Rationales*

1. Reduce environmental stimuli. Assign private room, if possible, with soft lighting, low noise level, and simple room decor. *In hyperactive state, the patient is extremely distractible, and responses to even the slightest stimuli are exaggerated.*
2. Limit group activities. Help the patient try to engage in one-to-one interaction. *The patient's ability to interact with others is often impaired during an acute manic state. One-to-one interaction reduces environmental stimuli and facilitates managing patient safety.*
3. Remove hazardous objects and substances from the patient's environment (including smoking materials). *The patient's hyperactivity, impulsivity, and distractibility increase the risk for inadvertent self-harm. Patient safety is a nursing priority.*
4. Stay with the patient to offer support and provide a feeling of security as agitation grows and hyperactivity increases.
5. Provide structured schedule of activities that includes established rest periods throughout the day. *A structured schedule provides a feeling of security for the patient.*
6. Provide structured physical activities as an outlet for hyperactivity (e.g., brisk walks, housekeeping chores, dance therapy, aerobics). *Physical exercise provides a safe and effective means of relieving pent-up tension.*
7. Administer tranquilizing medication, as ordered by physician. Antipsychotic drugs are commonly prescribed for rapid relief of agitation and hyperactivity. Atypical forms commonly used include olanzapine, ziprasidone, quetiapine, risperidone, asenapine, and aripiprazole. Haloperidol, a typical antipsychotic, is indicated in the treatment of bipolar

mania. Observe for effectiveness and evidence of adverse side effects (see Chapter 26).

8. Redirect the patient to other activities when agitation and other manic behaviors begin to escalate. *In an acute manic state, the patient is highly distractible, so redirection and distraction can be effective in diffusing escalating, potentially harmful behavior. Reducing stimulation in the environment may also decrease severity of manic symptoms.*

Outcome Criteria

1. The patient is no longer exhibiting signs of physical agitation.
2. The patient exhibits no evidence of physical injury obtained while experiencing hyperactive behavior.

■ RISK FOR SELF-DIRECTED OR OTHER-DIRECTED VIOLENCE

Definition: Susceptible to behaviors in which an individual demonstrates that he or she can be physically, emotionally, and/or sexually harmful [either to self or to others] (NANDA-I, 2018, pp. 416–417)

Risk Factors ("related to")

[Manic excitement]
[Biochemical alterations]
[Threat to self-concept]
[Suspicion of others]
[Paranoid ideation]
[Delusions]
[Hallucinations]
[Rage reactions]
Negative body language (e.g., rigid posture, clenching of fists and jaw, hyperactivity, pacing, breathlessness, threatening stances)
[History or threats of violence toward self or others or of destruction to the property of others]
Impulsivity
Suicidal ideation, plan, available means
[Repetition of verbalizations (continuous complaints, requests, and demands)]

Goals/Objectives

Short-term Goals

1. The patient's agitation will be maintained at manageable level. Within [a specified time], the patient will recognize signs of increasing anxiety and agitation and report to staff (or other care provider) for assistance with intervention.
2. The patient will not harm self or others.

Long-term Goal

The patient will not harm self or others.

Interventions With *Selected Rationales*

1. Maintain low level of stimuli in the patient's environment (low lighting, few people, simple decor, low noise level). *Anxiety and agitation rise in a stimulating environment. A suspicious, agitated patient may perceive others as threatening.*
2. Observe the patient's behavior frequently. Do this while carrying out routine activities so as to avoid creating suspiciousness in the individual. *Close observation is required so that intervention can occur if needed to ensure the patient's (and others') safety.*
3. Remove all dangerous objects from the patient's environment (sharp objects, glass or mirrored items, belts, ties, smoking materials) *so that in his or her agitated, hyperactive state, the patient may not use them to harm self or others.*
4. Try to redirect the violent behavior with physical outlets for the patient's hostility (e.g., walking, push-ups). *Physical exercise is a safe and effective way of relieving pent-up tension.*
5. Intervene at the first sign of increased anxiety, agitation, or verbal or behavioral aggression. Offer empathetic response to the patient's feelings: "You seem anxious (or frustrated, or angry) about this situation. How can I help?" *Validation of the patient's feelings conveys a caring attitude, and offering assistance reinforces trust.*
6. It is important to maintain a calm attitude toward the patient. Respond in a matter-of-fact manner to verbal hostility. *Anxiety is contagious and can be transmitted from staff to patient.*
7. As the patient's anxiety increases, offer some alternatives: participating in a physical activity (e.g., physical exercise), talking about the situation, taking some antianxiety medication. *Offering alternatives to the patient demonstrates a patient-centered approach and affords the patient a greater sense of control over the situation.*
8. Have sufficient staff available to indicate a show of strength to the patient if it becomes necessary. *This conveys to the patient evidence of control over the situation and provides some physical security for staff.*
9. Administer tranquilizing medications, as ordered by physician. Monitor medication for effectiveness and for adverse side effects.
10. If the patient is not calmed by "talking down" or by medication, use of mechanical restraints may be necessary. The avenue of the "least restrictive alternative" must be selected when planning interventions for a violent patient. Restraints should be used only as a last resort, after all other interventions have been unsuccessful and the patient is clearly at risk of harm to self or others.

11. If restraint is deemed necessary, ensure that sufficient staff is available to assist. Follow protocol established by the institution. Assess the patient in restraints at least every 15 minutes to ensure that circulation to extremities is not compromised (check temperature, color, pulses); to assist the patient with needs related to nutrition, hydration, and elimination; and to position the patient so that comfort is facilitated and aspiration can be prevented. Some institutions may require continuous one-to-one monitoring of restrained the patients, particularly those who are highly agitated, and for whom there is a high risk of self- or accidental injury. *Patient safety is a nursing priority.*

12. As agitation decreases, assess the patient's readiness for restraint removal or reduction. Remove one restraint at a time while assessing the patient's response. *This procedure minimizes the risk of injury to patient and staff.*

Outcome Criteria

1. The patient is able to verbalize anger in an appropriate manner.
2. There is no evidence of violent behavior to self or others.
3. The patient is no longer exhibiting hyperactive behaviors.

■ IMBALANCED NUTRITION, LESS THAN BODY REQUIREMENTS

Definition: Intake of nutrients insufficient to meet metabolic needs (NANDA-I, 2018, p. 157)

Possible Contributing Factors ("related to")

[Refusal or inability to sit still long enough to eat meals]
[Lack of appetite]
[Excessive physical agitation]
[Physical exertion in excess of energy produced through caloric intake]
[Lack of interest in food]

Defining Characteristics ("evidenced by")

Loss of weight
Pale mucous membranes
Poor muscle tone
Insufficient interest in food
[Amenorrhea]
[Poor skin turgor]
[Anemia]
[Electrolyte imbalances]

Goals/Objectives

Short-term Goal

The patient will consume sufficient foods and between-meal snacks to meet recommended daily allowances of nutrients.

Long-term Goal

The patient will exhibit no signs or symptoms of malnutrition.

Interventions With *Selected Rationales*

1. In collaboration with dietitian, determine number of calories required to provide adequate nutrition for maintenance or re-alistic (according to body structure and height) weight gain.
2. Provide patient with high-protein, high-calorie, nutritious finger foods and drinks that can be consumed "on the run." *Because of hyperactive state, the patient has difficulty sitting still long enough to eat a meal. The likelihood is greater that he or she will consume food and drinks that can be carried around and eaten with little effort.*
3. Have juice and snacks available on the unit at all times. *Nutritious intake is required on a regular basis to compensate for increased caloric requirements due to hyperactivity.*
4. Maintain accurate record of intake, output, and calorie count. *This information is necessary to make an accurate nutritional assessment and maintain the patient's safety.*
5. Weigh the patient daily. *Weight loss or gain is important nutritional assessment information.*
6. Determine the patient's likes and dislikes, and collaborate with dietitian to provide favorite foods. *The patient is more likely to eat foods that he or she particularly enjoys.*
7. Administer vitamin and mineral supplements, as ordered by physician, *to improve nutritional state.*
8. Pace or walk with the patient as finger foods are taken. As agitation subsides, sit with the patient during meals. Offer support and encouragement. Assess and record amount consumed. *Presence of a trusted individual may provide feeling of security and decrease agitation. Encouragement and positive reinforcement increase self-esteem and foster repetition of desired behaviors.*
9. Monitor laboratory values, and report significant changes to physician. *Laboratory values provide objective nutritional assessment data.*
10. Explain the importance of adequate nutrition and fluid intake. *The patient may have inadequate or inaccurate knowledge regarding the contribution of good nutrition to overall wellness.*

Outcome Criteria

1. The patient has gained (maintained) weight during hospitalization.
2. Vital signs, blood pressure, and laboratory serum studies are within normal limits.

3. The patient is able to verbalize importance of adequate nutrition and fluid intake.

■ DISTURBED THOUGHT PROCESSES

Definition: Disruption in cognitive operations and activities (Note: This diagnosis has been retired by NANDA-I but is retained in this text because of its appropriateness in describing these specific behaviors.)

Possible Contributing Factors ("related to")

[Biochemical alterations]
[Electrolyte imbalance]
[Psychotic process]
[Sleep deprivation]

Defining Characteristics ("evidenced by")

[Inaccurate interpretation of environment]
[Hypervigilance]
[Altered attention span—distractibility]
[Egocentricity]
[Decreased ability to grasp ideas]
[Impaired ability to make decisions, solve problems, reason]
[Delusions of grandeur]
[Delusions of persecution]
[Suspiciousness]

Goals/Objectives

Short-term Goal

Within 1 week, patient will be able to recognize and verbalize when thinking is not reality-based.

Long-term Goal

By time of discharge from treatment, patient's verbalizations will reflect reality-based thinking with no evidence of delusional ideation.

Interventions With *Selected Rationales*

1. Convey acceptance of patient's need for the false belief, while letting him or her know that you do not share the delusion. *A positive response would convey to the patient that you accept the delusion as reality.*
2. Do not argue or deny the belief. Use *reasonable doubt* as a therapeutic technique: "I understand that you believe this is true, but I personally find it hard to accept." *Arguing with the patient or denying the belief serves no useful purpose because delusional ideas*

are not eliminated by this approach, and the development of a trusting relationship may be impeded.

3. Use the techniques of *consensual validation* and *seeking clarification* when communication reflects alteration in thinking (e.g., "Is it that you mean . . . ?" or "I don't understand what you mean by that. Would you please explain?"). *These techniques reveal to the patient how he or she is being perceived by others, and the responsibility for not understanding is accepted by the nurse.*

4. Reinforce and focus on reality. Talk about real events and real people. Use real situations and events to divert patient away from long, tedious, repetitive verbalizations of false ideas.

5. Give positive reinforcement as patient is able to differentiate between reality-based and nonreality-based thinking. *Positive reinforcement enhances self-esteem and encourages repetition of desirable behaviors.*

6. Teach patient to intervene, using thought-stopping techniques, when irrational thoughts prevail. Thought stopping involves using the command "Stop!" or a loud noise (such as hand clapping) to interrupt unwanted thoughts. *This noise or command distracts the individual from the undesirable thinking, which often precedes undesirable emotions or behaviors.*

7. Use touch cautiously, particularly if thoughts reveal ideas of persecution. *Patients who are suspicious may perceive touch as threatening and may respond with aggression.*

Outcome Criteria

1. Thought processes reflect an accurate interpretation of the environment.

2. Patient is able to recognize thoughts that are not based in reality and intervene to stop their progression.

■ DISTURBED SENSORY PERCEPTION

Definition: Change in the amount or patterning of incoming stimuli [either internally or externally initiated] accompanied by a diminished, exaggerated, distorted, or impaired response to such stimuli (Note: This diagnosis has been retired by NANDA-I but is retained in this text because of its appropriateness in describing these specific behaviors.)

Possible Contributing Factors ("related to")

[Biochemical imbalance]
[Electrolyte imbalance]
[Sleep deprivation]
[Psychotic process]

Defining Characteristics ("evidenced by")

[Change in usual response to stimuli]
[Hallucinations]
[Disorientation]
[Inappropriate responses]
[Rapid mood swings]
[Exaggerated emotional responses]
[Visual and auditory distortions]
[Talking and laughing to self]
[Listening pose (tilting head to one side as if listening)]
[Stops talking in middle of sentence to listen]

Goals/Objectives

Short-term Goal

The patient will be able to recognize and verbalize when he or she is interpreting the environment inaccurately.

Long-term Goal

The patient will be able to define and test reality, eliminating the occurrence of sensory misperceptions.

Interventions With *Selected Rationales*

1. Observe the patient for signs of hallucinations (listening pose, laughing or talking to self, stopping in midsentence). *Early intervention may prevent aggressive responses to command hallucinations.*
2. Avoid touching the patient and request the patient's permission beforehand. *The patient may perceive touch as threatening and respond in an aggressive manner.*
3. An attitude of acceptance will encourage the patient to share the content of the hallucination with you. *This is important in order to prevent possible injury to the patient or others from command hallucinations.*
4. Do not reinforce the hallucination. Use words such as "the voices" instead of "they" when referring to the hallucination. *Words like "they" validate that the voices are real.*

> **CLINICAL PEARL** Let the patient who is "hearing voices" know that you do not share the perception. Say, "Even though I realize that the voices are real to you, I do not hear any voices speaking." The nurse must be honest with the patient so that he or she may realize that the hallucinations are not real.

5. Try to connect the times of the misperceptions to times of increased anxiety. Help the patient to understand this connection. *If the patient can learn to interrupt the escalating anxiety, reality orientation may be maintained.*

6. Try to distract the patient away from the misperception. *Involvement in interpersonal activities and explanation of the actual situation may bring the patient back to reality.*

Outcome Criteria

1. The patient is able to differentiate between reality and unrealistic events or situations.
2. The patient is able to refrain from responding to false sensory perceptions.

■ IMPAIRED SOCIAL INTERACTION

Definition: Insufficient or excessive quantity or ineffective quality of social exchange (NANDA-I, 2018, p. 301)

Possible Contributing Factors ("related to")

Disturbed thought processes
[Delusions of grandeur]
[Delusions of persecution]
Self-concept disturbance

Defining Characteristics ("evidenced by")

Discomfort in social situations
Inability to receive or communicate a satisfying sense of social engagement (e.g., belonging, caring, interest, or shared history)
Use of unsuccessful social interaction behaviors
Dysfunctional interaction with others
[Excessive use of projection—does not accept responsibility for own behavior]
[Verbal manipulation]
[Inability to delay gratification]

Goals/Objectives

Short-term Goal

The patient will verbalize which of his or her interaction behaviors are appropriate and which are inappropriate within 1 week.

Long-term Goal

The patient will demonstrate use of appropriate interaction skills as evidenced by reality-based communication with socially acceptable behaviors and boundaries.

Interventions With *Selected Rationales*

1. Explain the rules and expectations for interaction within the unit environment (therapeutic milieu) as well as consequences

for inappropriate behavior and communication. *Clarifying expectations is foundational in establishing a trusting relationship and in reinforcing consequences when the patient violates established boundaries. Maintaining patient safety is a nursing priority.*

2. Set limits and enforce identified consequences. Terms of the limitations and consequences must be agreed on by all staff who will be working with the patient. *When the patient is unable to establish safe and appropriate limits, this must be done for him or her. Consistency in limit setting reinforces expectations for appropriate behavior and communication.*

3. Do not argue, bargain, or try to reason with the patient. Merely state the limits and expectations. Individuals with mania can be very charming in their efforts to fulfill their own desires. Confront the patient as soon as possible when interactions with others are manipulative or exploitative. Follow through with established consequences for unacceptable behavior. *Consistency in enforcing the consequences is essential if positive outcomes are to be achieved. Inconsistency creates confusion and encourages testing of limits.*

4. Provide positive reinforcement for socially acceptable behaviors. Explore feelings, and help the patient seek more appropriate ways of dealing with them. *Positive reinforcement enhances self-esteem and promotes repetition of desirable behaviors.*

5. Help the patient recognize that he or she must accept the consequences of own behaviors and refrain from attributing them to others. *The patient must accept responsibility for own behaviors before adaptive change can occur.*

6. Help the patient identify positive aspects about self and recognize accomplishments. *As self-esteem is increased, the patient will feel less need to manipulate or exploit others for own gratification.*

7. As the manic episode is resolving, encourage the patient (and the family when possible) to identify early warning signs of an impending manic episode and management strategies to minimize negative outcomes. *Increased sexual promiscuity, financial overspending, and other behaviors common in an acute manic episode can create hardship for the patient and his or her family and fracture interpersonal relationships. Engaging the patient and family in identifying symptoms and management strategies may strengthen the support system and minimize consequences associated with manic behavior and communication.*

Outcome Criteria

1. The patient is able to verbalize positive aspects of self.
2. The patient accepts responsibility for own behaviors.
3. The patient does not manipulate others for gratification of own needs.

■ INSOMNIA

Definition: A disruption in amount and quality of sleep that impairs functioning (NANDA-I, 2018, p. 213)

Possible Contributing Factors ("related to")

[Excessive hyperactivity]
[Agitation]
[Biochemical alterations]

Defining Characteristics ("evidenced by")

Reports difficulty falling asleep
[Pacing in hall during sleeping hours]
[Sleeping only short periods at a time]
[Numerous periods of wakefulness during the night]
[Awakening and rising extremely early in the morning; exhibiting signs of restlessness]

Goals/Objectives

Short-term Goal

Within 3 days, with the aid of a sleeping medication, the patient will sleep 4 to 6 hours without awakening.

Long-term Goal

By time of discharge from treatment, the patient will be able to acquire 6 to 8 hours of uninterrupted sleep without sleeping medication.

Interventions With *Selected Rationales*

1. Provide a quiet environment with a low level of stimulation. *Hyperactivity increases and ability to achieve sleep and rest are hindered in a stimulating environment.*
2. Monitor sleep patterns. Provide structured schedule of activities that includes established times for naps or rest. *Accurate baseline data are important in planning care to help the patient with this problem. A structured schedule, including time for naps, will help the hyperactive patient achieve much-needed rest.*
3. Assess the patient's activity level. The patient may ignore or be unaware of feelings of fatigue. Observe for signs such as increasing restlessness; fine tremors; slurred speech; and puffy, dark circles under eyes. *The patient can collapse from exhaustion if hyperactivity is uninterrupted and rest is not achieved.*
4. Before bedtime, provide nursing measures that promote sleep, such as warm bath; warm, nonstimulating drinks; soft music; and relaxation exercises.

5. Prohibit intake of caffeinated drinks, such as tea, coffee, and colas. *Caffeine is a central nervous system stimulant and may interfere with the patient's achievement of rest and sleep.*
6. Administer sedative medications, as ordered, to assist the patient to achieve sleep until normal sleep pattern is restored.

Outcome Criteria

1. The patient is sleeping 6 to 8 hours per night without sleeping medication.
2. The patient is able to fall asleep within 30 minutes of retiring.
3. The patient is dealing openly with fears and feelings rather than manifesting denial of them through hyperactivity.

@ INTERNET REFERENCES

Additional information about bipolar disorders, including psychosocial and pharmacological treatment of these disorders, may be located at the following Web sites:

- www.dbsalliance.org
- www.mentalhealth.com
- https://www.nami.org
- www.mental-health-matters.com
- https://www.mentalhelp.net
- https://medlineplus.gov
- https://www.drugs.com
- www.mentalhealthamerica.net

Movie Connections

Lust for Life (Bipolar disorder) • *Call Me Anna* (Bipolar disorder) • *Blue Sky* (Bipolar disorder) • *A Woman Under the Influence* (Bipolar disorder) • *Mr. Jones* (Bipolar disorder) • *Frances* (Bipolar disorder) • *The Whole Wide World* (Bipolar disorder) • *Pollock* (Bipolar disorder) • *Silver Linings Playbook* (Bipolar disorder) • *Touched With Fire* (Bipolar disorder)

CHAPTER 8

Anxiety, Obsessive-Compulsive, and Related Disorders

■ BACKGROUND ASSESSMENT DATA

Anxiety may be defined as apprehension, tension, or uneasiness from anticipation of danger, the source of which is largely unknown or unrecognized. Anxiety may be regarded as pathological when it interferes with social and occupational functioning, achievement of desired goals, or emotional comfort. Anxiety disorders are among the most common of all psychiatric illnesses. They are more common in women than in men, with the exception of social anxiety and obsessive compulsive disorders, which are equally prevalent among men and women (ADAA, 2018).

The manifestations of obsessive-compulsive disorder (OCD) include the presence of obsessions, compulsions, or both, the severity of which is significant enough to cause distress or impairment in social, occupational, or other important areas of functioning (American Psychiatric Association [APA], 2013). Obsessions are defined as recurrent and persistent thoughts, impulses, or images experienced as intrusive and stressful. Compulsions are identified as repetitive, ritualistic behaviors that the individual feels compelled and driven to perform in an effort to decrease feelings of anxiety and discomfort. Related disorders (OCD-types) include body dysmorphic disorder, hoarding disorder, trichotillomania (hair-pulling disorder), and excoriation (skin-picking) disorder.

Selected types of anxiety, obsessive-compulsive, and related disorders are presented in the following sections.

Panic Disorder

Panic disorder is characterized by recurrent panic attacks, the onset of which are unpredictable, and which are manifested by intense apprehension, fear, or terror, often associated with feelings of impending doom, and accompanied by intense physical discomfort. The symptoms come on unexpectedly; that is, they do not occur immediately before or on exposure to a situation that usually causes anxiety (as in specific phobia). They are not triggered by situations in which the person is the focus of others' attention (as in social anxiety disorder). The attacks usually last minutes or, more rarely, hours. The individual often experiences varying degrees of nervousness and apprehension between attacks. Symptoms of depression are common.

Generalized Anxiety Disorder

This disorder is characterized by persistent, unrealistic, and excessive anxiety and worry, which have occurred more days than not for at least 6 months. The symptoms cause clinically significant distress or impairment in social, occupational, or other important areas of functioning. The anxiety and worry are associated with muscle tension, restlessness, or feeling "keyed up" or "on edge" (APA, 2013).

Agoraphobia

The individual with agoraphobia experiences fear of being in places or situations from which escape might be difficult or in which help might not be available in the event that panic symptoms should occur. It is possible that the individual may have experienced the symptom(s) in the past and is preoccupied with fears of their recurrence. Sadock, Sadock, and Ruiz report that "in the United States, most researchers of panic disorder believe that agoraphobia almost always develops as a complication in patients with panic disorder" (2015, p. 398). Impairment can be severe. In extreme cases, the individual is unable to leave his or her home without being accompanied by a friend or relative. If this is not possible, the person may become totally confined to his or her home.

Social Anxiety Disorder (Social Phobia)

Social anxiety disorder is an excessive fear of situations in which a person might do something embarrassing or be evaluated negatively by others. The individual has extreme concerns about being exposed to possible scrutiny by others and fears social or performance situations in which embarrassment may occur (APA, 2013). In some instances, the fear may be quite defined, such as the fear of speaking or eating in a public place, fear of using a public restroom, or fear of writing in the presence of others. In other cases, the social phobia may involve general social situations, such as saying things or answering questions in a manner that would provoke laughter on the part of others. Exposure to the phobic situation usually results in feelings of panic anxiety, with sweating, tachycardia, and dyspnea.

Specific Phobia

Specific phobia is identified by fear of specific objects or situations that could conceivably cause harm (e.g., snakes, heights), but the person's reaction to them is excessive, unreasonable, and inappropriate. Exposure to the phobic stimulus produces overwhelming symptoms of panic, including palpitations, sweating, dizziness, and difficulty breathing. A diagnosis of specific phobia is made only when the irrational fear restricts the individual's activities and interferes with his or her daily living.

Obsessive-Compulsive Disorder

OCD is characterized by involuntary recurring thoughts or images that the individual is unable to ignore and by the recurring impulse to perform a seemingly purposeless, ritualistic activity. These obsessions and compulsions serve to reduce anxiety on the part of the individual. The disorder is equally common among men and women. It may begin in childhood but more often begins in adolescence or early adulthood. The course is usually chronic and may be complicated by depression or substance abuse.

Body Dysmorphic Disorder

Body dysmorphic disorder is characterized by the exaggerated belief that the body is deformed or defective in some specific way. While the preoccupation may involve any area of the body or multiple areas, the most common foci are perceived skin defects, hair (thinning, excessive, or facial hair), or size and shape of the nose (APA, 2013).Other complaints may have to do with some aspect of the ears, eyes, mouth, lips, or teeth. Some patients may present with complaints involving other parts of the body, and in some instances, a true defect is present. The significance of the defect is unrealistically exaggerated, however, and the person's concern is grossly excessive.

Trichotillomania (Hair-Pulling Disorder)

The *Diagnostic and Statistical Manual of Mental Disorders, Fifth Edition (DSM-5)* defines this disorder as the recurrent pulling out of one's hair, which results in hair loss (APA, 2013). The impulse is preceded by an increasing sense of tension and results in a sense of release or gratification from pulling out the hair. The most common sites for hair pulling are the scalp, eyebrows, and eyelashes, but hair pulling may occur in any area of the body on which hair grows. These areas of hair loss are often found on the opposite side of the body from the dominant hand. Pain is seldom reported to accompany the hair pulling, although tingling and pruritus in the area are not uncommon. The disorder is relatively rare but occurs more often in women than it does in men.

Hoarding Disorder

The *DSM-5* defines the essential feature of hoarding disorder as "persistent difficulties discarding or parting with possessions, regardless of their actual value" (APA, 2013, p. 248) Additionally, the diagnosis may be specified as "with excessive acquisition," which identifies the excessive need for continual acquiring of items (either by buying them or by other means). In previous editions of the *DSM*, hoarding was considered a symptom of OCD. However, in the *DSM-5*, it has been reclassified as a diagnostic disorder.

Individuals with this disorder collect items until virtually all surfaces within the home are covered. There may be only narrow pathways, winding through stacks of clutter, in which to walk. Some individuals also hoard food and animals, keeping dozens or hundreds of pets, often in unsanitary conditions (Mayo Clinic, 2019).

Prevalence statistics for hoarding disorder are difficult to clarify because many people with this disorder do not seek treatment. Based on community surveys, the prevalence of clinically significant hoarding is estimated to be approximately 2% to 6% (APA, 2013). More men than women are diagnosed with the disorder, and it is almost three times more prevalent in older adults (ages 55 to 94) than in younger adults (ages 34 to 44) (APA, 2013). The severity of the symptoms, regardless of when they begin, appears to increase with each decade of life. Associated symptoms include perfectionism, indecisiveness, anxiety, depression, distractibility, and difficulty planning and organizing tasks (APA, 2013). Some experts have identified a connection between unresolved grief and hoarding behavior.

Anxiety Disorder Due to Another Medical Condition

The symptoms of this disorder are judged to be the direct physiological consequence of another medical condition. Symptoms may include prominent generalized anxiety symptoms, panic attacks, or obsessions or compulsions. Medical conditions that have been known to cause anxiety disorders include endocrine, cardiovascular, respiratory, metabolic, and neurological disorders.

Substance/Medication-Induced Anxiety Disorder

The *DSM-5* describes the essential features of this disorder as prominent anxiety symptoms that are judged to be caused by the direct physiological effects of a substance (i.e., a drug of abuse, a medication, or toxin exposure). The symptoms may occur during substance intoxication or withdrawal from alcohol, amphetamines, cocaine, hallucinogens, sedatives, hypnotics, anxiolytics, caffeine, cannabis, or other substances (APA, 2013).

■ PREDISPOSING FACTORS TO ANXIETY, OCD, AND RELATED DISORDERS

1. Physiological
   a. **Biochemical:** Increased levels of norepinephrine have been noted in panic and generalized anxiety disorders. Gamma-aminobutyric acid (GABA) dysfunction has been associated with anxiety disorders, especially panic disorder

(Sadock et al, 2015). Abnormal elevations of blood lactate have also been noted in patients with panic disorder. Decreased levels of serotonin have been implicated in the etiology of OCD. Alterations in the serotonin and endogenous opioid systems have been noted with trichotillomania. The serotonergic system may also be a factor in the etiology of body dysmorphic disorder. This can be reflected in a high incidence of comorbidity with major mood disorder and anxiety disorder and the positive responsiveness of the condition to the serotonin-specific drugs. Studies of serotonin's role in anxiety disorders, though, have had mixed results (Sadock et al, 2015), and some anxiety disorders have been associated with too much serotonin.

b. **Genetics:** Studies suggest that anxiety disorders are prevalent within the general population. It has been shown that they are more common among first-degree biological relatives of people with the disorders than among the general population. Trichotillomania has commonly been associated with OCDs among first-degree relatives, leading researchers to conclude that the disorder has a possible hereditary or familial predisposition.

c. **Neuroanatomical:** Structural brain imaging studies in patients with panic disorder have implicated pathological involvement in the temporal lobes, particularly the hippocampus (Sadock et al, 2015). Neuroimaging and neurocognitive assessment have identified impairment in motor inhibition responses (the ability to stop an action once initiated) in patients with OCD and trichotillomania (Kaplan, 2012). Functional neuroimaging techniques have shown increased metabolic rates and blood flow in the basal ganglia, frontal lobes, and cingulum as well as bilaterally smaller caudates in individuals with OCD (Sadock et al, 2015). In individuals with hoarding disorder, neuroimaging studies have indicated less activity in the cingulate cortex (the area of the brain that connects the emotional part of the brain with the parts that control higher-level thinking), which may account for deficits in attention and decision making that are common in this population (Sadock et al, 2015).

d. **Medical or Substance-Induced:** Anxiety disorders may be caused by a variety of medical conditions or the ingestion of various substances. (Refer to previous section on categories of anxiety disorders.)

2. Psychosocial

a. **Psychodynamic Theory:** The psychodynamic view focuses on the inability of the ego to intervene when conflict occurs between the id and the superego, producing anxiety. For various reasons (unsatisfactory parent-child relationship, conditional love, or provisional gratification), ego development is delayed. If developmental defects in ego functions compromise the capacity to modulate anxiety, the individual resorts to unconscious mechanisms to resolve the conflict. Overuse or ineffective use of ego defense mechanisms results in maladaptive responses to anxiety.

b. **Cognitive Theory:** The main thesis of the cognitive view is that faulty, distorted, or counterproductive thinking patterns accompany or precede maladaptive behaviors and emotional disorders (Sadock et al, 2015). If there is a disturbance in this central mechanism of cognition, there is a consequent disturbance in feeling and behavior. Because of distorted thinking, anxiety is maintained by erroneous or dysfunctional appraisal of a situation. There is a loss of ability to reason regarding the problem, whether it is physical or interpersonal. The individual feels vulnerable in a given situation, and the distorted thinking results in an irrational appraisal, fostering a negative outcome.

c. **Learning Theory:** Phobias may be acquired by direct learning or imitation (modeling) (e.g., a mother who exhibits fear toward an object will provide a model for the child, who may also develop a phobia of the same object). They may be maintained as conditioned responses when reinforcements occur. In the case of phobias, when the individual avoids the phobic object, he or she escapes fear, which is indeed a powerful reinforcement.

d. **Life Experiences:** Certain early experiences may set the stage for phobic reactions later in life. Some researchers believe that phobias, particularly specific phobias, are symbolic of original anxiety-producing objects or situations that have been repressed.

Examples include the following:

- A child who is punished by being locked in a closet develops a phobia for elevators or other closed places.
- A child who falls down a flight of stairs develops a phobia for high places.
- A young woman who, as a child, survived a plane crash in which both her parents were killed has a phobia of airplanes.

In general, anxiety disorders appear to be largely multidetermined and, as such, may include a combination of genetic vulnerability, neuroanatomical and neurobiochemical changes, and environmental factors.

■ SYMPTOMATOLOGY (SUBJECTIVE AND OBJECTIVE DATA)

An individual may experience a panic attack under any of the following conditions:

- As the predominant disturbance, with no apparent precipitant
- When exposed to a phobic stimulus

- When attempts are made to curtail ritualistic behavior
- Following a psychologically stressful event

Symptoms of a panic attack include the following (APA, 2013):

- Palpitations, pounding heart, or accelerated heart rate
- Sweating
- Trembling or shaking
- Sensations of shortness of breath or smothering
- Feelings of choking
- Chest pain or discomfort
- Nausea or abdominal distress
- Feeling dizzy, unsteady, lightheaded, or faint
- Chills or heat sensations
- Paresthesia (numbness or tingling sensations)
- Derealization (feelings of unreality) or depersonalization (feelings of being detached from oneself)
- Fear of losing control or going crazy
- Fear of dying

Other symptoms of anxiety, OCD, or related disorders include the following:

1. Restlessness, feeling "on edge," excessive worry, being easily fatigued, difficulty concentrating, irritability, and sleep disturbances (generalized anxiety disorder).
2. Repetitive, obsessive thoughts, common ones being related to violence, contamination, and doubt; repetitive, compulsive performance of purposeless activity, such as hand washing, counting, checking, touching (OCD).
3. Marked and persistent fears of specific objects or situations (specific phobia), social or performance situations (social anxiety disorder), or being in a situation from which one has difficulty escaping (agoraphobia).
4. Repetitive pulling out of one's own hair (trichotillomania).
5. Persistent difficulty discarding or parting with possessions (hoarding disorder).
6. Having the exaggerated belief that the body is deformed or defective in some specific way (body dysmorphic disorder).

Common Nursing Diagnoses and Interventions

(Interventions are applicable to various health-care settings, such as inpatient and partial hospitalization, community outpatient clinic, home health, and private practice.)

■ ANXIETY (Panic)

Definition: Vague, uneasy feeling of discomfort or dread accompanied by an autonomic response (the source often nonspecific or unknown to the individual); a feeling of apprehension caused by anticipation of danger. It is an alerting signal that warns of impending danger and enables the individual to take measures to deal with threat (NANDA International [NANDA-I], 2018, p. 324)

Possible Contributing Factors ("related to")

Unconscious conflict about essential values and goals of life
Situational and maturational crises
[Real or perceived] threat to self-concept
[Real or perceived] threat of death
Unmet needs
[Being exposed to a phobic stimulus]
[Attempts at interference with ritualistic behaviors]

Defining Characteristics ("evidenced by")

Increased respiration
Increased pulse
Decreased or increased blood pressure
Nausea
Confusion
Increased perspiration
Faintness
Trembling or shaking
Restlessness
Insomnia
[Fear of dying, going crazy, or doing something uncontrolled during an attack]

Goals/Objectives

Short-term Goal

The patient will verbalize ways to intervene in escalating anxiety within 1 week.

Long-term Goal

By time of discharge from treatment, the patient will be able to recognize symptoms of onset of anxiety and intervene before reaching panic stage.

Interventions With *Selected Rationales*

1. Maintain a calm, nonthreatening manner while working with the patient. *Anxiety is contagious and may be transferred from staff to patient or vice versa. Patients develop feeling of security in presence of calm staff person.*
2. Reassure the patient of his or her safety and security. This can be conveyed by physical presence of nurse. Do not leave the patient alone at this time. *The patient may fear for his or her life. Presence of a trusted individual provides the patient with feeling of security and assurance of personal safety.*

3. Use simple words and brief messages, spoken calmly and clearly, to explain hospital experiences to the patient. *In an intensely anxious situation, the patient is unable to comprehend anything but the most elementary communication.*

4. Hyperventilation may occur during periods of extreme anxiety. Hyperventilation causes the amount of carbon dioxide (CO_2) in the blood to decrease, possibly resulting in lightheadedness, rapid heart rate, shortness of breath, numbness or tingling in the hands or feet, and syncope. If hyperventilation occurs, assist the patient to breathe into a small paper bag held over the mouth and nose. The patient should take 6 to 12 natural breaths, alternating with short periods of diaphragmatic breathing. This technique should not be used with patients who have coronary or respiratory disorders, such as coronary artery disease, asthma, or chronic obstructive pulmonary disease.

5. Keep the immediate surroundings low in stimuli (dim lighting, few people, simple decor). *A stimulating environment may increase level of anxiety.*

6. Administer tranquilizing medication, as ordered by physician. Assess medication for effectiveness and for adverse side effects.

7. When level of anxiety has been reduced, explore with the patient possible reasons for occurrence. *Recognition of precipitating factor(s) is the first step in teaching the patient to interrupt escalation of the anxiety.*

8. Teach the patient signs and symptoms of escalating anxiety and ways to interrupt its progression (e.g., relaxation techniques, deep-breathing exercises, physical exercises, brisk walks, jogging, meditation). The patient will determine which method is most appropriate for him or her. *Relaxation techniques result in a physiological response opposite that of the anxiety response, and physical activities discharge excess energy in a healthful manner.*

Outcome Criteria

1. The patient is able to maintain anxiety at level in which problem-solving can be accomplished.

2. The patient is able to verbalize signs and symptoms of escalating anxiety.

3. The patient is able to demonstrate techniques for interrupting the progression of anxiety to the panic level.

■ FEAR

Definition: Response to perceived threat that is consciously recognized as a danger (NANDA-I, 2018, p. 337)

Possible Contributing Factors ("related to")

Phobic stimulus
[Being in place or situation from which escape might be difficult]
[Causing embarrassment to self in front of others]

Defining Characteristics ("evidenced by")

[Refuses to leave own home alone]
[Refuses to eat in public]
[Refuses to speak or perform in public]
[Refuses to expose self to (specify phobic object or situation)]
Identifies object of fear
[Symptoms of apprehension or sympathetic stimulation in presence of phobic object or situation]

Goals/Objectives

Short-term Goal

The patient will discuss the phobic object or situation with the health-care provider within (time specified).

Long-term Goal

By time of discharge from treatment, the patient will be able to function in the presence of the phobic object or situation without experiencing panic anxiety.

Interventions With *Selected Rationales*

1. Reassure the patient of his or her safety and security. *At panic level of anxiety, the patient may fear for own life.*
2. Explore the patient's perception of threat to physical integrity or threat to self-concept. *It is important to understand the patient's perception of the phobic object or situation in order to assist with the desensitization process.*
3. Discuss reality of the situation with the patient to help the patient recognize aspects that can be changed and those that cannot. *The patient must accept the reality of the situation (aspects that cannot change) before the work of reducing the fear can progress.*
4. Include the patient in making decisions related to selection of alternative coping strategies (e.g., the patient may choose either to avoid the phobic stimulus or attempt to eliminate the fear associated with it). *Encouraging the patient to make choices promotes feelings of empowerment and serves to increase feelings of self-worth.*
5. If the patient elects to work on elimination of the fear, the techniques of desensitization may be employed. This is a systematic plan of behavior modification, designed to expose the individual gradually to the situation or object (either in reality or through fantasizing) until the fear is no longer experienced.

This is also sometimes accomplished through implosion therapy, in which the individual is "flooded" with stimuli related to the phobic situation or object (rather than in gradual steps) until anxiety is no longer experienced in relation to the object or situation. *Fear is decreased as the physical and psychological sensations diminish in response to repeated exposure to the phobic stimulus under nonthreatening conditions.*

6. Encourage the patient to explore underlying feelings that may be contributing to irrational fears. Help the patient to understand how facing these feelings, rather than suppressing them, can result in more adaptive coping abilities. *Verbalization of feelings in a nonthreatening environment may help the patient come to terms with unresolved issues.*

Outcome Criteria

1. The patient does not experience disabling fear when exposed to phobic object or situation.
   or
2. The patient verbalizes ways in which he or she will be able to avoid the phobic object or situation with minimal change in lifestyle.
3. The patient is able to demonstrate adaptive coping techniques that may be used to maintain anxiety at a tolerable level.

■ INEFFECTIVE COPING

Definition: A pattern of invalid appraisal of stressors, with cognitive and/or behavioral efforts, that fails to manage demands related to well-being (NANDA-I, 2018, p. 327)

Possible Contributing Factors ("related to")

[Underdeveloped ego; punitive superego]
[Fear of failure]
Situational crises
Maturational crises
[Personal vulnerability]
[Inadequate support systems]
[Unmet dependency needs]

Defining Characteristics ("evidenced by")

[Ritualistic behavior]
[Obsessive thoughts]
Inability to meet basic needs
Inability to meet role expectations
Inadequate problem-solving
[Alteration in societal participation]

Goals/Objectives

Short-term Goal

Within 1 week, the patient will decrease participation in ritualistic behavior by half.

Long-term Goal

By time of discharge from treatment, the patient will demonstrate ability to cope effectively without resorting to obsessive-compulsive behaviors or increased dependency.

Interventions With *Selected Rationales*

1. Assess the patient's level of anxiety. Try to determine the types of situations that increase anxiety and result in ritualistic behaviors. *Recognition of precipitating factors is the first step in teaching the patient to interrupt the escalating anxiety.*
2. Initially meet the patient's dependency needs as required. Encourage independence and give positive reinforcement for independent behaviors. *Sudden and complete elimination of all avenues for dependency would create intense anxiety on the part of the patient. Positive reinforcement enhances self-esteem and encourages repetition of desired behaviors.*
3. In the beginning of treatment, allow plenty of time for rituals. Do not be judgmental or verbalize disapproval of the behavior. *To deny the patient this activity may precipitate panic level of anxiety.*
4. Support the patient's efforts to explore the meaning and purpose of the behavior. *The patient may be unaware of the relationship between emotional problems and compulsive behaviors. Knowledge and recognition of this fact is important before change can occur.*
5. Provide structured schedule of activities for the patient, including adequate time for completion of rituals. *Structure provides a feeling of security for the anxious patient.*
6. Gradually begin to limit amount of time allotted for ritualistic behavior as the patient becomes more involved in other activities. *Anxiety is minimized when the patient is able to replace ritualistic behaviors with more adaptive ones.*
7. Give positive reinforcement for nonritualistic behaviors. *Positive reinforcement enhances self-esteem and encourages repetition of desired behaviors.*
8. Encourage recognition of situations that provoke obsessive thoughts or ritualistic behaviors. Explain ways of interrupting these thoughts and patterns of behavior (e.g., thought-stopping techniques, relaxation techniques, physical exercise, or other constructive activity with which the patient feels comfortable). *Knowledge and practice of coping techniques that are more adaptive will help the patient change and let go of maladaptive responses to anxiety.*

Outcome Criteria

1. The patient is able to verbalize signs and symptoms of increasing anxiety and intervene to maintain anxiety at manageable level.
2. The patient demonstrates ability to interrupt obsessive thoughts and refrain from ritualistic behaviors in response to stressful situations.

■ DISTURBED BODY IMAGE

Definition: Confusion in mental picture of one's physical self (NANDA-I, 2018, p. 276)

Possible Contributing Factors ("related to")

[Severe level of anxiety, repressed]
[Low self-esteem]
[Unmet dependency needs]

Defining Characteristics ("evidenced by")

[Preoccupation with real or imagined change in bodily structure or function]
[Verbalizations about physical appearance that are out of proportion to any actual physical abnormality that may exist]
Reports fear of reaction by others
Reports negative feelings about body
Change in social involvement

Goals/Objectives

Short-term Goal

The patient will verbalize understanding that changes in bodily structure or function are exaggerated out of proportion to the change that actually exists. (Time frame for this goal must be determined according to individual patient's situation.)

Long-term Goal

The patient will verbalize perception of own body that is realistic to actual structure or function by time of discharge from treatment.

Interventions With *Selected Rationales*

1. Establish trusting relationship with the patient. *Trust enhances therapeutic interactions between nurse and patient.*
2. If there is actual change in structure or function, encourage the patient to progress through stages of grieving. Assess level of knowledge and provide information regarding normal grieving

process and associated feelings. *Knowledge of acceptable feelings facilitates progression through the grieving process.*

3. Identify misperceptions or distortions the patient has regarding body image. Correct inaccurate perceptions in a matter-of-fact, nonthreatening manner. Withdraw attention when preoccupation with distorted image persists. *Lack of attention may encourage elimination of undesirable behaviors.*

4. Help the patient recognize personal body boundaries. *Use of touch may help him or her recognize acceptance of the individual by others and reduce fear of rejection because of changes in bodily structure or function.*

5. Encourage independent self-care activities, providing assistance as required. *Self-care activities accomplished independently enhance self-esteem and also create the necessity for the patient to confront reality of his or her bodily condition.*

6. Provide positive reinforcement for the patient's expressions of realistic bodily perceptions. *Positive reinforcement enhances self-esteem and encourages repetition of desired behaviors.*

Outcome Criteria

1. The patient verbalizes realistic perception of body.
2. The patient demonstrates acceptance of changes in bodily structure or function (if they exist), as evidenced by expression of positive feelings about body, ability or willingness to perform self-care activities independently, and a focus on personal achievements rather than preoccupation with distorted body image.

■ INEFFECTIVE IMPULSE CONTROL

Definition: A pattern of performing rapid, unplanned reactions to internal or external stimuli without regard for the negative consequences of these reactions to the impulsive individual or to others (NANDA-I, 2018, p. 258)

Possible Contributing Factors ("related to")

Altered cognitive functioning
Mood disturbance
Ineffective coping
Disorder of personality
[Genetic vulnerability]
[Possible childhood abuse or neglect]

Defining Characteristics ("evidenced by")

Acting without thinking
[Inability to control impulse to pull out own hair]

Goals/Objectives

Short-term Goal

The patient will verbalize adaptive ways to cope with stress by means other than pulling out own hair (time dimension to be individually determined).

Long-term Goal

The patient will be able to demonstrate adaptive coping strategies in response to stress and a discontinuation of pulling out own hair (time dimension to be individually determined).

Interventions With *Selected Rationales*

1. Support the patient in his or her effort to stop hair pulling. Help the patient understand that it is possible to discontinue the behavior. The patient realizes that the behavior is maladaptive but feels helpless to stop. *Support from the nurse builds trust.*

2. Ensure that a nonjudgmental attitude is conveyed and criticism of the behavior is avoided. *An attitude of acceptance promotes feelings of dignity and self-worth.*

3. Assist the patient with Habit Reversal Training (HRT), *which has been shown to be an effective tool in treatment of hair-pulling disorder.* Three components of HRT include the following:

   a. **Awareness Training:** Help the patient become aware of times when the hair pulling most often occurs (e.g., the patient learns to recognize urges, thoughts, or sensations that precede the behavior; the therapist points out to the patient each time the behavior occurs). *This helps the patient identify situations in which the behavior occurs or is most likely to occur. Awareness gives the patient a feeling of increased self-control.*

   b. **Competing Response Training:** In this step, the patient learns to substitute another response to the urge to pull his or her hair. For example, when a patient experiences a hair-pulling urge, suggest that the individual clasp his or her hands together so as to make hair pulling impossible at that moment. *Substituting an incompatible behavior may help to extinguish the undesirable behavior.*

   c. **Social Support:** Encourage family members to participate in the therapy process and to offer positive feedback for attempts at habit reversal. *Positive feedback enhances self-esteem and increases the patient's desire to continue with the therapy. It also provides cues for family members to use in their attempts to help the patient in treatment.*

4. Once the patient has become aware of hair-pulling times, reinforce that occupying the hands (such as holding an item) when hair-pulling is anticipated, can help prevent automatic behaviors from occurring. *This deters behaviors outside of the patient's awareness.*

5. Practice stress management techniques: deep breathing, meditation, stretching, physical exercise, listening to soft music. *Hair pulling is thought to occur at times of increased anxiety.*

6. Offer support and encouragement when setbacks occur. Help the patient to understand the importance of not quitting when it seems that change is not happening as quickly as he or she would like. Although some people see a decrease in behavior within a few days, most will take several months to notice the greatest change.

@ INTERNET REFERENCES

Additional information about anxiety disorders and medications to treat these disorders may be located at the following Web sites:
- https://adaa.org
- www.mentalhealth.com
- https://medlineplus.gov
- https://www.nami.org
- http://mental-health-matters.com/psychological-disorders
- https://www.drugs.com

Movie Connections

As Good As It Gets (OCD) • *The Aviator* (OCD) • *What About Bob?* (Phobias) • *Copycat* (Agoraphobia) • *Analyze This* (Panic disorder) • *Vertigo* (Specific phobia) • *Dirty Filthy Love* (OCD, trichotillomania)

CHAPTER 9

Trauma- and Stressor-Related Disorders

■ BACKGROUND ASSESSMENT DATA

"Trauma is an emotional response to a terrible event like an accident, rape or natural disaster. Immediately after the event, shock and denial are typical. Longer term reactions include unpredictable emotions, flashbacks, strained relationships and even physical symptoms like headaches or nausea. While these feelings are normal, some people have difficulty moving on with their lives" (American Psychological Association, 2019). These symptoms are not related to common experiences such as uncomplicated bereavement, marital conflict, or chronic illness but are associated with events that would be markedly distressing to almost anyone. The individual may experience the trauma alone or in the presence of others.

About 60% of men and 50% of women are exposed to a traumatic event in their lifetime (Department of Veterans Affairs, 2018). Women are more likely to experience sexual assault and childhood sexual abuse, whereas men are more likely to experience accidents, physical assaults, combat, or to witness death or injury. Although the exposure to trauma is high, less than 10% of trauma victims develop post-traumatic stress disorder (PTSD) (Department of Veterans Affairs, 2018). The disorder appears to be more common in women than in men.

Historically, individuals who experienced stress reactions that followed exposure to an extreme traumatic event were given the diagnosis of PTSD. Stress reactions from "normal" daily events (e.g., divorce, failure, rejection) were characterized as adjustment disorders rather than PTSD. An adjustment disorder is characterized by a maladaptive reaction to an identifiable stressor or stressors that results in the development of clinically significant emotional or behavioral symptoms (APA, 2013). The response occurs within 3 months after onset of the stressor and has persisted for no longer than 6 months after the stressor or its consequences have ended.

A number of studies have indicated that adjustment disorders are probably quite common. Sadock, Sadock, and Ruiz (2015) report:

> Adjustment disorders are one of the most common psychiatric diagnoses for disorders of patients hospitalized for medical and surgical problems. In one study, 5% of people admitted to a hospital over a 3-year period were classified as having an adjustment disorder. Up to 50% of people with specific medical problems or stressors have been diagnosed with adjustment disorders. (p. 446)

Adjustment disorders can occur at any age and while they are more often associated with negative experiences, they can also occur in response to positive events. Adjustment to change is stressful for most people but the APA (2013) differentiates an adjustment disorder as one in which the distress and functional impairment is greater than what would be expected.

■ TYPES OF TRAUMA- AND STRESSOR-RELATED DISORDERS

Post-traumatic Stress Disorder

The *Diagnostic and Statistical Manual of Mental Disorders, Fifth Edition (DSM-5)*, describes the essential feature of PTSD as "the development of characteristic symptoms following exposure to one or more traumatic events" (APA, 2013, p. 274). The trauma may be experienced by the individual or witnessed as it occurred to others, or the symptoms may be in response to having learned about a traumatic event having occurred to a significant other. Symptoms of the disturbance have been endured for more than 1 month; or, in the event of delayed expression, the full diagnostic criteria may not have occurred until at least 6 months after the trauma.

Acute Stress Disorder

Acute stress disorder (ASD) is described by the *DSM-5* as a trauma-related disorder similar to PTSD. The similarities between the two disorders occur in terms of precipitating traumatic events and symptomatology; however, in ASD, the symptoms are time limited, up to 1 month following the trauma. By definition, if the symptoms last longer than 1 month, the diagnosis would be PTSD.

Adjustment Disorder

An adjustment disorder is characterized by a maladaptive reaction to an identifiable stressor or stressors that results in the development of clinically significant emotional or behavioral symptoms (APA, 2013). The response occurs within 3 months after onset of the stressor and has persisted for no longer than 6 months after the stressor or its consequences have ended. A number of clinical presentations are associated with adjustment disorders. The following categories, identified by the *DSM-5* (APA, 2013), are distinguished by the predominant features of the maladaptive response.

Adjustment Disorder With Depressed Mood

This category is the most commonly diagnosed adjustment disorder. The clinical presentation is one of predominant mood disturbance, although less pronounced than that of major depressive disorder. The symptoms, such as depressed mood, tearfulness, and feelings of hopelessness, exceed what is an expected or normative response to an identified stressor.

Adjustment Disorder With Anxiety

This category denotes a maladaptive response to a stressor in which the predominant manifestation is anxiety. For example, the symptoms may reveal nervousness, worry, and jitteriness. The clinician must differentiate this diagnosis from those of anxiety disorders.

Adjustment Disorder With Mixed Anxiety and Depressed Mood

The predominant features of this category include disturbances in mood (depression, feelings of hopelessness and sadness) and manifestations of anxiety (nervousness, worry, jitteriness) that are more intense than what would be expected or considered to be a normative response to an identified stressor.

Adjustment Disorder With Disturbance of Conduct

This category is characterized by conduct in which there is violation of the rights of others or of major age-appropriate societal norms and rules. Examples include truancy, vandalism, reckless driving, fighting, and defaulting on legal responsibilities. Differential diagnosis must be made from conduct disorder or antisocial personality disorder.

Adjustment Disorder With Mixed Disturbance of Emotions and Conduct

The predominant features of this category include emotional disturbances (e.g., anxiety or depression) as well as disturbances of conduct in which there is violation of the rights of others or of major age-appropriate societal norms and rules (e.g., truancy, vandalism, fighting).

Adjustment Disorder Unspecified

This subtype is used when the maladaptive reaction is not consistent with any of the other categories. The individual may have physical complaints, withdraw from relationships, or exhibit impaired work or academic performance but without significant disturbance in emotions or conduct.

■ PREDISPOSING FACTORS TO TRAUMA- AND STRESSOR-RELATED DISORDERS

PTSD and ASD

1. **Biological Theory:** Exposure to trauma has been associated with hyperarousal of the sympathetic nervous system, excessive amygdala activity, and decreased hippocampus volume, all of

which are neurobiological reactions to heightened stress. Dysfunctions occurring in the hypothalamic-pituitary-adrenal axis, either from chronic stress or exposure to an extreme stressor, have been linked to many psychiatric illnesses, including PTSD, depression, Alzheimer's disease, and substance abuse as well as many medical conditions, such as inflammatory disorders and cardiovascular disease (Valentino & Van Bockstaele, 2015). In addition, many neuroendocrine abnormalities, including serotonin, glutamate, thyroid, and endogenous opioids (among others), have been associated with stress responses and PTSD. Adverse childhood experiences (ACEs), traumas occurring before the age of 18, have been linked to several chronic health conditions, risky health behaviors, substance abuse, and early death (CDC, 2019).

Valentino and Van Bockstaele (2015) identify that the activation of endogenous opioids both reduces stress and mimics the stress response depending on which opioid receptors are activated. Studies have shown that opioids, when administered shortly after exposure to a trauma, reduced the incidence of PTSD, suggesting that opioids may have a protective effect. Chronic activation, however, may sensitize neurons in a way that increases vulnerability to stress-induced relapse. Lanius (2013) discusses the effects of repeated activation of mu opioid receptors, including increasing one's addiction potential to other drugs or even to the learned experience of relief when traumatic stress is reexperienced. He identifies that opiate antagonists, such as naltrexone, have demonstrated effectiveness in treatment.

2. **Psychosocial Theory:** One psychosocial model that has become widely accepted seeks to explain why certain persons exposed to massive trauma develop trauma-related disorders and others do not. Variables include characteristics that relate to (1) the traumatic experience, (2) the individual, and (3) the recovery environment.

> **The Traumatic Experience:** Specific characteristics relating to the trauma have been identified as crucial elements in the determination of an individual's long-term response to stress. They include:

- Severity and duration of the stressor
- Extent of anticipatory preparation for the event
- Exposure to death
- Numbers affected by life threat
- Amount of control over recurrence
- Location where the trauma was experienced (e.g., familiar surroundings, at home, in a foreign country)

> **The Individual:** Variables that are considered important in determining an individual's response to trauma include:

- Degree of ego strength
- Effectiveness of coping resources

- Presence of preexisting psychopathology
- Outcomes of previous experiences with stress or trauma
- Behavioral tendencies (temperament)
- Current psychosocial developmental stage
- Demographic factors (e.g., age, socioeconomic status, education)

    The Recovery Environment: It has been suggested that the quality of the environment in which the individual attempts to work through the traumatic experience is correlated with the outcome. Environmental variables include:

- Availability of social supports
- The cohesiveness and protectiveness of family and friends
- The attitudes of society regarding the experience
- Cultural and subcultural influences

In research with Vietnam veterans, it was shown that the best predictors of PTSD were the severity of the stressor and the degree of psychosocial isolation in the recovery environment.

3. **Cognitive Theory:** Most individuals hold positive beliefs of the world as a source of benevolence and joy and of the self as worthy and in control of his or her life. An individual is vulnerable to trauma-related disorders when his or her fundamental beliefs about the self and the world are invalidated by a trauma that cannot be comprehended and a sense of helplessness and hopelessness prevail.

Adjustment Disorder

1. **Biological Theory:** Chronic disorders, such as neurocognitive or intellectual developmental disorders, are thought to impair the ability of an individual to adapt to stress, causing increased vulnerability to adjustment disorder. Sadock and associates (2015) suggest that genetic factors also may influence individual risks for maladaptive response to stress.

2. **Psychosocial Theories:** Some proponents of psychoanalytic theory view adjustment disorder as a maladaptive response to stress that is caused by early childhood trauma, increased dependency, and retarded ego development. Other psychoanalysts put considerable weight on the constitutional factor, or birth characteristics that contribute to the manner in which individuals respond to stress. In many instances, adjustment disorder is precipitated by a specific meaningful stressor having found a point of vulnerability in an individual of otherwise adequate ego strength.

    Some studies relate a predisposition to adjustment disorder to factors such as developmental stage, timing of the stressor, and available support systems. When a stressor occurs and the individual does not have the developmental maturity, available support systems, or adequate coping strategies to adapt, normal functioning is disrupted, resulting in psychological or somatic symptoms. The disorder also may be related to a dysfunctional grieving process. The individual may remain in the denial or anger stage, with inadequate defense mechanisms to complete the grieving process.

3. **Stress-Adaptation Model:** This model considers the type of stressor the individual experiences, the situational context in which it occurs, and intrapersonal factors in the predisposition to adjustment disorder. It has been found that continuous stressors (those to which an individual is exposed over an extended period of time) are more commonly cited than sudden-shock stressors (those that occur without warning) as precipitants to maladaptive functioning.

The situational context in which the stressor occurs may include factors such as personal and general economic conditions; occupational and recreational opportunities; the availability of social supports, such as family, friends, and neighbors; and the availability of cultural or religious support groups. Intrapersonal factors that have been implicated in the predisposition to adjustment disorder include birth temperament, learned social skills and coping strategies, the presence of psychiatric illness, degree of flexibility, and level of intelligence.

■ SYMPTOMATOLOGY (SUBJECTIVE AND OBJECTIVE DATA)

PTSD and ASD

1. Re-experiencing the traumatic event
2. Sustained high level of anxiety or arousal
3. A general numbing of responsiveness
4. Intrusive recollections
5. Nightmares of the event
6. Inability to remember certain aspects of the trauma
7. Depression
8. Survivor's guilt
9. Substance abuse
10. Anger and aggressive behavior
11. Relationship problems
12. Panic attacks

Adjustment Disorder

1. Depressed mood
2. Tearfulness
3. Hopelessness
4. Nervousness
5. Worry
6. Restlessness
7. Ambivalence

8. Anger, expressed inappropriately
9. Increased dependency
10. Violation of the rights of others
11. Violation of societal norms and rules, such as truancy, vandalism, reckless driving, fighting
12. Inability to function occupationally or academically
13. Manipulative behavior
14. Social isolation
15. Physical complaints, such as headache, backache, other aches and pains, fatigue

Trauma-Informed Care

Experts highlight the importance of trauma-informed care as essential to improving the quality of care for patients both in and outside of behavioral health-care settings (Hopper, Bassuk, & Olivet, 2010; Substance Abuse and Mental Health Services Administration [SAMHSA], 2015). The National Center for Trauma-Informed Care (SAMHSA, 2015) calls national attention to the importance of this critical approach. Trauma-informed care generally describes a philosophical approach that values awareness and understanding of trauma when assessing, planning, and implementing care. SAMHSA advances the following principles in defining this approach. Trauma-informed care:

- Realizes the widespread impact of trauma and various paths for recovery.
- Recognizes the signs and symptoms of trauma in patients, families, staff, and all those involved with the system.
- Responds by fully integrating knowledge about trauma in policies, procedures, and practices.
- Seeks to actively resist retraumatization.

Health-care providers may unwittingly retraumatize patients if they do not fully understand the impact of previous trauma on the patient's current health concerns. Even interventions such as seclusion and restraint, which have been designed to protect patients' safety when they are at imminent risk of harm to themselves or others, may be retraumatizing to a patient with a history of trauma.

Common Nursing Diagnoses and Interventions

(Interventions are applicable to various health-care settings, such as inpatient and partial hospitalization, community outpatient clinic, home health, and private practice.)

■ POSTTRAUMA SYNDROME

Definition: Sustained maladaptive response to a traumatic, overwhelming event (NANDA International [NANDA-I], 2018, p. 316)

Possible Contributing Factors ("related to")

Being held prisoner of war
Criminal victimization
Disasters; epidemics
Physical or psychological abuse
Serious accidents
Serious threat to or injury of loved ones or self
Sudden destruction of one's home or community
Torture
Tragic occurrence involving multiple deaths
War
Witnessing mutilation or violent death

Defining Characteristics ("evidenced by")

[Physical injuries related to trauma]
Avoidance
Repression
Difficulty concentrating
Grieving; guilt
Intrusive thoughts
Neurosensory irritability
Palpitations
Anger and/or rage; aggression
Intrusive dreams; nightmares; flashbacks
Panic attacks; fear
Gastric irritability
Psychogenic amnesia
Substance abuse

Goals/Objectives

Short-term Goals

1. The patient will begin a healthy grief resolution, initiating the process of psychological healing (within time frame specific to individual).
2. The patient will demonstrate ability to deal with emotional reactions in an individually appropriate manner.

Long-term Goal

The patient will integrate the traumatic experience into his or her persona, renew significant relationships, and establish meaningful goals for the future.

Interventions With *Selected Rationales*

1. Assign the same staff as often as possible. Use a nonthreatening, matter-of-fact, but friendly approach. Respect the patient's wishes regarding interaction with individuals of opposite gender at this

time (especially important if the trauma was rape). Be consistent and keep all promises, and convey an attitude of unconditional acceptance. *A posttrauma patient may be suspicious of others in his or her environment. These interventions serve to facilitate a trusting relationship.*

2. Stay with the patient during periods of flashbacks and night-mares. Offer reassurance of safety and security and that these symptoms are not uncommon following a trauma of the magnitude he or she has experienced. *The presence of a trusted individual may help to calm fears for personal safety and reassure the anxious patient that he or she is not "going crazy."*

3. Obtain an accurate history from significant others about the trauma and the patient's specific response. *Various types of traumas elicit different responses in patients. For example, human-engendered traumas often generate a greater degree of humiliation and guilt in victims than do traumas associated with natural disasters.*

4. Encourage the patient to talk about the trauma at his or her own pace. Provide a nonthreatening, private environment, and include a significant other if the patient wishes. Acknowledge and validate the patient's feelings as they are expressed. *This debriefing process is the first step in the progression toward resolution.*

5. Discuss coping strategies used in response to the trauma, as well as those used during stressful situations in the past. Determine those that have been most helpful, and discuss alternative strategies for the future. Include available support systems, including religious and cultural influences. Identify maladaptive coping strategies, such as substance use or psychosomatic responses, and practice more adaptive coping strategies for possible future posttrauma responses. *Resolution of the posttrauma response is largely dependent on the effectiveness of the coping strategies employed.*

6. Assist the individual to try to comprehend the trauma if possible. Discuss feelings of vulnerability and the individual's "place" in the world following the trauma. *Posttrauma response is largely a function of the shattering of basic beliefs the survivor holds about self and world. Assimilation of the event into one's persona requires that some degree of meaning associated with the event be incorporated into the basic beliefs, which will affect how the individual eventually comes to reappraise self and world* (Epstein, 1991).

■ COMPLICATED GRIEVING

Definition: A disorder that occurs after the death of a significant other [or any other loss of significance to the individual], in which the experience of distress accompanying bereavement fails to follow normative expectations and manifests in functional impairment (NANDA-I, 2018, p. 340)

Possible Contributing Factors ("related to")

[Having experienced a trauma outside the range of usual human experience]
[Survivor's guilt]
[Real or perceived loss of any concept of value to the individual]
[Bereavement overload (cumulative grief from multiple unresolved losses)]
[Thwarted grieving response to a loss]
[Absence of anticipatory grieving]
[Feelings of guilt generated by ambivalent relationship with lost concept]
Insufficient social support

Defining Characteristics ("evidenced by")

[Verbal expression of distress at loss]
[Idealization of lost concept]
[Denial of loss]
[Excessive anger, expressed inappropriately]
[Developmental regression]
[Altered activities of daily living (ADLs)]
[Diminished sense of control]
[Persistent anxiety]
Depression
Self-blame
Traumatic distress

Goals/Objectives

Short-term Goals

1. By end of 1 week, the patient will express anger toward loss of valuable entity.
2. By end of 1 week, the patient who has experienced a trauma will verbalize feelings (guilt, anger, self-blame, hopelessness) associated with the trauma.

Long-term Goal

The patient will demonstrate progress in dealing with stages of grief and will verbalize a sense of optimism and hope for the future.

Interventions With *Selected Rationales*

1. Acknowledge feelings of guilt or self-blame that the patient may express. Guilt at having survived a trauma in which others died is common. *The patient needs to discuss these feelings and recognize that he or she is not responsible for what happened but must take responsibility for own recovery.*
2. Assess stage of grief in which the patient is fixed. Discuss normalcy of feelings and behaviors related to stages of grief.

Knowledge of grief stage is necessary for accurate intervention. Guilt may be generated if the patient believes it is unacceptable to have these feelings. Knowing they are normal can provide a sense of relief.

3. Assess impact of the trauma on the patient's ability to resume regular ADLs. Consider employment, marital relationship, and sleep patterns. *Following a trauma, individuals are at high risk for physical injury because of disruption in ability to concentrate and solve problems and because of lack of sufficient sleep. Isolation and avoidance behaviors may interfere with interpersonal relatedness.*

4. Assess for self-destructive ideas and behavior. *The trauma may result in feelings of hopelessness and worthlessness, leading to high risk for suicide.*

5. Assess for maladaptive coping strategies, such as substance abuse. *These behaviors interfere with and delay the recovery process.*

6. Identify available community resources from which the individual may seek assistance if problems with complicated grieving persist. Support groups for victims of various types of traumas exist within most communities. *The presence of support systems in the recovery environment has been identified as a major predictor in the successful recovery from trauma.*

7. Help the patient solve problems as he or she attempts to determine methods for more adaptive coping with the experienced loss. Provide positive feedback for strategies identified and decisions made. *Positive reinforcement enhances self-esteem and encourages repetition of desirable behaviors.*

8. Encourage the patient to reach out for spiritual support during this time in whatever form is desirable to him or her. Assess spiritual needs of the patient, and assist as necessary in the fulfillment of those needs. *Spiritual support can enhance successful adaptation to painful life experiences for some individuals.*

■ RISK FOR SELF-DIRECTED OR OTHER-DIRECTED VIOLENCE

Definition: Susceptible to behaviors in which an individual demonstrates that he/she can be physically, emotionally, and/or sexually harmful either to self or to others (NANDA-I, 2018, pp. 416–417)

Risk Factors ("related to")

[Negative role modeling]
[Dysfunctional family system]
[Low self-esteem]
[Unresolved grief]
[Psychic overload]
[Extended exposure to stressful situation]

[Lack of support systems]
[Biological factors, such as organic changes in the brain]
Body language (e.g., rigid posture, clenching of fists and jaw, hyperactivity, pacing, breathlessness, threatening stances)
[History or threats of violence toward self or others or of destruction to the property of others]
Impulsivity
Suicidal ideation, plan, available means
[Anger; rage]
[Increasing anxiety level]
[Depressed mood]

Goals/Objectives

Short-term Goals

1. The patient will seek out staff member when hostile or suicidal feelings occur.
2. The patient will verbalize adaptive coping strategies for use when hostile or suicidal feelings occur.

Long-term Goals

1. The patient will demonstrate adaptive coping strategies for use when hostile or suicidal feelings occur.
2. The patient will not harm self or others.

Interventions With *Selected Rationales*

1. Observe the patient's behavior frequently. Do this through routine activities and interactions; avoid appearing watchful and suspicious. Close observation is required so that intervention can occur if required to ensure the patient's (and others') safety.
2. Observe for suicidal behaviors: verbal statements, such as "I'm going to kill myself" and "Very soon my mother won't have to worry herself about me any longer," and nonverbal behaviors, such as giving away cherished items and mood swings. *Patients who are contemplating suicide often give clues regarding their potential behavior. The clues may be very subtle and require keen assessment skills by the nurse.*
3. Determine suicidal intent and available means. Ask direct questions, such as "Do you plan to kill yourself?," "How do you plan to do it?," and "How strong is your intention to die?" These questions should be part of an ongoing collaborative assessment of risks and warning signs for suicide. *The risk of suicide is greatly increased if the patient has developed a plan, has strong intentions to die, and particularly if means exist for the patient to execute the plan.*
4. Help the patient recognize when anger occurs and to accept those feelings as his or her own. Encourage the patient to keep an "anger notebook," in which feelings of anger experienced

during a 24-hour period are recorded. Information regarding source of anger, behavioral response, and the patient's perception of the situation should also be noted. Discuss entries with the patient and suggest alternative behavioral responses for those identified as maladaptive.

5. Act as a role model for appropriate expression of angry feelings, and give positive reinforcement to the patient for attempting to conform. *It is vital that the patient learns how to appropriately express angry feelings, because suicide and other self-destructive behaviors are often viewed as the result of anger turned inward on the self.*

6. Remove all dangerous objects from the patient's environment (e.g., sharp items, belts, ties, straps, breakable items, smoking materials). *Patient safety is a nursing priority.*

7. Try to redirect violent behavior by means of physical outlets for the patient's anxiety (e.g., exercising, jogging). *Physical exercise is a safe and effective way of relieving pent-up tension.*

8. Be available to stay with the patient as anxiety level and tensions begin to rise. *Presence of a trusted individual provides a feeling of security and may help to prevent rapid escalation of anxiety.*

9. Staff should maintain and convey a calm attitude to the patient. *Anxiety is contagious and can be transmitted from staff members to the patient.*

10. Have sufficient staff available to indicate a show of strength to the patient if necessary. *This conveys to the patient evidence of control over the situation and provides some physical security for staff.*

11. Administer tranquilizing medications as ordered by physician, or obtain an order if necessary. Monitor patient response for effectiveness of the medication and for adverse side effects. *Short-term use of tranquilizing medications such as anxiolytics or antipsychotics can induce a calming effect on the patient and may prevent aggressive behaviors.*

12. Use of mechanical restraints or isolation room may be required if less restrictive interventions are unsuccessful. Follow policy and procedure prescribed by the institution in executing this intervention. Assess the patient in restraints at least every 15 minutes to ensure that circulation to extremities is not compromised (check temperature, color, pulses); to assist the patient with needs related to nutrition, hydration, and elimination; and to position the patient so that comfort is facilitated and aspiration is prevented. Continuous one-to-one monitoring may be necessary for the patient who is highly agitated or for whom there is a high risk of self- or accidental injury. *Patient safety is a nursing priority.*

13. As agitation decreases, assess the patient's readiness for restraint removal or reduction. Remove one restraint at a time, while assessing the patient's response. *This minimizes risk of injury to the patient and staff.*

Outcome Criteria

1. Anxiety is maintained at a level at which the patient feels no need for aggression.
2. The patient denies any ideas of self-destruction.
3. The patient demonstrates use of adaptive coping strategies when feelings of hostility or suicide occur.
4. The patient verbalizes community support systems from which assistance may be requested when personal coping strategies are not successful.

■ ANXIETY (Moderate to Severe)

Definition: Vague uneasy feeling of discomfort or dread accompanied by an autonomic response (the source often nonspecific or unknown to the individual); a feeling of apprehension caused by anticipation of danger. It is an alerting signal that warns of impending danger and enables the individual to take measures to deal with threat. (NANDA-I, 2018, p. 324)

Possible Contributing Factors ("related to")

Situational and maturational crises
[Low self-esteem]
[Complicated grieving]
[Feelings of powerlessness and lack of control in life situation]
[Having experienced a trauma outside the range of usual human experience]

Defining Characteristics ("evidenced by")

Increased tension
[Increased helplessness]
Overexcited
Apprehensive; fearful
Restlessness
Poor eye contact
Feelings of inadequacy
Insomnia
Focus on the self
Increased cardiac and respiratory rates
Diminished ability to problem-solve and learn
Scanning; hypervigilance

Goals/Objectives

Short-term Goal

The patient will demonstrate use of relaxation techniques to maintain anxiety at manageable level within 1 week.

Long-term Goal

By time of discharge from treatment, the patient will be able to recognize events that precipitate anxiety and intervene to prevent disabling behaviors.

Interventions With *Selected Rationales*

1. Be available to stay with the patient. Remain calm and provide assurance of safety. *Patient safety and security is a nursing priority.*
2. Help the patient identify situation that precipitated onset of anxiety symptoms. *The patient may be unaware that emotional issues are related to symptoms of anxiety. Recognition may be the first step in elimination of this maladaptive response.*
3. Review the patient's methods of coping with similar situations in the past. Discuss ways in which the patient may assume control over these situations. *In seeking to create change, it would be helpful for the patient to identify past responses and to determine whether they were successful and if they could be employed again. A measure of control reduces feelings of powerlessness in a situation, ultimately decreasing anxiety. Patient strengths should be identified and used to his or her advantage.*
4. Provide quiet environment. Reduce stimuli: low lighting, few people. *Anxiety level may be decreased in calm atmosphere with few stimuli.*
5. Administer antianxiety medications as ordered by physician, or obtain order if necessary. Monitor the patient's response for effectiveness of the medication as well as for adverse side effects. *Short-term use of antianxiety medications (e.g., lorazepam, chlordiazepoxide, alprazolam) provide relief from the immobilizing effects of anxiety and facilitate the patient's cooperation with therapy.*
6. Discuss with the patient signs of increasing anxiety and ways of intervening to maintain the anxiety at a manageable level (e.g., exercise, walking, jogging, relaxation techniques). *Anxiety and tension can be reduced safely and with benefit to the patient through physical activities.*

Outcome Criteria

1. The patient is able to verbalize events that precipitate anxiety and to demonstrate techniques for its reduction.
2. The patient is able to verbalize ways in which he or she may gain more control of the environment and thereby reduce feelings of powerlessness.

■ INEFFECTIVE COPING

Definition: A pattern of invalid appraisal of stressors, with cognitive and/or behavioral efforts, that fails to manage demands related to well-being (NANDA-I, 2018, p. 327)

Possible Contributing Factors ("related to")

Situational crises
Maturational crises
[Inadequate support systems]
[Low self-esteem]
[Unresolved grief]
[Inadequate coping strategies]

Defining Characteristics ("evidenced by")

Inability to meet role expectations
[Alteration in societal participation]
Inadequate problem solving
[Increased dependency]
[Manipulation of others in the environment for purposes of
    fulfilling own desires]
[Refusal to follow rules]

Goals/Objectives

Short-term Goal

By the end of 1 week, the patient will comply with behavioral expectations and refrain from manipulating others to fulfill own desires.

Long-term Goal

By time of discharge from treatment, the patient will identify, develop, and use socially acceptable coping skills.

Interventions With *Selected Rationales*

1. Discuss with the patient expectations for behavior and consequences of nonadherence. Carry out the consequences
matter-of-factly if expectations for appropriate behavior are
violated. *Negative consequences may work to decrease manipulative
behaviors.*
2. Do not debate, argue, rationalize, or bargain with the patient regarding limit setting on manipulative behaviors. *Ignoring these attempts may work to decrease manipulative behaviors. Consistency among
all staff members is essential if this intervention is to be successful.*
3. Encourage discussion of angry feelings. Help the patient identify the true object of the hostility. Facilitate physical outlets
for healthy release of the hostile feelings (e.g., exercise, individualized occupational therapy activities). *Verbalization of feelings with a trusted individual may help the patient work through
unresolved issues. Physical exercise provides a safe and effective means
of releasing pent-up tension.*
4. Take care not to reinforce dependent behaviors. Encourage the
patient to perform as independently as possible, and provide positive feedback. *Independent accomplishment and positive reinforcement
enhance self-esteem and encourage repetition of desirable behaviors.*

5. Help the patient recognize some aspects of his or her life over which a measure of control is maintained. *Recognition of personal control, however minimal, diminishes the feeling of powerlessness and decreases the need for manipulation of others.*
6. Identify the stressor that precipitated the maladaptive coping. If a major life change has occurred, encourage the patient to express fears and feelings associated with the change. Assist the patient through the problem-solving process:
   a. Identify possible alternatives that indicate positive adaptation.
   b. Discuss benefits and consequences of each alternative.
   c. Select the most appropriate alternative.
   d. Implement the alternative.
   e. Evaluate the effectiveness of the alternative.
   f. Recognize areas of limitation, and make modifications. Request assistance with this process, if needed.
7. Provide positive reinforcement for application of adaptive coping skills and evidence of successful adjustment. *Positive reinforcement enhances self-esteem and encourages repetition of desirable behaviors.*

Outcome Criteria

1. The patient is able to verbalize alternative, socially acceptable, and lifestyle-appropriate coping skills he or she plans to use in response to stress.
2. The patient is able to solve problems and fulfill ADLs independently.
3. The patient does not manipulate others for own gratification.

■ RISK-PRONE HEALTH BEHAVIOR

Definition: Impaired ability to modify lifestyle and/or actions in a manner that improves the level of wellness (NANDA-I, 2018, p. 149)

Possible Contributing Factors ("related to")

[Low self-esteem]
[Intense emotional state]
[Negative attitudes toward health behavior]
[Absence of intent to change behavior]
Multiple stressors
[Absence of social support for changed beliefs and practices]
[Disability or health status change requiring change in lifestyle]
[Lack of motivation to change behaviors]
[Use of alcohol or other substances of abuse]

Defining Characteristics ("evidenced by")

Minimizes health status change
Failure to achieve optimal sense of control

Failure to take actions that prevent health problems or improve level of wellness

Demonstrates nonacceptance of health status change

Goals/Objectives

Short-term Goals

1. The patient will discuss with primary nurse the kinds of lifestyle changes that will occur to improve the level of wellness.
2. With the help of primary nurse, the patient will formulate a plan of action for incorporating those changes into his or her lifestyle.
3. The patient will demonstrate movement toward independence, considering change in health status.

Long-term Goal

The patient will demonstrate competence to function independently to his or her optimal ability by time of discharge from treatment.

Interventions With *Selected Rationales*

1. Encourage the patient to talk about lifestyle and its impact on level of wellness. Discuss coping mechanisms that were used at stressful times in the past. *It is important to identify the patient's strengths so that they may be used to facilitate adaptation to the change or loss that has occurred.*
2. Encourage the patient to discuss changes in health status or loss and particularly to express anger associated with it. *Some individuals may not realize that anger is a normal stage in the grieving process. If it is not released in an appropriate manner, it may be turned inward on the self, leading to pathological depression.*
3. Encourage the patient to express fears associated with the change or loss or alteration in lifestyle that the change or loss has created. *Change often creates a feeling of disequilibrium, and the individual may respond with fears that are irrational or unfounded. He or she may benefit from feedback that corrects misperceptions about how life will be with the change in health status.*
4. Provide assistance with ADLs as required, but encourage independence to the limit that the patient's ability will allow. Give positive feedback for activities accomplished independently. *Independent accomplishments and positive feedback enhance self-esteem and encourage repetition of desired behaviors. Successes also provide hope that adaptive functioning is possible and decrease feelings of powerlessness.*
5. Help the patient with decision making regarding incorporation of change or loss into lifestyle. Identify problems that the change or loss is likely to create. Discuss alternative solutions, weighing potential benefits and consequences of each alternative. Support the patient's decision in the selection of an alternative. *The great amount of anxiety that usually accompanies a major lifestyle change*

often interferes with an individual's ability to solve problems and to make appropriate decisions. The patient may need assistance with this process in an effort to progress toward successful adaptation.

6. Use role-playing of potential stressful situations that might occur in relation to the health status change. *Role-playing decreases anxiety and provides a feeling of security by providing the patient with a plan of action for responding in an appropriate manner when a stressful situation occurs.*

7. Ensure that the patient and family are fully knowledgeable regarding the physiology of the change in health status and its necessity for optimal wellness. Encourage them to ask questions, and provide printed material explaining the change to which they may refer following discharge. *Increased knowledge enhances successful adaptation.*

8. Help the patient identify resources within the community from which he or she may seek assistance in adapting to the change in health status. Examples include self-help or support groups and public health nurse, counselor, or social worker. Encourage the patient to keep follow-up appointments with physician and to call physician's office prior to follow-up date if problems or concerns arise.

Outcome Criteria

1. The patient is able to perform ADLs independently.
2. The patient is able to make independent decisions regarding lifestyle considering change in health status.
3. The patient is able to express hope for the future with consideration of change in health status.

■ RELOCATION STRESS SYNDROME*

Definition: Physiological and/or psychosocial disturbance following transfer from one environment to another (NANDA-I, 2018, p. 320)

Possible Contributing Factors ("related to")

Move from one environment to another
[Losses involved with decision to move]
Feelings of powerlessness
Lack of adequate support system
[Little or no preparation for the impending move]
Impaired psychosocial health [status]
Decreased [physical] health status

---

*This diagnosis would be appropriate for the individual with adjustment disorder if the precipitating stressor was relocation to a new environment.

Defining Characteristics ("evidenced by")

Anxiety
Depression
Loneliness
Reports unwillingness to move
Sleep pattern disturbance
Increased physical symptoms
Dependency
Insecurity
Withdrawal
Anger; fear

Goals/Objectives

Short-term Goal

The patient will verbalize at least one positive aspect regarding relocation to new environment within (realistic time period).

Long-term Goal

The patient will demonstrate positive adaptation to new environment, as evidenced by involvement in activities, expression of satisfaction with new acquaintances, and elimination of previously evident physical and psychological symptoms associated with the relocation (time dimension to be determined individually).

Interventions With *Selected Rationales*

1. Encourage the individual to discuss feelings (concerns, fears, anger) regarding relocation. *Exploration of feelings with a trusted individual may help the individual perceive the situation more realistically and come to terms with the inevitable change.*
2. Encourage the individual to discuss how the change will affect his or her life. Ensure that the individual is involved in decision making and problem-solving regarding the move. *Taking responsibility for making choices regarding the relocation will increase feelings of control and decrease feelings of powerlessness.*
3. Help the individual identify positive aspects about the move. *Anxiety associated with the opposed relocation may interfere with the individual's ability to recognize anything positive about it. Assistance may be required.*
4. Help the individual identify resources within the new community from which assistance with various types of services may be obtained. *Because of anxiety and depression, the individual may not be able to identify these resources alone. Assistance with problem-solving may be required.*
5. Identify groups within the community that specialize in helping individuals adapt to relocation. Examples include Newcomers Club, Welcome Wagon Club, senior citizens groups, school and

church organizations. *These groups offer support from individuals who may have encountered similar experiences. Adaptation may be enhanced by the reassurance, encouragement, and support of peers who exhibit positive adaptation to relocation stress.*

6. Refer the individual or family for professional counseling if deemed necessary. *An individual who is experiencing complicated grieving over loss of previous residence may require therapy to achieve resolution of the problem. It may be that other unresolved issues are interfering with successful adaptation to the relocation.*

Outcome Criteria

1. The individual no longer exhibits signs of anxiety, depression, or somatic symptoms.
2. The individual verbalizes satisfaction with the new environment.
3. The individual willingly participates in social and vocational activities within his or her new environment.

@ INTERNET REFERENCES

Additional information about trauma- and stressor-related disorders may be located at the following Web sites:

- www.mentalhealth.com/rx/p23-aj01.html
- www.psyweb.com/Mdisord/jsp/adjd.jsp
- http://athealth.com/adjustment-disorder
- https://medlineplus.gov/ency/article/000932.htm
- https://www.nimh.nih.gov/health/topics/post-traumatic-stress-disorder-ptsd/index.shtml
- https://www.ptsd.va.gov/professional/treat/essentials/acute_stress_disorder.asp

Movie Connections

The Deer Hunter (PTSD) • *Hell and Back Again* (PTSD) • *Jackknife* (PTSD) • *Brothers* (PTSD) • *The War at Home* (PTSD) • *Fearless* (PTSD) • *The Fisher King* (PTSD) • *Changeover* (PTSD and comorbid mental health issues)

CHAPTER 10

Somatic Symptom and Related Disorders

■ BACKGROUND ASSESSMENT DATA

Somatic symptom disorders are characterized by physical symptoms suggesting medical disease but without demonstrable organic pathology or known pathophysiological mechanism to account for them. For this reason, most patients with a somatic symptom or related disorder are seen in primary care and hospital settings rather than in mental health-care settings. It is important to note that the inability of modern medicine to determine the existence of pathophysiology to explain a patient's symptoms is not sufficient to diagnose him or her with a mental illness. Somatic symptom and related disorders are classified as mental disorders, by the *Diagnostic and Statistical Manual of Mental Disorders, Fifth Edition (DSM-5)*, when the excessive focus on somatic symptoms is beyond any medical explanation *and* it causes significant distress and impairment in one's functioning (American Psychiatric Association [APA], 2013). The APA (2013) identifies the following categories of somatic symptom disorders.

Somatic Symptom Disorder

Somatic symptom disorder is a syndrome of multiple somatic symptoms that cannot be explained medically and are associated with psychosocial distress and frequent visits to health-care professionals to seek assistance. Symptoms may be vague, dramatized, or exaggerated in presentation, and an excessive amount of time and energy is devoted to worry and concern about the symptoms. Individuals with somatic symptom disorder are so convinced that their symptoms are related to organic pathology that they adamantly reject and are often irritated by any implication that stress or psychosocial factors play a role in their conditions. The disorder is chronic, with symptoms beginning before age 30. Anxiety and depression are frequently manifested, and, as such, there is an increased risk for suicide attempts (Yates, 2019).

The disorder usually runs a fluctuating course, with periods of remission and exacerbation. Patients often receive medical care from several physicians, sometimes concurrently, leading to the possibility of dangerous treatment combinations. There may be a risk of seeking relief through overmedicating with prescribed analgesics or antianxiety agents. Drug abuse and dependence are common complications of somatic symptom disorder.

Illness Anxiety Disorder

Illness anxiety disorder is defined as an unrealistic or inaccurate interpretation of physical symptoms or sensations, leading to preoccupation about and fear of having a serious disease. The fear becomes disabling and persists despite appropriate reassurance that no organic pathology can be detected. Symptoms may be minimal or absent, but the individual is highly anxious about and suspicious of the presence of an undiagnosed, serious medical illness (APA, 2013).

Individuals with illness anxiety disorder are extremely conscious of bodily sensations and changes and may become convinced that a rapid heart rate indicates they have heart disease or that a small sore is skin cancer. They are profoundly preoccupied with their bodies and are totally aware of even the slightest change in feeling or sensation. The response to these small changes, however, is usually unrealistic and exaggerated.

Some individuals with illness anxiety disorder have a long history of "doctor shopping" and are convinced that they are not receiving the proper care. Others avoid seeking medical assistance because to do so would increase their anxiety to intolerable levels. Depression is common, and obsessive-compulsive traits frequently accompany the disorder. Preoccupation with the fear of serious disease may interfere with social or occupational functioning. Some individuals are able to function appropriately on the job, however, while limiting their physical complaints to non-work time.

Individuals with illness anxiety disorder are so apprehensive and fearful that they become alarmed at the slightest intimation of serious illness. Even reading about a disease or hearing that someone they know has been diagnosed with an illness precipitates alarm.

Both somatic symptom disorder and illness anxiety disorder have similar features to what was previously referred to as *hypochondriasis,* but the *DSM-5* identifies two separate disorders to distinguish between individuals who are primarily preoccupied with perceived physical symptoms (somatic symptom disorder) and those who are primarily focused on fear of illness in general (illness anxiety disorder).

Conversion Disorder (Functional Neurological Symptom Disorder)

Conversion disorder is a loss of or change in body function that cannot be explained by any known medical disorder or pathophysiological mechanism. There is likely a psychological component involved in the initiation, exacerbation, or perpetuation of the symptom, although it may or may not be identifiable.

Conversion symptoms affect voluntary motor or sensory functioning suggestive of neurological disease. Examples include paralysis, aphonia (inability to produce voice), seizures, coordination disturbance, difficulty swallowing, urinary retention, akinesia, blindness, deafness, double vision, anosmia (inability to perceive smell), loss of pain sensation, and hallucinations.

Abnormal limb shaking with impaired or loss of consciousness that resembles epileptic seizures is another type of conversion disorder symptom, referred to as *psychogenic* or *nonepileptic seizures*. Pseudocyesis (false pregnancy) is a conversion symptom and may represent a strong desire to be pregnant.

The *DSM-5* clarifies that "although the diagnosis [of conversion disorder] requires that the symptom is not explained by neurological disease, it should not be made simply because results from investigations are normal or because the symptom is 'bizarre.' There must be clear evidence of incompatibility with neurological disease" (APA, 2013, p. 319). For example, if a patient appears to be having a seizure but the EEG is normal, the eyes are closed and resist opening, and there is no urinary incontinence, conversion disorder may be diagnosed. Multiple causes likely play a role in etiology.

While not diagnostic of a conversion disorder, some patients display an apparent indifference to symptoms that seem very serious to others. This feature is coined *la belle indifférence*. Most symptoms of conversion disorder resolve within a few weeks.

Psychological Factors Affecting Other Medical Conditions

Psychological factors play a role in virtually all medical conditions. In this disorder, it is evident that psychological or behavioral factors have been implicated in the development, exacerbation, or delayed recovery from a medical condition.

Factitious Disorder

Factitious disorders involve conscious, intentional feigning of physical or psychological symptoms. Individuals with factitious disorder pretend to be ill in order to receive emotional care and support commonly associated with the role of "patient." Even though the behaviors are deliberate and intentional, there may be an associated compulsive element that diminishes personal control. Individuals with this disorder characteristically become so skilled at presenting their "symptoms" that they successfully gain admission to hospitals and treatment centers. Individuals may aggravate existing symptoms, induce new ones, or even inflict painful injuries on themselves (Sadock et al, 2015). The disorder may also be identified as *Munchausen syndrome*, and symptoms may be psychological, physical, or a combination of both.

The disorder may be imposed on oneself, or on another person (previously called *factitious disorder by proxy*). In the latter case, physical symptoms are intentionally imposed on a person under the care of the perpetrator. Diagnosis of factitious disorder can be difficult, as individuals become very inventive in their quest to produce symptoms. "The most common case of factitious disorder by proxy involves a mother who deceives medical personnel into believing her child is ill" (Sadock et al, 2015, p. 492). This may be accomplished by lying about the child's medical history, manipulating data such as by contaminating laboratory samples, and inducing illness or injury in the child through use of substances or other physical assaults.

■ PREDISPOSING FACTORS TO SOMATIC SYMPTOM DISORDERS

1. Physiological
   a. **Genetics:** Studies have shown an increased incidence of somatic symptom disorder, conversion disorder, and illness anxiety disorder in first-degree relatives, implying a possible inheritable predisposition (Sadock et al, 2015).
   b. **Biochemical:** Understanding of the biochemical underpinnings of somatic symptom disorders is preliminary but the response of symptoms in illness anxiety disorder to SSRIs has supported the theory that low levels of serotonin are a contributing factor (Kahn, 2018). Decreased levels of serotonin and endorphins may also play a role in the sensation of pain. Autonomic arousal, associated with the effects of endogenous noradrenergic compounds (such as tachycardia and gastric hypermotility), may also be a contributing factor in some patients with somatization (Yates, 2019).
   c. **Neuroanatomical:** Brain dysfunction has been proposed by some researchers as a factor in factitious disorders (Sadock et al, 2015). The hypothesis is that impairment in information processing contributes to the aberrant behaviors associated with the disorder. Sadock and associates report that "brain imaging studies have found hypometabolism in the dominant hemisphere and hypermetabolism in the nondominant hemisphere and have implicated impaired hemispheric communication in the cause of conversion disorder" (2015, p. 474). Other reports of brain imaging studies have identified that there is reduced volume of the amygdala as well as reduced connectivity between the amygdala and brain centers controlling executive and motor functions in one or more somatic symptom disorders (Yates, 2019).
2. Psychosocial
   a. **Psychodynamic Theory:** Psychodynamic theorists view illness anxiety disorder as an ego defense mechanism. They suggest that physical complaints are the expression of low

self-esteem and feelings of worthlessness and that the individual believes it is easier to feel something is wrong with the body than to feel something is wrong with the self. Another psychodynamic view of illness anxiety disorder (as well as somatic symptom disorder, predominantly pain) is related to a defense against guilt. The individual views the self as "bad," based on real or imagined past misconduct, and views physical suffering as the deserved punishment required for atonement. This view has also been related to individuals with factitious disorders.

The psychodynamic theory of conversion disorder proposes that emotions associated with a traumatic event that the individual cannot express because of moral or ethical unacceptability are "converted" into physical symptoms. The unacceptable emotions are repressed and converted to a somatic hysterical symptom that is symbolic in some way of the original emotional trauma.

Some reports suggest that individuals with factitious disorders were victims of child abuse or neglect. Frequent childhood hospitalizations provided a reprieve from the traumatic home situation and a loving and caring environment that was absent in the child's family. This theory proposes that the individual with factitious disorder is attempting to recapture the only positive support he or she may have known by seeking out the environment in which it was received as a child. Regarding factitious disorder imposed on another, Sadock and associates stated, "One apparent purpose of the behavior is for the caretaker to indirectly assume the sick role; another is to be relieved of the caretaking role by having the child hospitalized" (2015, p. 492).

b. **Family Dynamics:** Another view suggests that in families who have difficulty resolving conflicts, a child's illness creates a shift in focus from the unresolved conflicts to the child's illness. This provides a reprieve from the instability posed by issues that the family cannot confront openly, and the child in turn receives positive reinforcement for the illness. *Somatization* becomes reinforced as a way to shift the focus away from family issues and discord. The stabilization of the family achieved by somatizing is referred to as a *tertiary gain*.

c. **Learning Theory:** Somatic complaints are often reinforced when the sick role relieves the individual from the need to deal with a stressful situation, whether it be within society or within the family. The sick person learns that he or she may avoid stressful obligations, may postpone unwelcome challenges, and is excused from troublesome duties (primary gain); becomes the prominent focus of attention because of the illness (secondary gain); or relieves conflict within the family as concern is shifted to the ill person and away from the real issue (tertiary gain). These types of positive rein-forcements virtually guarantee repetition of the response.

d. **Past Experience With Physical Illness:** Past experience with serious or life-threatening physical illness, either per-sonal or that of close family members, can predispose an individual to illness anxiety disorder. Once an individual has experienced a threat to biological integrity, he or she may develop a fear of recurrence. This generates an exag-gerated response to minor physical changes, leading to excessive anxiety and health concerns.

■ SYMPTOMATOLOGY (SUBJECTIVE AND OBJECTIVE DATA)

1. Any physical symptom for which there is no organic basis but for which evidence exists for the implication of psychological factors.
2. Depressed mood is common.
3. Loss or alteration in physical functioning, with no organic basis. Examples include the following:
   a. Blindness or tunnel vision
   b. Paralysis
   c. Anosmia (inability to smell)
   d. Aphonia (inability to speak)
   e. Seizures
   f. Coordination disturbances
   g. Pseudocyesis (false pregnancy)
   h. Akinesia or dyskinesia
   i. Anesthesia or paresthesia
4. "Doctor shopping."
5. Excessive use of analgesics.
6. Requests for surgery.
7. Assumption of an invalid role.
8. Impairment in social or occupational functioning because of preoccupation with physical complaints.
9. Psychosexual dysfunction (impotence, dyspareunia [painful coitus], sexual indifference).
10. Excessive dysmenorrhea.
11. Excessive anxiety and fear of having a serious illness.
12. Objective evidence that a general medical condition has been precipitated by or is being perpetuated by psychological or behavioral circumstances.
13. Conscious, intentional feigning of physical or psychological symptoms (may be imposed on the self or on another person).

Common Nursing Diagnoses and Interventions

(Interventions are applicable to various health-care settings, such as inpatient and partial hospitalization, community outpatient clinic, home health, and private practice.)

■ INEFFECTIVE COPING

Definition: A pattern of invalid appraisal of stressors, with cognitive and/or behavioral efforts, that fails to manage demands related to well-being (NANDA International [NANDA-I], 2018, p. 327)

Possible Contributing Factors ("related to")

[Severe level of anxiety, repressed]
[Low self-esteem]
[Unmet dependency needs]
[History of self or loved one having experienced a serious illness or disease]
[Regression to, or fixation in, an earlier level of development]
[Retarded ego development]
[Inadequate coping skills]
[Possible child abuse or neglect]

Defining Characteristics ("evidenced by")

[Numerous physical complaints verbalized, in the absence of any pathophysiological evidence]
[Total focus on the self and physical symptoms]
[History of doctor shopping]
[Demanding behaviors]
[Refuses to attend therapeutic activities]
[Does not correlate physical symptoms with psychological problems]
[Feigning of physical or psychological symptoms to gain attention]
Inability to meet basic needs
Inability to meet role expectations
Inadequate problem-solving
Sleep pattern disturbance

Goals/Objectives

Short-term Goal

Within (specified time), the patient will verbalize understanding of correlation between physical symptoms and psychological problems.

Long-term Goal

By time of discharge from treatment, the patient will demonstrate ability to cope with stress by means other than preoccupation with physical symptoms.

Interventions With *Selected Rationales*

1. Monitor physician's ongoing assessments, laboratory reports, and other data to maintain assurance that possibility of organic

pathology is clearly ruled out. Review findings with the patient. *Accurate medical assessment is vital for the provision of adequate and appropriate care. Honest explanation may help the patient understand the psychological implications.*

2. Recognize and accept that the physical complaint is indeed real to the individual, even though no organic etiology can be identified. *Denial of the patient's feelings is nontherapeutic and interferes with establishment of a trusting relationship.*

3. Provide pain medication as prescribed by the physician. *Patient comfort and safety are nursing priorities.*

4. Identify gains that the physical symptoms are providing for the patient: increased dependency, attention, and distraction from other problems. *Identification of underlying motivation is important in assisting the patient with problem resolution.*

5. Initially, fulfill the patient's most urgent dependency needs. *Failure to do this may cause the patient to become extremely anxious, with an increase in maladaptive behaviors.*

6. Gradually withdraw attention to physical symptoms. Minimize time given in response to physical complaints. *Lack of positive response will discourage repetition of maladaptive behaviors.*

7. Explain to the patient that any new physical complaints will be referred to the physician, and give no further attention to them. Follow up on physician's assessment of the complaint. *The possibility of organic pathology must always be considered. Failure to do so could jeopardize the patient's safety.*

8. Encourage the patient to verbalize fears and anxieties. Explain that attention will be withdrawn if rumination about physical complaints begins, and follow through. *Without consistency of limit setting, change will not occur.*

9. Help the patient recognize the connection between physical symptoms and specific stressors. Discuss alternative coping strategies that the patient may use in response to stress (e.g., relaxation exercises, physical activities, assertiveness skills). The patient may need help with problem-solving.

10. Give positive reinforcement for adaptive coping strategies. *Positive reinforcement encourages repetition of desired behaviors.*

11. Have the patient keep a diary of appearance, duration, and intensity of physical symptoms. A separate record of situations that the patient finds especially stressful should also be kept. *Comparison of these records may provide objective data from which to observe the relationship between physical symptoms and stress.*

12. Help the patient identify ways to achieve recognition from others without resorting to physical symptoms. *Positive recognition from others enhances self-esteem and minimizes the need for attention through maladaptive behaviors.*

13. Explore how interpersonal relationships are affected by the patient's self-obsessed behavior. *The patient may not realize how he or she is perceived by others.*

14. Provide instruction in relaxation techniques and assertiveness skills. *These approaches decrease anxiety and increase self-esteem, which facilitate adaptive responses to stressful situations.*

Outcome Criteria

1. The patient is able to demonstrate techniques that may be used in response to stress to prevent the occurrence or exacerbation of physical symptoms.
2. The patient verbalizes an understanding of the relationship between emotional problems and physical symptoms.

■ DISTURBED SENSORY PERCEPTION

Definition: Change in the amount or patterning of incoming stimuli [either internally or externally initiated] accompanied by a diminished, exaggerated, distorted, or impaired response to such stimuli (Note: This diagnosis has been retired by NANDA-I but is retained in this text because of its appropriateness in describing these specific behaviors.)

Possible Contributing Factors ("related to")

[Severe level of anxiety, repressed]
[Low self-esteem]
[Unmet dependency needs]
[Regression to or fixation in an earlier level of development]
[Retarded ego development]
[Inadequate coping skills]
Psychological stress [narrowed perceptual fields caused by anxiety]

Defining Characteristics ("evidenced by")

[Loss or alteration in physical functioning suggesting a physical disorder (often neurological in nature) but for which organic pathology is not evident. Common alterations include paralysis, anosmia, aphonia, deafness, blindness]

Goals/Objectives

Short-term Goal

The patient will verbalize understanding of emotional problems as a contributing factor to the alteration in physical functioning (within time limit appropriate for specific individual).

Long-term Goal

The patient will demonstrate recovery of lost or altered function.

Interventions With *Selected Rationales*

1. Monitor the physician's ongoing assessments, laboratory reports, and other data to maintain assurance that possibility of organic

pathology is clearly ruled out. *Failure to do so may jeopardize the patient's safety.*

2. Identify primary or secondary gains that the physical symptom is providing for the patient (e.g., increased dependency, attention, protection from experiencing a stressful event). *These are considered to be etiological factors and may be used to assist in problem resolution.*

3. Fulfill the patient's needs related to activities of daily living (ADLs) with which the physical symptom is interfering. *Patient comfort and safety are nursing priorities.*

4. Do not focus on the disability, and encourage the patient to be as independent as possible. Intervene only when the patient requires assistance. *Positive reinforcement would encourage continual use of the maladaptive response for secondary gains, such as dependency.*

5. Maintain a nonjudgmental attitude when providing assistance with self-care activities to the patient. *The physical symptom is not within the patient's conscious control and is very real to him or her.*

6. Encourage the patient to participate in therapeutic activities to the best of his or her ability. Do not enable the patient to use the disability as a manipulative tool. Withdraw attention if the patient continues to focus on physical limitation. Reinforce reality as required, but ensure maintenance of a nonthreatening environment.

7. Encourage the patient to verbalize fears and anxieties. Help the patient to recognize that the physical symptom appears at a time of extreme stress and is a mechanism used for coping. *The patient may be unaware of the relationship between physical symptom and emotional stress.*

8. Help the patient identify coping mechanisms that he or she could use when faced with stressful situations rather than retreating from reality with a physical disability.

9. Explain assertiveness techniques and practice use of same through role-playing. *Use of assertiveness techniques enhances self-esteem and minimizes anxiety in interpersonal relationships.*

10. Help the patient identify a satisfactory support system within the community from which he or she may seek assistance as needed to cope with overwhelming stress.

Outcome Criteria

1. The patient is no longer experiencing symptoms of altered physical functioning.

2. The patient verbalizes an understanding of the relationship between extreme psychological stress and loss of physical functioning.

3. The patient is able to verbalize adaptive ways of coping with stress and identify community support systems to which he or she may go for help.

■ DEFICIENT KNOWLEDGE (Psychological Factors Affecting Medical Condition)

Definition: Absence of cognitive information related to a specific topic, or its acquisition (NANDA-I, 2018, p. 259)

Possible Contributing Factors ("related to")

Lack of interest in learning
[Severe level of anxiety]
[Low self-esteem]
[Regression to earlier level of development]
Cognitive limitation
Information misinterpretation

Defining Characteristics ("evidenced by")

[Denial of emotional problems]
[Statements such as, "I don't know why the doctor put me on the psychiatric unit. I have a physical problem"]
[Evidence of a general medical condition that is being precipitated by psychological or behavioral circumstances]
[History of numerous exacerbations of physical illness]
[Noncompliance with psychiatric treatment]
Inappropriate or exaggerated behaviors (e.g., hysterical, hostile, agitated, apathetic)

Goals/Objectives

Short-term Goal

The patient will cooperate with plan for teaching provided by primary nurse.

Long-term Goal

By time of discharge from treatment, the patient will be able to verbalize psychological factors affecting his or her medical condition.

Interventions With *Selected Rationales*

1. Assess the patient's level of knowledge regarding effects of psychological problems on the body. *An adequate database is necessary for the development of an effective teaching plan.*
2. Assess the patient's level of anxiety and readiness to learn. *Learning does not occur beyond the moderate level of anxiety.*
3. Discuss physical examinations and laboratory tests that have been conducted. Explain purpose and results of each. *Fear of the unknown may contribute to elevated level of anxiety. The patient has the right to know about and accept or refuse any medical treatment.*

4. Explore the patient's feelings and fears. Go slowly. These feelings may have been suppressed or repressed for so long that their disclosure may be very painful. Be supportive. *Expression of feelings in a nonthreatening environment and with a trusting individual may encourage the individual to confront unresolved issues.*

5. Have the patient keep a diary of appearance, duration, and intensity of physical symptoms. A separate record of situations the patient finds especially stressful should also be kept. *Comparison of these records may provide objective data from which to observe the relationship between physical symptoms and stress.*

6. Help the patient identify needs that are being met through the sick role. Together, formulate more adaptive means for fulfilling these needs. Practice by role-playing. *Repetition through practice serves to reduce discomfort in the actual situation.*

7. Provide instruction in assertiveness techniques, especially the ability to recognize the differences among passive, assertive, and aggressive behaviors, and the importance of respecting the human rights of others while protecting one's own basic human rights. *These skills will preserve the patient's self-esteem while also improving his or her ability to form satisfactory interpersonal relationships.*

8. Discuss adaptive methods of stress management such as relaxation techniques, physical exercise, meditation, breathing exercises, and autogenics. *Use of these adaptive techniques may decrease appearance or exacerbation of physical symptoms in response to stress.*

Outcome Criteria

1. The patient verbalizes an understanding of the relationship between psychological stress and exacerbation (or perpetuation) of physical illness.

2. The patient demonstrates the ability to use adaptive coping strategies in the management of stress.

■ FEAR (Of Having a Serious Illness)

Definition: Response to perceived threat that is consciously recognized as a danger (NANDA-I, 2018, p. 337)

Possible Contributing Factors ("related to")

[Past experience with life-threatening illness, either personal or that of close family members]

Defining Characteristics ("evidenced by")

[Preoccupation with and unrealistic interpretation of bodily signs and sensations]
[Excessive anxiety over health concerns]

Goals/Objectives

Short-term Goal

The patient will verbalize that fears associated with bodily sensations are irrational (within time limit deemed appropriate for specific individual).

Long-term Goal

The patient interprets bodily sensations correctly.

Interventions With *Selected Rationales*

1. Monitor the physician's ongoing assessments and laboratory reports. *Organic pathology must be clearly ruled out.*
2. Refer all new physical complaints to the physician. *To ignore all physical complaints could place the patient's safety in jeopardy.*
3. Assess the function the patient's illness is fulfilling for him or her (e.g., unfulfilled needs for dependency, nurturing, caring, attention, or control). *This information may provide insight into reasons for maladaptive behavior and provide direction for planning patient care.*
4. Identify times during which the preoccupation with physical symptoms worsens. Determine the extent of correlation of physical complaints with times of increased anxiety. *The patient may be unaware of the psychosocial implications of the physical complaints. Knowledge of the relationship is the first step in the process for creating change.*
5. Convey empathy. Let the patient know that you understand how a specific symptom may conjure up fears of previous life-threatening illness. *Unconditional acceptance and empathy promote a therapeutic nurse-patient relationship.*
6. Initially allow the patient a limited amount of time (e.g., 10 minutes each hour) to discuss physical symptoms. *Because this has been his or her primary method of coping for so long, complete prohibition of this activity would likely raise the patient's anxiety level significantly, further exacerbating the behavior.*
7. Help the patient determine what techniques may be most useful for him or her to implement when fear and anxiety are exacerbated (e.g., relaxation techniques, mental imagery, thought-stopping techniques, physical exercise). *All of these techniques are effective in reducing anxiety and may assist the patient in the transition from focusing on fear of physical illness to the discussion of honest feelings.*
8. Gradually increase the limit on amount of time spent each hour in discussing physical symptoms. If the patient violates the limits, withdraw attention. *Lack of positive reinforcement may help to extinguish the maladaptive behavior.*
9. Encourage the patient to discuss feelings associated with fear of serious illness. *Verbalization of feelings in a nonthreatening*

environment facilitates expression and resolution of disturbing emotional issues. When the patient can express feelings directly, there is less need to express them through physical symptoms.

10. Role-play the patient's plan for dealing with the fear the next time it assumes control and before anxiety becomes disabling. *Anxiety and fears are minimized when the patient has achieved a degree of comfort through practicing a plan for dealing with stressful situations in the future.*

@ INTERNET REFERENCES

Additional information about somatic symptom disorders may be located at the following Web sites:

- www.psyweb.com/Mdisord/somatd.html
- https://emedicine.medscape.com/article/290955-overview#a5
- http://emedicine.medscape.com/article/805361-overview
- http://emedicine.medscape.com/article/291304-overview
- https://emedicine.medscape.com/article/294908-overview

Movie Connections

Bandits (Illness anxiety disorder) • *Hannah and Her Sisters* (Illness anxiety disorder) • *Send Me No Flowers* (Illness anxiety disorder) • *Dead Again* (Amnesia) • *Mirage* (Amnesia) • *Suddenly Last Summer* (Amnesia) • *Sybil* (DID) • *The Three Faces of Eve* (DID) • *Identity* (DID)

CHAPTER 11

Dissociative Disorders

■ BACKGROUND ASSESSMENT DATA

Dissociative disorders are disturbances of or alteration in the usually integrated functions of consciousness, memory, and identity. During periods of intolerable stress, the individual blocks off part of his or her life from consciousness. This process is defined as an unconscious defense mechanism in which there is separation of identity, memory, and cognition from affect (Sadock, Sadock, & Ruiz, 2015). The following categories are defined in the *Diagnostic and Statistical Manual of Mental Disorders, Fifth Edition (DSM-5)* (American Psychiatric Association [APA], 2013):

1. **Dissociative Amnesia:** An inability to recall important personal information, usually of a traumatic or stressful nature. The extent of the disturbance is too great to be explained by ordinary forgetfulness. Types of impairment in recall include the following:
   a. **Localized Amnesia:** Inability to recall all incidents associated with a traumatic event. It may be broader than just a single event, however, such as being unable to remember months or years of child abuse (APA, 2013).
   b. **Selective Amnesia:** Inability to recall only certain incidents associated with a traumatic event for a specific period following the event.
   c. **Generalized Amnesia:** Inability to recall all events encompassing one's entire life, including one's identity.
   Dissociative amnesia sometimes, although rarely, is accompanied by a *dissociative fugue*. Dissociative fugue is characterized by sudden, unexpected travel away from customary places of daily activities or by bewildered wandering, with the inability to recall some or all of one's past. An individual in a fugue state may not be able to recall personal identity and sometimes assumes a new identity. Dissociative fugue is more common in dissociative identity disorder.

2. **Dissociative Identity Disorder (DID):** The existence within the individual of two or more distinct identity states, each of which is dominant at a particular time. The individual usually is not aware (at least initially) of the existence of subpersonalities. When there are more than two subpersonalities, however, they

are usually aware of each other. Transition from one subpersonality to another is usually sudden and often associated with psychosocial stress. The course tends to be more chronic than in the other dissociative disorders. This disorder was previously called *multiple personality disorder*. Dr. David Spiegel, a psychiatrist who was involved in promoting the American Psychiatric Association's adoption of DID as the preferred term for this condition, is quoted in Haberman's review (2014) as saying that the term *multiple personality* "carries with it the implication that they really have more than one personality. The problem is fragmentation of identity, not that you really are 12 people . . . that you have not more than one but less than one personality."

3. **Depersonalization-Derealization Disorder:** Characterized by a temporary change in the quality of self-awareness, which often takes the form of feelings of unreality, changes in body image, feelings of detachment from the environment, or a sense of observing oneself from outside the body. *Depersonalization* (a disturbance in the perception of oneself) is differentiated from *derealization*, which describes an alteration in the perception of the external environment. Both of these phenomena also occur in a variety of psychiatric illnesses such as schizophrenia, depression, anxiety states, and neurocognitive disorders.

■ PREDISPOSING FACTORS TO DISSOCIATIVE DISORDERS

1. Physiological
   a. **Genetics:** The overwhelming majority of adults with DID (85% to 97%) have a history of physical and sexual abuse. Although genetic factors are being studied, current evidence does not support a significant genetic influence.
   b. **Neurobiological:** Some clinicians have suggested a possible correlation between neurological alterations and dissociative disorders. Although available information is inadequate, it is possible that dissociative amnesia may be related to neurophysiological dysfunction. Areas of the brain that have been associated with memory include the hippocampus, amygdala, fornix, mammillary bodies, thalamus, and frontal cortex. Depersonalization has been evidenced with migraines and with marijuana use, responds to selective serotonin reuptake inhibitors (SSRIs), and is seen in cases where L-tryptophan, a serotonin precursor, is depleted. These facts suggest some level of serotonergic involvement in this dissociative symptom (Sadock et al, 2015). Some studies have suggested a possible link between DID and certain neurological conditions, such as temporal lobe epilepsy and

severe migraine headaches. Electroencephalographic abnormalities have been observed in some patients with DID.

2. Psychosocial

a. **Psychodynamic Theory:** Freud (1962) believed that dissociative behaviors occurred when individuals repressed distressing mental contents from conscious awareness. Current psychodynamic explanations of dissociation are based on Freud's concepts. The repression of mental contents is perceived as a coping mechanism for protecting the patient from emotional pain that has arisen from either disturbing external circumstances or anxiety-provoking internal urges and feelings. In the case of depersonalization and derealization, the pain and anxiety are expressed as feelings of unreality or detachment from the environment of the painful situation.

b. **Psychological Trauma:** A growing body of evidence points to the etiology of DID as a set of traumatic experiences that overwhelms the individual's capacity to cope by any means other than dissociation. These experiences usually take the form of severe physical, sexual, and/or psychological abuse by a parent or significant other in the child's life. The most widely accepted explanation for DID is that it begins as a survival strategy to help children cope with horrifying sexual, physical, or psychological abuse and evolves into a fragmented identity as the victim struggles to integrate conflicting aspects of personality into a cohesive whole. Dissociative amnesia is frequently related to acute and extreme trauma but may also develop in the clinical presentation of DID or in response to combat trauma during wartimes.

Symptomatology (Subjective and Objective Data)

1. Impairment in recall.
   a. Inability to remember specific incidents.
   b. Inability to recall any part of one's past life, including one's identity.
2. Sudden travel away from familiar surroundings; assumption of new identity with inability to recall past.
3. Assumption of fragmented identities within the personality; behavior involves transition from one identity to another as a method of dealing with stressful situations.
4. Feeling of unreality; detachment from a stressful situation—may be accompanied by light-headedness, depression, obsessive rumination, somatic concerns, anxiety, fear of going insane, and a disturbance in the subjective sense of time (APA, 2013).

Common Nursing Diagnoses and Interventions

(Interventions are applicable to various health-care settings, such as inpatient and partial hospitalization, community outpatient clinic, home health, and private practice.)

■ INEFFECTIVE COPING

Definition: A pattern of invalid appraisal of stressors, with cognitive and/or behavioral efforts, that fails to manage demands related to well-being (NANDA International [NANDA-I], 2018, p. 327)

Possible Contributing Factors ("related to")

[Severe level of anxiety, repressed]
[Childhood trauma]
[Childhood abuse]
[Low self-esteem]
[Unmet dependency needs]
[Regression to or fixation in an earlier level of development]
[Inadequate coping skills]

Defining Characteristics ("evidenced by")

[Dissociating self from painful situation by experiencing:
    Memory loss (partial or complete)
    Sudden travel away from home with inability to recall previous identity
    The presence of more than one personality within the individual
    Detachment from reality]
Inadequate problem-solving
Inability to meet role expectations
[Inappropriate use of defense mechanisms]

Goals/Objectives

Short-term Goals

1. The patient will verbalize understanding that he or she is employing dissociative behaviors in times of psychosocial stress.
2. The patient will verbalize more adaptive ways of coping in stressful situations than resorting to dissociation.

Long-term Goal

The patient will demonstrate ability to cope with stress (employing means other than dissociation).

Interventions With *Selected Rationales*

1. Reassure the patient of safety and security by your presence. Dissociative behaviors may be frightening to the patient. *Presence of a trusted individual provides feeling of security and assurance of freedom from harm.*
2. Identify stressor that precipitated severe anxiety. *This information is necessary to the development of an effective plan of patient care and problem resolution.*

3. Explore feelings that the patient experienced in response to the stressor. Help the patient understand that the disequilibrium felt is acceptable—even expected—in times of severe stress. *The patient's self-esteem is preserved by the knowledge that others may experience these behaviors in similar circumstances.*

4. As anxiety level decreases (and memory returns), use exploration and an accepting, nonthreatening environment to encourage the patient to identify repressed traumatic experiences that contribute to chronic anxiety.

5. Have the patient identify methods of coping with stress in the past and determine whether the response was adaptive or maladaptive. *In times of extreme anxiety, the patient is unable to evaluate appropriateness of response. This information is necessary for the patient to develop a plan of action for the future.*

6. Help the patient define more adaptive coping strategies. Make suggestions of alternatives that might be tried. Examine benefits and consequences of each alternative. Assist the patient in the selection of those that are most appropriate for him or her. *Depending on current level of anxiety, the patient may require assistance with problem-solving and decision making.*

7. Provide positive reinforcement for the patient's attempts to change. *Positive reinforcement enhances self-esteem and encourages repetition of desired behaviors.*

8. Identify community resources to which the individual may go for support if past maladaptive coping patterns return.

Outcome Criteria

1. The patient is able to demonstrate techniques that may be used in response to stress to prevent dissociation.
2. The patient verbalizes an understanding of the relationship between severe anxiety and the dissociative response.

■ IMPAIRED MEMORY

Definition: Persistent inability to remember or recall bits of information or skills (NANDA-I, 2018, p. 261)

Possible Contributing Factors ("related to")

[Severe level of anxiety, repressed]
[Childhood trauma]
[Childhood abuse]
[Threat to physical integrity]
[Threat to self-concept]

Defining Characteristics ("evidenced by")

[Memory loss—inability to recall selected events related to a stressful situation]

[Memory loss—inability to recall events associated with entire life]

[Memory loss—inability to recall own identity]

Goals/Objectives

Short-term Goal

The patient will verbalize understanding that loss of memory is related to a stressful situation and begin discussing stressful situation with nurse or therapist.

Long-term Goal

The patient will recover deficits in memory and develop more adaptive coping mechanisms to deal with stressful situations.

Interventions With *Selected Rationales*

1. Obtain as much information as possible about the patient from family and significant others, if possible. Consider likes, dislikes, important people, activities, music, and pets. *A comprehensive baseline assessment is important for the development of an effective plan of care.*

2. Do not confront the patient with information he or she does not appear to remember. *Individuals who are exposed to painful information from which the amnesia is providing protection may decompensate even further into a psychotic state.*

3. Instead, expose the patient to stimuli that represent pleasant experiences from the past, such as smells associated with enjoyable activities, beloved pets, and music the patient enjoys.

4. As memory begins to return, engage the patient in activities that may provide additional stimulation. *Recall often occurs during activities that simulate life experiences.*

5. Encourage the patient to discuss situations that have been especially stressful and to explore the feelings associated with those times. *Verbalization of feelings in a nonthreatening environment may help the patient come to terms with unresolved issues that may be contributing to the dissociative process.*

6. Identify specific conflicts that remain unresolved, and help the patient to identify possible solutions. *Unless these underlying conflicts are resolved, any improvement in coping behaviors must be viewed as temporary.*

7. Provide instruction regarding more adaptive ways to respond to anxiety *so that dissociative behaviors are no longer needed.*

8. Provide positive feedback for decisions made. Respect the patient's right to make those decisions independently, and

refrain from attempting to influence him or her toward those that may seem more logical. *Independent choice provides a feeling of control, decreases feelings of powerlessness, and increases self-esteem.*

Outcome Criteria

1. The patient has recovered lost memories for events of past life.
2. The patient is able to demonstrate adaptive coping strategies that may be used in response to severe anxiety to avert amnestic behaviors.

■ DISTURBED PERSONAL IDENTITY

Definition: Inability to maintain an integrated and complete perception of self (NANDA-I, 2018, p. 269)

Possible Contributing Factors ("related to")

[Severe level of anxiety, repressed]
[Childhood trauma]
[Childhood abuse]
[Threat to physical integrity]
[Threat to self-concept]

Defining Characteristics ("evidenced by")

[Presence of more than one personality within the individual]

Goals/Objectives

Short-term Goals

1. The patient will verbalize understanding of the existence of multiple personalities within the self.
2. The patient will be able to recognize stressful situations that precipitate transition from one personality to another.

Long-term Goals

1. The patient will verbalize understanding of the reasons for fragmented identity.
2. The patient will enter into and cooperate with long-term therapy, with the ultimate goal of integration into one personality.

Interventions With *Selected Rationales*

1. The nurse must develop a trusting relationship with the original personality and with each of the subpersonalities. *Trust is the basis of a therapeutic relationship. Each of the subpersonalities views itself as a separate entity and must initially be treated as such.*
2. Help the patient understand the existence of the subpersonalities. *The patient may be unaware of this dissociative response to stressful situations.*

3. Help the patient identify the need each subpersonality serves in the personal identity of the individual. *Knowledge of the needs each personality fulfills is the first step in the integration process and the patient's ability to face unresolved issues without dissociation.*

4. Help the patient identify stressful situations that precipitate the transition from one personality to another. Carefully observe and record these transitions. *This knowledge is required to assist the patient in responding more adaptively and eliminating the need for transition to another identity.*

5. Use nursing interventions necessary to deal with maladaptive behaviors associated with individual subpersonalities. For example, if one identity is suicidal, precautions must be taken to guard against the patient's self-harm. If another aspect of the patient's identity has a tendency toward physical hostility, precautions must be taken for the protection of others. *Safety of the patient and others is a nursing priority.*

6. Help subpersonalities to understand that their "being" will not be destroyed but integrated into a unified identity within the individual. *Because subpersonalities function as separate entities, the idea of total elimination generates fear and defensiveness.*

> **CLINICAL PEARL** It may be possible to seek assistance from one of the identities. For example, a strong-willed subpersonality may help to control the behaviors of a "suicidal" aspect of their identity. "Helping the identities to be aware of one another as legitimate parts of the self and to negotiate and resolve their conflicts is at the very core of the therapeutic process" (International Society for the Study of Trauma and Dissociation, 2011, p. 132).

7. Provide support during disclosure of painful experiences and reassurance when the patient becomes discouraged with lengthy treatment.

Outcome Criteria

1. The patient recognizes the existence of more than one personality.
2. The patient is able to verbalize the purpose these personalities serve.
3. The patient verbalizes the intention of seeking long-term outpatient psychotherapy.

■ DISTURBED SENSORY PERCEPTION (Visual/Kinesthetic)

Definition: Change in the amount or patterning of incoming stimuli [either internally or externally initiated] accompanied by a diminished, exaggerated, distorted, or impaired response to such stimuli (Note: This nursing diagnosis has been retired by NANDA. It is retained in this text because of its appropriateness to the specific behaviors described.)

Possible Contributing Factors ("related to")

[Severe level of anxiety, repressed]
[Childhood trauma]
[Childhood abuse]
[Threat to physical integrity]
[Threat to self-concept]

Defining Characteristics ("evidenced by")

[Alteration in the perception or experience of the self]
[Loss of one's own sense of reality]
[Loss of the sense of reality of the external world]

Goals/Objectives

Short-term Goal

The patient will verbalize adaptive ways of coping with stress.

Long-term Goal

By time of discharge from treatment, the patient will demonstrate the ability to perceive stimuli correctly and maintain a sense of reality during stressful situations.

Interventions With *Selected Rationales*

1. Provide support and encouragement during times of depersonalization. The patient manifesting these symptoms may express fear and anxiety. He or she does not understand the response and may express a fear of "going insane." *Support and encouragement from a trusted individual provide a feeling of security when fears and anxieties are manifested.*

2. Explain the depersonalization behaviors and the purpose they usually serve for the patient. *This knowledge may help to minimize fears and anxieties associated with their occurrence.*

3. Explain the relationship between severe anxiety and depersonalization behaviors. *The patient may be unaware that the occurrence of depersonalization behaviors is related to severe anxiety.*

4. Help the patient relate these behaviors to times of severe psychological stress that he or she has experienced personally. *Knowledge of this relationship is the first step in the process of behavioral change.*

5. Explore past experiences and possibly repressed painful situations such as trauma or abuse. *It is thought that traumatic experiences predispose individuals to dissociative disorders.*

6. Discuss these painful experiences with the patient and encourage him or her to deal with the feelings associated with these situations. Work to resolve the conflicts these repressed feelings have nurtured. *Conflict resolution will serve to decrease the need for the dissociative response to anxiety.*

7. Discuss ways the patient may more adaptively respond to stress, and use role-play to practice using these new methods. *Having practiced through role-play helps to prepare the patient to face stressful situations by using these new behaviors when they occur in real life.*

Outcome Criteria

1. The patient perceives stressful situations correctly and is able to maintain a sense of reality.
2. The patient demonstrates use of adaptive strategies for coping with stress.

@ INTERNET REFERENCES

Additional information about dissociative disorders may be located at the following Web sites:
- https://www.nami.org/Learn-More/Mental-Health-Conditions/Dissociative-Disorders
- www.isst-d.org
- https://mental-health-matters.com/psychological-disorders/ http://emedicine.medscape.com/article/294508-overview

Movie Connections

Dead Again (Amnesia) • *Mirage* (Amnesia) • *Suddenly Last Summer* (Amnesia) • *The Three Lives of Karen* (Dissociative fugue) • *Sybil* (DID) • *The Three Faces of Eve* (DID) • *Identity* (DID) • *Shutter Island* (DID)

CHAPTER 12

Sexual Disorders and Gender Dysphoria

■ BACKGROUND ASSESSMENT DATA

The *Diagnostic and Statistical Manual of Mental Disorders, Fifth Edition (DSM-5)* (American Psychiatric Association [APA], 2013), identifies three categories of disorders associated with sexuality: gender dysphoria, sexual dysfunctions, and paraphilic disorders. *Gender dysphoria* refers to the "distress that may accompany the incongruence between one's experienced or expressed gender and one's assigned gender" (APA, 2013, p. 451). Not all individuals with a transgender identity will experience clinically significant distress and, as such, it is important to note that the focus of this diagnostic category is on dysphoria as the clinical problem rather than identity per se (APA, 2013). *Sexual dysfunction disorders* can be described as an impairment or disturbance in any of the phases of the sexual response cycle. These include disorders of desire, arousal, orgasm, and disorders that relate to the experience of genital pain during intercourse. The term *paraphilia* is defined in the DSM-5 (APA, 2013) as "any intense and persistent sexual interest other than sexual interest in genital stimulation or preparatory fondling with phenotypically normal, physically mature, consenting human partners" (p. 685). In a *paraphilic disorder*, these sexual fantasies or behaviors are recurrent over a period of at least 6 months and cause the individual clinically significant distress or impairment in social, occupational, or other important areas of functioning (APA, 2013).

■ GENDER DYSPHORIA

Gender *identity* is the sense of knowing to which gender one belongs—that is, the awareness of one's masculinity or femininity. Gender *dysphoria* is the distress that may accompany the incongruence between one's experienced and expressed gender and one's assigned or natal gender (APA, 2013). The *DSM-5* identifies two categories of gender dysphoria: gender dysphoria in children and gender dysphoria in adolescents and adults.

Intervention with adolescents and adults with gender dysphoria is multifaceted. Adolescents rarely have the desire or motivation to alter their cross-gender roles. Some adults seek therapy to learn how to cope with their sexual identity, whereas others have direct and immediate request for hormonal therapy and surgical sex reassignment. Treatment of the adult with gender dysphoria is a complex process. If the transgendered individual intensely desires to have the genitalia and physical appearance of the assigned gender changed to conform to his or her gender identity, this change requires a great deal more than surgical alteration of physical features. In most cases, the individual must undergo extensive psychological testing and counseling, as well as live in the role of the desired gender for up to 2 years before surgery.

Treatment of children with gender dysphoria may be initiated when the behaviors cause significant distress and when the patient desires it. Determining whether a child is truly experiencing gender dysphoria should be done cautiously, as gender-related behaviors vary widely in this age group. When the issue is identified as real gender dysphoria (e.g., the child is manifesting significant distress, symptoms of clinical depression, or suicidal ideation associated with transgender identity concerns), treatment should include evaluation and management of concurrent mental health problems, social support systems, and in later childhood, nonjudgmental exploration of the individual's desires with regard to sexual reassignment.

Some practitioners still engage in treatment models that attempt to "repair" or change the person's gender identity, but this approach is contrary to position statements by the American Psychiatric Association (Byne et al, 2012) and the practice guidelines established by The American Academy of Child and Adolescent Psychiatry (Adelson, 2012), The American Psychological Association (2015), and The Endocrine Society (2017).

Another treatment model suggests that children who have differing gender identity are dysphoric only because of their image within the culture. This model stresses that children should be accepted as they see themselves—different from their assigned gender—and supported in their efforts to live as the gender in which they feel most comfortable. One option for treatment is pubertal delay for adolescents aged 12 to 16 years who have suffered with extreme lifelong gender dysphoria and who have supportive parents who encourage the child to pursue a desired change in gender (Adelson, 2012; Byne et al, 2012). A gonadotropin-releasing hormone agonist is administered to suppress changes associated with puberty. The treatment is reversible if the adolescent later decides not to pursue the gender change. When the medication is withdrawn, external sexual development proceeds, and the individual has avoided permanent surgical intervention. If he or she decides as an adult to advance to surgical intervention, pubertal delay may facilitate transition, since there have not been clearly established secondary sex characteristics. The type of treatment one chooses (if any) is a matter of personal choice. However, issues associated with mental health concerns, such as depression, risk for suicide, anxiety, social isolation, anger, self-esteem, and parental conflict, must be addressed.

Children who demonstrate gender-nonconforming behaviors are often targets of bullying and violence. Nurses can play a key role in educating families and providing support to identify safe, supportive peer groups for these children.

Predisposing Factors Associated With Gender Dysphoria

1. Biological Factors
    The etiology of transgender identity is unknown. However, in a review of the research on biological influences in gender identity (Saraswat, Weinand, & Safer, 2015) the authors conclude that "current evidence suggests a biological etiology for transgender identity," most notably neuroanatomical differences in gray and white matter. However, the authors note that all of the studies exploring etiological influences are small so results should be interpreted with caution.
2. Psychosocial Factors
    Gender roles are certainly culturally influenced, as parents encourage masculine or feminine behaviors in their children. However, there is no clear evidence that psychological factors or family dynamics cause someone to identify as transgender. Parents may present with anxiety over their child's gender-nonconforming behavior based on their attitudes and perceptions. Likewise, children may present with symptoms of anxiety and depression related to negative attitudes toward their gender-nonconforming behaviors. Interestingly, researchers have observed that many children who show gender-nonconforming behavior do not grow up to become transgender, and many people who identify themselves as transgender in adulthood were not identified as gender-nonconforming in childhood (Sadock, Sadock, & Ruiz, 2015).

Symptomatology (Subjective and Objective Data)

In Children or Adolescents:

1. Insistence that one is of the opposite gender and emotional distress associated with his or her gender identity.
2. Interference with social or other areas of functioning that is associated with gender identity distress.
3. Verbalized or observed signs of mood disturbance related to gender identity concerns.

4. Expresses suicidal ideation or other risk factors and warning signs for suicide.

In Adults:

1. Persistent discomfort or mood disturbance associated with his or her gender identity.
2. Expressed impairment in social or other areas of functioning related to gender identity concerns.

Common Nursing Diagnoses and Interventions for Gender Dysphoria

(Interventions are applicable to various health-care settings, such as in-patient and partial hospitalization, community outpatient clinic, home health, and private practice.)

■ DISTURBED PERSONAL IDENTITY

Definition: Inability to maintain an integrated and complete perception of self (NANDA-I, 2018, p. 269)

Possible Contributing Factors ("related to")

Low self-esteem
Cultural incongruence
Perceived prejudice or discrimination

Defining Characteristics ("evidenced by")

[Statements that gender identity is a source of internal distress]
Ineffective coping strategies
Impaired relationships

Goals/Objectives

Short-term Goals

1. The patient will verbalize effective coping strategies to enhance self-esteem and satisfying interpersonal relationships.
2. The patient will not harm self.

Long-term Goals

1. The patient will express satisfaction in social and other areas of functioning.
2. The patient will remain free from self-harm.

Interventions With *Selected Rationales*

1. Spend time with the patient and show positive regard. *Trust and unconditional acceptance are essential to the establishment of a therapeutic nurse-patient relationship.*

2. Be aware of own feelings and attitudes toward this patient and his or her behavior. *Attitudes influence behavior. The nurse must not allow negative attitudes to interfere with the effectiveness of interventions.*
3. Allow the patient to describe his or her perception of the problem. *It is important to know how the patient perceives the problem before attempting to correct misperceptions.*
4. Behavioral change is attempted with the child's best interests in mind—that is, to help him or her with cultural and societal integration while maintaining individuality. *To preserve self-esteem and enhance self-worth, the child must know that he or she is accepted unconditionally as a unique and worthwhile individual.*

Outcome Criteria

1. The patient verbalizes and demonstrates self-satisfaction with gender identity.
2. The patient demonstrates use of effective coping mechanisms to maintain self-esteem and remain free from self-harm.

■ IMPAIRED SOCIAL INTERACTION

Definition: Insufficient or excessive quantity or ineffective quality of social exchange (NANDA-I, 2018, p. 301)

Possible Contributing Factors ("related to")

[Social victimization, bullying from peer group]
[Disrupted communication with family or significant others]
[Low self-esteem]

Defining Characteristics ("evidenced by")

Discomfort in social situations
Inability to receive or communicate a satisfying sense of belonging, caring, interest, or shared history
Use of unsuccessful social interaction behaviors
Dysfunctional interaction with others

Goals/Objectives

Short-term Goal

The patient will verbalize possible reasons for ineffective interactions with others.

Long-term Goal

The patient will interact with others in mutually satisfying relationships.

Interventions With *Selected Rationales*

1. Explore positive coping strategies. Once the patient feels comfortable with new coping skills in role-playing or one-to-one nurse-patient interactions, the new behaviors may be tried in group situations. If possible, remain with the patient during initial interactions with others. *Presence of a trusted individual provides security for the patient in a new situation. It also provides the potential for feedback to the patient about his or her behavior.*

2. Observe patient behaviors and the responses he or she elicits from others. Give social attention (e.g., smile, nod) to desired behaviors. Follow up these "practice" sessions with one-to-one processing of the interaction. Give positive reinforcement for efforts. *Positive reinforcement encourages repetition of desirable behaviors. One-to-one processing provides time for discussing the appropriateness of specific behaviors and why they should or should not be repeated.*

3. Offer support if the patient is feeling hurt from peer ridicule. Encourage the patient to discuss feelings and explore positive coping strategies. *Validation of the patient's feelings is important.*

4. Create a trusting, nonthreatening atmosphere for the patient in an attempt to promote effective coping skills and improve social interactions.

Outcome Criteria

1. The patient expresses satisfaction with his or her responses in social interaction.
2. The patient verbalizes and demonstrates comfort with gender identity in interactions with others.

■ LOW SELF-ESTEEM

Definition: Negative evaluation and/or feelings about one's own capabilities (NANDA-I, 2018, pp. 272–275)

Possible Contributing Factors ("related to")

[Rejection by peers]
Lack of approval and/or affection
Repeated negative reinforcement
[Lack of personal satisfaction with assigned gender]

Defining Characteristics ("evidenced by")

[Inability to form close, personal relationships]
[Negative view of self]

[Expressions of worthlessness]
[Social isolation]
[Hypersensitivity to slight or criticism]
Reports feelings of shame or guilt
Self-negating verbalizations
Lack of eye contact

Goals/Objectives

Short-term Goal

The patient will verbalize positive statements about self, including past accomplishments and future prospects.

Long-term Goal

The patient will verbalize and demonstrate behaviors that indicate self-satisfaction with gender identity, ability to interact with others, and a sense of self as a worthwhile person.

Interventions With *Selected Rationales*

1. To enhance the child's self-esteem:
   a. Encourage the child to engage in activities in which he or she is likely to achieve success.
   b. Help the child to focus on aspects of his or her life for which positive feelings exist. Discourage rumination about situations that are perceived as failures or over which the patient has no control. Give positive feedback for these behaviors.
2. Help the child identify behaviors or aspects of life he or she would like to change. If realistic, assist the child in problem-solving ways to bring about the change. *Having some control over his or her life may decrease feelings of powerlessness and increase feelings of self-worth and self-satisfaction.*
3. Offer to be available for support to the child if he or she is feeling rejected by peers. Explore opportunities for enhancing peer acceptance. *Having an available support person who does not judge the child's behavior and who provides unconditional acceptance assists the child to progress toward acceptance of self as a worthwhile person.*
4. Assess risk factors and warning signs for suicide and collaboratively engage the patient in developing a plan for personal safety. *Patient safety is a nursing priority.*

Outcome Criteria

1. The patient verbalizes positive perception of self.
2. The patient verbalizes self-satisfaction about accomplishments and demonstrates behaviors that reflect self-worth.
3. The patient remains free from self-harm.

■ SEXUAL DYSFUNCTIONS

Sexual dysfunctions may occur in any phase of the sexual response cycle. Types of sexual dysfunctions include the following:

1. Sexual Interest/Arousal Disorders
   a. **Female Sexual Interest/Arousal Disorder:** This disorder is characterized by a reduced or absent interest or pleasure in sexual activity (APA, 2013). The individual typically does not initiate sexual activity and is commonly unreceptive to partner's attempts to initiate. There is an absence of sexual thoughts or fantasies and absent or reduced arousal in response to sexual or erotic cues. The condition has persisted for at least 6 months and causes the individual significant distress.
   b. **Male Hypoactive Sexual Desire Disorder:** This disorder is defined by the *DSM-5* as a persistent or recurrent deficiency or absence of sexual fantasies and desire for sexual activity. In making the judgment of deficiency or absence, the clinician considers factors that affect sexual functioning, such as age and circumstances of the person's life (APA, 2013). The condition has persisted for at least 6 months and causes the individual significant distress.
   c. **Erectile Disorder:** Erectile disorder is characterized by marked difficulty in obtaining or maintaining an erection during sexual activity or a decrease in erectile rigidity that interferes with sexual activity (APA, 2013). The problem has persisted for at least 6 months and causes the individual significant distress. *Primary erectile disorder* refers to cases in which the man has never been able to have intercourse; *secondary erectile disorder* refers to cases in which the man has difficulty getting or maintaining an erection but has been able to have vaginal or anal intercourse at least once.

2. Orgasmic Disorders
   a. **Female Orgasmic Disorder:** Female orgasmic disorder is defined by the *DSM-5* as a marked delay in, infrequency of, or absence of orgasm during sexual activity (APA, 2013). It may also be characterized by a reduced intensity of orgasmic sensation. The condition, which is sometimes referred to as *anorgasmia*, has lasted at least 6 months and causes the individual significant distress. Women who can achieve orgasm through noncoital clitoral stimulation but are not able to experience it during coitus in the absence of manual clitoral stimulation are not necessarily categorized as anorgasmic. A woman is considered to have *primary orgasmic disorder* when she has never experienced orgasm by any kind of stimulation. *Secondary orgasmic disorder* exists if the woman has experienced at least one

orgasm, regardless of the means of stimulation, but no longer does so.

  b. **Delayed Ejaculation:** Delayed ejaculation is characterized by marked delay in ejaculation or marked infrequency or absence of ejaculation during partnered sexual activity (APA, 2013). The condition has lasted for at least 6 months and causes the individual significant distress. With this disorder, the man is unable to ejaculate, even though he has a firm erection and has had more than adequate stimulation. The severity of the problem may range from only occasional problems ejaculating *(secondary disorder)* to a history of never having experienced an orgasm *(primary disorder)*. In the most common version, the man cannot ejaculate during coitus but may be able to ejaculate as a result of other types of stimulation.

  c. **Premature (Early) Ejaculation:** The *DSM-5* describes premature (early) ejaculation as persistent or recurrent ejaculation occurring within 1 minute of beginning partnered sexual activity and before the person wishes it (APA, 2013). The condition has lasted at least 6 months and causes the individual significant distress. The diagnosis should take into account factors that affect the duration of the excitement phase, such as the person's age, the uniqueness of the sexual partner, and frequency of sexual activity (Sadock et al, 2015). Premature (early) ejaculation is the most common sexual disorder for which men seek treatment. It is particularly common among young men who have a very high sex drive and have not yet learned to control ejaculation.

3. Sexual Pain Disorders

  a. **Genito-Pelvic Pain/Penetration Disorder:** With this disorder, the individual experiences considerable difficulty with vaginal intercourse and attempts at penetration. Pain is felt in the vagina, around the vaginal entrance and clitoris, or deep in the pelvis. There is fear and anxiety associated with anticipation of pain or vaginal penetration. A tensing and tightening of the pelvic floor muscles occurs during attempted vaginal penetration (APA, 2013). The condition may be *lifelong* (present since the individual became sexually active) or *acquired* (began after a period of relatively normal sexual function). It has persisted for at least 6 months and causes the individual clinically significant distress.

4. Substance/Medication-Induced Sexual Dysfunction

  a. With these disorders, the sexual dysfunction developed after substance intoxication or withdrawal or after exposure to a medication (APA, 2013). The dysfunction may involve pain, impaired desire, impaired arousal, or impaired orgasm. Some substances/medications that can interfere with sexual functioning include alcohol, amphetamines, cocaine, opioids, sedatives, hypnotics, anxiolytics, antidepressants, antipsychotics, antihypertensives, and others.

Predisposing Factors to Sexual Dysfunctions

1. Physiological
   a. **Sexual Interest/Arousal Disorders:** Studies have correlated decreased levels of serum testosterone with hypoactive sexual desire disorder in men. Evidence also suggests a relationship between serum testosterone and increased female libido (Sadock et al, 2015). Diminished libido has been observed in both men and women with elevated levels of serum prolactin (Wisse, 2015). Various medications, such as antihypertensives, antipsychotics, antidepressants, anxiolytics, and anticonvulsants, as well as chronic use of drugs such as alcohol and cocaine, have also been implicated in sexual desire disorders, especially after chronic use. Problems with sexual arousal may occur in response to decreased estrogen levels in postmenopausal women. Medications such as antihistamines and cholinergic blockers may produce similar results. Erectile dysfunction in men may be attributed to arteriosclerosis, diabetes, temporal lobe epilepsy, multiple sclerosis, some medications (e.g., antihypertensives, antidepressants, anxiolytics), spinal cord injury, pelvic surgery, and chronic use of alcohol.
   b. **Orgasmic Disorders:** In women, these may be attributed to some medical conditions (hypothyroidism, diabetes, and depression) and certain medications (antihypertensives, antidepressants). Medical conditions that may interfere with male orgasm include genitourinary surgery (e.g., prostatectomy), Parkinson's disease, and diabetes. Various medications have also been implicated, including antihypertensives, antidepressants, and antipsychotics. Transient cases of the disorder may occur with excessive alcohol intake. Although early ejaculation is commonly caused by psychological factors, general medical conditions or substance use may also be contributing influences. Particularly in cases of secondary dysfunction, in which a man at one time had ejaculatory control but later lost it, physical factors may be involved. Examples include a local infection such as prostatitis or a degenerative neural disorder such as multiple sclerosis.
   c. **Sexual Pain Disorders:** In women, sexual pain disorders may be caused by intact hymen, episiotomy scar, vaginal or urinary tract infection, ligament injuries, endometriosis, or ovarian cysts or tumors. Painful intercourse in men may be attributed to penile infections, phimosis, urinary tract infections, or prostate problems.

2. Psychosocial
   a. **Sexual Interest/Arousal Disorders:** A variety of individual and relationship factors may contribute to hypoactive sexual desire or sexual arousal disorders. Individual factors include fears associated with sex; history of sexual abuse and trauma; chronic stress, anxiety, depression; and aging-related concerns (e.g., changes in physical appearance). Among the relationship causes are interpersonal conflicts; current physical, verbal, or sexual abuse; extramarital affairs; and desire or practices that differ from those of one's partner. In general, the presence of sexual desire is influenced by sexual drives, self-esteem, accepting oneself as a sexual person, good stress management, and good relationship skills; disruption in any of these areas can contribute to lower desire (Sadock et al, 2015).
   b. **Orgasmic Disorders:** Numerous psychological factors are associated with inhibited female orgasm. They include fears of becoming pregnant or damage to the vagina, rejection by the sexual partner, hostility toward men, and feelings of guilt regarding sexual impulses (Sadock et al, 2015). Various developmental factors may also have relevance to orgasmic dysfunction. Examples include negative messages about sexuality from family, religion and culture, unwanted sexual experiences, or punishment for childhood sexual experimentation (Donahey, 2016).

      Psychological factors are also associated with inhibited male orgasm (delayed ejaculation). In the primary disorder (in which the man has never experienced orgasm), the man often comes from a rigid, puritanical background. He perceives sex as sinful and the genitals as dirty, and he may have conscious or unconscious incest wishes and associated guilt (Sadock et al, 2015). In the case of secondary disorder (previously experienced orgasms that have now stopped), interpersonal difficulties are usually implicated. Premature (early) ejaculation may be related to a lack of physical awareness on the part of a sexually inexperienced man. The ability to control ejaculation occurs as a gradual maturing process with a sexual partner in which foreplay becomes more give-and-take "pleasuring" rather than strictly goal-oriented. The man becomes aware of the sensations and learns to delay the point of ejaculatory inevitability. Relationship problems such as a stressful marriage, negative cultural conditioning, anxiety over intimacy, and lack of comfort in the sexual relationship may also contribute to this disorder.
   c. **Sexual Pain Disorders:** Penetration disorders may occur after having experienced painful intercourse for any organic reason, after which involuntary constriction of the vagina occurs in anticipation and fear of recurring pain. The diagnosis

does not apply if the etiology is determined to be due to another medical condition. A variety of psychosocial factors have been identified in patients with sexual pain disorder. Clinicians report that frequently an individual with this disorder has been raised in a strict religious environment where sex was associated with sin (Sadock et al, 2015). Early traumatic sexual experiences (e.g., rape or incest) may also contribute to penetration disorder. Other etiological factors that may be important include painful childhood experiences with surgical, dental, or pelvic examination; phobias associated with pregnancy, sexually transmitted infections or cancer; and catastrophizing or fear of pain (Bergeron, Rosen, & Corsini-Munt, 2016; Dreyfus, 2012; King & Regan 2014; Sadock et al, 2015).

Symptomatology (Subjective and Objective Data)

1. Absence of sexual fantasies and desire for sexual activity.
2. Discrepancy between partners' levels of desire for sexual activity.
3. Inability to produce adequate lubrication for sexual activity.
4. Absence of a subjective sense of sexual excitement during sexual activity.
5. Failure to attain or maintain penile erection until completion of sexual activity.
6. Inability to achieve orgasm (in men, to ejaculate) following a period of sexual excitement judged adequate in intensity and duration to produce such a response.
7. Ejaculation occurs with minimal sexual stimulation or before, on, or shortly after penetration and before the individual wishes it.
8. Genital pain occurring before, during, or after sexual intercourse.
9. Fear or anxiety in anticipation of vaginal penetration, with tensing or tightening of the pelvic floor muscles.

Common Nursing Diagnoses and Interventions for Sexual Dysfunctions

(Interventions are applicable to various health-care settings, such as inpatient and partial hospitalization, community outpatient clinic, home health, and private practice.)

■ SEXUAL DYSFUNCTION

Definition: A state in which an individual experiences a change in sexual function during the sexual response phases of desire, excitation, and/or orgasm, which is viewed as unsatisfying, unrewarding, or inadequate (NANDA International [NANDA-I], 2018, p. 305)

Possible Contributing Factors ("related to")

Ineffectual or absent role models
Physical [or sexual] abuse
Psychosocial abuse
Values conflict
Lack of privacy
Lack of significant other
Altered body structure or function (pregnancy, recent childbirth, drugs, surgery, anomalies, disease process, trauma, radiation)
Misinformation or deficient knowledge
[Depression]
[Pregnancy phobia]
[Sexually transmitted disease phobia]
[Cancer phobia]
[Previous painful experience]
[Severe anxiety]
[Relationship difficulties]

Defining Characteristics ("evidenced by")

[Verbalization of problem:
  • Absence of desire for sexual activity
  • Absence of lubrication or subjective sense of sexual excitement during sexual activity
  • Failure to attain or maintain penile erection during sexual activity
  • Inability to achieve orgasm or ejaculation
  • Premature ejaculation
  • Genital pain during intercourse
  • Constriction of the vagina that prevents penile penetration]
Inability to achieve desired satisfaction

Goals/Objectives

Short-term Goals

1. The patient will identify stressors that may contribute to loss of sexual function within 1 week.
or
2. The patient will discuss pathophysiology of disease process that contributes to sexual dysfunction within 1 week.
For the patient with permanent dysfunction due to disease process:
3. The patient will verbalize willingness to seek professional assistance from a sex therapist in order to learn alternative ways of achieving sexual satisfaction with partner by (time is individually determined).

Long-term Goal

The patient will resume sexual activity at level satisfactory to self and partner by (time is individually determined).

Interventions With *Selected Rationales*

1. Assess the patient's sexual history and previous level of satisfaction in his or her sexual relationship. *This establishes a database from which to work and provides a foundation for goal setting.*
2. Assess the patient's perception of the problem. *The patient's idea of what constitutes a problem may differ from that of the nurse. It is the patient's perception on which the goals of care must be established.*
3. Help the patient determine time dimension associated with the onset of the problem and discuss what was happening in his or her life situation at that time. *Stress in all areas of life can affect sexual functioning. The patient may be unaware of correlation between stress and sexual dysfunction.*
4. Assess the patient's mood and level of energy. *Depression and fatigue decrease desire and enthusiasm for participation in sexual activity.*
5. Review medication regimen; observe for side effects. *Many medications can affect sexual functioning. Evaluation of the drug and the individual's response is important to ascertain whether the drug may be contributing to the problem.*
6. Encourage the patient to discuss the disease process that may be contributing to sexual dysfunction. Ensure that the patient is aware that alternative methods of achieving sexual satisfaction exist and can be learned through sex counseling if he or she and the partner desire to do so. *The patient may be unaware that satisfactory changes can be made in his or her sex life. He or she may also be unaware of the availability of sex counseling.*
7. Provide information regarding sexuality and sexual functioning. *Increasing knowledge and correcting misconceptions can decrease feelings of powerlessness and anxiety and facilitate problem resolution.*
8. Make a referral for additional counseling or sex therapy, if required. The patient may even request that an initial appointment be made for him or her. *Complex problems are likely to require assistance from an individual who is specially trained to treat problems related to sexuality. The patient and partner may be somewhat embarrassed to seek this kind of assistance. Support from a trusted nurse can provide the impetus for them to pursue the help they need.*

Outcome Criteria

1. The patient is able to correlate physical or psychosocial factors that interfere with sexual functioning.
2. The patient is able to communicate with partner about their sexual relationship without discomfort.
3. The patient and partner verbalize willingness and desire to seek assistance from a professional sex therapist.

or

4. The patient verbalizes resumption of sexual activity at level satisfactory to self and partner.

■ PARAPHILIC DISORDERS

Paraphilic disorders are characterized by recurrent and intense sexual arousal of at least 6 months' duration involving any of the following:

1. The preference for use of a nonhuman object.
2. Repetitive sexual activity with humans involving real or simulated suffering or humiliation.
3. Repetitive sexual activity with nonconsenting partners.

The individual has acted on these sexual urges, or the urges or fantasies cause clinically significant distress or impairment in social, occupational, or other important areas of functioning (APA, 2013). Many paraphilic behaviors are illegal sex acts, so an individual may come to the attention of legal authorities before he or she is introduced to psychiatric treatment for this disorder. It is not uncommon for individuals with paraphilias to exhibit multiple paraphilias (APA, 2013).

Types of paraphilic disorders include the following:

1. **Exhibitionistic Disorder:** The major symptoms include recurrent, intense sexual urges, behaviors, or sexually arousing fantasies, of at least 6 months' duration, involving the exposure of one's genitals to an unsuspecting stranger (APA, 2013). Masturbation may occur during the exhibitionism. Most individuals with exhibitionistic disorder are men, and the behavior is generally established in adolescence.
2. **Fetishistic Disorder:** Fetishistic disorder involves recurrent, intense sexual urges, behaviors, or sexually arousing fantasies, of at least 6 months' duration, involving the use of nonliving objects, a specific nongenital body part, or a combination of both (APA, 2013). Commonly, the sexual focus is on objects intimately associated with the human body (e.g., shoes, gloves, stockings) or on a nongenital body part (e.g., feet, hair). The fetish object is generally used during masturbation or incorporated into sexual activity with another person to produce sexual excitation.
3. **Frotteuristic Disorder:** This disorder is defined as the recurrent preoccupation with intense sexual urges or fantasies, of at least 6 months' duration, involving touching or rubbing against a nonconsenting person (APA, 2013). Sexual excitement is derived from the actual touching or rubbing, not from the coercive nature of the act. The disorder is significantly more common in men than in women.
4. **Pedophilic Disorder:** The *DSM-5* describes the essential feature of pedophilic disorder as recurrent sexual urges, behaviors, or sexually arousing fantasies, of at least 6 months' duration, involving sexual activity with a prepubescent child. The age of the molester is 16 years or older, and he or she is at least 5 years

older than the child. This category of paraphilic disorder is the most common of sexual assaults.

5. **Sexual Masochism Disorder:** The identifying feature of this disorder is recurrent, intense sexual urges, behaviors, or sexually arousing fantasies, of at least 6 months' duration, involving the act of being humiliated, beaten, bound, or otherwise made to suffer (APA, 2013). These masochistic activities may be fantasized, solitary, or with a partner. Examples include becoming sexually aroused by self-inflicted pain or by being restrained, raped, or beaten by a sexual partner.

6. **Sexual Sadism Disorder:** The essential feature of sexual sadism disorder is identified as recurrent, intense, sexual urges, behaviors, or sexually arousing fantasies, of at least 6 months' duration, of acts involving the psychological or physical suffering of another person (APA, 2013). The sadistic activities may be fantasized or acted on with a nonconsenting partner. In all instances, sexual excitation occurs in response to the suffering of the victim. Examples include rape, beating, torture, or even killing.

7. **Voyeuristic Disorder:** This disorder is identified by recurrent, intense sexual urges, behaviors, or sexually arousing fantasies, of at least 6 months' duration, involving the act of observing an unsuspecting person who is naked, in the process of disrobing, or engaging in sexual activity (APA, 2013). Sexual excitement is achieved through the act of looking, and no contact with the person is attempted. Masturbation usually accompanies the "window peeping" but may occur later as the individual fantasizes about the voyeuristic act.

8. **Transvestic Disorder:** This disorder involves recurrent and intense sexual arousal (as manifested by fantasies, urges, or behaviors of at least 6 months' duration) from dressing in the clothes of the opposite gender. The individual is commonly a heterosexual man who keeps a collection of women's clothing that he intermittently uses to dress in when alone. The sexual arousal may be produced by an accompanying fantasy of the individual as a woman with female genitalia or merely by the view of himself fully clothed as a woman without attention to the genitalia. Transvestism is identified as a *disorder* when it causes marked distress to the individual, or interferes with social, occupational, or other important areas of functioning.

Predisposing Factors to Paraphilic Disorders

1. Physiological
   a. **Biological:** Many studies have identified biologic abnormalities in individuals with paraphilias. Two common findings are that 74% have abnormal hormone levels and 24% have chromosomal abnormalities (Sadock et al, 2015).

Temporal lobe diseases, such as psychomotor seizures or tumors, have been implicated in some individuals with paraphilic disorder. Abnormal levels of androgens also may contribute to inappropriate sexual arousal. The majority of studies have involved violent sex offenders, and the results cannot accurately be generalized.

2. Psychosocial
   a. **Psychoanalytic Theory:** The psychoanalytic approach defines an individual with paraphilic disorder as one who has failed the normal developmental process toward heterosexual adjustment (Sadock et al, 2015). This occurs when the individual fails to resolve the Oedipal crisis and either identifies with the parent of the opposite gender or selects an inappropriate object for libido cathexis.
   b. **Behavioral Theory:** The behavioral model hypothesizes that whether or not an individual engages in paraphilic behavior depends on the type of reinforcement he or she receives following the behavior. The initial act may be committed for various reasons. Some examples include recalling memories of experiences from an individual's early life (especially the first shared sexual experience), modeling behavior of others who have carried out paraphilic acts, mimicking sexual behavior depicted in the media, and recalling past trauma, such as one's own molestation (Sadock et al, 2015).
   c. Once the initial act has been committed, the individual with paraphilic disorder consciously evaluates the behavior and decides whether to repeat it. A fear of punishment or perceived harm or injury to the victim, or a lack of pleasure derived from the experience, may extinguish the behavior. However, when negative consequences do not occur, when the act itself is highly pleasurable, or when the person with the paraphilic disorder immediately escapes and thereby avoids seeing any negative consequences experienced by the victim, the activity is more likely to be repeated.

Symptomatology (Subjective and Objective Data)

1. Exposure of one's genitals to a stranger.
2. Sexual arousal in the presence of nonliving objects.
3. Touching and rubbing one's genitals against a nonconsenting person.
4. Sexual attraction to or activity with a prepubescent child.
5. Sexual arousal from being humiliated, beaten, bound, or otherwise made to suffer (through fantasy, self-infliction, or by a sexual partner).
6. Sexual arousal by inflicting psychological or physical suffering on another individual (either consenting or nonconsenting).

7. Sexual arousal from dressing in the clothes of the opposite gender.
8. Sexual arousal from observing unsuspecting people either naked or engaged in sexual activity.
9. Masturbation often accompanies the activities described when they are performed solitarily.
10. The individual is markedly distressed by these activities.

Common Nursing Diagnoses for Patients With Paraphilic Disorders

(Interventions are applicable to various health-care settings, such as inpatient and partial hospitalization, community outpatient clinic, home health, and private practice.)

■ INEFFECTIVE SEXUALITY PATTERN

Definition: Expressions of concern regarding own sexuality (NANDA-I, 2018, p. 306)

Possible Contributing Factors ("related to")

Lack of significant other
Ineffective or absent role models
Conflicts with sexual orientation or variant preferences
[Delayed sexual adjustment]

Defining Characteristics ("evidenced by")

Reports difficulties, limitations, or changes in sexual behaviors or activities
[Expressed dissatisfaction with sexual behaviors]
[Reports that sexual arousal can only be achieved through variant practices, such as pedophilia, fetishism, masochism, sadism, frotteurism, exhibitionism, voyeurism]
[Desires to experience satisfying sexual relationship with another individual without need for arousal through variant practices]

Goals/Objectives

(Time elements to be determined by individual situation.)

Short-term Goals

1. The patient will verbalize aspects about sexuality that he or she would like to change.
2. The patient and partner will communicate with each other ways in which each believes their sexual relationship could be improved.

Long-term Goals

1. The patient will express satisfaction with own sexuality pattern.
2. The patient and partner will express satisfaction with sexual relationship.

Interventions With *Selected Rationales*

1. Take sexual history, noting the patient's expression of areas of dissatisfaction with his or her sexual pattern. *Knowledge of what the patient perceives as the problem is essential for providing the type of assistance he or she may need.*
2. Assess areas of stress in the patient's life and examine the relationship with his or her sexual partner. *Variant sexual behaviors are often associated with added stress in the patient's life. The relationship with his or her partner may deteriorate as individual eventually gains sexual satisfaction only from variant practices.*
3. Note cultural, social, ethnic, racial, and religious factors that may contribute to conflicts regarding variant sexual practices. *The patient may be unaware of the influence these factors exert in creating feelings of discomfort, shame, and guilt regarding sexual attitudes and behavior.*
4. Be accepting and nonjudgmental. *Sexuality is a very personal and sensitive subject. The patient is more likely to share this information if he or she does not fear being judged by the nurse.*
5. Assist the therapist in a plan of behavior modification to help the patient who desires to decrease variant sexual behaviors. *Individuals with paraphilic disorders are treated by specialists who have experience in modifying variant sexual behaviors. Nurses can intervene by providing assistance with implementation of the plan for behavior modification.*
6. Explain to the patient that sexuality is a normal human response and does not relate exclusively to the sex organs or sexual behavior. Sexuality involves complex interrelationships among one's self-concept, body image, personal history, family and cultural influences, and all interactions with others. *If the patient feels "abnormal" or very unlike everyone else, the self-concept is likely to be very low—he or she may even feel worthless. To promote feelings of self-worth and desire to change behavior, help him or her to understand that even though the behavior is variant, feelings and motivations are common.*

Outcome Criteria

1. The patient is able to verbalize fears about abnormality and inappropriateness of sexual behaviors.
2. The patient expresses desire to change variant sexual behavior and cooperates with plan of behavior modification.
3. The patient expresses satisfaction with own sexuality pattern or satisfying sexual relationship with another.

@ INTERNET REFERENCES

Additional information about sexual disorders and gender dysphoria may be located at the following Web sites:

- www.priory.com/sex.htm
- http://emedicine.medscape.com/article/293890-overview
- http://emedicine.medscape.com/article/291419-overview

Movie Connections

Mystic River (Pedophilic disorder) • *Blue Velvet* (Sexual masochism disorder) • *Looking for Mr. Goodbar* (Sadism/masochism disorders) • *Normal* (Transvestic disorder) • *Transamerica* (Gender dysphoria)

CHAPTER 13

Eating Disorders

■ BACKGROUND ASSESSMENT DATA

The *Diagnostic and Statistical Manual of Mental Disorders, Fifth Edition (DSM-5)* (American Psychiatric Association [APA], 2013), states that eating disorders are characterized by "a persistent disturbance of eating or eating-related behavior that results in the altered consumption or absorption of food and that significantly impairs physical health or psychosocial functioning" (p. 329). Three such disorders that are described in the *DSM-5* include anorexia nervosa, bulimia nervosa, and binge-eating disorder. Obesity is not classified as a psychiatric disorder per se; however, because of the strong emotional factors associated with it, it is suggested that obesity may be considered within the category of *Psychological Factors Affecting Medical Condition.* Obesity is also considered as a factor associated with binge-eating disorder.

Anorexia Nervosa

Defined

Anorexia nervosa is a clinical syndrome in which the person has a morbid fear of obesity. It is characterized by the individual's gross distortion of body image, preoccupation with food, and refusal to eat. The disorder occurs predominantly in females 12 to 30 years of age. Once thought to be rare among males, more recent data (Woolridge & Lemberg, 2016) identifies that men account for 25% of those with anorexia and bulimia and 36% of those with binge eating disorders. Without intervention, death from starvation can occur.

Symptomatology (Subjective and Objective Data)

1. Morbid fear of obesity. Preoccupied with body size. Reports "feeling fat" even when in an emaciated condition.
2. Refusal to eat. Reports "not being hungry," although it is thought that the actual feelings of hunger do not cease until late in the disorder.
3. Preoccupation with food. Thinks and talks about food at great length. Prepares enormous amounts of food for friends and family members but refuses to eat any of it. Amenorrhea is common, often appearing even before noticeable weight loss has occurred.

4. Other physical symptoms include hypothermia, bradycardia, hypotension with orthostatic changes, peripheral edema, metabolic changes, and lanugo (fine neonatal like hair growth).
5. Delayed psychosexual development.
6. Compulsive behavior, such as excessive hand washing, may be present.
7. Extensive exercising is common.
8. Feelings of depression and anxiety often accompany this disorder.
9. May engage in the binge-and-purge syndrome from time to time (see following section on bulimia nervosa).

Bulimia Nervosa

Defined

Bulimia nervosa is an eating disorder (commonly called the *binge-and-purge syndrome*) characterized by extreme overeating, followed by self-induced vomiting and abuse of laxatives and diuretics. The disorder occurs predominantly in females and begins in adolescence or early adult life.

Symptomatology (Subjective and Objective Data)

1. Binges are usually solitary and secret, and the individual may consume thousands of calories in one episode.
2. After the binge has begun, there is often a feeling of loss of control or inability to stop eating.
3. Following the binge, the individual engages in inappropriate compensatory measures to avoid gaining weight (e.g., self-induced vomiting; excessive use of laxatives, diuretics, or enemas; fasting; and extreme exercising).
4. Eating binges may be viewed as pleasurable but are followed by intense self-criticism and depressed mood.
5. Individuals with bulimia are usually within normal weight range—some a few pounds underweight, some a few pounds overweight.
6. Obsession with body image and appearance is a predominant feature of this disorder. Individuals with bulimia display undue concern with sexual attractiveness and how they will appear to others.
7. Binges usually alternate with periods of normal eating and fasting.
8. Excessive vomiting may lead to problems with dehydration and electrolyte imbalance.
9. Gastric acid in the vomitus may contribute to the erosion of tooth enamel.

Predisposing Factors to Anorexia Nervosa and Bulimia Nervosa

1. Physiological
   a. **Genetics:** A hereditary predisposition to eating disorders has been hypothesized on the basis of family histories and an apparent association with other disorders for which the

likelihood of genetic influences exist. Some studies identify higher concordance rates in monozygotic than in dizygotic twins (Sadock, Sadock, & Ruiz, 2015). Anorexia nervosa is more common among sisters of those with the disorder than among the general population. Family studies find that a history of anorexia nervosa confers up to 11 times the risk for family members (Call et al, 2017), and those with a family history of bulimia nervosa, mood disorders, substance use disorders, or obesity are at greater risk for developing bulimia.

b. **Neurobiological Influences:** Neurochemical influences in bulimia and anorexia nervosa may be associated with the neurotransmitters serotonin and norepinephrine. Neurobiological changes that occur in starvation, including depression and obsessional thinking, may contribute to maintaining the illness (Call et al, 2017). This hypothesis has been supported by the positive response these individuals have shown to therapy with the selective serotonin reuptake inhibitors (SSRIs). Some studies have found high levels of endogenous opioids in the spinal fluid of patients with anorexia, promoting the speculation that these chemicals may contribute to denial of hunger (Sadock et al, 2015). Some individuals with anorexia nervosa have been shown to gain weight when given naloxone, an opioid antagonist. Questions still remain as to whether neurochemical changes are causal or are an outcome of the body's reaction to changes in nutrition and mood.

2. Psychosocial

a. **Psychodynamic Theory:** Psychodynamic theories suggest that the development of an eating disorder is rooted in an unfulfilled sense of separation-individuation. When events occur that threaten the vulnerable ego, feelings of lack of control over one's body (self) emerge. Behaviors associated with food and eating provide feelings of control over one's life.

b. **Family Dynamics:** Historically, parents of children with eating disorders have been presumed to be overcontrolling and perfectionistic, causing pathology in their children. This theory has been problematic, at least in part, since not all siblings in the same family develop eating disorders. There is *not* sufficient evidence to support these claims, and they may have contributed to a resistance toward seeking health care based on parents' fear that they will be judged as "the cause of the problem." The Academy for Eating Disorders published a position statement (2009) that includes the following:

> The AED stands firmly against any model of eating disorders in which family influences are seen as the primary cause of eating disorders, condemns statements that blame families for

their child's illness, and recommends that families be included in the treatment of younger patients, unless this is clearly ill advised on clinical grounds.

Certainly conflicts arise in a family when a child is starving himself or herself, but it has become clear that family members need to be involved in treatment rather than shunned or blamed. Family-based approaches, such as the Maudsley approach, are supported by clinical evidence.

Obesity
Defined
The following formula is used to determine the degree of obesity in an individual:

$$\text{Body mass index (BMI)} = \frac{\text{weight (kg)}}{\text{height (m)}^2}$$

The BMI range for normal weight is 20 to 24.9. Studies by the National Center for Health Statistics indicate that *overweight* is defined as a BMI of 25.0 to 29.9 (based on U.S. Dietary Guidelines for Americans). Based on criteria of the World Health Organization, *obesity* is defined as a BMI of 30.0 or greater. These guidelines, which were released by the National Heart, Lung, and Blood Institute in July 1998, markedly increased the number of Americans considered to be overweight. The average American woman has a BMI of 26, and fashion models typically have BMIs of 18. Anorexia nervosa is characterized by a BMI of 17 or lower. In extreme anorexia nervosa, the BMI may be less than 15.

Binge-Eating Disorder
Binge-eating disorder is characterized by recurrent episodes of binge eating; that is, eating in a discrete period of time an excessive amount of food and feeling a sense that the episode of eating is beyond the individual's control. The eating usually takes place in isolation, and the individual feels disgusted with himself or herself, depressed, or very guilty afterward (APA, 2013). Binge-eating disorder differs from bulimia nervosa in that the individual does not engage in compensatory behaviors (e.g., self-induced vomiting, laxatives, diuretics) following the binge to rid the body of the excess calories. Therefore, obesity becomes a factor in the disorder.

The etiology of binge-eating disorder is unknown. Brain imaging studies of people with binge-eating disorder reveal increased activity in the orbitofrontal cortex, which are the centers associated with reward and pleasure responses such as those seen in response to substances of abuse (Balodis, Grilo, & Potenza, 2015). This finding has supported the hypothesis that binge-eating disorder may be an illness of addiction.

Obesity is known to contribute to a number of health problems, including hyperlipidemia, diabetes mellitus, osteoarthritis, and increased workload on the heart and lungs.

Predisposing Factors to Obesity

1. Physiological
   a. **Genetics:** Genetics have been implicated in the development of obesity in that 80% of offspring of two obese parents are obese (Sadock et al, 2015). This hypothesis has also been supported by studies of twins reared by normal-weight and overweight parents.
   b. **Physical:** Overeating and/or obesity have also been associated with lesions in the appetite and satiety centers of the hypothalamus, hypothyroidism, decreased insulin production in diabetes mellitus, and increased cortisone production in Cushing's disease.
   c. **Lifestyle:** On a more basic level, obesity can be viewed as the ingestion of a greater number of calories than are expended. Weight gain occurs when caloric intake exceeds caloric output in terms of basal metabolism and physical activity. Many overweight individuals lead sedentary lifestyles, making it very difficult to burn off calories.
2. Psychosocial
   a. **Psychoanalytic Theory:** This theory suggests that obesity is the result of unresolved dependency needs, with the individual being fixed in the oral stage of psychosexual development. The symptoms of obesity are viewed as depressive equivalents, attempts to regain "lost" or frustrated nurturance and caring. Obesity is often comorbid with eating disorders, especially binge-eating disorder, as well as substance use disorders, schizophrenia, mood and anxiety disorders, personality disorders, and others (Sadock et al, 2015).

Common Nursing Diagnoses and Interventions (for Anorexia Nervosa and Bulimia Nervosa)

(Interventions are applicable to various health-care settings, such as inpatient and partial hospitalization, community outpatient clinic, home health, and private practice.)

■ IMBALANCED NUTRITION: LESS THAN BODY REQUIREMENTS

Definition: Intake of nutrients insufficient to meet metabolic needs (NANDA International [NANDA-I], 2018, p. 157)

Possible Contributing Factors ("related to")

[Refusal to eat]
[Ingestion of large amounts of food, followed by self-induced vomiting]
[Abuse of laxatives, diuretics, and/or diet pills]
[Physical exertion in excess of energy produced through caloric intake]

Defining Characteristics ("evidenced by")

[Loss of 15% of expected body weight (anorexia nervosa)]
Pale mucous membranes
Poor muscle tone
Excessive loss of hair [or increased growth of hair on body (lanugo)]
[Amenorrhea]
[Poor skin turgor]
[Electrolyte imbalances]
[Hypothermia]
[Bradycardia]
[Hypotension]
[Cardiac irregularities]
[Edema]

Goals/Objectives

Short-term Goal

The patient will gain _____ pounds per week (amount to be established by the patient, nurse, and dietitian).

Long-term Goal

By time of discharge from treatment, the patient will exhibit no signs or symptoms of malnutrition.

Interventions With *Selected Rationales*

1. If the patient is unable or unwilling to maintain adequate oral intake, physician may order a liquid diet to be administered via nasogastric tube. Nursing care of the individual receiving tube feedings should be administered according to established hospital procedures. *The patient's physical safety is a nursing priority, and without adequate nutrition, a life-threatening situation exists.*

For oral diet:

2. In collaboration with dietitian, determine number of calories required to provide adequate nutrition and realistic (according to body structure and height) weight gain. *Adequate calories are required to affect a weight gain of 2 to 3 pounds per week.*

3. Monitor lab values for phosphate, potassium, calcium, and magnesium while nutrition is being restored. **Refeeding syndrome,** a series of negative intracellular electrolyte shifts associated with aggressive renourishment in a malnourished patient, poses a risk for hypophosphatemia, hypokalemia, hypocalcemia, and hypomagnesemia. Cardiovascular collapse, arrhythmias, altered mental status, and death can occur in untreated refeeding syndrome. Electrolyte supplementation may be indicated (Toulany & Katzman, 2019).

4. Explain to the patient details of behavior modification program as outlined by physician. Explain benefits of compliance with prandial routine and consequences for noncompliance. *Behavior modification bases privileges granted or restricted directly on weight gain and loss. Focus is placed on emotional issues rather than on food and eating specifically.*

5. Sit with the patient during mealtimes for support and to observe amount ingested. A limit (usually 30 minutes) should be imposed on time allotted for meals. *Without a time limit, meals can become lengthy, drawn-out sessions, providing the patient with attention based on food and eating.*

6. The patient should be observed for at least 1 hour following meals. *This time may be used by the patient to discard food stashed from tray or to engage in self-induced vomiting.*

7. The patient may need to be accompanied to bathroom *if self-induced vomiting is suspected.*

8. Strict documentation of intake and output. *This information is required to promote patient safety and plan nursing care.*

9. Weigh the patient daily immediately on arising and following first voiding. Always use same scale, if possible. *Patient care, privileges, and restrictions will be based on accurate daily weights.* If weight loss occurs, enforce restrictions. *Restrictions and limits must be established and carried out consistently to avoid power struggles and to encourage patient compliance with therapy.*

10. Do not discuss food or eating with the patient once protocol has been established. However, do offer support and positive reinforcement for obvious improvements in eating behaviors. *Discussing food with the patient provides positive feedback for maladaptive behaviors.*

11. The patient must understand that if, because of poor oral intake, nutritional status deteriorates, tube feedings will be initiated to ensure the patient's safety. *Staff must be consistent and firm with this action, using a matter-of-fact, nonpunitive approach regarding the tube insertion and subsequent feedings.*

12. As nutritional status improves and eating habits are established, begin to explore with the patient the feelings associated with his or her extreme fear of gaining weight. *Emotional issues must be resolved if maladaptive responses are to be eliminated.*

Outcome Criteria

1. The patient has achieved and maintained at least 85% of expected body weight.
2. Vital signs, blood pressure, and laboratory serum studies are within normal limits.
3. The patient verbalizes importance of adequate nutrition.

■ DEFICIENT FLUID VOLUME

Definition: Decreased intravascular, interstitial, and/or intracellular fluid. This refers to dehydration, water loss alone without change in sodium (NANDA-I, 2018, p. 184)

Possible Contributing Factors ("related to")

[Decreased fluid intake]
[Abnormal fluid loss caused by self-induced vomiting]
[Excessive use of laxatives or enemas]
[Excessive use of diuretics]
[Electrolyte or acid-base imbalance brought about by malnourished condition or self-induced vomiting]

Defining Characteristics ("evidenced by")

Decreased urine output
Increased urine concentration
Elevated hematocrit
Decreased blood pressure
Increased pulse rate
Increased body temperature
Dry skin
Decreased skin turgor
Weakness
Change in mental status
Dry mucous membranes

Goals/Objectives

Short-term Goal

The patient will drink 125 mL of fluid each hour during waking hours.

Long-term Goal

By time of discharge from treatment, the patient will exhibit no signs or symptoms of dehydration (as evidenced by quantity of urinary output sufficient to the individual patient; normal specific gravity; vital signs within normal limits; moist, pink mucous membranes; good skin turgor; and immediate capillary refill).

Interventions With *Selected Rationales*

1. Keep strict record of intake and output. Teach the patient the importance of daily fluid intake of 2000 to 3000 mL. *This information is required to promote patient safety and plan nursing care.*

2. Weigh the patient daily immediately on arising and following first voiding. Always use same scale, if possible. *An accurate daily weight is needed to plan nursing care for the patient.*

3. Assess and document the condition of skin turgor and any changes in skin integrity. *Condition of the skin provides valuable data regarding patient hydration.*

4. Discourage the patient from bathing every day if skin is very dry. *Hot water and soap are drying to the skin.*

5. Monitor laboratory serum values and vital signs, and notify physician of significant alterations. *Laboratory data and vital signs (temperature, pulse, blood pressure, and respirations) provide an objective measure for evaluating adequate hydration.*

6. The patient should be observed for at least 1 hour following meals and may need to be accompanied to the bathroom if self-induced vomiting is suspected. *Vomiting causes active loss of body fluids and can precipitate fluid volume deficit.*

7. Assess and document moistness and color of oral mucous membranes. *Dry, pale mucous membranes may be indicative of malnutrition or dehydration.*

8. Encourage frequent oral care *to moisten mucous membranes, reducing discomfort from dry mouth, and to decrease bacterial count, minimizing risk of tissue infection.*

9. Help the patient identify true feelings and fears that contribute to maladaptive eating behaviors. *Emotional issues must be resolved if maladaptive behaviors are to be eliminated.*

Outcome Criteria

1. The patient's vital signs, blood pressure, and laboratory serum studies are within normal limits.

2. No abnormalities of skin turgor and dryness of skin and oral mucous membranes are evident.

3. The patient verbalizes knowledge regarding consequences of fluid loss due to self-induced vomiting and importance of adequate fluid intake.

■ INEFFECTIVE ADOLESCENT EATING DYNAMICS

Definition: Altered eating attitudes and behaviors resulting in over or under eating patterns that compromise nutritional health (NANDA-I, 2018, p. 163)

Possible Contributing Factors ("related to")

[Delayed ego development]
[Unfulfilled tasks of trust and autonomy]
Altered family dynamics
Depression
Eating disorder
Anxiety
Media influence on eating behaviors [and perpetuation of unhealthy
    expectations for body image]
Media influence on knowledge of high-caloric unhealthy foods
[Unmet dependency needs]
[Feelings of helplessness and lack of control in life situation]
[Possible chemical imbalance caused by malfunction of hypo-
    thalamus]
[Unrealistic perceptions]

Defining Characteristics ("evidenced by")

[Preoccupation with extreme fear of obesity, and distortion of own
    body image]
[Refusal to eat]
[Obsessed with talking about food]
[Compulsive behavior (e.g., excessive hand washing)]
[Excessive overeating, followed by self-induced vomiting and/or
    abuse of laxatives and diuretics]
Frequently eating processed and fast foods
[Poor self-esteem]
[Chronic fatigue]
Minimizes symptoms

Goals/Objectives

Short-term Goal

The patient will verbalize understanding of the correlation be-
    tween emotional issues and maladaptive eating behaviors
    (within time deemed appropriate for individual patient).

Long-term Goal

By time of discharge from treatment, the patient will demonstrate
    the ability to discontinue use of maladaptive eating behaviors
    and to cope with emotional issues in a more adaptive manner.

Interventions With *Selected Rationales*

1. Establish a trusting relationship with the patient by being honest, accepting, and available and by keeping all promises. Convey unconditional positive regard. *The therapeutic nurse-patient
   relationship is built on trust.*

2. Acknowledge the patient's anger at feelings of loss of control brought about by the established eating regimen associated with the program of behavior modification. *Anger is a normal human response and should be expressed in an appropriate manner. Feelings that are not expressed remain unresolved and add an additional component to an already serious situation.*

3. When nutritional status has improved, begin to explore with the patient the feelings associated with his or her extreme fear of gaining weight. *Emotional issues must be resolved if maladaptive behaviors are to be eliminated.*

4. Avoid arguing or bargaining with the patient who is resistant to treatment. State matter-of-factly which behaviors are unacceptable and how privileges will be restricted for noncompliance. *It is essential that all staff members are consistent with this intervention if positive change is to occur.*

5. Explore family dynamics. Involve the family in treatment as much as possible and as appropriate. *Family-based approaches to treatment such as the Maudsley approach have demonstrated efficacy in treating anorexia nervosa in children and adolescents. The patient must recognize how maladaptive eating behaviors are related to emotional problems and impact family dynamics.*

6. Explore with the patient ways in which he or she may feel in control within the environment without resorting to maladaptive eating behaviors. *When the patient feels control over major life issues, the need to gain control through maladaptive eating behaviors will diminish.*

7. Educate families about dangers associated with adolescent's unmonitored use of internet sites. *Several internet sites dedicated to unhealthy eating behaviors not only describe ways to accomplish rapid weight loss but also how to conceal weight loss from health-care professionals (e.g., drinking lots of fluids before getting weighed or adding weights to pocketed garments).*

Outcome Criteria

1. The patient verbalizes understanding of the correlation between emotional issues and maladaptive eating behaviors.

2. The patient demonstrates the use of adaptive coping strategies unrelated to eating behaviors.

■ ANXIETY (Moderate to Severe)

Definition: Vague uneasy feeling of discomfort or dread accompanied by an autonomic response (the source often nonspecific or unknown to the individual); a feeling of apprehension caused by anticipation of danger. It is an alerting signal that warns of impending danger and enables the individual to take measures to deal with that threat (NANDA-I, 2018, p. 324)

Possible Contributing Factors ("related to")

Situational and maturational crises
[Unmet dependency needs]
[Low self-esteem]
[Feelings of helplessness and lack of control in life situation]
[Unfulfilled tasks of trust and autonomy]

Defining Characteristics ("evidenced by")

Increased tension
Increased helplessness
Overexcited
Apprehensive; fearful
Restlessness
Poor eye contact
[Increased difficulty taking oral nourishment]
[Inability to learn]

Goals/Objectives

Short-term Goal

The patient will demonstrate use of relaxation techniques to maintain anxiety at manageable level within 1 week.

Long-term Goal

By time of discharge from treatment, the patient will be able to recognize events that precipitate anxiety and intervene to prevent disabling behaviors.

Interventions With *Selected Rationales*

1. Be available to stay with the patient. Remain calm and provide reassurance of safety. *Patient safety and security is a nursing priority.*
2. Help the patient identify the situation that precipitated onset of anxiety symptoms. *The patient may be unaware that emotional issues are related to symptoms of anxiety. Recognition may be the first step in elimination of this maladaptive response.*
3. Review the patient's methods of coping with similar situations in the past. *In seeking to create change, it is helpful for the patient to identify past responses and determine whether they were successful and whether they could be employed again. Patient strengths should be identified and used to his or her advantage.*
4. Provide quiet environment. Reduce stimuli: low lighting, few people. *Anxiety level may be decreased in calm atmosphere with few stimuli.*
5. Administer antianxiety medications, as ordered by physician. Monitor for effectiveness of medication as well as for adverse side effects. *Short-term use of antianxiety medications (e.g., lorazepam, chlordiazepoxide, alprazolam) provides relief from the*

immobilizing effects of anxiety and facilitates the patient's cooperation with therapy.
6. Teach the patient to recognize signs of increasing anxiety and ways to intervene for maintaining the anxiety at a manageable level (e.g., exercise, walking, jogging, relaxation techniques). *Anxiety and tension can be reduced safely and with benefit to the patient through physical activities and relaxation techniques.*

Outcome Criteria

1. The patient is able to verbalize events that precipitate anxiety and demonstrate techniques for its reduction.
2. The patient is able to verbalize ways in which he or she may gain more control of the environment and thereby reduce feelings of helplessness.

■ DISTURBED BODY IMAGE/LOW SELF-ESTEEM

Definition: Disturbed body image is defined as confusion in mental picture of one's physical self (NANDA-I, 2018, p. 276). Low self-esteem is defined as negative evaluation and/or feelings about one's own capabilities (pp. 272–275)

Possible Contributing Factors ("related to")

[Lack of positive feedback]
[Perceived failures]
[Unrealistic expectations (on the part of self and others)]
[Delayed ego development]
[Unmet dependency needs]
[Morbid fear of obesity]
[Perceived loss of control in some aspect of life]

Defining Characteristics ("evidenced by")

[Distorted body image, views self as fat, even in the presence of normal body weight or severe emaciation]
[Denial that problem with low body weight exists]
[Difficulty accepting positive reinforcement]
[Not taking responsibility for self-care (self-neglect)]
[Nonparticipation in therapy]
[Self-destructive behavior (self-induced vomiting; abuse of laxatives or diuretics; refusal to eat)]
Lack of eye contact
[Depressed mood and self-deprecating thoughts following episode of binging and purging]
[Preoccupation with appearance and how others perceive them]

Goals/Objectives

Short-term Goal

The patient will verbally acknowledge misperception of body image as "fat" within specified time (depending on severity and chronicity of condition).

Long-term Goal

The patient will demonstrate an increase in self-esteem as manifested by verbalizing positive aspects of self and exhibiting less preoccupation with own appearance as a more realistic body image is developed by time of discharge from therapy.

Interventions With *Selected Rationales*

1. Help the patient reexamine negative perceptions of self and recognize positive attributes. Encourage reframing of irrational thinking about body image and self-worth. *The patient's own identification of strengths and positive attributes can increase sense of self-worth.*

2. Offer positive reinforcement for independently made decisions influencing the patient's life. *Positive reinforcement enhances self-esteem and may encourage the patient to continue functioning more independently.*

3. Offer positive reinforcement when honest feelings related to autonomy and dependence issues remain separated from maladaptive eating behaviors.

4. Help the patient develop a realistic perception of body image and relationship with food. *The patient needs to recognize that his or her perception of body image is unhealthy and that maintaining control through maladaptive eating behaviors is dangerous—even life threatening.*

5. Promote feelings of control within the environment through participation and independent decision making. Through positive feedback, help the patient learn to accept self as is, including weaknesses as well as strengths. *The patient must come to understand that he or she is a capable, autonomous individual who can perform outside the family unit and who is not expected to be perfect. Control of his or her life must be achieved in other ways besides dieting and weight loss.*

6. Help the patient realize that perfection is unrealistic, and explore this need with him or her. *As the patient begins to feel better about self, identifies positive self-attributes, and develops the ability to accept certain personal inadequacies, the need for unrealistic achievements should diminish.*

7. Help the patient claim ownership of angry feelings and recognize that expressing them is acceptable if done so in an appropriate manner. Be an effective role model. *Unexpressed anger is often turned inward on the self, resulting in depreciation of self-esteem.*

Outcome Criteria

1. The patient is able to verbalize positive aspects about self.
2. The patient expresses interest in welfare of others and less preoccupation with own appearance.
3. The patient verbalizes that image of body as "fat" was misperception and demonstrates ability to take control of own life without resorting to maladaptive eating behaviors.

Common Nursing Diagnoses and Interventions (for Obesity)

(Interventions are applicable to various health-care settings, such as inpatient and partial hospitalization, community outpatient clinic, home health, and private practice.)

■ OBESITY

Definition: A condition in which an individual accumulates excessive fat for age and gender that exceeds overweight (NANDA-I, 2018, p. 169)

Possible Contributing Factors ("related to")

[Compulsive eating]
Excessive intake in relation to metabolic needs
[Sedentary lifestyle]
[Genetics]
[Unmet dependency needs—fixation in oral developmental stage]

Defining Characteristics ("evidenced by")

Weight 20% over ideal for height and frame
[Body mass index of 30 or more]

Goals/Objectives

Short-term Goal

The patient will verbalize understanding of what must be done to lose weight.

Long-term Goal

The patient will demonstrate change in eating patterns resulting in a steady weight loss.

Interventions With *Selected Rationales*

1. Encourage the patient to keep a diary of food intake. *A food diary provides the opportunity for the patient to gain a realistic picture of the amount of food ingested and provides data on which to base the dietary program.*

2. Discuss feelings and emotions associated with eating. *This helps to identify when the patient is eating to satisfy an emotional need rather than a physiological one.*

3. With input from the patient, formulate an eating plan that includes food from the required food groups with emphasis on low-fat intake. It is helpful to keep the plan as similar to the patient's usual eating pattern as possible. *Diet must eliminate calories while maintaining adequate nutrition. The patient is more likely to stay on the eating plan if he or she is able to participate in its creation and if it deviates as little as possible from usual types of foods.*

4. Identify realistic increment goals for weekly weight loss. *Reasonable weight loss (1 to 2 pounds per week) results in more lasting effects. Excessive, rapid weight loss may result in fatigue and irritability and may ultimately lead to failure in meeting goals for weight loss. Motivation is more easily sustained by meeting "stair-step" goals.*

5. Plan a progressive exercise program tailored to individual goals and choice. *Exercise may enhance weight loss by burning calories and reducing appetite, increasing energy, toning muscles, and enhancing a sense of well-being and accomplishment. Walking is an excellent choice for overweight individuals.*

6. Discuss the probability of reaching plateaus when weight remains stable for extended periods. *The patient should know that this is likely to happen as changes in metabolism occur. Plateaus cause frustration, and the patient may need additional support during these times to remain on the weight-loss program.*

7. Provide instruction about medications to assist with weight loss if ordered by the physician. *Appetite-suppressant drugs (e.g., lorcaserin, phentermine) and others that have weight loss as a side effect (e.g., fluoxetine, topiramate) may be helpful to someone who is severely overweight. Drugs should be used for this purpose for only a short period while the individual attempts to adjust to the new pattern of eating.*

Outcome Criteria

1. The patient has established a healthy pattern of eating for weight control with weight loss progressing toward a desired goal.

2. The patient verbalizes plans for future maintenance of weight control.

■ DISTURBED BODY IMAGE/LOW SELF-ESTEEM

Definition: Disturbed body image is defined as confusion in mental picture of one's physical self (NANDA-I, 2018, p. 276). Low self-esteem is defined as negative evaluation and/or feelings about one's own capabilities (pp. 272–275)

Possible Contributing Factors ("related to")

Altered self-perception
Impaired psychosocial functioning
Exposure to trauma
[Dissatisfaction with appearance]
[Unmet dependency needs]

Defining Characteristics ("evidenced by")

Negative feelings about body (e.g., feelings of helplessness, hopelessness, or powerlessness)
[Verbalization of desire to lose weight]
[Failure to take responsibility for self-care (self-neglect)]
Lack of eye contact
[Expressions of low self-worth]

Goals/Objectives

Short-term Goal

The patient will begin to accept self based on self-attributes rather than on appearance.

Long-term Goal

The patient will pursue loss of weight as desired.

Interventions With *Selected Rationales*

1. Assess the patient's feelings and attitudes about being obese. *Obesity and compulsive eating behaviors may have deep-rooted psychological implications, such as compensation for lack of love and nurturing or a defense against intimacy.*
2. Ensure that the patient has privacy during self-care activities. *The obese individual may be sensitive or self-conscious about his or her body.*
3. Have the patient recall coping patterns related to food in family of origin, and explore how these may affect current situation. *Parents are role models for their children. Maladaptive eating behaviors are learned within the family system and are supported through positive reinforcement. Food may be substituted by the parent for affection and love, and eating is associated with a feeling of satisfaction, becoming the primary defense.*
4. Determine the patient's motivation for weight loss and set goals. *The individual may harbor repressed feelings of hostility, which may be expressed inward on the self. Because of a poor self-concept, the person often has difficulty with relationships. When the motivation is to lose weight for someone else, successful weight loss is less likely to occur.*
5. Help the patient identify positive self-attributes. Focus on strengths and past accomplishments unrelated to physical

appearance. *It is important that self-esteem not be tied solely to size of the body. The patient needs to recognize that obesity need not interfere with positive feelings regarding self-concept and self-worth.*
6. Refer the patient to a support or therapy group. *Support groups can provide companionship, increase motivation, decrease loneliness and social ostracism, and give practical solutions to common problems. Group therapy can be helpful in dealing with underlying psychological concerns.*

Outcome Criteria

1. The patient verbalizes self-attributes not associated with physical appearance.
2. The patient attends regular support group for social interaction and for assistance with weight management.

@ INTERNET REFERENCES

Additional information about anorexia nervosa, bulimia nervosa, and binge-eating disorder may be located at the following Web sites:

- www.anad.org
- http://healthymindsnetwork.org/research
- https://www.nationaleatingdisorders.org
- https://www.nimh.nih.gov/health/publications/eating-disorders/index.shtml
- https://medlineplus.gov/eatingdisorders.html
- http://www.mayoclinic.org/diseases-conditions/binge-eating-disorder/home/ovc-20182926
- https://www.eatingdisorderhope.com/information/help-overcome-eating-disorders/beda
- https://psychcentral.com/disorders/eating_disorders

Additional information about obesity may be located at the following Web sites:

- https://shapeupus.org
- www.obesity.org
- https://medlineplus.gov/obesity.html
- https://obesitymedicine.org/
- https://www.niddk.nih.gov/health-information/weight-management/binge-eating-disorder

Movie Connections

The Best Little Girl in the World (Anorexia nervosa)
• *Kate's Secret* (Bulimia nervosa) • *For the Love of Nancy* (Anorexia nervosa)
• *Super Size Me* (Obesity) • *To the Bone* (Anorexia nervosa)

CHAPTER 14

Personality Disorders

■ BACKGROUND ASSESSMENT DATA

The *Diagnostic and Statistical Manual of Mental Disorders, Fifth Edition (DSM-5)* (American Psychiatric Association [APA], 2013), defines *personality disorder* as "an enduring pattern of inner experience and behavior that deviates markedly from the expectations of the individual's culture, is pervasive and inflexible, has an onset in adolescence or early adulthood, is stable over time, and leads to distress or impairment" (p. 645). The most common symptoms occurring in personality disorders are impairment in interpersonal relationship functions (41%), dysfunctions in cognition (30%), affect (18%), and impulse control (6%) (Bornstein et al, 2014).

The *DSM-5* groups the personality disorders into three clusters. These clusters, and the disorders classified under each, are described as follows:

1. **Cluster A:** Behaviors described as odd or eccentric
   a. Paranoid personality disorder
   b. Schizoid personality disorder
   c. Schizotypal personality disorder
2. **Cluster B:** Behaviors described as dramatic, emotional, or erratic
   a. Antisocial personality disorder
   b. Borderline personality disorder (BPD)
   c. Histrionic personality disorder
   d. Narcissistic personality disorder
3. **Cluster C:** Behaviors described as anxious or fearful
   a. Avoidant personality disorder
   b. Dependent personality disorder
   c. Obsessive-compulsive personality disorder

A description of these personality disorders is presented in the following sections.

1. Cluster A
   a. **Paranoid Personality Disorder:** The essential feature is a pervasive and unwarranted suspiciousness and mistrust of people. There is a general expectation of being exploited or harmed by others in some way. Symptoms include guardedness in relationships with others, pathological jealousy, hypersensitivity, inability to relax, lack of emotion, and lack of

a sense of humor. These individuals are very critical of others but have much difficulty accepting criticism themselves.

b. **Schizoid Personality Disorder:** This disorder is characterized by an inability to form close, personal relationships; often seen by others as eccentric, isolated, or lonely (Sadock, Sadock, & Ruiz, 2015). Symptoms include social isolation; absence of warm, tender feelings for others; indifference to praise, criticism, or the feelings of others; and flat, dull affect (appears cold and aloof).

c. **Schizotypal Personality Disorder:** This disorder is characterized by peculiarities of ideation, appearance, and behavior and by deficits in interpersonal relatedness that are not severe enough to meet the criteria for schizophrenia. Schizotypal personality is marked by symptoms that look more like schizophrenia than those in schizoid personality in that the former individuals show significant peculiarities in thinking, behavior, and appearance. Symptoms include magical thinking; ideas of reference; social isolation; illusions; odd speech patterns; aloof, cold, suspicious behavior; and undue social anxiety.

2. Cluster B

a. **Antisocial Personality Disorder:** This disorder is characterized by a pattern of socially irresponsible, exploitative, and guiltless behavior, as evidenced by the tendency to fail to conform to the law, to sustain consistent employment, to exploit and manipulate others for personal gain, to deceive, and to fail to develop stable relationships. The individual must be at least 18 years of age and have a history of conduct disorder before the age of 15. The *DSM-5* currently identifies antisocial personality and psychopathy as synonymous terms, but recent research reveals that these are better understood as distinct disorders (Hatchett, 2015; Thompson, Ramos, & Willett, 2014). Substance use disorder is commonly identified as a comorbid disorder. (Symptoms of this disorder are identified later in this chapter, along with predisposing factors and nursing care.)

b. **Borderline Personality Disorder:** BPD is characterized by a pattern of intense and chaotic relationships, with affective instability and fluctuating attitudes toward other people. These individuals are impulsive, are directly and indirectly self-destructive, and lack a clear sense of identity. (Symptoms of this disorder are identified later in this chapter, along with predisposing factors and nursing care.)

c. **Histrionic Personality Disorder:** The essential feature of this disorder is described by the *DSM-5* as a "pervasive pattern of excessive emotionality and attention-seeking behavior" (APA, 2013, p. 667). Individuals with histrionic personality disorder often exhibit seductive, flirtatious behavior in efforts to reassure themselves of their attractiveness and to gain approval. Symptoms include exaggerated expression of emotions, incessant drawing of attention to oneself, overreaction to minor events, constantly seeking approval from others, egocentricity, vain and demanding behavior, extreme concern with physical appearance, and inappropriately sexually seductive appearance or behavior.

  d. **Narcissistic Personality Disorder:** This disorder is characterized by a grandiose sense of self-importance; preoccupation with fantasies of success, power, brilliance, beauty, or ideal love; a constant need for admiration and attention; exploitation of others for fulfillment of own desires; lack of empathy; response to criticism or failure with indifference or humiliation and rage; and preoccupation with feelings of envy.

3. Cluster C

  a. **Avoidant Personality Disorder:** This disorder is characterized by social withdrawal brought about by extreme sensitivity to rejection. Symptoms include unwillingness to enter into relationships unless given unusually strong guarantees of uncritical acceptance; low self-esteem; and social withdrawal in spite of a desire for affection and acceptance. Depression and anxiety are common. Social phobia may be a complication of this disorder.

  b. **Dependent Personality Disorder:** Individuals with this disorder passively allow others to assume responsibility for major areas of life because of their inability to function independently. They lack self-confidence, are unable to make decisions, perceive themselves as helpless and stupid, possess fear of being alone or abandoned, and seek constant reassurance and approval from others.

  c. **Obsessive-Compulsive Personality Disorder:** This disorder is characterized by a pervasive pattern of perfectionism and inflexibility. Interpersonal relationships have a formal and serious quality, and others often perceive these individuals as stilted or "stiff." Other symptoms include difficulty expressing tender feelings, insistence that others submit to his or her way of doing things, excessive devotion to work and productivity to the exclusion of pleasure, indecisiveness, perfectionism, preoccupation with details, depressed mood, and being judgmental of self and others. Recurrent obsessions and compulsions are absent in this personality disorder, and patients who present with such symptoms are diagnosed with obsessive-compulsive *disorder* rather than obsessive compulsive *personality disorder* (Sadock et al, 2015).

The behaviors associated with personality disorders may be manifested by virtually anyone from time to time. It is only when personality traits or styles are pervasive, repeatedly interfere with an individual's ability to function within age-appropriate cultural and developmental expectations, disrupt interpersonal relationships, and distort a person's pattern of perception and thinking about the environment that a diagnosis of personality disorder is assigned.

Individuals with personality disorders may be encountered in all types of treatment settings. They are not often treated in acute care settings, but because suicide ideation and attempts are common in the individual with BPD, hospitalization is necessary from time to time. The individual with antisocial personality disorder also may be hospitalized as an alternative to imprisonment when a legal determination is made that psychiatric intervention may be helpful. Since hospitalization may occur for patients with borderline or antisocial personality disorder, suggestions for inpatient care are included in this chapter. The interventions may be used in other types of treatment settings as well. Since personality disorder symptoms and behaviors interfere with communication and relationship building, the nurse's use of clear communication skills, a nonjudgmental approach, and the ability to maintain professional and therapeutic boundaries is essential.

■ BORDERLINE PERSONALITY DISORDER

Defined

This personality disorder is characterized by instability of affect, behavior, object relationships, and self-image. The term *borderline* came into being because these patients' emotionally unstable behavior seems to fall *on the border* between neurotic and psychotic. Transient psychotic symptoms appear during periods of extreme stress. The disorder is diagnosed more commonly in women than in men.

Predisposing Factors to Borderline Personality Disorder

1. Physiological
   a. **Biochemical:** Patients with BPD have a high incidence of major depressive episodes, and antidepressants have demonstrated benefits in some cases (Sadock et al, 2015). This fact and supporting information from brain imaging studies have led to the hypothesis that serotonin and/or norepinephrine dysregulation may contribute to the development of BPD. As stated elsewhere, questions remain about whether these dysfunctions contribute to the development of such disorders or whether they are a neurochemical response to intense emotional states.
   b. **Genetics:** An increased prevalence of major depression and substance use disorders in first-degree relatives of individuals with borderline personality suggest that there may be complex genetic vulnerabilities as well as environmental influences (Sadock et al, 2015). Patients with BPD are five times more likely to have a first-degree relative with BPD, and many studies have shown personality traits such as impulsivity, affect lability, and neuroticism to be heritable traits (MacIntosh,

Godbout, & Dubash, 2015). Borderline personality disorder shares many common features with bipolar disorder, including that they share the same genetic variances (Rodriguez, 2017). Epigenetic studies have identified changes to the oxytocin system (related to being a carrier of a specific allele) as associated with negative perceptions of others, increased stress markers, decreased empathy, confidence, and positivity (Pier et al, 2016). Treatment with oxytocin has demonstrated some benefits but requires more research.

c. **Neurobiological:** Magnetic resonance imaging studies to assess anatomical and functional activities in the brain have identified several factors associated with BPD. Decreases in the volume of the left amygdala and right hippocampus are apparent. The left amygdala, left hippocampus, and posterior cingulate cortex show heightened activation and the prefrontal cortex shows decreased activation during the processing of negative emotions (Pier et al, 2016).

2. Psychosocial

a. **Childhood Trauma:** Studies have shown that many individuals with BPD were raised in families with chaotic environments. Lubit (2013) states, "Risk factors [for BPD] include family environments characterized by trauma, neglect, and/or separation; exposure to sexual and physical abuse; and serious parental psychopathology such as substance abuse and antisocial personality disorder." Seventy percent of patients with BPD report a history of physical and/or sexual abuse (Gunderson, 2011). In some instances, this disorder has been likened to post-traumatic stress disorder (PTSD) in response to childhood trauma and abuse. Ford and Courtois (2014) cite several studies identifying a 30% to 40% comorbidity of PTSD and BPD and a prevalence of about 85% of those diagnosed with BPD having been initially diagnosed with PTSD. However, the BPD symptoms persisted after remission of PTSD symptoms. As mentioned previously, borderline personality disorder also shares many common symptoms with bipolar disorder and a history of childhood trauma is commonly found in both. Comorbid substance use disorders may also complicate the differentiation of symptoms and treatment needs. Thorough assessment to identify the multiple psychosocial influences in BPD is clearly essential.

b. **Theory of Object Relations:** According to Mahler's theory of object relations (Mahler, Pine, & Bergman, 1975), the infant passes through six phases from birth to 36 months, when a sense of separateness from the parenting figure is finally established (see Appendix A). Between the ages of 16 to 24 months (phase 5, the rapprochement phase), children become acutely aware of their separateness, and because this is frightening, they look to the mother for "emotional refueling" and to maintain a sense of security while, at the same time, begin to explore their separateness and independence. The theory of object relations suggests that the individual with borderline personality is fixed in the rapprochement phase of development. This fixation occurs when the mother begins to feel threatened by the increasing autonomy of her child and so withdraws her emotional support during those times, *or* she may instead reward clinging, dependent behaviors. Consequently, the child develops a deep fear of abandonment that persists into adulthood.

Other research looking at attachment issues in childhood suggest that childhood maltreatment, particularly neglect, may be associated with reactive attachment disorder, which results in the development of neurocognitive deficits, particularly temporal limbic dysfunction; the symptoms of BPD with regard to unhealthy attachment in relationships may be related, at least in part, to these neurocognitive deficits rooted in childhood development disruptions (Minzenberg, Poole, & Vinogradov, 2008; Pier et al, 2016).

Symptomatology (Subjective and Objective Data)

Individuals with borderline personality always seem to be in a state of crisis. Their affect is one of extreme intensity, and their behavior reflects frequent changeability. These changes can occur within days, hours, or even minutes. Often these individuals exhibit a single, dominant affective tone, such as depression, which may give way periodically to anxious agitation or inappropriate outbursts of anger.

Common symptoms include the following:

1. **Mood Swings:** Depression is so common in patients with this disorder that before the inclusion of BPD in the *DSM*, many of these patients were diagnosed as depressed. Underlying the depression is a sense of anxiety and rage that is sporadically turned inward on the self and externally on the environment. It is not uncommon for this individual to express intense, impulsive anger and rage toward their closest friends and family. Seldom is the individual aware of the true source of these feelings until well into long-term therapy.

2. **Inability to Be Alone:** Patients with BPD have little tolerance for being alone. They prefer a frantic search for companionship, no matter how unsatisfactory, to being alone with feelings of loneliness, emptiness, and boredom (Sadock et al, 2015). This often manifests in short, fleeting relationships with strangers and sometimes promiscuous behavior.

3. **Clinging and Distancing:** The patient with BPD commonly exhibits a pattern of interaction with others that is characterized

by clinging and distancing behaviors. When patients are clinging to another individual, they may exhibit helpless, dependent, or even childlike behaviors. They overidealize a single individual with whom they want to spend all their time, with whom they express a frequent need to talk, or from whom they seek constant reassurance. Acting-out behaviors, even self-mutilation, may result when they cannot be with this chosen individual. Distancing behaviors are characterized by hostility, anger, and devaluation of others, arising from a feeling of discomfort with closeness. "I hate you, please don't leave me" is an apt description of the mixed messages that are communicated when this patient engages in clinging and distancing behaviors. Distancing behaviors also occur in response to separations, confrontations, or attempts to limit certain behaviors. Devaluation of others is manifested by discrediting or undermining their strengths and personal significance.

4. **Splitting:** Splitting is a form of manipulation that is common in people with BPD. It may arise from their lack of achievement of object constancy and is manifested by an inability to integrate and accept both positive and negative feelings. In relationships, this individual often pits one person against another (e.g., "You're a good nurse and she's a bad nurse") in an effort to manipulate others and meet their own needs.

5. **Manipulation:** In their efforts to prevent the separation they so desperately fear, patients with this disorder become masters of manipulation. Splitting, lying, and threatening others are common manifestations, but virtually any behavior becomes an acceptable means of achieving the desired result: relief from separation anxiety and fear of abandonment.

6. **Self-destructive Behaviors:** Repetitive, self-mutilative behaviors, such as cutting, scratching, and burning, are classic manifestations of BPD. About 75% of individuals with BPD have a history of at least one deliberate act of self-harm and a prevalence rate of around 9% for death by suicide (Lubit, 2016). Although these acts can be fatal, most commonly they are manipulative gestures designed to elicit a rescue response from significant others. Suicide attempts often follow separation or perceived abandonment from another person.

7. **Impulsivity:** Individuals with BPD have poor impulse control. Common manifestations include substance abuse, gambling, promiscuity, reckless driving, and binging and purging (APA, 2013). Many times, these acting-out behaviors occur in response to real or perceived feelings of abandonment.

8. **Temporary Psychosis:** Transient episodes of extreme stress can precipitate periods of dissociation or paranoia. These symptoms are almost always specific, limited, and fleeting (Sadock et al, 2015).

Common Nursing Diagnoses and Interventions

(Interventions are applicable to various health-care settings, such as inpatient and partial hospitalization, community outpatient clinic, home health, and private practice.)

■ RISK FOR SELF-MUTILATION/RISK FOR SELF-DIRECTED OR OTHER-DIRECTED VIOLENCE

Definition: Risk for self-mutilation is defined as susceptible to deliberate self-injurious behavior causing tissue damage with the intent of causing nonfatal injury to attain relief of tension (NANDA International [NANDA-I], 2018, p. 420). Risk for self- or other-directed violence is defined as susceptible to behaviors in which an individual demonstrates that he or she can be physically, emotionally, and/or sexually harmful to self or others (pp. 416–417)

Risk Factors ("related to")

[Extreme fears of abandonment]
[Feelings of unreality]
[Depressed mood]
[Use of suicidal gestures for manipulation of others]
[Unmet dependency needs]
[Unresolved grief]
[Rage reactions]
[Physically self-damaging acts (cutting, burning, drug overdose, etc.)]
Body language (e.g., rigid posture, clenching of fists and jaw, hyperactivity, pacing, breathlessness, threatening stances)
History or threats of violence toward self or others or of destruction to the property of others
Impulsivity
Suicidal ideation, plan, available means
History of suicide attempts
Low self-esteem
Irresistible urge to [injure] self
[Childhood abuse]

Goals/Objectives

Short-term Goals

1. The patient will seek out staff member if feelings of harming self or others emerge.
2. The patient will not harm self or others.

Long-term Goal

The patient will not harm self or others.

Interventions With *Selected Rationales*

1. Observe the patient's behavior frequently. Do this through routine activities and interactions; avoid appearing watchful and suspicious. *Close observation is required so that intervention can occur if required to ensure the patient's (and others') safety.*

2. Encourage the patient to seek out a staff member when the urge for self-mutilation is experienced. *Discussing feelings of self-harm with a trusted individual provides some relief to the patient and encourages exploration of alternative ways to reduce anxiety. An attitude of acceptance of the patient as a worthwhile individual is conveyed.*

3. If self-mutilation occurs, care for the patient's wounds in a matter-of-fact manner. Do not give positive reinforcement to this behavior by offering sympathy or additional attention. *Lack of attention to the maladaptive behavior may decrease repetition of its use.*

4. Encourage the patient to talk about feelings he or she was having just before this behavior occurred. *To problem-solve the situation with the patient, knowledge of the precipitating factors is important.*

5. Act as a role model for appropriate expression of angry feelings, and give positive reinforcement to the patient when attempts to conform are made. *It is vital that the patient expresses angry feelings, because suicide and other self-destructive behaviors may be a result of anger turned inward on the self.*

6. Remove all dangerous objects from the patient's environment *so that he or she may not purposefully or inadvertently use them to inflict harm to self or others. Patient safety is a nursing priority.*

7. Try to redirect violent behavior with physical outlets for the patient's anxiety (e.g., exercise bike, jogging). *Physical exercise is a safe and effective way of relieving pent-up tension.*

8. Have sufficient staff available to indicate a show of strength to the patient if necessary. *This conveys to the patient evidence of control over the situation and provides some physical security for staff.*

9. Administer tranquilizing medications as ordered by the physician or obtain an order if necessary. Monitor the patient for effectiveness of the medication and for the appearance of adverse side effects. Some patients show disinhibition with this class of drugs (Sadock et al, 2015). *Tranquilizing medications such as anxiolytics or antipsychotics may have a calming effect on the patient and may prevent aggressive behaviors.*

10. If the patient is not calmed by "talking down" or by medication, use of mechanical restraints may be necessary. The avenue of the "least restrictive alternative" must be selected when planning interventions for a violent patient. Restraints should be used only as a last resort, after all other interventions have

been unsuccessful, and the patient is clearly at risk of harm to self or others.

11. If restraint is deemed necessary, ensure that sufficient staff is available to assist. Follow protocol established by the institution. Assess the patient in restraints at least every 15 minutes to ensure that circulation to extremities is not compromised (check temperature, color, pulses); to assist the patient with needs related to nutrition, hydration, and elimination; and to position the patient so that comfort is facilitated and aspiration is prevented. Some institutions may require continuous one-to-one monitoring of restrained patients, particularly those who are highly agitated and for whom there is a high risk of self- or accidental injury.

12. As agitation decreases, assess the patient's readiness for restraint removal or reduction. Remove one restraint at a time while assessing the patient's response. *This minimizes the risk of injury to patient and staff.*

13. If warranted by high acuity of the situation, staff may need to be assigned on a one-to-one basis. *Because of their extreme fear of abandonment, patients with BPD should not be left alone at a stressful time, as it may cause an acute rise in anxiety and agitation levels.*

Outcome Criteria

1. The patient has not harmed self or others.
2. Anxiety is maintained at a level in which the patient feels no need for aggression.
3. The patient denies any ideas of self-harm.
4. The patient verbalizes community support systems from which assistance may be requested when personal coping strategies are unsuccessful.

■ ANXIETY (Severe to Panic)

Definition: Vague uneasy feeling of discomfort or dread accompanied by an autonomic response (the source is often nonspecific or unknown to the individual); a feeling of apprehension caused by anticipation of danger. It is an alerting signal that warns of impending danger and enables the individual to take measures to deal with threat (NANDA-I, 2018, p. 324)

Possible Contributing Factors ("related to")

Threat to self-concept
Unmet needs
[Extreme fear of abandonment]
Unconscious conflicts [associated with fixation in earlier level of development]

Defining Characteristics ("evidenced by")

[Transient psychotic symptoms in response to severe stress, manifested by disorganized thinking, confusion, altered communication patterns, disorientation, misinterpretation of the environment]

[Excessive use of projection (attributing own thoughts and feelings to others)]

[Depersonalization (feelings of unreality)]

[Derealization (a feeling that the environment is unreal)]

[Acts of self-mutilation in an effort to find relief from feelings of unreality]

Goals/Objectives

Short-term Goal

The patient will demonstrate use of relaxation techniques to maintain anxiety at manageable level.

Long-term Goal

The patient will be able to recognize events that precipitate anxiety and intervene to prevent disabling behaviors.

Interventions With *Selected Rationales*

1. Encourage discussion of events, thoughts, and feelings associated with disruptive or self-harming behavior to promote insight in the connection of these behaviors to feelings of anxiety. Explore alternative strategies to reduce anxiety. *Patients with BPD often resort to manipulative behaviors, self-mutilating, or other self-harming behavior to relieve anxiety. Symptoms of depersonalization often occur at panic-level anxiety and may increase risk for self-harming behaviors.* If injury occurs, care for the wounds in a matter-of-fact manner without providing reinforcement for this behavior. *Lack of reinforcement may discourage repetition of the maladaptive behavior.*

2. During periods of panic anxiety, stay with the patient and provide reassurance of safety and security. Orient the patient to the reality of the situation. *Patient comfort and safety are nursing priorities.*

3. Administer tranquilizing medications as ordered by physician, or obtain order if necessary. Monitor the patient for effectiveness of the medication as well as for adverse side effects. Some patients show disinhibition with this class of drugs (Sadock et al, 2015). *Antianxiety medications (e.g., lorazepam, chlordiazepoxide, alprazolam) provide relief from the immobilizing effects of anxiety and facilitate the patient's cooperation with therapy.*

4. Correct misinterpretations of the environment as expressed by the patient. *Confronting misinterpretations honestly, with a caring and accepting attitude, provides a therapeutic orientation to reality and preserves the patient's feelings of dignity and self-worth.*

5. Encourage the patient to talk about true feelings. Help him or her recognize ownership of these feelings rather than projecting them onto others in the environment. *Exploration of feelings with a trusted individual may help the patient perceive the situation more realistically and come to terms with unresolved issues.*

6. Collaborate with other team members to establish that more than one nurse will develop a therapeutic relationship with the patient. Reinforce the importance of staff maintaining open communication and consistency in the provision of care for these individuals. *Individuals with BPD have a tendency to cling to one staff member, if allowed, transferring their maladaptive dependency to that individual. This dependency can be avoided if the patient is able to establish therapeutic relationships with two or more staff members who encourage independent self-care activities and provide consistency in communicating expectations.*

Outcome Criteria

1. The patient is able to verbalize events that precipitate anxiety and demonstrate techniques for its reduction.
2. The patient manifests no symptoms of depersonalization.
3. The patient interprets the environment realistically.

■ COMPLICATED GRIEVING

Definition: A disorder that occurs after the death of a significant other [or any other loss of significance to the individual], in which the experience of distress accompanying bereavement fails to follow normative expectations and manifests in functional impairment (NANDA-I, 2018, p. 340)

Possible Contributing Factors ("related to")

[Maternal deprivation during rapprochement phase of development (internalized as a loss, with fixation in the anger stage of the grieving process)]
[Loss of self-esteem as a result of childhood trauma]

Defining Characteristics ("evidenced by")

Persistent emotional distress
[Anger]
[Internalized rage]
Depression
[Labile affect]
[Extreme fear of being alone (fear of abandonment)]
[Acting-out behaviors, such as sexual promiscuity, suicidal gestures, temper tantrums, substance abuse]

[Difficulty expressing feelings]
[Altered activities of daily living]
[Reliving of past experiences with little or no reduction of intensity of the grief]
[Feelings of inadequacy; dependency]

Goals/Objectives

Short-term Goal
The patient will discuss with nurse or therapist maladaptive patterns of expressing anger.

Long-term Goal
The patient will be able to identify the true source of angry feelings, accept ownership of these feelings, and express them in a socially acceptable manner, in an effort to satisfactorily progress through the grieving process.

Interventions With *Selected Rationales*

1. Convey an accepting attitude—one that creates a nonthreatening environment for the patient to express feelings. Be honest and keep all promises. *An accepting attitude conveys to the patient that you believe he or she is a worthwhile person. Trust is enhanced.*
2. Identify the function that anger, frustration, and rage serve for the patient. Allow the patient to express these feelings within reason. *Verbalization of feelings in a nonthreatening environment may help the patient come to terms with unresolved issues.*
3. Encourage the patient to discharge pent-up anger through participation in large motor activities (e.g., brisk walks, jogging, physical exercises, volleyball, exercise bike). *Physical exercise provides a safe and effective method for discharging pent-up tension.*
4. Explore with the patient the true source of the anger. This is painful exploration that often leads to regression as the patient deals with the feelings of early abandonment or abuse. It seems that sometimes the patient must "get worse before he or she can get better." *Reconciliation of the feelings associated with this stage is necessary before progression through the grieving process can continue.*
5. As anger is displaced onto the nurse, caution must be taken to guard against the negative effects of countertransference. *These behaviors have the capacity for eliciting a whole array of negative feelings from the nurse. The existence of negative feelings by the nurse must be acknowledged, but they must not be allowed to interfere with the therapeutic process.*
6. Explain the behaviors associated with the normal grieving process. Help the patient to recognize his or her position in this process. *Knowledge of the acceptability of the feelings associated with normal grieving may help to relieve some of the guilt that these responses generate.*

7. Help the patient understand appropriate ways of expressing anger. Give positive reinforcement for behaviors used to express anger appropriately. Act as a role model. *Positive reinforcement enhances self-esteem and encourages repetition of desirable behaviors. It is appropriate to let the patient know when he or she has done something that has generated angry feelings in you. Role modeling ways to express anger in an appropriate manner is a powerful learning tool.*

8. Clearly identify expected behaviors within the milieu and set limits on those that are in violation of stated expectations. Clearly communicate consequences of violating stated expectations. Be supportive, yet consistent and firm, in caring for this patient. *The patient lacks sufficient self-control to limit maladaptive behaviors, so assistance is required from staff. Without consistency on the part of all staff members working with this patient, a positive outcome will not be achieved.*

Outcome Criteria

1. The patient is able to verbalize how anger and acting-out behaviors are associated with maladaptive grieving.

2. The patient is able to discuss the original source of the anger and demonstrates socially acceptable ways of expressing the emotion.

■ IMPAIRED SOCIAL INTERACTION

Definition: Insufficient or excessive quantity or ineffective quality of social exchange (NANDA-I, 2018, p. 301)

Possible Contributing Factors ("related to")

[Fixation in rapprochement phase of development]
[Extreme fears of abandonment and unhealthy fixation or over-prioritizing of relationship (engulfment)
[Lack of personal identity]

Defining Characteristics ("evidenced by")

[Alternating clinging and distancing behaviors]
[Inability to form satisfactory intimate relationship with another person]
Use of unsuccessful social interaction behaviors
[Use of primitive dissociation (splitting) in their relationships (viewing others as all good or all bad)]
[Manipulative behaviors]

Goals/Objectives

Short-term Goal

The patient will discuss with nurse behaviors that impede the development of satisfactory interpersonal relationships.

Long-term Goal

By time of discharge from treatment, the patient will interact appropriately with others in the treatment setting in both social and therapeutic activities (evidencing a discontinuation of splitting and clinging and distancing behaviors).

Interventions With *Selected Rationales*

1. Approach the patient with unconditional positive regard. *Patient behaviors, such as manipulating, lying, and splitting, violate the nurse's sense of success in establishing a trusting relationship with this individual and may culminate in negative or distancing behaviors from the nurse. Understanding the disorder and the impact of childhood trauma on the dynamics of the patient's behavior assists in developing an approach of compassion and conveying hopefulness that this is a treatable rather than an untreatable condition.*

2. Encourage the patient to examine splitting or clinging behaviors (to recognize that they are occurring) and associated feelings. *Patient may be unaware of their pattern of interaction with others and may not be aware of their connection to feelings of anxiety or fears of abandonment. Recognition must take place before change can occur.*

3. Help the patient understand that you will be available, without reinforcing dependent behaviors. *Knowledge of your availability may provide needed security for the patient.*

4. Give positive reinforcement for independent behaviors. *Positive reinforcement enhances self-esteem and encourages repetition of desirable behaviors.*

5. Engage multiple staff members in working with the patient in order to avoid the patient's developing dependence on one particular staff member. Maintain consistency with preestablished expectations to minimize opportunities for the patient to manipulate or split staff members. *The patient must learn to relate to more than one staff member in an effort to decrease use of splitting and to diminish fears of abandonment.*

6. Develop a clear model of communication and intervention among team members for the hospitalized patient with BPD. *Consistency in intervention helps to model healthy interpersonal skills for the patient and may minimize successful efforts at splitting staff members.*

> **CLINICAL PEARL** Recognize when the patient is playing one staff member against another. Remember that splitting is the primary defense mechanism of individuals with these disorders, and the impressions they have of others as either "good" or "bad" are a manifestation of this defense. Do not engage the patient in discussions that are attempts to degrade other staff members. Suggest instead that the patient discuss problems directly with staff person involved.

7. With the patient, explore feelings that relate to fears of abandonment and engulfment. Help the patient understand that clinging and distancing behaviors are engendered by these fears. *Exploration of feelings with a trusted individual may help the patient come to terms with unresolved issues.*

8. Help the patient understand how these behaviors interfere with satisfactory relationships. *The patient may be unaware of how others perceive these behaviors and why they are not acceptable.*

9. Assist the patient to work toward achievement of object constancy. Be available, without promoting dependency. *This may help the patient resolve fears of abandonment and develop the ability to establish satisfactory intimate relationships. Even brief encounters with a patient during short hospital stays provide an opportunity to convey connectedness and a sense that they are valued.*

10. Collaborate with the patient and other members of the health-care team (social worker, psychologist, psychiatric nurse practitioner, psychiatrist) to consider longer term outpatient treatment options such as dialectical behavior therapy. *Dialectical behavior therapy is an evidence-based treatment approach that has demonstrated benefits for patients with borderline personality disorder.*

11. Provide education, support, and referral resources for family members and significant others who may also experience anger and frustration at failed attempts to navigate interpersonal relationships with the patient. *Research has shown that family members of these patients often report feeling excluded and discriminated against by health-care providers* (Lawn, Diped, & McMahon, 2015).

Outcome Criteria

1. The patient is able to interact with others in both social and therapeutic activities in a socially acceptable manner.
2. The patient does not use splitting or clinging and distancing behaviors in relationships and is able to relate the use of these behaviors to failure of past relationships.

■ DISTURBED PERSONAL IDENTITY

Definition: Inability to maintain an integrated and complete perception of self (NANDA-I, 2018, p. 269)

Possible Contributing Factors ("related to")

[Failure to complete tasks of separation/individuation stage of development]
[Underdeveloped ego]
[Unmet dependency needs]
[Absence of or rejection by parental gender-role model]

Defining Characteristics ("evidenced by")

[Excessive use of projection]
[Vague self-image]
[Unable to tolerate being alone]

[Feelings of depersonalization and derealization]
[Self-mutilation (cutting, burning) to validate existence of self]
Gender confusion
Feelings of emptiness
Uncertainties about goals and values

Goals/Objectives

Short-term Goal

The patient will describe characteristics that make him or her a unique individual.

Long-term Goal

The patient will be able to distinguish own thoughts, feelings, behaviors, and image from those of others as the initial step in the development of a healthy personal identity.

Interventions With *Selected Rationales*

1. Help the patient recognize the reality of his or her separateness. Do not attempt to translate his or her thoughts and feelings into words. *Because of the blurred ego boundaries, the patient may believe you can read his or her mind.* For this reason, caution should be taken in the expression of empathetic understanding. For example, avoid statements such as "I know how you must feel about that."

2. Help the patient recognize separateness from nurse by clarifying which behaviors and feelings belong to whom. If deemed appropriate, allow the patient to touch your hand or arm. *Touch and physical presence provide reality for the patient and serve to strengthen weak ego boundaries.*

3. Encourage the patient to discuss thoughts and feelings. Help the patient recognize ownership of these feelings rather than projecting them onto others in the environment. *Verbalization of feelings in a nonthreatening environment may help the patient come to terms with unresolved issues.*

4. Confront statements that project the patient's feelings onto others. Ask the patient to validate that others possess those feelings. The expression of *reasonable doubt* as a therapeutic technique may be helpful ("I find that hard to believe").

5. Always call the patient by his or her name. If the patient experiences feelings of depersonalization or derealization, orientation to the environment and correction of misperceptions may be helpful. *These interventions help to preserve the patient's feelings of dignity and self-worth.*

6. Help the patient identify more adaptive ways of reducing anxiety than self-mutilation. *Patient safety is a nursing priority.*

7. Work with the patient to clarify values. Discuss beliefs, attitudes, and feelings underlying his or her behaviors. Help the

patient to identify those values that have been (or are intended to be) incorporated as his or her own. Care must be taken by the nurse to avoid imposing his or her own value system on the patient. *Underdeveloped ego and fixation in an early developmental level may contribute to the patient's not having established his or her own value system. In order to accomplish this, ownership of beliefs and attitudes must be identified and clarified.*

8. Use of photographs of the patient may help to establish or clarify ego boundaries. *Photographs may help to increase the patient's awareness of self as separate from others.*

Outcome Criteria

1. The patient is able to distinguish between own thoughts and feelings and those of others.
2. The patient claims ownership of those thoughts and feelings and does not use projection in relationships with others.

■ CHRONIC LOW SELF-ESTEEM

Definition: Negative evaluation and/or feelings about one's own capabilities, lasting at least 3 months (NANDA-I, 2018, p. 272)

Possible Contributing Factors ("related to")

[Lack of positive feedback]
[Unmet dependency needs]
[Retarded ego development]
[Repeated negative feedback, resulting in diminished self-worth]
[Dysfunctional family system]
[Fixation in earlier level of development]
[Childhood trauma]

Defining Characteristics ("evidenced by")

[Difficulty accepting positive reinforcement]
[Self-destructive behavior]
[Frequent use of derogatory and critical remarks against the self]
Lack of eye contact
[Manipulation of one staff member against another in an attempt to gain special privileges]
[Inability to form close, personal relationships]
[Inability to tolerate being alone]
[Degradation of others in an attempt to increase own feelings of self-worth]
Hesitant to try new things or situations [because of fear of failure]
Excessively seeks reassurance

Goals/Objectives

Short-term Goals

1. The patient will discuss fear of failure with nurse or therapist.
2. The patient will verbalize things he or she likes about self.

Long-term Goals

1. The patient will exhibit increased feelings of self-worth as evidenced by verbal expression of positive aspects about self, past accomplishments, and future prospects.
2. The patient will exhibit increased feelings of self-worth by setting realistic goals and trying to reach them, thereby demonstrating a decrease in fear of failure.

Interventions With *Selected Rationales*

1. Promote setting goals that are realistic. It is important for the patient to achieve something, so plan for activities in which success is likely. *Success increases self-esteem.*
2. Convey unconditional positive regard for the patient. Promote understanding of your acceptance of him or her as a worthwhile human being. *Acceptance by others increases feelings of self-worth.*
3. Set limits on manipulative behavior. Identify the consequences for violation of those limits. Minimize negative feedback to the patient. Enforce the limits and impose the consequences for violations in a matter-of-fact manner. Consistency among all staff members is essential. *Negative feedback can be extremely threatening to a person with low self-esteem and possibly aggravate the problem. Consequences should convey unacceptability of the behavior but not the person.*
4. Encourage independence in the performance of personal responsibilities, as well as in decision making related to the patient's self-care. Offer recognition and praise for accomplishments. *Positive reinforcement enhances self-esteem and encourages repetition of desirable behaviors.*
5. Help the patient increase level of self-awareness through critical examination of feelings, attitudes, and behaviors. *Self-exploration in the presence of a trusted individual may help the patient come to terms with unresolved issues.*
6. Help the patient identify positive self-attributes as well as those aspects of the self he or she finds undesirable. Discuss ways to effect change in these areas. *Individuals with low self-esteem often have difficulty recognizing their positive attributes. They may also lack problem-solving ability and require assistance to formulate a plan for implementing the desired changes.*
7. Discuss the patient's future. Assist the patient in the establishment of short-term and long-term goals. What are his or her strengths? How can he or she best use those strengths to achieve those goals? Encourage the patient to perform at a level

realistic to his or her ability. Offer positive reinforcement for decisions made.

Outcome Criteria

1. The patient verbalizes positive aspects about self.
2. The patient demonstrates the ability to make independent decisions regarding management of own self-care.
3. The patient expresses some optimism and hope for the future.
4. The patient sets realistic goals for self and demonstrates willingness to reach them.

■ ANTISOCIAL PERSONALITY DISORDER

Defined

Antisocial personality is a disorder diagnosed in adults who have demonstrated a pattern of antisocial behavior that began before the age of 15. These behaviors violate the rights of others, and individuals with this disorder display no evidence of guilt feelings at having done so. Individuals with antisocial personality have a very low tolerance for frustration, act impulsively, and are unable to delay gratification. They are restless and easily bored, often taking chances and seeking thrills, as if they were immune to danger. Their pattern of impulsivity may be manifested in failure to plan ahead, culminating in sudden job, residence, or relationship changes (APA, 2013). There is often a long history of involvement with law-enforcement agencies. Substance abuse is not uncommon. The disorder is more frequently diagnosed in men than in women. Individuals with antisocial personalities are often labeled *sociopathic* or *psychopathic* in the lay literature.

Predisposing Factors to Antisocial Personality Disorder

1. Physiological
   a. **Genetics:** Twin and adoptive studies have implicated the role of genetics in antisocial personality disorder, especially for the personality traits of callousness and unemotional responses, which may be more definitive of psychopathy (Thompson et al, 2014). Other antisocial behaviors among twins seemed to be more environmentally influenced. Recent research has suggested that a particular gene (MAOA) may be altered after a certain amount of exposure to violence such as child maltreatment or physical or sexual abuse (Oullett-Morin et al, 2016). Alteration of this gene is believed to be associated with the eventual development of differential features of antisocial personality.
   b. **Neurobiology:** Brain imaging studies have identified deficits in prefrontal cortex gray matter, which regulates cognitive control and inhibition, and decreased activity in the amygdala, which is responsible for modulating fearful

or threatening stimuli. Other studies have identified dys-regulation of neurotransmitters (dopamine and serotonin) and endocrine abnormalities (testosterone and cortisol), as present in individuals with antisocial personality disorder, and these dysregulations may be related to the symptoms of impulsivity (Thompson et al, 2014). Neuropsychological studies have demonstrated an increased reactivity to environmental irritants and cues that may be triggers for disinhibition (Verona & Patrick, 2015).

c. **Temperament:** Characteristics of temperament, such as temper tantrums in the infant, may be significant in the predisposition to antisocial personality. As these children mature, they commonly develop a bullying attitude toward other children. Parents report that they are undaunted by punishment, take risks that may lead to physical harm, and seem unaffected by pain. The likelihood of developing antisocial personality disorder is increased if the individual had attention-deficit/hyperactivity disorder and conduct disorder as a child (APA, 2013).

2. Psychosocial

a. **Family Dynamics:** Antisocial personality disorder frequently arises from a chaotic home environment. Parental deprivation during the first 5 years of life appears to be a critical predisposing factor in the development of antisocial personality disorder. Separation due to parental delinquency appears to be more highly correlated with the disorder than is parental loss from other causes. Studies have shown that antisocial personality disorder in adulthood is highly associated with physical abuse and neglect, teasing, and lack of parental bonding in childhood (Kolla et al, 2013; Krastins et al, 2014). Severe physical abuse was found to be particularly correlated to violent offending, triggering the development of a pattern of reactive aggression that is persistent over one's lifetime (Kolla et al, 2013). Abuse also contributes to the development of antisocial behavior in that it provides a model for behavior, and it may result in injury to the child's central nervous system, thereby impairing the child's ability to function appropriately.

Symptomatology (Subjective and Objective Data)

1. Extremely low self-esteem (abuses other people in an attempt to validate his or her own superiority).
2. Inability to sustain satisfactory job performance.
3. Inability to function as a responsible parent.
4. Failure to follow social and legal norms; repeated performance of antisocial acts that are grounds for arrest (whether arrested or not).

5. Inability to develop satisfactory, enduring, intimate relationship with a partner.
6. Aggressive behaviors; repeated physical fights; spouse or child abuse.
7. Extreme impulsivity.
8. Repeated lying for personal benefit.
9. Reckless driving; driving while intoxicated.
10. Inability to learn from punishment.
11. Socially extroverted and uses charm to manipulate and exploit others.
12. Lack of guilt or remorse felt in response to exploitation of others.
13. Pattern of difficulties with interpersonal relationships.
14. Repeated failure to honor financial obligations.

Common Nursing Diagnoses and Interventions

(Interventions are applicable to various health-care settings, such as inpatient and partial hospitalization, community outpatient clinic, home health, and private practice.)

■ RISK FOR OTHER-DIRECTED VIOLENCE

Definition: Susceptible to behaviors in which an individual demonstrates that he or she can be physically, emotionally, and/or sexually harmful to others (NANDA-I, 2018, p. 416)

Risk Factors ("related to")

[Rage reactions]
History of witnessing family violence
Neurological impairment (e.g., positive EEG)
[Suspiciousness of others]
[Interruption of patient's attempt to fulfill own desires]
[Inability to tolerate frustration]
[Learned behavior within patient's subculture]
[Vulnerable self-esteem]
Body language (e.g., rigid posture, clenching of fists and jaw, hyperactivity, pacing, breathlessness, threatening stances)
[History or threats of violence toward self or others or of destruction to the property of others]
Impulsivity
Availability of weapon(s)
[Substance abuse or withdrawal]
[Provocative behavior: Argumentative, dissatisfied, overreactive, hypersensitive]
History of childhood abuse

Goals/Objectives

Short-term Goals

1. The patient will discuss angry feelings and situations that precipitate hostility.
2. The patient will not harm others.

Long-term Goal

The patient will not harm others.

Interventions With *Selected Rationales*

1. Convey an accepting attitude toward this patient. Feelings of rejection are undoubtedly familiar to him or her. Work on development of trust. Be honest, keep all promises, and convey the message to the patient that it is not *him* or *her* but the *behavior* that is unacceptable. Be alert, however, to the tendency of this patient to manipulate others. Do not misconstrue charm or compliments as indicative of mutual trust. Maintaining clear, professional boundaries is essential. *An attitude of acceptance promotes feelings of self-worth. Trust is the basis of a therapeutic relationship. Clear understanding of professional boundaries is essential to maintaining a therapeutic relationship.*
2. Maintain a low level of stimuli in the patient's environment (low lighting, few people, simple decor, low noise level). *A stimulating environment may increase agitation and promote aggressive behavior.*
3. Observe the patient's behavior frequently. Do this through routine activities and interactions; avoid appearing watchful and suspicious. *Close observation is required so that intervention can occur if needed to ensure the patient's (and others') safety.*
4. Remove all dangerous objects from the patient's environment so that he or she may not purposefully or inadvertently use them to inflict harm to self or others. *Patient safety is a nursing priority.*
5. Help the patient identify the true object of his or her hostility (e.g., "You seem to be upset with ..."). *Because of weak ego development, the patient may be misusing the defense mechanism of displacement. Helping him or her recognize this in a nonthreatening manner may help reveal unresolved issues so that they may be confronted.*
6. Encourage the patient to gradually verbalize hostile feelings. *Verbalization of feelings in a nonthreatening environment may help the patient come to terms with unresolved issues.*
7. Explore with the patient alternative ways of handling frustration (e.g., large motor skills that channel hostile energy into socially acceptable behavior). *Physically demanding activities help to relieve pent-up tension.*
8. Screen for substance use and abuse. *Substance use disorders are a common comorbidity and must be addressed as part of a comprehensive care plan.*
9. Staff should maintain and convey a calm attitude toward the patient. *Anxiety is contagious and can be transferred from staff to*

patient. *A calm attitude provides the patient with a feeling of safety and security.*

10. Have sufficient staff available to present a show of strength to the patient if necessary. *This conveys to the patient evidence of control over the situation and provides some physical security for staff.*

11. Administer tranquilizing medications as ordered by the physician or obtain an order if necessary. Monitor the patient for effectiveness of the medication as well as for appearance of adverse side effects. *Antianxiety agents (e.g., lorazepam, chlordiazepoxide, oxazepam) produce a calming effect and may help to allay hostile behaviors.* (Note: Medications are often not prescribed for patients with antisocial personality disorder because of these individuals' strong susceptibility to addictions.)

12. If the patient is not calmed by "talking down" or by medication, use of mechanical restraints may be necessary. The avenue of the "least restrictive alternative" must be selected when planning interventions for a violent patient. Restraints should be used only as a last resort, after all other interventions have been unsuccessful, and the patient is clearly at risk of harm to self or others.

13. If restraint is deemed necessary, ensure that sufficient staff is available to assist. Follow protocol established by the institution. Assess the patient in restraints at least every 15 minutes to ensure that circulation to extremities is not compromised (check temperature, color, pulses); to assist the patient with needs related to nutrition, hydration, and elimination; and to position the patient so that comfort is facilitated and aspiration is prevented. Some institutions may require continuous one-to-one monitoring of restrained patients, particularly those who are highly agitated and for whom there is a high risk of self- or accidental injury.

14. As agitation decreases, assess the patient's readiness for restraint removal or reduction. Remove one restraint at a time while assessing the patient's response. *This minimizes the risk of injury to the patient and staff.*

Outcome Criteria

1. The patient is able to rechannel hostility into socially acceptable behaviors.
2. The patient is able to discuss angry feelings and verbalize ways to tolerate frustration appropriately.

■ DEFENSIVE COPING

Definition: Repeated projection of falsely positive self-evaluation based on a self-protective pattern that defends against underlying perceived threats to positive self-regard (NANDA-I, 2018, p. 326)

Possible Contributing Factors ("related to")

[Inadequate support systems]
[Inadequate coping method]
[Underdeveloped ego]
[Underdeveloped superego]
[Dysfunctional family system]
[Negative role modeling]
[Absent, erratic, or inconsistent methods of discipline]
[History of abuse and trauma]

Defining Characteristics ("evidenced by")

[Disregard for societal norms and laws]
[Absence of guilt feelings]
[Inability to delay gratification]
Denial of obvious problems
Grandiosity
Hostile laughter
Projection of blame and responsibility
Ridicule of others
Superior attitude toward others

Goals/Objectives

Short-term Goals

1. Within 24 hours after admission, the patient will verbalize understanding of treatment setting rules and regulations and the consequences for violation of them.
2. The patient will verbalize personal responsibility for difficulties experienced in interpersonal relationships within (time period reasonable for the patient).

Long-term Goals

1. By the time of discharge from treatment, the patient will be able to cope more adaptively by delaying gratification of own desires and following rules and regulations of the treatment setting.
2. By the time of discharge from treatment, the patient will demonstrate ability to interact with others without becoming defensive, rationalizing behaviors, or expressing grandiose ideas.

Interventions With *Selected Rationales*

1. From the onset, the patient should be made aware of which behaviors are acceptable and which are not. Explain consequences of violation of the limits. Consequences must involve something of value to the patient. All staff must be consistent in enforcing these limits. Consequences should be administered in a matter-of-fact manner immediately following the infraction. *Because the patient cannot (or will not) impose own limits on maladaptive behaviors,*

these behaviors must be delineated and enforced by staff. Undesirable consequences may help to decrease repetition of these behaviors.

2. Do not attempt to coax or convince the patient to do the "right thing." Do not use the words "You should (or shouldn't) …"; instead, use "You will be expected to… ." The ideal would be for this patient to eventually internalize societal norms, beginning with this step-by-step, "either/or" approach on the unit (*either you do [don't do] this, or this will occur*). *Explanations must be concise, concrete, and clear, with little or no capacity for misinterpretation.*

3. Provide positive feedback or reward for acceptable behaviors. *Positive reinforcement enhances self-esteem and encourages repetition of desirable behaviors.*

4. *In an attempt to assist the patient to delay gratification,* begin to increase the length of time requirement for acceptable behavior in order to achieve the reward. For example, 2 hours of acceptable behavior may be exchanged for a phone call; 4 hours of acceptable behavior for 2 hours of television; 1 day of acceptable behavior for a recreational therapy bowling activity; 5 days of acceptable behavior for a weekend pass.

5. A milieu unit provides an appropriate environment for the patient with antisocial personality. *The democratic approach, with specific rules and regulations, community meetings, and group therapy sessions, emulates the type of societal situation in which the patient must learn to live. Feedback from peers is often more effective than confrontation from an authority figure. The patient learns to follow the rules of the group as a positive step in the progression toward internalizing the rules of society.*

6. Help the patient gain insight into his or her own behavior. Often, these individuals rationalize to such an extent that they deny that their behavior is inappropriate (e.g., thinking may be reflected in statements such as, "The owner of this store has so much money, he'll never miss the little bit I take. He has everything, and I have nothing. It's not fair! I deserve to have some of what he has"). *The patient must come to understand that certain behaviors are not tolerated within the society and that severe consequences are imposed on those individuals who refuse to comply. The patient must want to change his or her behavior before he or she can be helped. One of the difficulties posed in interventions for personality disorders is that often the behaviors are ego-syntonic; in other words, the patient may not perceive these behaviors as requiring change.*

7. Talk about past behaviors with the patient. Discuss which behaviors are acceptable by societal norms and which are not. Help the patient identify ways in which he or she has exploited others and the benefits versus consequences of previous behavior. Explore the patient's insight into feelings associated with his or her behavior. *An attempt may be made to enlighten the patient to the sensitivity of others by promoting self-awareness in an effort to help the patient gain insight into his or her own behavior.*

8. Throughout the relationship with the patient, maintain attitude of "It is not *you*, but your *behavior*, that is unacceptable." *An attitude of acceptance promotes feelings of dignity and self-worth.*

Outcome Criteria

1. The patient follows rules and regulations of the milieu environment.
2. The patient is able to verbalize which of his or her behaviors are not acceptable.
3. The patient shows regard for the rights of others by delaying gratification of own desires when appropriate.

■ CHRONIC LOW SELF-ESTEEM

Definition: Negative evaluation and/or feelings about one's own capabilities, lasting at least three months (NANDA-I, 2018, p. 272)

Possible Contributing Factors ("related to")

[Lack of positive feedback]
[Unmet dependency needs]
[Retarded ego development]
[Repeated negative feedback, resulting in diminished self-worth]
[Dysfunctional family system]
[Absent, erratic, or inconsistent parental discipline]
[Extreme poverty]
[History of childhood abuse]

Defining Characteristics ("evidenced by")

[Denial of problems obvious to others]
[Projection of blame or responsibility for problems]
[Grandiosity]
[Aggressive behavior]
[Frequent use of derogatory and critical remarks against others]
[Manipulation of others to fulfill own desires]
[Inability to form close, personal relationships]

Goals/Objectives

Short-term Goal

The patient will verbalize an understanding that derogatory and critical remarks against others reflect feelings of self-contempt.

Long-term Goal

The patient will experience an increase in self-esteem, as evidenced by verbalizations of positive aspects of self and the lack of manipulative behaviors toward others.

Interventions With *Selected Rationales*

1. Ensure that goals are realistic. It is important for the patient to achieve something, so plan for activities in which success is likely. *Success increases self-esteem.*

2. Identify ways in which the patient is manipulating others. Set limits on manipulative behavior. *Because the patient is unable (or unwilling) to limit own maladaptive behaviors, assistance is required from staff.*

3. Explain the consequences of manipulative behavior. All staff must be consistent and follow through with consequences in a matter-of-fact manner. *From the onset, the patient must be aware of the consequences of his or her maladaptive behaviors. Without consistency of follow-through from all staff, a positive outcome cannot be achieved.*

4. Encourage the patient to talk about his or her behavior, the limits, and consequences for violation of those limits. *Discussion of feelings regarding these circumstances may help the patient achieve some insight into his or her situation.*

5. Discuss how manipulative behavior interferes with formation of close, personal relationships. *The patient may be unaware of others' perception of him or her and of why these behaviors are not acceptable to others.*

6. Help the patient identify more adaptive interpersonal strategies. Provide positive feedback for nonmanipulative behaviors. *The patient may require assistance with solving problems. Positive reinforcement enhances self-esteem and encourages repetition of desirable behaviors.*

7. Encourage the patient to confront the fear of failure by attending therapy activities and undertaking new tasks. Offer recognition of successful endeavors.

8. Help the patient identify positive aspects of the self and develop ways to change the characteristics that are socially unacceptable. *Individuals with low self-esteem often have difficulty recognizing their positive attributes. They may also lack problem-solving ability and require assistance to formulate a plan for implementing the desired changes.*

9. Minimize negative feedback to the patient. Enforce limit setting in a matter-of-fact manner, imposing previously established consequences for violations. *Negative feedback can be extremely threatening to a person with low self-esteem, possibly aggravating the problem. Consequences should convey unacceptability of the behavior but not the person.*

10. Encourage independence in the performance of personal responsibilities and in decision making related to own self-care. Offer recognition and praise for accomplishments. *Positive reinforcement enhances self-esteem and encourages repetition of desirable behaviors.*

11. Help the patient increase level of self-awareness through critical examination of feelings, attitudes, and behaviors. Help the patient understand that it is perfectly acceptable for attitudes and behaviors to differ from those of others, as long as they do not become intrusive. *As the patient becomes more aware and accepting of himself or herself, the need for judging the behavior of others will diminish.*

12. Teach the patient assertiveness techniques, especially the ability to recognize the differences among passive, assertive, and aggressive behaviors and the importance of respecting the human rights of others while protecting one's own basic human rights. *These techniques promote self-esteem while enhancing the ability to form satisfactory interpersonal relationships.*

Outcome Criteria

1. The patient verbalizes positive aspects about self.
2. The patient does not manipulate others in an attempt to increase feelings of self-worth.
3. The patient considers the rights of others in interpersonal interactions.

■ IMPAIRED SOCIAL INTERACTION

Definition: Insufficient or excessive quantity or ineffective quality of social exchange (NANDA-I, 2018, p. 301)

Possible Contributing Factors ("related to")

Self-concept disturbance
[Unmet dependency needs]
[Retarded ego development]
[Retarded superego development]
[Negative role modeling]
Knowledge deficit about ways to enhance mutuality

Defining Characteristics ("evidenced by")

Discomfort in social situations
Inability to receive or communicate a satisfying sense of social engagement (e.g., belonging, caring, interest, shared history)
Use of unsuccessful social interaction behaviors
Dysfunctional interaction with others
[Exploitation of others for the fulfillment of own desires]
[Inability to develop satisfactory, enduring, intimate relationship with a sexual partner]
[Physical and verbal hostility toward others when fulfillment of own desires is thwarted]

Goals/Objectives

Short-term Goal

The patient will demonstrate appropriate communication (no evidence of manipulation or exploitation) with nurse or therapist within 1 week.

Long-term Goal

The patient will interact appropriately with others, demonstrating concern for the needs of others as well as for his or her own needs, by time of discharge from treatment.

Interventions With *Selected Rationales*

1. Develop therapeutic rapport with the patient. Establish trust by always being honest; keep all promises; convey acceptance of person, separate from unacceptable behaviors ("It is not *you*, but your *behavior*, that is unacceptable."). *An attitude of acceptance promotes feelings of self-worth. Trust is the basis of a therapeutic relationship.*

2. Offer to remain with the patient during initial interactions with others. *Presence of a trusted individual increases feelings of security during uncomfortable situations.*

3. Provide constructive criticism and positive reinforcement for efforts. *Positive feedback enhances self-esteem and encourages repetition of desirable behaviors.*

4. Confront the patient as soon as possible when interactions with others are manipulative or exploitative. Establish consequences for unacceptable behavior, and always follow through. *Because of the strong id influence on the patient's behavior, he or she should receive immediate feedback when behavior is unacceptable. Consistency in enforcing the consequences is essential if positive outcomes are to be achieved. Inconsistency creates confusion and encourages testing of limits.*

5. Act as a role model for the patient through appropriate interactions with him or her and with others. *Role modeling is a powerful and effective form of learning.*

6. Provide group situations for the patient. *It is through these group interactions with positive and negative feedback from his or her peers that the patient will learn socially acceptable behavior.*

Outcome Criteria

1. The patient willingly and appropriately participates in group activities.

2. The patient has satisfactorily established and maintained one interpersonal relationship with nurse or therapist, without evidence of manipulation or exploitation.

3. The patient demonstrates ability to interact appropriately with others, showing respect for self and others.

4. The patient is able to verbalize reasons for inability to form close interpersonal relationships with others in the past.

■ DEFICIENT KNOWLEDGE (Of Self-Care Activities to Achieve and Maintain Optimal Wellness)

Definition: Absence of cognitive information related to a specific topic, or its acquisition (NANDA-I, 2018, p. 259)

Possible Contributing Factors ("related to")

Lack of interest in learning
[Low self-esteem]
[Denial of need for information]
[Denial of risks involved with maladaptive lifestyle]
Unfamiliarity with information sources

Defining Characteristics ("evidenced by")

[History of substance abuse]
[Statement of lack of knowledge]
[Statement of misconception]
[Request for information]
[Demonstrated lack of knowledge regarding basic health practices]
[Reported or observed inability to take the responsibility for meeting basic health practices in any or all functional pattern areas]
[History of lack of health-seeking behavior]
Inappropriate or exaggerated behaviors (e.g., hysterical, hostile, agitated, apathetic)

Goals/Objectives

Short-term Goal

The patient will verbalize understanding of knowledge required to fulfill basic health needs following implementation of teaching plan.

Long-term Goal

The patient will be able to demonstrate skills learned for fulfillment of basic health needs by time of discharge from therapy.

Interventions With *Selected Rationales*

1. Assess the patient's level of knowledge regarding positive self-care practices. *An adequate database is necessary for the development of an effective teaching plan.*
2. Assess the patient's level of anxiety and readiness to learn. *Learning does not occur beyond the moderate level of anxiety.*

3. Incorporate motivational interviewing to determine the patient's motivation to change and to determine the method of learning most appropriate for the patient (e.g., discussion, question and answer, use of audio or visual aids, oral, written). Be sure to consider level of education and development. *Teaching will be ineffective if presented at a level or by a method inappropriate to the patient's ability to learn. Readiness to learn is foundational to successful education and behavior change.*

4. Develop a teaching plan, including measurable objectives for the learner. Provide information regarding healthful strategies for activities of daily living as well as about harmful effects of substance abuse on the body. Include suggestions for community resources to assist the patient when adaptability is impaired. *The patient needs this information to promote effective health maintenance.*

5. Include significant others in the learning activity, if possible. *Input from individuals who are directly involved in the potential change increases the likelihood of a positive outcome.*

6. Implement the teaching plan at a time that facilitates and in a place that is conducive to optimal learning (e.g., in the evening when family members visit; in an empty, quiet classroom or group therapy room). *Learning is enhanced by an environment with few distractions.*

7. Begin with simple concepts and progress to the more complex. *Retention is increased if introductory material is easy to understand.*

8. Provide activities for the patient and significant others in which to actively participate during the learning exercise. *Active participation increases retention.*

9. Ask the patient and significant others to demonstrate knowledge gained by verbalizing information regarding positive self-care practices. *Verbalization of knowledge gained is a measurable method of evaluating the teaching experience.*

10. Provide positive feedback for participation, as well as for accurate demonstration of knowledge gained. *Positive feedback enhances self-esteem and encourages repetition of desirable behaviors.*

Outcome Criteria

1. The patient is able to verbalize information regarding positive self-care practices.
2. The patient is able to verbalize available community resources for obtaining knowledge about and help with deficits related to health care.

INTERNET REFERENCES

Additional information about personality disorders may be located at the following Web sites:

- www.mentalhealth.com/home/dx/paranoidpersonality.html
- www.mentalhealth.com/home/dx/schizoidpersonality.html
- www.mentalhealth.com/home/dx/schizotypalpersonality.html
- www.mentalhealth.com/home/dx/antisocialpersonality.html
- www.mentalhealth.com/home/dx/borderlinepersonality.html
- www.mentalhealth.com/home/dx/histrionicpersonality.html
- www.mentalhealth.com/home/dx/narcissicpersonality.html
- www.mentalhealth.com/home/dx/avoidantpersonality.html
- www.mentalhealth.com/home/dx/dependentpersonality.html
- www.mentalhealth.com/home/dx/obsessivepersonality.html
- https://www.mayoclinic.org/diseases-conditions/personality-disorders/symptoms-causes/syc-20354463

 Movie Connections

Taxi Driver (Schizoid personality) • *One Flew Over the Cuckoo's Nest* (Antisocial) • *The Boston Strangler* (Antisocial) • *Just Cause* (Antisocial) • *The Dream Team* (Antisocial) • *Goodfellas* (Antisocial) • *Fatal Attraction* (Borderline) • *Play Misty for Me* (Borderline) • *Girl, Interrupted* (Borderline) • *Gone With the Wind* (Histrionic) • *Wall Street* (Narcissistic) • *The Odd Couple* (Obsessive-compulsive) • *As Good As It Gets* (Obsessive-compulsive) • *Silver Linings Playbook* (Borderline, bipolar, and obsessive compulsive disorders)

SPECIAL TOPICS IN PSYCHIATRIC-MENTAL HEALTH NURSING

CHAPTER **15**

Problems Related to Abuse or Neglect

■ BACKGROUND ASSESSMENT DATA

Abuse and neglect includes intimate partner violence, completed or attempted rape, stalking, and physical violence. Although women experience violence more often than men, men are also at times victims of intimate partner violence.

Child abuse and related fatalities continue to be a significant health concern. It is well documented that adverse childhood experiences (ACEs) such as abuse and neglect can have a major impact on health and well-being throughout one's life. ACE studies have found that as the number of ACE events increases, so do risks for heart disease, asthma, diabetes, cancer, depression, anxiety, posttraumatic stress disorder (PTSD), disability, unemployment, sexually transmitted diseases, and other health problems (CDC, 2019). The impact of trauma on physical, mental, emotional, and spiritual health is one of the primary reasons that nurses need to assess for trauma and provide **trauma-informed care.**

Categories of Abuse and Neglect
Physical Abuse of a Child

Physical abuse of a child includes "any nonaccidental physical injury (ranging from minor bruises to severe fractures or death) as a result of punching, beating, kicking, biting, shaking, throwing, stabbing, choking, hitting (with a hand, stick, strap, or other object), burning, or any other method that is inflicted by a parent, caregiver, or other individual who has responsibility for the child" (American Psychiatric Association [APA], 2013, p. 717). The most obvious way to detect it is by outward physical signs. However, behavioral indicators may also be evident.

Sexual Abuse of a Child

This category is defined as "employment, use, persuasion, inducement, enticement, or coercion of any child to engage in, or assist any other person to engage in, any sexually explicit conduct or any simulation of such conduct for the purpose of producing any visual depiction of such conduct; or the rape, and in cases of caretaker or interfamilial relationships, statutory rape, molestation, prostitution, or other form of sexual exploitation of children, or incest with children" (Child Welfare Information Gateway, 2013). *Incest* is the occurrence of sexual contacts or interaction between, or sexual exploitation of, close relatives, or between participants who are related to each other by a kinship bond that is regarded as a prohibition to sexual relations (e.g., caretakers, stepparents, stepsiblings) (Sadock, Sadock, & Ruiz, 2015).

Human trafficking, which includes sex trafficking, is another form of child abuse that is a significant public health concern. Federal law defines human trafficking as: a commercial sex act [that] is induced by force, fraud, or coercion, or in which the person induced to perform such act has not attained 18 years of age or, the recruitment, harboring, transportation, provision, or obtaining of a person for labor or services, through the use of force, fraud, or coercion for the purpose of subjection to involuntary servitude, peonage, debt bondage, or slavery (U.S. Department of Education, 2013).

Neglect of a Child

Physical neglect of a child includes refusal of or delay in seeking health care, abandonment, expulsion from the home or refusal to allow a runaway to return home, and inadequate supervision. *Emotional neglect* refers to a chronic failure by the parent or caretaker to provide the child with the hope, love, and support necessary for the development of a sound, healthy personality.

Physical Abuse of an Adult

Physical abuse of an adult may be defined as behavior used with the intent to cause harm and to establish power and control over another person. It may include slaps, punches, biting, hair pulling, choking, kicking, stabbing or shooting, or forcible restraint.

Sexual Abuse of an Adult

Sexual abuse of an adult may be defined as the expression of power and dominance by means of a sexual act most commonly by men over women, although men may also be victims of sexual assault. Sexual assault is identified by forcible execution against the victim's will.

Elder Abuse

Elder abuse and neglect are also significant problems. The CDC (2017) estimates that 1 in 10 people older than age 60 and living at home are victims of abuse, neglect, or financial exploitation. There is general agreement that these statistics underestimate the scope of the problem. Despite mandatory reporting laws in most states and the recent trend toward more reporting of abuse, adult protective services vary markedly among states. One study estimated that for every case that these agencies know about, 24 have not been reported (National Center on Elder Abuse, no date).

Predisposing Factors (That Contribute to Patterns of Abuse)

1. Physiological
   a. **Neurophysiological:** Disordered brain physiology especially in the limbic system has been linked to episodic violence (Sadock et al, 2015).
   b. **Biochemical:** Evidence supports that low 5-hydroxytryptamine (5HT) and 5-hydroxyindoleacetic acid (5HIAA) serotonin levels and turnover are associated with impulsive aggression, but these findings should not be interpreted as simplistic conclusions (Victoroff, 2017) The role of testosterone, which has been classically associated with aggression, may actually be better understood as a complex interaction with other hormones such as serotonin and cortisol. Finally, GABA and more than 20 peptide hormones have been implicated in various aspects of aggression. Research is ongoing to explore the mechanisms of these biochemicals and their interactions in the brain as well as the role of environmental factors.
   c. **Genetics:** Some studies have implicated heredity as a component in the predisposition to aggressive behavior. Both direct genetic links and the genetic karyotype XYY have been investigated as possibilities. Evidence remains inconclusive.
   d. **Disorders of the Brain:** Various disorders of the brain, including tumors, trauma, and certain diseases (e.g., encephalitis and epilepsy), have been implicated in the predisposition to aggressive behavior.
2. Psychosocial
   a. **Psychodynamic Theory:** The psychodynamic theorists imply that unmet needs for satisfaction and security result in an underdeveloped ego and a weak superego. It is thought that when frustration occurs, aggression and violence supply this individual with a dose of power and prestige that boosts

the self-image and validates significance to his or her life that is lacking. The immature ego cannot prevent dominant id behaviors from occurring, and the weak superego is unable to produce feelings of guilt.

b. **Learning Theory:** This theory postulates that aggressive and violent behaviors are learned from prestigious and influential role models. Individuals who were abused as children or whose parents disciplined with severe physical punishment are more likely to behave in a violent manner as adults.

c. **Societal Influences:** Social scientists believe that aggressive behavior is primarily a product of one's culture and social structure. Societal influences may contribute to violence when individuals believe that their needs and desires cannot be met through conventional means, and they resort to delinquent behaviors in an effort to obtain desired ends. Poverty and substance abuse are risk factors for both perpetrators and victims of aggressive violence.

Symptomatology (Subjective and Objective Data)

1. Signs of physical abuse may include the following:
   a. Bruises over various areas of the body (including suspicious and symmetrical injuries). They may present with different colors of bluish-purple to yellowish-green (indicating various stages of healing).
   b. Bite marks, skin welts, burns.
   c. Fractures, scars, serious internal injuries, brain damage.
   d. Lacerations, abrasions, or unusual bleeding.
   e. Bald spots indicative of severe hair pulling.
   f. In a child, regressive behaviors (such as thumb-sucking and enuresis) are common.
   g. Extreme anxiety and mistrust of others.
2. Signs of neglect of a child may include the following:
   a. Soiled clothing that does not fit and may be inappropriate for the weather.
   b. Poor hygiene.
   c. Always hungry, with possible signs of malnutrition (e.g., emaciated with swollen belly).
   d. Listless and tired much of the time.
   e. Unattended medical problems.
   f. Social isolation; unsatisfactory peer relationships.
   g. Poor school performance and attendance record.
3. Signs of sexual abuse of a child include the following:
   a. Frequent urinary infections.
   b. Difficulty or pain in walking or sitting.
   c. Rashes or itching in the genital area; scratching the area a great deal or fidgeting when seated.
   d. Frequent vomiting.

  e. Seductive behavior; compulsive masturbation; provocative sex play.
  f. Excessive anxiety and mistrust of others.
  g. Sexually abusing another child.
4. Signs of sexual abuse of an adult include the following (Burgess, 2010):
  a. Contusions and abrasions about various parts of the body.
  b. Headaches, fatigue, sleep-pattern disturbances.
  c. Stomach pains, nausea, and vomiting.
  d. Vaginal discharge and itching, burning on urination, rectal bleeding and pain.
  e. Rage, humiliation, embarrassment, desire for revenge, self-blame.
  f. Fear of physical violence and death.

Common Nursing Diagnoses and Interventions
(Interventions are applicable to various health-care settings, such as inpatient and partial hospitalization, community outpatient clinic, home health, and private practice.)

■ RAPE-TRAUMA SYNDROME

Definition: Sustained maladaptive response to a forced, violent sexual penetration against the victim's will and consent (NANDA International [NANDA-I], 2018, p. 319)

Possible Contributing Factors ("related to")
[Having been the victim of sexual violence executed with the use of force and against one's personal will and consent]

Defining Characteristics ("evidenced by")
Disorganization
Change in relationships
Confusion
Physical trauma (e.g., bruising, tissue irritation)
Suicide attempts
Denial; guilt
Paranoia; humiliation, embarrassment
Aggression; muscle tension and/or spasms
Mood swings
Dependence
Powerlessness; helplessness
Nightmares and sleep disturbances
Sexual dysfunction

Revenge; phobias
Loss of self-esteem
Impaired decision making
Substance abuse; depression
Anger; anxiety; agitation
Shame; shock; fear

Goals/Objectives

Short-term Goal

The patient's physical wounds will heal without complication.

Long-term Goal

The patient will begin a healthy grief resolution, initiating the process of physical and psychological healing (time to be individually determined).

Interventions With *Selected Rationales*

1. It is important to communicate the following to the individual who has been sexually assaulted:
   a. You are safe here.
   b. I'm sorry that it happened.
   c. I'm glad that you survived.
   d. It's not your fault. No one deserves to be treated this way.
   e. You did the best that you could.
   The individual who has been sexually assaulted fears for his or her life and must be reassured of safety. He or she may also be overwhelmed with self-doubt and self-blame, and these statements instill trust and validate self-worth.

2. Explain every assessment procedure that will be conducted and why it is being conducted. Ensure that data collection is conducted in a caring, nonjudgmental manner *to decrease fear and anxiety and increase trust.*

3. Engage the services of a sexual assault nurse examiner (SANE) whenever possible. *Specialized skills in assessing and maintaining the viability of evidence supports the patient should he or she decide to pursue legal action.*

4. Ensure that the patient has adequate privacy for all immediate postcrisis interventions. Try to have as few people as possible providing the immediate care or collecting immediate evidence. *The post-trauma patient is extremely vulnerable. Additional people in the environment increase this feeling of vulnerability and serve to escalate anxiety.*

5. Encourage the patient to give an account of the assault. Listen, but do not probe. *Nonjudgmental listening provides an avenue for catharsis that the patient needs to begin healing. A detailed account may be required for legal follow-up, and a caring nurse, as a patient advocate, may help to lessen the trauma of evidence collection.*

6. Discuss with the patient whom to call for support or assistance. Provide information about referrals for aftercare. *Because of severe anxiety and fear, the patient may need assistance from others during this immediate postcrisis period. Provide referral information in writing for later reference (e.g., psychotherapist, mental health clinic, community advocacy group).*

Outcome Criteria

1. The patient is no longer experiencing panic anxiety.
2. The patient demonstrates a degree of trust in the primary nurse.
3. The patient has received immediate attention to physical injuries.
4. The patient has initiated behaviors consistent with the grief response.

■ POWERLESSNESS

Definition: The lived experience of lack of control over a situation, including a perception that one's actions do not significantly affect an outcome (NANDA-I, 2018, p. 343)

Possible Contributing Factors ("related to")

[Lifestyle of helplessness]
[Low self-esteem]
[Living with, or in a long-term relationship with, an individual who victimizes by inflicting physical pain or injury with the intent to cause harm and continues to do so over a long period of time]
[Lack of support network of caring others]
[Lack of financial independence]

Defining Characteristics ("evidenced by")

Reports lack of control [over situation or outcome]
[Reluctance to express true feelings]
[Passivity]
[Verbalizations of abuse]
[Lacerations over areas of body]
[Fear for personal and children's safety]
[Verbalizations of no way to get out of relationship]

Goals/Objectives

Short-term Goal

The patient will recognize and verbalize choices that are available, thereby perceiving some control over life situation (time dimension to be individually determined).

Long-term Goal

The patient will exhibit control over life situation by making decision about what to do regarding living with cycle of abuse (time dimension to be individually determined).

Interventions With *Selected Rationales*

1. In collaboration with physician, ensure that all physical wounds, fractures, and burns receive immediate attention. Take photographs if the victim will permit. *Patient safety is a nursing priority. Photographs may be called in as evidence if charges are filed.*
2. Take the patient to a private area to do the interview. *If the patient is accompanied by the person who did the battering, he or she is not likely to be truthful about the injuries.*
3. If she has come alone or with her children, assure her of her safety. *(Author's note: Female gender is used here because most intimate partner violence [IPV] is directed by men toward women, although it is understood that men are also victims of IPV.)* Encourage her to discuss the battering incident. Ask questions about whether this has happened before, whether the abuser takes drugs, whether the woman has a safe place to go, and whether she is interested in pressing charges. *Some women will attempt to keep secret how their injuries occurred in an effort to protect the partner or because they are fearful that the partner will kill them if they tell.*
4. Ensure that "rescue" efforts are not attempted by the nurse. Offer support, but remember that the final decision must be made by the patient. *Making her own decision will give the patient a sense of control over her life situation. Imposing judgments and giving advice are nontherapeutic.*
5. Stress to the victim the importance of safety. She must be made aware of the variety of resources that are available to her. These may include crisis hotlines, community groups for women who have been abused, shelters, counseling services, and information regarding the victim's rights in the civil and criminal justice system. Following a discussion of these available resources, the woman may choose for herself. If her decision is to return to the marriage and home, this choice also must be respected. *Knowledge of available choices can serve to decrease the victim's sense of powerlessness, but true empowerment comes only when she chooses to use that knowledge for her own benefit.*

Outcome Criteria

1. The patient has received immediate attention to physical injuries.
2. The patient verbalizes assurance of her immediate safety.
3. The patient discusses life situation with primary nurse.
4. The patient is able to verbalize choices available to her from which she may receive assistance.

■ RISK FOR DELAYED DEVELOPMENT (In Children)

Definition: Susceptible to delay of 25% or more in one or more of the areas of social or self-regulatory behavior, or in cognitive, language, gross or fine motor skills, which may compromise health (NANDA-I, 2018, p. 459)

Risk Factors ("related to")

[The infliction by caretakers of physical or sexual abuse, usually occurring over an extended period of time]
[The child's basic physiological needs are unmet]
[The child has been responded to with indifference and neglect]
[The child's social, educational, recreational, and developmental needs have been neglected]

Goals/Objectives

Short-term Goal

The patient will develop a trusting relationship with the nurse and report how evident injuries were sustained (time dimension to be individually determined).

Long-term Goal

The patient will demonstrate behaviors consistent with age-appropriate growth and development.

Interventions With *Selected Rationales*

1. Perform complete physical assessment of the child. Take particular note of bruises (in various stages of healing), lacerations, and patient complaints of pain in specific areas. Do not overlook or discount the possibility of sexual abuse. Assess for nonverbal signs of abuse: aggressive conduct, excessive fears, extreme hyperactivity, apathy, withdrawal, age-inappropriate behaviors. *An accurate and thorough physical assessment is required in order to provide appropriate care for the patient.*
2. Conduct an in-depth interview with the parent or adult who accompanies the child. Consider the following: If the injury is being reported as an accident, is the explanation reasonable? Is the injury consistent with the explanation? Is the injury consistent with the child's developmental capabilities? *Fear of imprisonment or loss of child custody may place the abusive parent on the defensive. Discrepancies may be evident in the description of the incident, and lying to cover up involvement is a common defense that may be detectable in an in-depth interview.*
3. Use games or play therapy to gain the child's trust. Use these techniques to assist in describing his or her side of the story.

Establishing a trusting relationship with an abused child is extremely difficult. The child may not even want to be touched. These types of play activities can provide a nonthreatening environment that may enhance the child's attempt to discuss these painful issues.

4. Determine whether the nature of the injuries warrants reporting to authorities. Specific state statutes must enter into the decision of whether to report suspected child abuse. Individual state statutes regarding what constitutes child abuse and neglect may be found at www.childwelfare.gov/systemwide/laws_policies/state. *A report is made if there is reason to suspect that a child has been injured as a result of physical, mental, emotional, or sexual abuse. "Reason to suspect" exists when there is evidence of a discrepancy or inconsistency in explaining a child's injury. Most states require that the following individuals report cases of suspected child abuse: all health-care workers, all mental health therapists, teachers, child-care providers, firefighters, emergency medical personnel, and law enforcement personnel. Reports are made to the Department of Health and Human Services or a law enforcement agency.*

Outcome Criteria

1. The patient has received immediate attention to physical injuries.
2. The patient demonstrates trust in the primary nurse by discussing abuse through the use of play therapy.
3. The patient is demonstrating a decrease in regressive behaviors.

■ POST-TRAUMA SYNDROME

Definition: "Sustained maladaptive response to a traumatic, overwhelming event, which may compromise health." (NANDA-I, 2018, p. 316)

Possible Contributing Factors ("related to")

Environment not conducive to needs
Insufficient social support
Homelessness
Current or historical exposure to physically or psychologically traumatic events

Defining Characteristics ("evidenced by")

Nightmares
Flashbacks
Dissociative amnesia
Withdrawal

Substance use
Hypervigilance
Cardiac or other physical symptoms

Goals/Objectives

Short-term goal

Patient will seek and receive trauma-informed support services.

Long-term goal

Patient will demonstrate adaptive coping mechanisms and report resolution of intrusive trauma-related symptoms

Interventions With *Selected Rationales*

1. Conduct a thorough biopsychosocial assessment including assessment for history of homelessness, trauma and evidence of current trauma-related symptoms. *Homeless individuals are a high-risk population for trauma either historically (such as victims of domestic violence) or by virtue of current unstable living conditions.*
2. Ask direct questions about patient history of traumatic events. *Traumatic events may have long- term consequences for both physical and emotional well-being. Awareness of past trauma also reduces the risk of retraumatization when providing health care.*
3. Provide opportunity for the patient to give accounts of past trauma, using a nonjudgmental approach and without probing. *Nonjudgmental listening provides an avenue for catharsis that the patient needs to begin healing. Empathic listening without probing reduces the risk of retraumatization.*
4. Provide trauma-informed care:
   a. Communicate with transparency and encourage patient collaboration in decisions around care and treatment. *Patients with a history of trauma may be hypervigilant and have difficulty establishing trust. Transparency and collaboration facilitate trust.*
   b. Ensure that the patient has adequate privacy for all immediate interventions and ask for the patient's permission for nursing interventions, particularly those that include touch. Try to have as few people as possible providing care or collecting assessment data. *These approaches empower the patient to participate in decision-making and reduce the risk of retraumatization.*
   c. Explore community resources available to assist with trauma recovery. *Accessing resources to assist with trauma recovery may prevent longer term consequences associated with unresolved trauma issues.*

Outcome Criteria

The patient demonstrates ability to establish trust with the nurse.
The patient verbalizes that acute post-trauma symptoms have resolved.

The patient identifies resources available to support ongoing recovery from trauma.

@ INTERNET REFERENCES

Additional information related to child abuse may be found at the following Web sites:

- https://www.childwelfare.gov
- https://medlineplus.gov/childabuse.html
- https://www.childhelp.org/child-abuse/

Additional information on human trafficking may be found at the following Web sites:

- https://www.dhs.gov/blue-campaign/what-human-trafficking
- https://www.fbi.gov/investigate/civil-rights/human-trafficking

Additional information related to sexual assault may be found at the following Web sites:

- https://medlineplus.gov/sexualassault.html

Additional information about elder abuse may be found at the following Web sites:

- https://www.nia.nih.gov/health/elder-abuse
- https://ncea.acl.gov (The National Center on Elder Abuse)
- https://www.cdc.gov/violenceprevention/elderabuse/definitions.html

Additional information related to intimate partner violence may be located at the following Web sites:

- www.thehotline.org
- www.nursingworld.org/MainMenuCategories/ANA Marketplace/ANAPeriodicals/OJIN/TableofContents/Volume72002/No1Jan2002/DomesticViolenceChallenge.html
- https://www.cdc.gov/violenceprevention/intimatepartnerviolence/index.html
- http://www.nursingworld.org/MainMenuCategories/ANAMarketplace/ANAPeriodicals/OJIN/TableofContents/Volume72002/No1Jan2002/IntimatePartnerViolence.html

---

🎬 Movie Connections

The Burning Bed (Domestic violence) • *Life With Billy* (Domestic violence) • *Two Story House* (Child abuse) • *The Prince of Tides* (Domestic violence) • *Radio Flyer* (Child abuse) • *Flowers in the Attic* (Child abuse) • *A Case of Rape* (Sexual assault) • *The Accused* (Sexual assault)

CHAPTER 16

Suicide Prevention

■ BACKGROUND ASSESSMENT DATA

In 2017, the most recent year for which statistics have been recorded, 47,173 people died by suicide in the United States (American Foundation for Suicide Prevention [AFSP], 2019). The numbers continue to climb despite nationwide attention to suicide prevention. This rate of suicide is the highest in more than 15 years.

These statistics have established suicide as the second-leading cause of death (behind unintentional injuries) among young Americans aged 10 to 34 years, the fourth-leading cause of death for individuals aged 35 to 54, the eighth-leading cause of death for individuals aged 55 to 64, and the tenth-leading cause of death overall (Centers for Disease Control and Prevention [CDC], 2019). Many more people attempt suicide than die by suicide (about 12:1), and even more people seriously contemplate the act without carrying it out. Because statistics about numbers of suicide attempts reflect only those who have entered a treatment setting, the numbers could be much higher. With a steady incline in suicide rates from 2000 to 2017, suicide has become a major health-care problem in the United States. Not only is the number of suicides increasing, but the demographics have changed. Historically, the highest rates of suicide were among the elderly, but the highest current rate of suicide occurs among middle-aged individuals aged 45 to 54 years, and the second-highest in those aged 85 and older (AFSP, 2019). In addition, the suicide rate has historically been lower among military personnel than among the general population. However, in some time periods since the Iraq War began—including in 2010 and 2011—more soldiers died by suicide than died in combat (Nock et al, 2013).

Most, although not all, people who are suicidal have a mental illness. Assessing for suicide risk is essential in every encounter with patients regardless of the health-care setting. Differentiating risk factors and warning signs is foundational to making clinical judgments about referral and the level of treatment required to maintain the patient's safety. One evidence-based tool to assist in evaluating the severity of suicide risk is the Columbia-Suicide Severity Rating Scale. A copy of this screening tool is included in Appendix S, Suicide Risk Assessment.

■ PREDISPOSING FACTORS: THEORIES ON SUICIDE
Psychological Theories
Anger Turned Inward

Freud (1957) believed that suicide was a response to intense self-hatred. The anger originates toward a love object but is ultimately turned inward against the self. In other words, Freud thought that suicide occurred as a result of an earlier repressed desire to kill someone else.

Hopelessness and Other Symptoms of Depression

Hopelessness has long been identified as a symptom of depression and an underlying factor in the predisposition to suicide. Because depression is often associated with suicidal ideation and attempts, any individual manifesting signs of clinical depression should be assessed for suicide risk. Although the many symptoms identified in suicide assessment tools attempt to assess for seriousness of suicidal ideation, current research is attempting to glean which symptoms might be more predictive of the move from ideation to attempts. In addition to hopelessness, the strength of the person's intention to die and the amount of suicide-specific rumination about suicide have also been identified as significant factors (Jobes, 2015, Rogers & Jobes, 2017).

History of Aggression and Violence

A history of violent behavior or impulsive acts has been associated with increased risk for suicide (Sadock et al, 2015), although recent evidence suggests that impulsive traits are higher in individuals with suicidal ideation but not necessarily associated with more attempts (Klonsky & May, 2015b).

Shame and Humiliation

Some individuals have viewed suicide as a "face-saving" mechanism—a way to prevent public humiliation after a social defeat such as a sudden loss of status or income. Often, these individuals are too embarrassed to seek treatment or other support systems. Both shame and humiliation may also interrupt one's sense of connectedness with others, and a sense of belonging and connectedness is considered protective against suicide. Evidence supports that the experience of shame is pronounced in trauma survivors (Taylor, 2015) and in females with borderline personality disorder (Wiklander et al, 2012). This research helps us understand some of the influencing factors for increased risk of suicide in these populations.

Sociological Theories
Durkheim's Theory

Durkheim's classic work (1951) studied the individual's interaction with the society in which he or she lived. He believed that the more cohesive the society and the more that the individual felt an integrated part of society, the less likely he or she was to carry out suicide. Durkheim described three social categories of suicide:

1. Egoistic suicide is the response of the individual who feels separate from the mainstream of society. Integration is lacking, and the individual does not feel a part of any cohesive group (such as a family or a church).
2. Altruistic suicide is the opposite of egoistic suicide. The individual who is prone to altruistic suicide is excessively integrated into the group. The group is often governed by cultural, religious, or political ties, and allegiance is so strong that the individual will sacrifice his or her life for the group.
3. Anomic suicide occurs in response to changes in an individual's life (e.g., divorce, loss of job) that disrupt feelings of relatedness to the group. An interruption in the customary norms of behavior instills feelings of separateness and fears of being without support from the formerly cohesive group.

Connectedness continues to be identified as an important protective factor for suicide prevention and may include a sense of closeness with individuals, groups, families, schools, faith communities, community organizations, or cultural group (Suicide Prevention Resource Center, 2019).

Interpersonal Theory of Suicide

Thomas Joiner's (2005) interpersonal theory of suicide supports some of the same principles advanced by Durkheim associating lack of a feeling of belonging with suicide risk. But Joiner's theory introduces the concept that suicidal ideation and suicide attempts need to be understood as distinct processes. He proposed that low connectedness and a high sense of burden interact with each other to increase suicidal thoughts and desires, but those features in the presence of high capability for suicide are strongly associated with the move from ideation to lethal attempts.

The Three-Step Theory

Klonsky and May (2015a), inspired by Joiner's theory and using their research finding that impulsivity is elevated in people who have made suicide attempts and those who have thoughts and have never made an attempt, sought to identify the factors that elevate suicidal ideation to an active risk for attempts. Their research supported the following three-step trajectory:

1. Pain (usually psychological pain) when combined with hopelessness, significantly increases suicidal ideation (for both men and women and across age groups).
2. Connectedness prevents suicidal ideation from escalating in those at risk, but when pain and hopelessness exceed one's sense of connectedness to others, suicidal ideation becomes active.
3. When strong, active suicidal ideation is present, it leads to an attempt only if one has the capacity to make an attempt.

Biological Theories
Genetics

Twin studies have shown a much higher concordance rate for monozygotic twins than for dizygotic twins. Some studies with people who have attempted suicide have focused on the genotypic variations in the gene for tryptophan hydroxylase, with results indicating significant association to suicidality (Sadock et al, 2015). Tryptophan hydroxylase is an enzyme associated with the synthesis of serotonin, and diminished serotonin has implications for both depression and suicidal behavior. Additional research has identified a genetic variation in prefrontal cortex tissue that may be a biomarker for suicide risk when vulnerable individuals are exposed to a significant stressor (Sudak, 2017). These findings suggest the potential for genetic predisposition toward suicidal behavior, but more research is needed to clarify this possible genetic link.

Neurochemical Factors

Some studies have revealed a deficiency of serotonin (measured as a decrease in the levels of 5-hydroxyindole acetic acid [5-HIAA] in the cerebrospinal fluid) in depressed patients who attempted suicide (Sadock et al, 2015). These studies, as well as postmortem studies, have supported the hypothesis that deficiencies in central nervous system serotonin are associated with suicide.

However, a recent meta-analysis examining biological factors found that they are, in general, weak predictors of a future suicide attempt or death by suicide (Chang et al, 2016). The only two biological factors that had statistical significance in this analysis were cytokines (anti-inflammatory response chemicals) and low levels of fish oil nutrients (including omega-3).

■ SYMPTOMATOLOGY (SUBJECTIVE AND OBJECTIVE DATA)

When nurses assess a patient's suicidal ideation, it is important to identify and distinguish ideas (thoughts), plans (intentions), and attempts (behavior). Each of these assessment factors can provide information about level of risk. When the patient has attempted self-injury, it is important to distinguish between *suicidal* self-injury and *nonsuicidal* self-injury. The latter injury is often used as a method to release emotions, but it may also be a way of communicating the severity of distress that the patient is experiencing (Nock et al, 2013).

The following basic items should be considered when conducting a suicidal assessment: demographics; medical-psychiatric diagnoses; suicidal ideas or acts; analysis of the suicidal crisis; psychiatric, medical, and family history; interpersonal support system; and coping strategies.

Demographics

Demographics provide information about groups that have been statistically associated with higher risks for suicide. Some examples include:

- *Age* – Highest rates are currently in the 45-54 year age group, and it is the second leading cause of death in children 10 to 14 and in adolescents.
- *Gender* – Men have statistically higher rates of death by suicide. Suicide rates in the transgender population, approaching 41%, identify this as a high-risk group.
- *Ethnicity/race* – Highest rates occur in Caucasians, followed by American Indian/Alaska Natives.
- *Marital Status* – Single, divorced, and widowed individuals are a statistically higher risk group for suicide, especially during periods of change in status.
- *Socioeconomic status* – Individuals in the highest and lowest socioeconomic classes have statistically higher risks for suicide than middle-class individuals.
- *Occupation* – Health-care professionals (especially physicians), law enforcement officers, dentists, artists, mechanics, lawyers, and insurance agents have all been identified as occupational groups incurring greater risks for suicide (Sadock et al, 2015).
- *Religion* – People with close, religious affiliations where suicide is prohibited have statistically lower rates of suicide.
- *Family History* – A family history of suicide increases an individual's risk for suicide.
- *Military History* – Both active duty and veterans in military services have statistically higher rates of suicide.

Medical-Psychiatric Diagnoses

Assessment data must be gathered regarding any psychiatric or physical condition for which a patient is being treated. Mood disorders (major depression and bipolar disorders) are the disorders most commonly associated with suicide. Substance use disorders are also associated with risk for suicide attempts. Other psychiatric disorders in which suicide risks have been identified include anxiety disorders, schizophrenia, anorexia nervosa, and borderline and antisocial personality disorders. Chronic and terminal physical illnesses have also been identified as potentiating risk factors.

Suicide Ideas or Acts

How serious is the patient's intent to die by suicide? How frequent are the thoughts about suicide? Does the person have a plan? If so, does he or she have the means? How lethal are the means? Does he or she intend to carry out this plan? Has the individual ever attempted suicide before? These questions must be asked by the person conducting the assessment of the patient who is expressing suicidal ideation.

Individuals may provide both behavioral and verbal clues about their intention to act. Examples of behavioral clues that may indicate a decision to carry out suicidal intent include giving away prized possessions, getting financial affairs in order, writing suicide notes, and sudden lift in mood.

Verbal clues may be both direct and indirect. Examples of direct statements include "I want to die" or "I'm going to kill myself." Examples of indirect statements include "This is the last time you'll see me," "I won't be around much longer for the doctor to worry about," or "I don't have anything worth living for anymore."

Recent research (Rogers & Joiner, 2017) provides evidence that suicide-specific rumination, that is, fixation on one's thoughts, intentions, and plans may be an important predictor of suicidal behavior. Asking how frequently the patient is thinking about suicide ideas, intentions, and plans helps to discern this level of risk.

The lethality of the method identified by an individual with suicidal ideation or by one who has already made an attempt provides meaningful information about the patient's intent to die. Use of firearms, hanging, and suffocation, for example, are considered highly lethal methods.

Other assessments include determining whether the individual has a plan, and if so, whether he or she has the means to carry out that plan. If the person states the suicide will be carried out with a gun, does he or she have access to a gun? Bullets? If pills are planned, what kind of pills? Are they accessible? Asking the patient, "How likely are you to carry out this plan?" may provide verbal confirmation of their level of intent.

Interpersonal Support Systems

Does the individual have support persons on whom he or she can rely during a crisis situation? Lack of a meaningful network of satisfactory relationships may implicate an individual as a high risk for suicide during an emotional crisis.

Analysis of the Suicidal Crisis

Three aspects of assessment that enhance understanding of the patient's current suicidal crisis are evaluation of the patient's precipitating stressors, relevant history, and life stage issues.

- *The precipitating stressor:* Adverse life events in combination with other risk factors, such as depression, may lead to suicide. Life stresses accompanied by an increase in emotional disturbance include the loss of a loved one either by death or by divorce, problems in major relationships, changes in social or occupational roles, or serious physical illness.

- ***Relevant history:*** Has the individual experienced numerous failures or rejections that would increase his or her vulnerability for a dysfunctional response to the current situation? Has the individual attempted suicide in the past? How recently? What was the method used in any previous attempts?
- ***Life stage issues:*** The ability to tolerate loss and disappointment is often compromised if those losses and disappointments occur during stages of life in which the individual struggles with developmental issues (e.g., adolescence, midlife).

Psychiatric, Medical, and Family History

The individual should be assessed with regard to previous psychiatric treatment for depression, substance use disorder, or previous suicide attempts. Medical history should be obtained to determine the presence of chronic, debilitating, or terminal illness. Is there a history of depressive disorder in the family, and has a close relative died by suicide in the past?

Coping Strategies

How has the individual handled previous crisis situations? How does this situation differ from previous ones?

Presenting Symptoms

Several acronyms have been developed as mnemonic devices to summarize important warning signs that suggest a person's more imminent risk for suicidal behavior. One is the acronym IS PATH WARM? (American Association of Suicidology, 2019b; Juhnke, Granello, & Lebrón-Striker, 2007). The assessment items and descriptors for each letter are as follows:

Ideation: Has suicide ideas that are current and active, especially with an identified plan

Substance abuse: Has current and/or excessive use of alcohol or other mood-altering drugs

Purposelessness: Expresses thoughts that there is no reason to continue living

Anger: Expresses uncontrolled anger or feelings of rage

Trapped: Expresses the belief that there is no way out of the current situation

Hopelessness: Expresses lack of hope and perceives little chance of positive change

Withdrawal: Expresses desire to withdraw from others or has begun withdrawing

Anxiety: Expresses anxiety, agitation, and/or changes in sleep patterns

Recklessness: Engages in reckless or risky activities with little thought of consequences

Mood: Expresses dramatic mood shifts

Although mnemonic devices such as IS PATH WARM? can be helpful in remembering what types of presenting symptoms to assess for, the overall assessment and management of suicidal behavior is far more complex and must consider available support systems, the patient's willingness to accept support, and the patient's ability to establish a trusting therapeutic alliance with health-care professionals intervening on his or her behalf. Ultimately a clinical judgment must be made about the patient's degree of risk so appropriate measures can be taken to prevent an attempt.

■ PROMOTING A THERAPEUTIC ALLIANCE

The nurse must approach discussion of suicide with a nonjudgmental attitude to promote the development of a therapeutic alliance with the patient. The Collaborative Assessment and Management of Suicidality (CAMS) model is an evidence-based approach that focuses on the importance of patient-centered, problem-focused intervention to build an alliance with patients for collaboration in reducing risk for suicidal behavior (Jobes, 2012). This model focuses on assessment, which necessarily includes asking the patient to identify what is driving the desire to take his or her own life so that alternatives (identifying and capitalizing on motivations to live) can be explored. For all health-care professionals, this work begins with developing skills in asking basic and direct questions such as "Are you having thoughts of hurting or killing yourself?"

One model for enhancing communication in suicide assessment is the CASE (Chronological Assessment of Suicide Events) approach. It is described as a flexible guide for interviewing that includes communication techniques designed to elicit and enhance detailed, valid feedback from patients about sensitive topics such as suicide. Several examples, as elaborated by Shea (2009), follow:

- *Normalizing* communicates that the patient is not the only one who experiences suicidal ideation.
  Example: "Sometimes when people are in a lot of emotional pain, they have thoughts of killing themselves. Have you had any thoughts like that?"
- *Asking about behavioral events* rather than the patient's opinions may elicit more concrete information.
  Example: "What did you do when you had those thoughts?" "How many pills did you take?" "What happened next?"
- *Gentle assumptions* encourage further discussion by assuming there is more to tell.
  Example: "What other times have you attempted suicide?"
- *Denial of the specific* is helpful when a patient generally denies suicidal ideation. This strategy encourages more

in-depth thought and response by asking questions that might trigger memories of specific events.

Example: After the patient denies suicidal ideation in response to a general question, the nurse asks more specifically, "Have you ever had thoughts of overdosing?" "Have you ever had thoughts about shooting yourself?"

• *Chronologically exploring* the presenting suicide event, recent suicide events, past suicide events, and finally, the immediate suicide events can broaden the nurse's understanding of the patient's immediate suicidal intent in the context of his or her behavior over time.

Common Nursing Diagnoses and Interventions for Suicide Prevention

(Interventions are applicable to a variety of health care settings such as inpatient, partial hospitalization, community outpatient clinics, home health, and private practice.)

■ RISK FOR SUICIDE

Definition: Susceptible to self-inflicted, life-threatening injury (NANDA-I, 2018, p. 422)

Risk Factors ("related to")

[Depressed mood]
Grief, hopelessness, social isolation
[Alienation from others; real or perceived]
[Purposelessness}
[Feeling trapped]
History of prior suicide attempts
Chronic or terminal illness, intractable pain
Psychiatric illness or substance abuse
Threatens to kill self
States a desire to die
[Has a suicide plan and the means to carry it out]
[Giving away possessions]

Goals/Objectives

Short-term Goals

The patient will seek out staff when feeling urge to harm self.
The patient will collaborate with a trusted staff member to identify a safety plan.
The patient will remain free of harm to self.

Long-term Goal

The patient will actively engage in his or her established plan to maintain personal safety.

Interventions With *Selected Rationales*

1. Ask the patient directly: "Have you thought about harming yourself in any way? If so, what do you plan to do? Do you have the means to carry out this plan? How strong are your intentions to die?" "How often do you think about suicide?" *The risk of suicide is greatly increased if the patient has developed a plan with lethal means and particularly if means are accessible for the patient to execute the plan. Suicide-specific rumination is associated with suicide attempts.*

2. Create a safe environment for the patient. Remove all potentially harmful objects from the patient's access (sharp objects, straps, belts, ties, glass items, alcohol). Supervise closely during meals and medication administration. Perform room searches as deemed necessary. *Patient safety is a priority.*

3. Maintain close observation of the patient. Depending on level of suicide precaution, provide one-to-one contact, constant visual observation, or every-15-minute checks at irregular intervals. Place the patient in a room close to nurse's station; do not assign to private room. Accompany to off-unit activities if attendance is indicated. May need to accompany to bathroom. *Close observation is necessary to ensure that the patient does not harm self in any way. Being alert for suicidal and escape attempts facilitates prevention or interruption of harmful behavior.*

4. Maintain special care in administration of medications. *Prevents saving up to overdose or discarding and not taking.*

5. Make rounds at frequent, irregular intervals (especially at night, toward early morning, at change of shift, or other predictably busy times for staff). *Prevents staff surveillance from becoming predictable. Being aware of the patient's location is important, especially when staff is busy and least available and observable.*

6. Encourage the patient to express honest feelings, including anger. Provide hostility release if needed. *Depression and suicidal behaviors may be viewed as anger turned inward on the self. If this anger can be verbalized in a nonthreatening environment, the patient may be able to eventually resolve these feelings.*

7. Establish a trusting, therapeutic relationship to encourage open discussion of suicide. *Establishing trust and open communications encourages the patient to share thoughts and feelings.*

8. Collaborate with the patient to develop a safety plan that includes recognition of warning signs, coping strategies, supportive people and places, resources and contact information for crisis management, and plans to restrict access to lethal means. *Actively engaging the patient in collaboration on the development of a safety plan promotes patient ownership and investment in the process.*

9. Assess verbal and nonverbal clues to identify the likelihood that the patient intends to follow through with the established safety plan and evaluate the patient's follow-through with safety plan measures while still hospitalized. *Assessment of patient safety includes analyzing congruence of verbal communication, nonverbal communication, and behavior.*

Outcome Criteria

The patient verbalizes no longer having thoughts of suicide.

The patient commits no acts of self-harm.

The patient verbalizes identified resources outside the hospital from whom he or she may request help if feeling suicidal.

■ HOPELESSNESS

Definition: Subjective state in which an individual sees limited or no alternatives or personal choices available and is unable to mobilize energy on own behalf (NANDA-I, 2018, p. 266)

Possible Contributing Factors ("related to")

Chronic stress
[Intractable pain]
Social isolation
Loss of spiritual or transcendent beliefs
[Perception of worthlessness]
[Absence of support systems]

Defining Characteristics ("evidenced by")

Hopelessness and despondency expressed in verbal cues
[Flat affect]
[Lack of initiative]
[Suicide ideas or attempts]

Goals/Objectives

Short-term Goal

The patient expresses hope, acceptance of life and of situations over which he or she has no control.

Long-term Goal

The patient demonstrates initiative in daily activities and identifies future-oriented goals.

Interventions with *Selected Rationales*

1. Identify stressors in the patient's life that precipitated current crisis. Include assessing degree of emotional pain and hopelessness in relationship to feelings of connectedness or lack of

connectedness with others. *It is important to identify contributing factors in order to assist the patient with stress management. Meaningful connections with others promotes hope and is identified as a protective factor against suicide.*

2. Determine coping behaviors previously used and the patient's perception of effectiveness then and now. *Identifying the patient's strengths encourages their use in the current crisis situation.*

3. Encourage the patient to explore and verbalize feelings and perceptions related to reasons for wanting to die as well as reasons for wanting to live. *Identification of feelings underlying behaviors helps the patient to begin the process of taking control of own life and enables the nurse to help the patient focus on maximizing his or her reasons for wanting to live.*

4. Provide expressions of hope to the patient in a positive, low-key manner (e.g., "I know you feel you cannot go on, but I believe that things can get better for you. What you are feeling is temporary. It is okay if you don't see it just now."). *The patient's current state of mind may prevent him or her from identifying anything positive in life. It is important to accept the patient's feelings nonjudgmentally and to affirm his or her personal worth and value.*

5. Help the patient identify areas of life situation that are under his or her own control. *The patient's emotional condition may interfere with the ability to problem-solve. Assistance may be required to perceive benefits and consequences of available alternatives accurately.*

6. Identify sources that the patient may use after discharge when crises occur or feelings of hopelessness and possible suicidal ideation prevail. *A collaboratively developed, concrete plan promotes hope in the face of a crisis situation.*

7. Assist the patient to explore and identify future-oriented goals. *Identifying goals encourages the patient to focus on hopefulness for the future.*

Outcome Criteria

1. The patient sets realistic goals and collaborates in the development and implementation of a personal safety plan.

2. The patient expresses optimism and hope for the future.

■ INEFFECTIVE COPING

Definition: A pattern of invalid appraisal of stressors with cognitive and/or behavioral efforts, that fails to manage demands related to well-being (NANDA-I, 2018, p, 327)

Possible Contributing Factors ("related to")

[Inability to identify aspects of one's situation under the person's
    control]
Inadequate social support
Altered mental status
[Feeling trapped or hopeless]
Poorly developed coping skills
[Impulsivity]

Defining Characteristics ("evidenced by")

Harmful behavior toward self
Recklessness
Substance abuse
Lack of goal-directed behavior

Goals/Objectives

Short-term goal

The patient identifies coping strategies and expresses commitment
    to incorporate these as part of a plan to maintain personal safety.

Long-term goal

The patient remains free from self-injury.

Interventions with *Selected Rationales*

1. Assist the patient to identify stressors and other warning signs
   that are associated with thoughts and plans for suicide. *Assisting
   the patient to develop awareness about factors contributing to suicide
   risk lays the foundation for collaborative development of a safety plan.*
2. Explore past coping skills that the patient identifies as effective.
   *Exploring the patient's perception of effective coping skills promotes
   active engagement in the process of identifying and carrying out a
   safety plan.*
3. Maintain a nonjudgmental attitude when discussing the
   patient's suicide ideas, plans, and intentions. *A nonjudgmental
   attitude promotes open communication and collaboration.*
4. Assist the patient to identify internal coping strategies for immediate response to a trigger event. *This promotes the patient's
   ability to develop a sense of personal control in response to suicide ideas.*
5. Assist the patient to identify support systems, resources, and
   social activities that the patient can use to support ongoing
   personal safety. *External coping strategies such as eliciting support
   from a family member or friend, community resources, and social
   activities (that may help the patient minimize rumination about*

suicide) are all positive coping skills essential to a comprehensive safety plan.

Outcome Criteria

1. The patient demonstrates use of effective coping strategies to maintain personal safety.
2. The patient remains free from self-injury.

@ INTERNET REFERENCES AND NATIONAL HOTLINE NUMBERS

- **National Suicide Hotline** 1-800-SUICIDE (24/7)
- **National Suicide Prevention Lifeline**
  www.suicidepreventionlifeline.org
  1-800-273-TALK (24/7)
- **American Association of Suicidology**
  www.suicidology.org
- **Depression and Bipolar Support Alliance (DBSA)**
  www.dbsalliance.org
- **American Foundation for Suicide Prevention**
  www.afsp.org
- **National Institute of Mental Health** www.nimh.nih.gov
- **National Alliance on Mental Illness** www.nami.org
- **American Psychiatric Association** www.psych.org
- **Mental Health America** www.mhanational.org
- **American Psychological Association** www.apa.org
- **Screening for Mental Health Stop a Suicide Today!**
  www.stopasuicide.org
- **Boys Town** www.boystown.org
  1-800-448-3000 (24/7 national hotline)
- **Centre for Suicide Prevention (Canada)**
  www.suicideinfo.ca
  1-833-456-4566 (24/7 helpline)
- **Samaritans (U.K. and Republic of Ireland)**
  www.samaritans.org
  116-123 (24/7 helpline)
- **Centers for Disease Control and Prevention: National Center for Injury Prevention and Control**
  https://www.cdc.gov/injury/index.html
- **SAVE (Suicide Awareness Voices of Education)**
  www.save.org
- **Alliance of Hope: For Suicide Loss Survivors**
  www.allianceofhope.org

Movie Connections

Dead Poet's Society • *It's Kind of a Funny Story* • *The Perks of Being a Wallflower* • *Girl, Interrupted* • *Cyberbully*

CHAPTER 17

Homelessness

■ BACKGROUND ASSESSMENT DATA

It is difficult to determine how many individuals are homeless in the United States. The National Alliance to End Homelessness (2019) reports that from 2007 to 2017, homelessness overall declined by 14.4%, with the most dramatic decreases among veterans. However, about 33% of the current homeless population have some form of severe mental illness (SMI) (NCH, 2017), and one of the cited contributing factors is limited access to inpatient psychiatric treatment. Homelessness among the mentally ill continues to be a significant concern for this vulnerable population.

Demographics

The Substance Abuse and Mental Health Services Administration (SAMHSA) (2019) provides the following demographics through statistics gathered from Projects for Assistance in Transition from Homelessness (PATH), which was specifically established for funding services to people with SMI.

1. **Age:** Approximately 20% of patients with SMI are younger than age 30; individuals between the ages of 31 and 61 make up the bulk of this population at 71.7%; about 7.2% are aged 62 years or older.
2. **Gender:** Male individuals with SMI comprise 59.2% of the homeless population, and 39.7% are female.
3. **Ethnicity and Race:** The homeless SMI population is estimated to be 55.7% Caucasian, 34.7% African American, 13.6% Hispanic, 3.8% American Indian or Alaska Native, and 3% other racial/ethnic groups. The ethnic makeup of homeless populations varies according to geographic location.

Mental Illness and Homelessness

Schizophrenia is frequently described as the most common diagnosis among the homeless with mental illness. Other prevalent disorders include bipolar disorder, substance addiction, depression, personality disorders, and neurocognitive disorders. SAMHSA (2019) identifies that in 2018, 40.9% of patients receiving PATH services had a co-occurring substance use disorder.

Predisposing Factors to Homelessness Among the Mentally Ill

1. **Deinstitutionalization:** Deinstitutionalization is frequently implicated as a contributing factor to homelessness among persons with mental illness. Deinstitutionalization began out of expressed concern by mental health professionals and others who described the "deplorable conditions" under which mentally ill individuals were housed. Some individuals believed that institutionalization deprived the mentally ill of their civil rights. Certainly another motivating factor for deinstitutionalization was the financial burden these patients placed on state governments.

2. **Poverty:** Cuts in various government entitlement programs have depleted the allotments available for individuals with severe and persistent mental illness living in the community. The job market is prohibitive for individuals whose behavior is incomprehensible or even frightening to many. The stigma and discrimination associated with mental illness may be diminishing slowly, but it is highly visible to those who suffer from its effects.

3. **Scarcity of Affordable Housing:** Single room occupancy (SRO) hotels have, in the past, provided a means of relatively inexpensive housing, and although some people believe that these facilities nurtured isolation, they provided adequate shelter from the elements for their occupants. The number of SRO hotels has diminished drastically. Persons with mental illness who were released from state and county mental hospitals and who did not have families with whom they could reside sought residence in board-and-care homes of varying quality. Halfway houses and supportive group living arrangements are helpful but scarce. Many of those with families return to their homes, but because families have received little if any instruction or support and the environment is often turbulent, individuals with mental illness leave these homes. So many SMI individuals frequent the homeless shelters that there is concern that the shelters are becoming mini-institutions for people with serious mental illness.

4. **Lack of Affordable Health Care:** For families barely able to scrape together enough money to pay for day-to-day living, a catastrophic illness can create the level of poverty that starts the downward spiral to homelessness.

5. **Domestic Violence:** According to a Family and Youth Services Bureau report (2016), up to 57% of homeless women identify domestic violence as the primary reason for homelessness. Other research found that 93% of homeless mothers had a history of trauma, 79% experienced trauma as children,

and 81% experienced multiple traumatic events (NCH, 2017). The need for trauma-informed care in this population cannot be overstated.

6. **Addiction Disorders:** Individuals with untreated alcohol or drug addictions are at increased risk for homelessness. The following have been cited as obstacles to addiction treatment for homeless persons: lack of health insurance, lack of documentation, waiting lists for treatment programs, scheduling difficulties, daily contact requirements, lack of transportation, ineffective treatment methods, lack of supportive services, and cultural insensitivity.

Symptomatology (Commonly Associated With Homelessness)

1. Mobility and migration (the penchant for frequent movement to various geographic locations)
2. Substance abuse
3. Nutritional deficiencies
4. Difficulty with thermoregulation
5. Increased incidence of tuberculosis
6. Increased incidence of sexually transmitted diseases
7. Increased incidence of gastrointestinal (GI) and respiratory disorders
8. Increased incidence of arrests and legal issues
9. Among homeless children (compared with control samples), increased incidence of:
   a. Ear infections
   b. GI and respiratory disorders
   c. Infestational ailments
   d. Developmental delays
   e. Psychological problems

Common Nursing Diagnoses and Interventions

(Interventions are applicable to various health-care settings, such as inpatient and partial hospitalization, community health clinic, "street clinic," and homeless shelters.)

■ INEFFECTIVE HEALTH MAINTENANCE

Definition: Inability to identify, manage, and/or seek out help to maintain well-being (NANDA International [NANDA-I], 2018, p. 150)

Possible Contributing Factors ("related to")

Perceptual/cognitive impairment
Deficient communication skills

Unachieved developmental tasks
Insufficient resources (e.g., housing, finances)
Inability to make appropriate judgments
Ineffective individual coping

Defining Characteristics ("evidenced by")

History of lack of health-seeking behavior
Impairment of personal support systems
Demonstrated lack of knowledge about basic health practices
Demonstrated lack of adaptive behaviors to environmental changes
Inability to take responsibility for meeting basic health practices

Goals/Objectives

Short-term Goal

The patient will seek and receive assistance with current health matters.

Long-term Goals

1. The patient will assume responsibility for own health-care needs within level of ability.
2. The patient will adopt lifestyle changes that support individual health-care needs.

Interventions With *Selected Rationales*

1. The triage nurse in the emergency department, street clinic, or shelter will begin the biopsychosocial assessment of the homeless patient. *An adequate assessment is required to ensure appropriate nursing care is provided.*
2. Assess developmental level of functioning and ability to communicate. Use language that the patient can comprehend. *This information is essential to ensure that the patient achieves an accurate understanding of information presented and that the nurse correctly interprets what the patient is attempting to convey.*
3. Assess the patient's use of substances, including use of tobacco. Discuss eating and sleeping habits. *These actions may be contributing to current health problems.*
4. Assess sexual practices *to determine level of personal risk.*
5. Assess oral hygiene practices *to determine specific self-care needs.*
6. Assess the patient's ability to make decisions. *The patient may need assistance in determining the type of care that is required, how to determine the most appropriate time to seek that care, and where to go to receive it.*
7. It is important to ask the following basic questions about illness management:
   a. Do you understand the symptoms and treatment options for your illness?
   b. How will you get your prescriptions filled?

c. Where are you going when you leave here, or where will you sleep tonight?
Answers to these questions at admission to a treatment setting will initiate discharge planning for the patient.

8. Teach the patient the basics of self-care (e.g., proper hygiene, facts about nutrition). *The patient must have this type of knowledge if he or she is to become more self-sufficient.*

9. Teach the patient about safe-sex practices *in an effort to avoid sexually transmitted diseases.*

10. Identify immediate problems and assist with crisis intervention. *Emergency departments, "storefront" clinics, or shelters may be the homeless patient's only resource in a crisis situation.*

11. Tend to physical needs immediately. Ensure that the patient has a thorough physical examination. *The patient cannot deal with psychosocial issues until physical problems have been addressed.*

12. Assess mental health status. *Many homeless individuals have some form of mental illness.* Ensure that appropriate psychiatric care is provided. If possible, inquire about possible long-acting medication injections for the patient. *The patient may be less likely to discontinue the medication if he or she does not have to take pills every day.*

13. Refer the patient to others who can provide assistance (e.g., case manager, social worker). *If the patient is to be discharged to a shelter, a case manager or social worker may be the best link between the patient and the health-care system to ensure that he or she obtains appropriate follow-up care.*

14. Implement trauma-informed care in assessment and intervention. *Trauma is a common experience in homeless individuals. Assessment and intervention that is sensitive to the impact of trauma enhances the effectiveness of nursing care.*

Outcome Criteria

1. The patient verbalizes understanding of information presented regarding optimal health maintenance.
2. The patient is able to verbalize signs and symptoms that should be reported to a health-care professional.
3. The patient verbalizes knowledge of available resources from which he or she may seek assistance as required.

■ POWERLESSNESS

Definition: The lived experience of lack of control over a situation, including a perception that one's actions do not significantly affect an outcome (NANDA-I, 2018, p. 343)

Possible Contributing Factors ("related to")

[Lifestyle of helplessness]
[Homelessness]
Inadequate interpersonal interactions

Defining Characteristics ("evidenced by")

Reports lack of control (e.g., over self-care, situation, outcome)
[Apathy]
[Inadequate coping patterns]

Goals/Objectives

Short-term Goal

The patient will identify areas over which he or she has control.

Long-term Goal

The patient will make decisions that reflect control over present situation and future outcome.

Interventions With *Selected Rationales*

1. Provide opportunities for the patient to make choices about his or her present situation. *Providing the patient with choices will increase his or her feeling of control.*
2. Avoid arguing or using logic with the patient who feels powerless. *Respecting and acknowledging the patient's subjective experience is foundational to developing trust and promoting patient-centered care.* Accept expressions of feelings, including anger and hopelessness. *An attitude of acceptance enhances feelings of trust and self-worth.*
3. Help the patient identify personal strengths and establish realistic life goals. *Unrealistic goals set the patient up for failure and reinforce feelings of powerlessness.*
4. Help the patient identify areas of life situation that he or she can control. *The patient's emotional condition interferes with his or her ability to solve problems. Assistance is required to accurately perceive the benefits and consequences of available alternatives.*
5. Help the patient identify areas of life situation that are not within his or her ability to control. Encourage verbalization of feelings related to this inability *in an effort to deal with unresolved issues (e.g., joblessness, homelessness) and accept what cannot be changed (e.g., living with a mental illness).*
6. Encourage the patient to seek out a support group or shelter resources. *Social isolation promotes feelings of powerlessness and hopelessness.*

Outcome Criteria

1. The patient verbalizes choices made in a plan to maintain control over his or her life situation.
2. The patient verbalizes honest feelings about life situations over which he or she has no control.
3. The patient is able to verbalize a system for problem solving as required to maintain hope for the future.

■ POST-TRAUMA SYNDROME

Definition: "Sustained maladaptive response to a traumatic, overwhelming event, which may compromise health." (NANDA-I, 2018, p. 316)

Possible Contributing Factors

Environment not conducive to needs
Insufficient social support
Homelessness
Current or historical exposure to physically or psychologically traumatic events

Defining Characteristics

Nightmares
Flashbacks
Dissociative amnesia
Withdrawal
Substance use
Hypervigilance
Cardiac or other physical symptoms

Goals/Objectives

Short-term goal

The patient will seek and receive trauma-informed support services.

Long-term goal

The patient will demonstrate adaptive coping mechanisms and report resolution of intrusive trauma-related symptoms

Interventions With *Selected Rationales*

1. Conduct a thorough biopsychosocial assessment including assessment for history of trauma and evidence of current trauma-related symptoms. *Homeless individuals are a high risk*

population for trauma either historically (such as victims of domestic violence) or by virtue of current unstable living conditions.

2. Ask direct questions about patient history of traumatic events. *Traumatic events may have long-term consequences for both physical and emotional well-being. Awareness of past trauma also reduces the risk of re-traumatization when providing health care.*

3. Provide opportunity for the patient to give accounts of past trauma, using a nonjudgmental approach and without probing. *Nonjudgmental listening provides an avenue for catharsis that the patient needs to begin healing. Empathic listening without probing reduces the risk of retraumatization.*

4. Communicate with transparency and encourage patient collaboration in decisions around care and treatment. *Patients with a history of trauma may be hypervigilant and have difficulty establishing trust. Transparency and collaboration facilitate trust.*

5. Ensure that the patient has adequate privacy for all immediate interventions and ask for the patient's permission for nursing interventions, particularly those that include touch. Try to have as few people as possible providing care or collecting assessment data. *These approaches empower the patient to participate in decision-making and reduce the risk of re-traumatization.*

6. Explore community resources available to assist with trauma recovery. *Accessing resources to assist with trauma recovery may prevent longer term consequences associated with unresolved trauma issues.*

Outcome Criteria

1. The patient demonstrates the ability to establish trust with the nurse.
2. The patient verbalizes that acute post-trauma symptoms have resolved.
3. The patient identifies resources available to support ongoing recovery from trauma.

@ INTERNET REFERENCES

Additional information related to homelessness may be located at the following Web sites:

- www.nationalhomeless.org
- https://endhomelessness.org
- https://www.projecthome.org/about/facts-homelessness

- https://www.hhs.gov/programs/social-services/homelessness/index.html
- https://www.samhsa.gov/homelessness-programs-resources
- https://www.americanbar.org/groups/public_services/homelessness_poverty.html

Movie Connections

The Soloist • *The Grapes of Wrath* • *Generosity* • *The Redemption* • *On the Streets* (documentary)

CHAPTER 18

Psychiatric Home Nursing Care

■ BACKGROUND ASSESSMENT DATA

Dramatic changes in the health-care delivery system and skyrocketing costs have created a need to find a way to provide quality, cost-effective care to psychiatric patients. Home care has become one of the fastest growing areas in the health-care system and is now recognized by many reimbursement agencies as a preferred method of community-based service. Just what is home health care? For psychiatric patients, it is a wide range of services including safety assessments, injections, patient and family education, counseling, and monitoring of an unstable illness. This service is typically provided to patients who are homebound for either psychiatric or physical reasons.

The psychiatric home-care nurse must have knowledge and skills to meet both the physical and psychosocial needs of the homebound patient. Serving health-care consumers in their home environment charges the nurse with the responsibility of providing holistic care.

Predisposing Factors

An increase in psychiatric home care may be associated with the following factors:

1. Earlier hospital discharges
2. Increased demand for home care as an alternative to institutional care
3. Broader third-party payment coverage
4. Greater physician acceptance of home care
5. The increasing need to contain health-care costs and the growth of managed care

Psychiatric home nursing care is provided through private home health agencies; private hospitals; public hospitals; government institutions, such as the Veterans Administration; and community mental health centers. Most often, home care is viewed as follow-up care to inpatient, partial, or outpatient hospitalization. The majority of home health care is paid for by Medicare. Other sources include Medicaid, private insurance, self-pay, and others.

An acute psychiatric diagnosis is not enough to qualify for the service. The patient must show that he or she is unable to leave the home without considerable difficulty or the assistance of another person. The plan of treatment and subsequent charting must explain why the patient's psychiatric disorder keeps him or her at home and justify the need for home services. Home care must be prescribed by a physician.

Although Medicare and Medicaid are the largest reimbursement providers, a growing number of health maintenance organizations (HMOs) and preferred provider organizations (PPOs) are recognizing the cost effectiveness of psychiatric home nursing care and are including it as part of their benefit packages. Most managed care agencies require that treatment, or even a specific number of visits, be preauthorized for psychiatric home nursing care.

Symptomatology (Subjective and Objective Data)

Homebound psychiatric patients most often have a diagnosis of depressive disorder, neurocognitive disorder, anxiety disorder, bipolar disorder, or schizophrenia. Psychiatric nurses also provide consultation for patients with primary medical disorders. Many elderly patients are homebound because of medical conditions that impair mobility and necessitate home care. Depression is a common comorbidity with several of these conditions, especially diabetes, cardiovascular conditions such as myocardial infarctions and strokes, and neurocognitive disorders. Psychiatric nurses may provide the following types of home nursing care:

- Education and consultation to assist the patient and caregivers in managing symptoms of psychiatric illness.
- Basic medical care, counseling, and education to patients who are homebound for medical conditions but have a psychiatric condition for which they have been receiving (and continue to need ongoing) treatment.
- Assessment and intervention for patients who are homebound and at risk for developing serious psychiatric symptoms without skilled care intervention. Table 18–1 identifies some of the conditions for which a psychiatric nursing home-care consultation may be sought.

The following components should be included in the comprehensive assessment of the homebound patient:

1. Patient's perception of the problem and need for assistance
2. Information regarding patient's strengths and personal habits
3. Health history, review of systems, and vital signs
4. Any recent changes (physical, psychosocial, environmental)
5. Availability of support systems
6. Current medication regimen (including patient's understanding about the medications and reason for taking)
7. Nutritional and elimination assessment

TABLE 18–1	Conditions That Warrant Psychiatric Nursing Consultation

- When a client has a new psychiatric diagnosis
- When a new psychotropic medication has been added to the regimen
- When the client's mental status exacerbates or causes deterioration in his or her medical condition
- When the client is suspected of abusing alcohol or drugs
- When a client is expressing suicidal ideation
- When a client is noncompliant with psychotropic medication
- When a client develops a fundamental change in mood or a thought disorder
- When a client is immobilized by severe depression or anxiety

Source: Adapted from Schroeder, B. (2013). *Getting started in home care*. *Nurse.com Nursing CE Courses*. Retrieved from http://ce.nurse.com/course/60085/getting-started-in-home-care.

8. Activities of daily living (ADLs) assessment
9. Substance use assessment
10. Neurological assessment
11. Mental status examination including risk of harm to self or others (see Appendices K and M)

Other important assessments include information about acute or chronic medical conditions, patterns of sleep and rest, solitude and social interaction, use of leisure time, education and work history, issues related to religion or spirituality, and adequacy of the home environment.

Nursing Diagnoses and Interventions Common to Homebound Psychiatric Patients

■ INEFFECTIVE HEALTH MANAGEMENT

Definition: Pattern of regulating and integrating into daily living a therapeutic regime for treatment of illness and its sequelae that is unsatisfactory for meeting specific health goals (NANDA International [NANDA-I], 2018, p. 151)

Possible Contributing Factors ("related to")

Perceived barriers
Social support deficit
Powerlessness
Perceived benefits
[Mistrust of regimen and/or health-care personnel]
Deficient knowledge
Complexity of therapeutic regimen

Defining Characteristics ("evidenced by")

Ineffective choices in daily living for meeting health goals
Failure to include treatment regimens in daily living
Failure to take action to reduce risk factors
Reports difficulty with prescribed regimens
Reports desire to manage the illness

Goals/Objectives

Short-term Goals

1. The patient will verbalize understanding of barriers to self-health management.
2. The patient will participate in problem-solving efforts toward adequate self-health management.

Long-term Goal

The patient will incorporate changes in lifestyle necessary to maintain effective self-health management.

Interventions With *Selected Rationales*

1. Assess the patient's knowledge of condition and treatment needs. *The patient may lack full comprehension of need for treatment regimen.*
2. Identify the patient's perception of treatment regimen. *The patient may be mistrustful of treatment regimen or of health-care system in general.*
3. Encourage the patient to participate in decision making while conveying genuine positive regard and honesty. *Incorporating these skills promotes a trusting relationship and patient-centered care.*
4. Assist the patient in recognizing strengths and past successes. *Recognition of strengths and past successes increases self-esteem and indicates to the patient that he or she can be successful in managing therapeutic regimen.*
5. Provide positive reinforcement for efforts. *Positive reinforcement promotes self-esteem and encourages repetition of desirable behaviors.*
6. Emphasize the benefits of adherence to treatment and/or medication. *Patients must understand that the consequence of lack of follow-through is possible decompensation.*
7. Help the patient develop plans for managing therapeutic regimen, such as attending support groups, integration in social and family systems, and seeking financial assistance. *Goal-directed plans and structure facilitate incorporating lifestyle changes that promote wellness.*

Outcome Criteria

1. The patient verbalizes understanding of information presented regarding management of therapeutic regimen.

2. The patient demonstrates desire and ability to perform strategies necessary to maintain adequate management of therapeutic regimen.
3. The patient verbalizes knowledge of available resources from which he or she may seek assistance as required.

■ RISK-PRONE HEALTH BEHAVIOR

Definition: Impaired ability to modify lifestyle and/or actions in a manner that improves the level of wellness (NANDA-I, 2018, p. 149)

Possible Contributing Factors ("related to")

Inadequate comprehension
Inadequate social support
Low self-efficacy
Inadequate financial resources
Multiple stressors
Negative attitude toward health care
[Intense emotional state]

Defining Characteristics ("evidenced by")

Demonstrates nonacceptance of health status change
Failure to achieve optimal sense of control
Failure to take action that prevents health problems
Minimizes health status change

Goals/Objectives

Short-term Goals

1. The patient will discuss with home health nurse the kinds of lifestyle changes that will occur because of the change in health status.
2. With the help of home health nurse, the patient will formulate a plan of action for incorporating those changes into his or her lifestyle.
3. The patient will demonstrate movement toward independence, considering change in health status.

Long-term Goal

The patient will demonstrate competence to function independently to his or her optimal ability, considering change in health status, by time of discharge from home health care.

Interventions With *Selected Rationales*

1. Encourage the patient to talk about lifestyle prior to the change in health status. Discuss coping mechanisms that were used at stressful times in the past. *It is important to identify the patient's*

strengths so that they may be used to facilitate adaptation to the change or loss that has occurred.

2. Encourage the patient to discuss the change or loss and particularly to express anger associated with it. *Some individuals may not realize that anger is a normal stage in the grieving process. If it is not released in an appropriate manner, it may be turned inward on the self, leading to pathological depression.*

3. Encourage the patient to express fears associated with the change or loss or alteration in lifestyle that the change or loss has created. *Change often creates a feeling of disequilibrium, and the individual may respond with fears that are irrational or unfounded. He or she may benefit from feedback that corrects misperceptions about how life will be with the change in health status.*

4. Provide assistance with ADLs as required, but encourage independence to the limit that the patient's ability will allow. Give positive feedback for activities accomplished independently. *Independent accomplishments and positive feedback enhance self-esteem and encourage repetition of desired behaviors. Successes also provide hope that adaptive functioning is possible and decrease feelings of powerlessness.*

5. Help the patient with decision making regarding incorporation of the change or loss into his or her lifestyle. Identify problems that the change or loss is likely to create. Discuss alternative solutions, weighing potential benefits and consequences of each alternative. Support the patient's decision in the selection of an alternative. *The great amount of anxiety that usually accompanies a major lifestyle change often interferes with an individual's ability to solve problems and to make appropriate decisions. Patient may need assistance with this process in an effort to progress toward successful adaptation. This approach incorporates concepts of motivational interviewing and patient-centered care, both of which have been identified as effective strategies for assisting a patient to explore behavior change.*

6. Use role-playing to decrease anxiety as the patient anticipates stressful situations that might occur in relation to the health status change. *Role-playing decreases anxiety and provides a feeling of security by arming the patient with a plan of action with which to respond in an appropriate manner when a stressful situation occurs.*

7. Ensure that the patient and family are fully knowledgeable regarding the physiology of the change in health status. Encourage them to ask questions, and provide printed material explaining the change to which they may refer following discharge. *Educating patients and families about the physiology associated with changes in health status empowers patients to be actively involved in their care and promotes confidence in caregivers who are providing supportive care.*

8. Help the patient identify resources within the community from which he or she may seek assistance in adapting to the change in health status. Examples include self-help or support groups, counselor, or social worker. Encourage the patient to keep follow-up

appointments with the physician or to call the physician's office prior to follow-up date if problems or concerns arise. *Assisting patients to identify relevant community resources empowers patients to become active participants in their ongoing care.*

Outcome Criteria

1. The patient is able to perform ADLs independently.
2. The patient is able to make independent decisions regarding lifestyle considering the change in health status.
3. The patient is able to express hope for the future with consideration of change in health status.

■ SOCIAL ISOLATION

Definition: Aloneness experienced by the individual and perceived as imposed by others and as a negative or threatening state (NANDA-I, 2018, p. 455)

Possible Contributing Factors ("related to")

Alterations in mental status
Inability to engage in satisfying personal relationships
Unaccepted social values
Unaccepted social behavior
Inadequate personal resources
Alterations in physical appearance
Altered state of wellness

Defining Characteristics ("evidenced by")

Reports feelings of aloneness imposed by others
Reports feelings of rejection
Developmentally inappropriate interests
Inability to meet expectations of others
Insecurity in public
Absence of supportive significant other(s)
Projects hostility
Withdrawn; uncommunicative
Preoccupation with own thoughts
Sad, dull affect

Goals/Objectives

Short-term Goal

The patient will verbalize willingness to be involved with others.

Long-term Goal

The patient will participate in interactions with others at level of ability or desire.

Interventions With *Selected Rationales*

1. Convey an accepting attitude by making regular visits. *An accepting attitude increases feelings of self-worth and facilitates trust.*
2. Show unconditional positive regard. *This conveys your belief in the patient as a worthwhile human being.*
3. Be honest and keep all promises. *Honesty and dependability promote a trusting relationship.*
4. Be cautious with touch until trust has been established. *A suspicious patient may perceive touch as a threatening gesture.*
5. Be with the patient to offer support during activities that may be frightening or difficult for him or her. *The presence of a trusted individual provides emotional security for the patient.*
6. Take walks with the patient. Help him or her perform simple tasks around the house. *Increased activity enhances both physical and mental status.*
7. Assess patient patterns of behavior in relationships and communication. Offer social skills education and feedback once a trusting relationship has been established. *Providing education and feedback related to communication and behavior provides a foundation for problem-solving and change.*
8. Help the patient identify present relationships that are satisfying and activities that he or she considers interesting. *Only the patient knows what he or she truly likes, and these personal preferences will facilitate success in reversing social isolation.*
9. Consider the feasibility of a pet. *There are many documented studies of the benefits of companion animals.*

Outcome Criteria

1. The patient demonstrates willingness and ability to socialize with others.
2. The patient independently pursues social activities with others.

■ RISK FOR CAREGIVER ROLE STRAIN

Definition: Susceptible to difficulty in fulfilling care responsibilities, expectations, and/or behaviors for family or significant others, which may compromise health (NANDA-I, 2018, p. 281)

Risk Factors

Caregiver's competing role commitments
Inadequate physical environment for providing care (e.g., housing, transportation, community services, equipment)
Unpredictable illness course or instability in the care receiver's health
Psychological or cognitive problems in care receiver
Presence of abuse or violence

Past history of poor relationship between caregiver and care receiver
Marginal caregiver's coping patterns
Lack of respite and recreation for caregiver
Substance abuse or codependency
Caregiver not developmentally ready for caregiver role
Illness severity of the care receiver
Duration of caregiving required
Family/caregiver isolation

Goals/Objectives

Short-term Goal

Caregivers will verbalize understanding of ways to facilitate the caregiver role.

Long-term Goal

Caregivers will demonstrate effective problem-solving skills and develop adaptive coping mechanisms to regain equilibrium.

Interventions With *Selected Rationales*

1. Assess caregivers' abilities to anticipate and fulfill the patient's unmet needs. Provide information to assist caregivers with this responsibility. Ensure that caregivers encourage the patient to be as independent as possible. *Caregivers may be unaware of what the patient can realistically accomplish. They may be unaware of the nature of the illness.*
2. Educate caregivers regarding symptoms of illness and management strategies. *Providing information about symptoms such as delusions, hallucinations, depression, and suicidal ideation and education about strategies for responding to these symptoms enhances the caregiver's skill and sense of competency to provide needed care.*
3. Ensure that caregivers are aware of available community support systems from which they can seek assistance when required. Examples include respite care services, day treatment centers, and adult day-care centers. *Caregivers require relief from the pressures and strain of providing 24-hour care for their loved one. Studies have shown that abuse arises out of caregiving situations that place overwhelming stress on the caregivers.*
4. Encourage caregivers to express feelings, particularly anger. *Release of these emotions can serve to prevent psychopathology, such as depression or psychophysiological disorders, from occurring.*
5. Encourage participation in support groups composed of members with similar life situations. Provide information about support groups that may be helpful:
   a. National Alliance on Mental Illness—https://www.nami.org/
   b. American Association on Intellectual and Developmental Disabilities—http://aaidd.org/
   c. Alzheimer's Association—http://aaidd.org/
   Hearing others who are experiencing the same problems discuss ways in which they have coped may help the caregiver adopt more adaptive

strategies. Individuals who are experiencing similar life situations provide empathy and support for each other.

Outcome Criteria

1. Caregivers are able to solve problems effectively regarding care of the patient.
2. Caregivers demonstrate adaptive coping strategies for dealing with stress of the caregiver role.
3. Caregivers openly express feelings.
4. Caregivers express desire to join a support group of other caregivers.

@ INTERNET REFERENCES

Additional information related to psychiatric home nursing care may be located at the following Web sites:

- https://www.cms.gov
- www.nahc.org
- https://www.aahomecare.org

CHAPTER **19**

Forensic Nursing

■ BACKGROUND ASSESSMENT DATA

Forensic nursing is broadly defined as a field of practice that integrates health care and consideration of relevant legal issues. Catalano (2020) offers the following:

> Forensic nursing is an emerging field that forms an alliance between nursing, law enforcement, and the forensic sciences. The term forensic means anything belonging to, or pertaining to, the law… Forensic nurses provide a continuum of care to victims and their families beginning in the emergency room or crime scene and leading to participation in the criminal investigation and the courts of law (p. 700).

The International Association of Forensic Nurses (IAFN) (2019) states:

> A forensic nurse is a nurse who provides specialized care for patients who are victims and/or perpetrators of trauma (both intentional and unintentional). Forensic nurses are NURSES first and foremost. However, the specialized role of forensic nurses goes far beyond medical care; forensic nurses also have a specialized knowledge of the legal system and skills in injury identification, evaluation and documentation. After attending to a patient's immediate medical needs, a forensic nurse often collects evidence, provides medical testimony in court, and consults with legal authorities.

The IAFN and American Nurses Association (ANA) (2015) defines the scope and standards of practice for forensic nursing. Areas of forensic nursing include:

1. Clinical forensic nursing (including interpersonal violence and death investigation)
2. Sexual assault nurse examiner (SANE)
3. Forensic mental health nursing (management of patient care for patients with concurrent legal issues which may include felony, manslaughter, or other charges)
4. Forensic correctional nursing

5. Legal nurse consultant
6. Forensic nurse death investigator
7. Nurses in general practice (including medical/social history, physical examination, and documentation of issues that may have legal ramifications)

Clinical Forensic Nursing in Trauma Care
Assessment

Forensic nurse examiners (FNEs) often practice in emergency departments. They are specially trained to perform services that will gather and protect the viability of evidence that may be needed in legal proceedings. These services include sexual assault examinations, formal assessments for abuse and neglect, forensic photography, wound identification, evidence collection, and expert testimony. All traumatic injuries in which liability is suspected are considered within the scope of forensic nursing. Reports to legal agencies are required to ensure follow-up investigation; however, the protection of patients' rights remains a nursing priority.

Several areas of assessment in which the clinical forensic nurse specialist in trauma care may become involved include the following:

1. **Preservation of Evidence:** Evidence from both crime-related and self-inflicted traumas must be safeguarded in a manner consistent with the investigation. Evidence such as clothing, bullets, blood stains, hairs, fibers, and small pieces of material such as fragments of metal, glass, paint, and wood should be saved and documented in all medical accident instances that have legal implications.
2. **Investigation of Wound Characteristics:** Wounds that the nurse must be able to identify include:
   a. **Sharp-Force Injuries:** Include stab wounds and other wounds resulting from penetration with a sharp object.
   b. **Blunt-Force Injuries:** Include cuts and bruises resulting from the impact of a blunt object against the body.
   c. **Dicing Injuries:** Multiple, minute cuts and abrasions caused by contact with shattered glass (e.g., often occur in motor vehicle accidents).
   d. **Patterned Injuries:** Specific injuries that reflect the pattern of the weapon used to inflict the injury.
   e. **Bite-Mark Injuries:** A type of patterned injury inflicted by human or animal.
   f. **Defense Wounds:** Injuries that reflect the victim's attempt to defend himself or herself from attack.

g. **Hesitation Wounds:** Usually superficial, sharp-force wounds; often found perpendicular to the lower part of the body and may reflect self-inflicted wounds.

h. **Fast-Force Injuries:** Usually gunshot wounds; may reflect various patterns of injury.

3. **Deaths in the Emergency Department:** When deaths occur in the emergency department as a result of abuse or accident, evidence must be retained, the death must be reported to legal authorities, and an investigation is conducted. It is therefore essential that the nurse carefully document the appearance, condition, and behavior of the victim upon arrival at the hospital. The information gathered from the patient and family (or others accompanying the patient) may serve to facilitate the postmortem investigation and may be used during criminal justice proceedings.

The critical factor is to be able to determine if the cause of death is natural or unnatural. *Natural* deaths occur because of disease pathology of the internal organs or the degenerative aging process (Lynch & Koehler, 2011). In the emergency department, most deaths are sudden and unexpected. Those that are considered natural most commonly involve the cardiovascular, respiratory, and central nervous systems. Deaths that are considered *unnatural* include those from trauma, from self-inflicted acts, or from injuries inflicted by another. Legal authorities must be notified of all deaths related to unnatural circumstances.

■ TRAUMA-INFORMED CARE

Understanding the need for trauma-informed care is essential when responding to a victim of assault. It will influence our ability to establish a trusting relationship and to collect accurate evidence. An individual's response to trauma is rooted in fight or flight mechanisms (the autonomic nervous system) that are designed to protect one's survival but when activated, disrupt normal functions of our body systems, including the brain. Notably, memories become fragmented and sensory experiences become intensified. When someone has also had previous traumas, the fight or flight response is easily reactivated.

Thus, when a patient is interviewed immediately following a traumatic event, the patient may have extreme difficulty recalling events in sequence so the nurse must recognize that collecting information will take time and may be shared in seemingly disconnected parts. Sensory experiences may be so intensified that any loud noise, smell, visual experience, or touch can retrigger intense fear.

Assuring patients of their safety and working to establish trust, empathy, and compassionate care is not only good patient

care in general but for the trauma victim it reduces the likelihood that fear, the fight or flight response, and its effects on
the body and brain will be re-triggered. This process is called
re-traumatization. Evidence suggests that when trauma is not
recognized or treated with compassionate intervention, the
effects on the entire body can become chronic, leading to a host
of disorders including PTSD, depression, anger, cardiac illness,
and chronic pain.

Common Nursing Diagnoses and Interventions
(for Forensic Nursing in Trauma Care)

■ POST-TRAUMA SYNDROME/RAPE-TRAUMA SYNDROME

Definition: Post-trauma syndrome is defined as sustained maladaptive
response to a traumatic, overwhelming event (NANDA International,
[NANDA-I], 2018, p. 316). Rape-trauma syndrome is defined as sustained
maladaptive response to a forced, violent sexual penetration against the
victim's will and consent (NANDA-I, 2018, p. 319)

Possible Contributing Factors ("related to")

Physical and/or psychosocial abuse
Tragic occurrence involving multiple deaths
Sudden destruction of one's home or community
Epidemics
Disasters
Serious accidents (e.g., industrial, motor vehicle)
Witnessing mutilation, violent death, [or other horrors]
Serious threat or injury to self or loved ones
Rape

Defining Characteristics ("evidenced by")

[Physical injuries related to trauma]
Avoidance
Repression
Difficulty concentrating
Grieving; guilt
Intrusive thoughts
Neurosensory irritability
Palpitations
Anger and/or rage; aggression
Intrusive dreams; nightmares; flashbacks

Panic attacks; fear
Gastric irritability
Psychogenic amnesia
Substance abuse

Goals/Objectives

Short-term Goals

1. The patient's physical wounds will heal without complication.
2. The patient will begin a healthy grief resolution, initiating the process of psychological healing.

Long-term Goal

The patient will demonstrate ability to deal with emotional reactions in an individually appropriate manner.

Interventions With Selected Rationales

1. It is important to communicate the following to the victim of sexual assault:
   a. You are safe here.
   b. I'm sorry that it happened.
   c. I am very glad you survived.
   d. It is not your fault. No one deserves to be treated this way.
   e. You did the best that you could.
   The person who has been sexually assaulted fears for his or her life and must be reassured of safety. She or he may also be overwhelmed with self-doubt and self-blame, and these statements instill trust and validate self-worth.
2. Provide trauma-informed care including:
   a. Provide time for the patient to describe events. The patient may have difficulty recalling events in sequence in the wake of trauma related to its effects on the brain.
   b. Minimize noise in the environment and ask for permission before touching the patient. *Sensory perceptions are intensified following trauma and can retraumatize the patient.*
   c. Empower the patient to collaborate in treatment and care decisions. *Trauma evokes feelings of helplessness and powerlessness. Authoritarian or unilateral decisions about treatment and care may retraumatize the patient.*
3. Explain every assessment procedure that will be conducted and why it is being conducted. Ensure that data collection is conducted in a caring, nonjudgmental manner *to decrease fear and anxiety and increase trust.*
4. Engage the services of a sexual assault nurse examiner whenever possible. *Specialized skills in assessing and maintaining the viability of evidence supports the patient should he or she decide to pursue legal action.*

5. Collect evidence taking appropriate measures to secure and maintain uncontaminated data. These measures include wearing unpowdered gloves (powder may contaminate DNA evidence) and using alternate light sources (some injuries such as bruising secondary to strangulation or other forceful holding may not be evident in standard light). *The U.S. Department of Justice (2013) has established a national protocol for sexual assault medical forensic examination with detailed information for first responders to victims of sexual violence.* Ledray (2009) suggests the following five essential components of a forensic examination of the sexual assault survivor in the emergency department:

   a. **Treatment and Documentation Injuries:** Samples of blood, semen, hair, and fingernail scrapings should be sealed in paper—not plastic—bags *to prevent the possible growth of mildew from accumulation of moisture inside the plastic container and the subsequent contamination of the evidence.*

   b. **Maintaining the Proper Chain of Evidence:** Samples must be properly labeled, sealed, and refrigerated when necessary and kept under observation or properly locked until rendered to the proper legal authority *in order to ensure the proper chain of evidence and freshness of the samples.*

   c. **Treatment and Evaluation of Sexually Transmitted Diseases (STDs):** If conducted within 72 hours of the attack, several tests and interventions are available for prophylactic treatment of certain STDs.

   d. **Pregnancy Risk Evaluation and Prevention:** Prophylactic regimens, such as the postcoital progestin-only contraceptive (Plan B One-Step; Next Choice), significantly reduce the risk of pregnancy, especially when administered within the first 24 hours. The effectiveness decreases as the time between the assault and the first dose increases.

   e. **Crisis Intervention and Arrangements for Follow-up Counseling:** *Because a survivor is often too ashamed or fearful to seek follow-up counseling*, it may be important for the nurse to obtain the individual's permission to allow a counselor to call her to make a follow-up appointment.

6. In the case of other types of trauma (e.g., gunshot victims; automobile/pedestrian hit-and-run victims), *ensure that any possible evidence is not lost.* Clothing that is removed from a victim should not be shaken, and each separate item of clothing should be placed carefully in a paper bag, which should sealed, dated, timed, and signed.

7. Ensure that the patient has adequate privacy for all i postcrisis interventions. Try to have as few peopl

providing the immediate care or collecting immediate evidence. *The post-trauma patient is extremely vulnerable. Additional people in the environment may increase this feeling of vulnerability and escalate anxiety.*

8. Encourage the patient to give an account of the trauma/assault. Listen, but do not probe. *Nonjudgmental listening provides an opportunity for catharsis that the patient needs to begin healing. A detailed account may be required for legal follow-up, and a caring nurse, as a patient advocate, may help to lessen the trauma of evidence collection.*

9. Discuss with the patient whom to call for support or assistance. Provide information about referrals for aftercare. *Because of severe anxiety and fear, the patient may need assistance from others during this immediate postcrisis period. Provide referral information in writing for later reference (e.g., psychotherapist, mental health clinic, community advocacy group).*

10. In the event of a sudden and unexpected death in the trauma care setting, the clinical forensic nurse may be called upon to present information associated with an anatomical donation request to the survivors. *The clinical forensic nurse specialist is an expert in legal issues and has the knowledge and sensitivity to provide coordination between the medical examiner and families who are grieving the loss of loved ones.*

Outcome Criteria

1. The patient is no longer experiencing panic anxiety.
2. The patient demonstrates a degree of trust in the primary nurse.
3. The patient has received immediate attention to physical injuries.
4. The patient has initiated behaviors consistent with the grief response.
5. Necessary evidence has been collected and preserved in order to proceed appropriately within the legal system.

Forensic Mental Health Nursing in Correctional Facilities
Assessment

It was believed that deinstitutionalization increased the freedom of mentally ill individuals in accordance with the principle of "least restrictive alternative." However, because of inadequate community-based services, many of these individuals drift into poverty and homelessness, increasing their vulnerability to criminalization. When a homeless mentally ill individual behaves in a manner that causes public disruption or presents risk of harm to self or others, law enforcement officials have the authority to protect the welfare of the public, as well as the safety of the individual, by initiating emergency hospitalization. However, legal criteria for commitment are so stringent in most cases that arrest becomes an easier way of getting the mentally ill person off the street if a criminal statute has been violated. The U.S. Department of Justice reported that U.S. prisons and jails held more than 2 million inmates in 2011 (Glaze & Parks, 2012). Khazan (2015) reports that 55% of all male inmates and 73% of female inmates have mental illness; the majority have depression (21%) or bipolar disorder (12%). Some of these individuals are incarcerated as a result of the increasingly popular "guilty but mentally ill" verdict. With this verdict, individuals are deemed mentally ill yet are held criminally responsible for their actions. The individual is incarcerated and receives special treatment, if needed, but it is no different from that available for and needed by any prisoner.

Psychiatric diagnoses commonly identified at the time of incarceration include schizophrenia, bipolar disorder, major depression, personality disorders (especially antisocial personality disorder), and substance use disorders, and many have dual diagnoses. Common psychiatric symptoms include hallucinations, suspiciousness, thought disorders, anger/agitation, and impulsivity. Denial of problems is also common in this population. Use of substances and nonadherence to medication regimen are common obstacles to rehabilitation. Denial is often used as a defense mechanism. Substance abuse has been shown to have a strong correlation with recidivism among the prison population. Many individuals report that they were under the influence of substances at the time of their criminal actions. Detoxification frequently occurs in jails and prisons, and some inmates have died from the withdrawal syndrome because of inadequate treatment during this process.

Common Nursing Diagnoses and Interventions (for Forensic Nursing in Correctional Facilities)

■ DEFENSIVE COPING

Definition: Repeated projection of falsely positive self-evaluation based on a self-protective pattern that defends against underlying perceived threats to positive self-regard (NANDA-I, 2018, p. 326)

Possible Contributing Factors ("related to")

Low level of self-confidence
[Retarded ego development]
[Underdeveloped superego]
[Negative role models]
[Lack of positive feedback]

[Absent, erratic, or inconsistent methods of discipline]
[Dysfunctional family system]

Defining Characteristics ("evidenced by")

Denial of obvious problems or weaknesses
Projection of blame or responsibility
Rationalization of failures
Hypersensitivity to criticism
Grandiosity
Superior attitude toward others
Difficulty establishing or maintaining relationships
Hostile laughter or ridicule of others
Difficulty in perception of reality testing
Lack of follow-through or participation in treatment or therapy

Goals/Objectives

Short-term Goal

The patient will verbalize personal responsibility for own actions, successes, and failures.

Long-term Goal

The patient will demonstrate ability to interact with others and adapt to lifestyle goals without becoming defensive, rationalizing behaviors, or expressing grandiose ideas.

Interventions With *Selected Rationales*

1. Recognize and support basic ego strengths. *Focusing on positive aspects of the personality may help to improve self-concept.*
2. Encourage the patient to recognize and verbalize feelings of inadequacy and need for acceptance from others and how these feelings provoke defensive behaviors, such as blaming others for own behaviors. *Recognition of the problem is the first step in the change process toward resolution.*
3. Provide immediate, matter-of-fact, nonthreatening feedback for unacceptable behaviors. *The patient may lack knowledge about how he or she is being perceived by others. Direct the behavior in a nonthreatening manner to a more acceptable behavior.*
4. Help the patient identify situations that provoke defensiveness and practice more appropriate responses through role-playing. *Role-playing provides confidence to deal with difficult situations when they actually occur.*
5. Provide immediate positive feedback for acceptable behaviors. *Positive feedback enhances self-esteem and encourages repetition of desirable behaviors.*
6. Help the patient set realistic, concrete goals and determine appropriate actions to meet those goals. *Success increases self-esteem.*

7. Evaluate with the patient the effectiveness of the new behaviors and discuss any modifications for improvement. *Because of limited problem-solving ability, assistance may be required to reassess and develop new strategies in the event that certain of the new coping methods prove ineffective.*
8. Use confrontation judiciously *to help the patient begin to identify defense mechanisms (e.g., denial and projection) that are hindering development of satisfying relationships and adaptive behaviors.*

Outcome Criteria

1. The patient verbalizes and accepts responsibility for own behavior.
2. The patient verbalizes correlation between feelings of inadequacy and the need to defend the ego through rationalization and grandiosity.
3. The patient does not ridicule or criticize others.
4. The patient interacts with others in group situations without taking a defensive stance.

■ COMPLICATED GRIEVING

Definition: A disorder that occurs after the death of a significant other [or any other loss of significance to the individual], in which the experience of distress accompanying bereavement fails to follow normative expectations and manifests in functional impairment (NANDA-I, 2018, p. 340)

Possible Contributing Factors ("related to")

[Loss of freedom]

Defining Characteristics ("evidenced by")

[Anger]
[Internalized rage]
Depression
[Labile affect]
[Suicidal ideation]
[Difficulty expressing feelings]
[Altered activities of daily living]
[Prolonged difficulty coping]

Goals/Objectives

Short-term Goal
The patient will verbalize feelings of grief related to loss of freedom.

Long-term Goal

The patient will progress satisfactorily through the grieving process.

Interventions With *Selected Rationales*

1. Convey an accepting attitude—one that creates a nonthreatening environment for the patient to express feelings. Be honest and keep all promises. *An accepting attitude conveys to the patient that you believe he or she is a worthwhile person. Trust is enhanced.*

2. Identify the function that anger, frustration, and rage serve for the patient. Allow the patient to express these feelings within reason. *Verbalization of feelings in a nonthreatening environment may help the patient come to terms with unresolved grief.*

3. Encourage the patient to discharge pent-up anger through participation in large motor activities (e.g., physical exercises, volleyball, jogging). *Physical exercise provides a safe and effective method for discharging pent-up tension.*

4. Anger may be displaced onto the nurse or therapist, and caution must be taken to guard against the negative effects of countertransference. These are very difficult patients who have the capacity for eliciting a whole array of negative feelings from the health-care professional. These feelings must be acknowledged but not allowed to interfere with the therapeutic process.

5. Explain the behaviors associated with the normal grieving process. Help the patient to recognize his or her position in this process. *This knowledge about normal grieving may help facilitate the patient's progression toward resolution of grief.*

6. Help the patient understand appropriate ways to express anger. Give positive reinforcement for behaviors used to express anger appropriately. Act as a role model. *Positive reinforcement enhances self-esteem and encourages repetition of desirable behaviors. It is appropriate to let the patient know when he or she has done something that has generated angry feelings in you. Role modeling ways to express anger in an appropriate manner is a powerful learning tool.*

7. Set limits on acting-out behaviors and explain consequences of violation of those limits. Be supportive, yet consistent and firm, in working with this patient. *The patient lacks sufficient self-control to limit maladaptive behaviors; therefore, assistance is required from staff. Without consistency on the part of all staff members working with the patient, a positive outcome will not be achieved.*

8. Provide a safe and protective environment for the patient against risk of self-directed violence. *Depression is the emotion that most commonly precedes suicidal attempts.*

Outcome Criteria

1. The patient is able to verbalize ways in which anger and acting-out behaviors are associated with maladaptive grieving.
2. The patient expresses anger and hostility outwardly in a safe and acceptable manner.
3. The patient has not harmed self or others.

■ RISK FOR INJURY

Definition: Susceptible to physical damage due to [internal or external] environmental conditions interacting with the individual's adaptive and defensive resources, which may compromise health (NANDA-I, 2018, p. 393)

Risk Factors ("related to")

[Substance use/detoxification at time of incarceration, exhibiting any of the following:
   Substance intoxication
   Substance withdrawal
   Disorientation
   Seizures
   Hallucinations
   Psychomotor agitation
   Unstable vital signs
   Delirium
   Flashbacks
   Panic level of anxiety]
Suicidal ideation

Goals/Objectives

Short-term Goal
The patient's condition will stabilize within 72 hours.

Long-term Goal
The patient will not experience physical injury.

Interventions With *Selected Rationales*

1. Assess the patient's level of disorientation to determine specific requirements for safety. *Knowledge of the patient's level of functioning is necessary to formulate an appropriate plan of care.*

2. Obtain a drug history, if possible, to determine:
   a. Type of substance(s) used.
   b. Time of last ingestion and amount consumed.
   c. Duration and frequency of consumption.
   d. Amount consumed on a daily basis.
3. Obtain a urine sample for laboratory analysis of substance content. *Subjective history often is not accurate. Knowledge regarding substance ingestion is important for accurate assessment of the patient's condition.*
4. Place the patient in a quiet room, if possible. *Excessive stimuli increase patient agitation.*
5. Institute necessary safety precautions. *Patient safety is a nursing priority.*
   a. Observe patient behaviors frequently; assign staff on a one-to-one basis if condition warrants it; accompany and assist the patient when ambulating; use a wheelchair for transporting long distances.
   b. Be sure that side rails are up when the patient is in bed.
   c. Pad headboard and side rails of bed with thick towels to protect the patient in case of a seizure.
   d. Use mechanical restraints as necessary to protect the patient if excessive hyperactivity accompanies the disorientation.
6. Ensure that smoking materials and other potentially harmful objects are stored outside the patient's access. *The patient may harm self or others in disoriented, confused state.*
7. Monitor vital signs every 15 minutes initially and less frequently as acute symptoms subside. *Vital signs provide the most reliable information regarding the patient's condition and need for medication during the acute detoxification period.*
8. Follow medication regimen, as ordered by the physician. Common medical interventions for detoxification from substances include the following:
   a. **Alcohol:** Benzodiazepines are the most widely used group of drugs for substitution therapy in alcohol withdrawal. The approach to treatment is to start with relatively high doses and reduce the dosage by 20% to 25% each day until withdrawal is complete. In patients with liver disease, accumulation of the longer-acting agents, such as chlordiazepoxide (Librium), may be problematic, and the use of the shorter-acting benzodiazepine, oxazepam (Serax), is more appropriate. Some physicians may order anticonvulsant medication to be used prophylactically; however, this is not a universal intervention. Multivitamin therapy, in combination with daily thiamine (either orally or by injection), is common protocol.

b. **Opioids:** Narcotic antagonists, such as naloxone (Narcan) or naltrexone (ReVia), are administered for opioid intoxication. Withdrawal is managed with rest and nutritional therapy. Substitution therapy may be instituted with methadone (Dolophine) to decrease withdrawal symptoms. In October 2002, the FDA approved two forms of the drug buprenorphine for treating opiate dependence. Buprenorphine is less powerful than methadone but is considered to be somewhat safer and causes fewer side effects, making it especially attractive for patients who are mildly or moderately addicted. Suboxone is a combination drug that includes both buprenorphine and naloxone.

c. **Depressants:** Substitution therapy may be instituted to decrease withdrawal symptoms using a long-acting barbiturate, such as phenobarbital (Luminal). Some physicians prescribe oxazepam (Serax) as needed for objective symptoms, gradually decreasing the dosage until the drug is discontinued. Long-acting benzodiazepines are commonly used for substitution therapy when the abused substance is a nonbarbiturate CNS depressant.

d. **Stimulants:** Treatment of stimulant intoxication is geared toward stabilization of vital signs. Intravenous antihypertensives may be used, along with intravenous diazepam (Valium) to control seizures. Minor tranquilizers, such as chlordiazepoxide, may be administered orally for the first few days while the patient is "crashing." Treatment is aimed at reducing drug craving and managing severe depression. Suicide precautions may be required. Therapy with antidepressant medication is not uncommon.

e. **Hallucinogens and Cannabinoids:** Medications are normally not prescribed for withdrawal from these substances. However, in the event of overdose or the occurrence of adverse reactions (e.g., anxiety or panic), benzodiazepines (e.g., diazepam or chlordiazepoxide) may be given as needed to decrease agitation. Should psychotic reactions occur, they may be treated with antipsychotics.

9. Assess the patient regularly for evidence of risk for suicide and initiate safety precautions as needed. *Patient safety is a nursing priority.*

Outcome Criteria

1. The patient is no longer exhibiting any signs or symptoms of substance intoxication or withdrawal.
2. The patient shows no evidence of physical injury obtained during substance intoxication or withdrawal.
3. The patient remains free from self-harm.

@ INTERNET REFERENCES

Additional information related to forensic nursing may be found at the following Web sites:

- https://nurse.org/resources/forensic-nurse/
- www.amrn.com
- http://journals.lww.com/forensicnursing/pages/default.aspx
- www.forensicnurses.org
- https://www.ncjrs.gov/pdffiles1/ovw/241903.pdf

CHAPTER 20

Complementary Therapies

■ INTRODUCTION

The connection between mind and body, and the influence of each on the other, is well recognized by all clinicians and particularly by psychiatrists. Conventional medicine as it is currently practiced in the United States is based solely on scientific methodology. Conventional, science-based medicine, also known as *allopathic* medicine, is the type of medicine historically taught in U.S. medical schools.

The term *alternative medicine* has come to be recognized as practices that differ from the usual traditional practices in the treatment of disease. "Alternative" refers to an intervention that is used *instead of* conventional treatment. "Complementary therapy" is an intervention that is different from, but used *in conjunction with*, traditional or conventional medical treatment. In the United States, over 30% of adults use some form of complementary or alternative therapy (National Center for Complementary and Integrative Health [NCCIH], 2019). The most commonly used complementary approaches are nonvitamin, nonmineral dietary supplements such as fish oil, probiotics, prebiotics, melatonin, and glucosamine chondroitin. According to the 2017 National Health Interview Survey (NHIS), the popularity of yoga has grown dramatically in recent years and the use of meditation increased more than three-fold from 4.1% in 2012 to 14.2% in 2017 (NCCIH, 2019). Approximately $34 billion a year is spent on these types of therapies in the United States.

In 1991, an Office of Alternative Medicine (OAM) was established by the National Institutes of Health (NIH) to study nontraditional therapies and to evaluate their usefulness and their effectiveness. Since that time, the name was changed to the National Center for Complementary and Alternative Medicine (NCCAM) and most recently has been changed to the National Center for Complementary and Integrative Health (NCCIH). The term *integrative health* has been used (in addition to the terms complementary and alternative medicine) to describe a holistic approach that incorporates complementary and conventional practices in a coordinated, comprehensive treatment plan. According to the mission statement of NCCIH:

> The mission of NCCIH is to define, through rigorous scientific investigation, the usefulness and safety of complementary and integrative health interventions and their roles in improving health and health care. (NIH, 2017a)

Some health insurance companies and health maintenance organizations (HMOs) appear to be bowing to public pressure by including alternative providers in their networks of providers for treatments such as acupuncture and massage therapy. Chiropractic care has been covered by some third-party payers for many years. Individuals who seek alternative therapy, however, are often reimbursed at lower rates than those who choose conventional practitioners.

Patient education is an important part of complementary care. Positive lifestyle changes are encouraged, and practitioners serve as educators as well as treatment specialists. Complementary medicine is viewed as *holistic* health care, which deals not only with the physical perspective but also with the emotional and spiritual components of the individual. Interest in holistic health care is increasing worldwide. A large number of U.S. medical schools—among them Harvard, Yale, Johns Hopkins, and Georgetown Universities—now offer coursework in holistic methods. In recent policy statements, the American Medical Association resolves to support the incorporation of complementary and alternative medicine (CAM) in medical education and continuing medical education curricula, covering CAM's benefits, risks, and efficacy (Cohen, 2018).

■ TYPES OF COMPLEMENTARY THERAPIES

Herbal Medicine

The use of plants to heal is probably as old as humankind. Virtually every culture in the world has relied on herbs and plants to treat illness. Clay tablets from about 4000 BC reveal that the Sumerians had apothecaries for dispensing medicinal herbs. At the root of Chinese medicine is the *Pen Tsao*, a text written around 3000 BC, which contained hundreds of herbal remedies. When the Pilgrims came to America in the 1600s, they brought a variety of herbs to be established and used for medicinal purposes. The new settlers soon discovered that Native Americans also had their own varieties of plants used for healing.

Many people are seeking a return to herbal remedies because they perceive these remedies as being less potent than prescription drugs and as being free of adverse side effects. However, because the Food and Drug Administration (FDA) classifies herbal remedies as dietary supplements or food additives, their labels cannot indicate medicinal uses. They are not subject to FDA approval, and they lack uniform standards of quality control.

Several organizations have been established to attempt regulation and control of the herbal industry. They include the Council for Responsible Nutrition, the American Herbal Products Association, and the American Botanical Council. The Commission E of the German Federal Health Agency is the group responsible for researching and regulating the safety and efficacy of herbs and plant medicines in Germany. All of the Commission E monographs of herbal medicines have been translated into English and compiled into one text (Blumenthal, 1998).

Until more extensive testing has been completed on humans and animals, the use of herbal medicines must be approached with caution and responsibility. *The notion that something being "natural" means it is therefore completely safe is a myth.* In fact, some of the plants from which prescription drugs are derived are highly toxic in their natural state. Also, because of lack of regulation and standardization, ingredients may be adulterated. A research study that reviewed FDA data on adulterated supplements from 2007 to 2016 found that 776 over-the-counter products from 146 companies contained adulterated ingredients (Tucker et al, 2018). Most of the adulterated products were marketed for sexual enhancement, weight loss, or muscle building and they were adulterated with sildenafil, sibutramine, or synthetic steroids, respectively—all of which are drugs that are regulated by the FDA (or certainly beyond that specified for dietary supplements). Their method of manufacture also may alter potency. For example, dried herbs lose potency rapidly because of exposure to air. In addition, it is often safer to use preparations that contain only one herb. There is a greater likelihood of unwanted side effects with combined herbal preparations.

Table 20–1 lists information about common herbal remedies, with possible implications for psychiatric/mental health nursing. Botanical names, medicinal uses, and safety profiles are included.

Acupressure and Acupuncture

Acupressure and acupuncture are healing techniques based on the ancient philosophies of traditional Chinese medicine dating back to 3000 BC. The main concept behind Chinese medicine is that healing energy (*qi*) flows through the body along specific pathways called *meridians*. It is believed that these meridians of qi connect various parts of the body in a way similar to the way in which lines on a road map link various locations. The pathways link a conglomerate of points, called *acupoints*. Therefore, it is possible to treat a part of the body distant to another if the two points are linked by a meridian.

In acupressure, the fingers, thumbs, palms, or elbows are used to apply pressure to the acupoints. This is thought to dissolve any

(Text continued on page 370)

TABLE 20–1	**Herbal Remedies**	
Common Name (Botanical Name)	**Medicinal Uses/ Possible Action**	**Safety Profile**
Black cohosh (*Cimicifuga racemosa*)	May provide relief of menstrual cramps; improved mood; calming effect. Extracts from the roots are thought to have action similar to estrogen.	Generally considered safe in low doses. Occasionally causes gastrointestinal (GI) discomfort. Toxic in large doses, causing dizziness, nausea, headaches, stiffness, and trembling. Should not take with heart problems, concurrently with antihypertensives, or during pregnancy.
Cascara sagrada (*Rhamnus purshiana*)	Relief of constipation	Generally recognized as safe; sold as over-the-counter drug in the United States. Should not be used during pregnancy. Contraindicated in bowel obstruction or inflammation.
Chamomile (*Matricaria chamomilla*)	As a tea, is effective as a mild sedative in the relief of insomnia. May also aid digestion, relieve menstrual cramps, and settle upset stomach.	Generally recognized as safe when consumed in reasonable amounts.
Echinacea (*Echinacea angustifolia* and *Echinacea purpurea*)	Stimulates the immune system; may have value in fighting infections and easing the symptoms of colds and flu.	Considered safe in reasonable doses. Observe for side effects or allergic reaction.
Fennel (*Foeniculum vulgare* or *Foeniculum officinale*)	Used to ease stomachaches and to aid digestion. Taken in a tea or in extracts to stimulate the appetites of people with anorexia (1–2 tsp seeds steeped in boiling water for making tea).	Generally recognized as safe when consumed in reasonable amounts.

TABLE 20–1	Herbal Remedies—cont'd	
Common Name (Botanical Name)	**Medicinal Uses/ Possible Action**	**Safety Profile**
Feverfew (*Tanacetum parthenium*)	Prophylaxis and treatment of migraine headaches. Effective in either the fresh leaf or freeze-dried forms (2–3 fresh leaves [or equivalent] per day).	A small percentage of individuals may experience the adverse effect of temporary mouth ulcers. Considered safe in reasonable doses.
Ginger (*Zingiber officinale*)	Ginger tea to ease stomachaches and to aid digestion. Two powdered gingerroot capsules have shown to be effective in preventing motion sickness.	Generally recognized as safe in designated therapeutic doses.
Ginkgo (*Ginkgo biloba*)	Used to treat insufficient blood flow to the brain, dementia, anxiety, and schizophrenia (in combination with antipsychotics). Has been shown to dilate blood vessels. Usual dosage is 120–240 mg/day.	Safety has been established with recommended dosages. Possible side effects include headache, GI problems, and dizziness. Contraindicated in pregnancy and lactation and in patients with bleeding disorder. Possible compound effect with concomitant use of aspirin or anticoagulants.
Ginseng (*Panax ginseng*)	The ancient Chinese saw this herb as one that increased wisdom and longevity. Current studies support a possible positive effect on the cardiovascular system. Action not known.	Generally considered safe. Side effects may include headache, insomnia, anxiety, skin rashes, diarrhea. Avoid concomitant use with anticoagulants.
Hops (*Humulus lupulus*)	Used in cases of nervousness, mild anxiety, and insomnia. Also may relieve the cramping associated with diarrhea. May be taken as a tea, in extracts, or capsules.	Generally recognized as safe when consumed in recommended dosages.

(Continued)

TABLE 20–1	Herbal Remedies—cont'd	
Common Name (Botanical Name)	**Medicinal Uses/ Possible Action**	**Safety Profile**
Kava-kava (*Piper methysticum*)	Used to reduce anxiety while promoting mental acuity. Dosage: 150–300 mg bid.	Scaly skin rash may occur when taken at high dosage for long periods. Motor reflexes and judgment when driving may be reduced while taking the herb. Concurrent use with central nervous system (CNS) depressants may produce additive tranquilizing effects. Reports of potential for liver damage. Investigations continue. Should not be taken for longer than 3 months without a doctor's supervision.
Passion flower (*Passiflora incarnata*)	Used in tea, capsules, or extracts to treat nervousness and insomnia. Depresses the CNS to produce a mild sedative effect.	Generally recognized as safe in recommended doses.
Peppermint (*Mentha piperita*)	Used as a tea to relieve upset stomachs and headaches and as a mild sedative. Pour boiling water over 1 tbsp dried leaves and steep to make a tea. Oil of peppermint is also used for inflammation of the mouth, pharynx, and bronchus.	Considered to be safe when consumed in designated therapeutic dosages.
Psyllium (*Plantago ovata*)	Psyllium seeds are a popular bulk laxative commonly used for chronic constipation. Also found to be useful in the treatment of hypercholesterolemia.	Approved as an over-the-counter drug in the United States.

TABLE 20–1	Herbal Remedies—cont'd	
Common Name (Botanical Name)	**Medicinal Uses/ Possible Action**	**Safety Profile**
Skullcap *(Scutellaria lateriflora)*	Used as a sedative for mild anxiety and nervousness.	Considered safe in reasonable amounts.
St. John's wort *(Hypericum perforatum)*	Used in the treatment of mild to moderate depression. May block reuptake of serotonin/ norepinephrine and have a mild monoamine oxidase–inhibiting effect. Effective dose: 900 mg/day. May also have antiviral, antibacterial, and anti-inflammatory properties.	Generally recognized as safe when taken at rec-ommended dosages. Side effects include mild GI irritation that is lessened with food; photosensitivity when taken in high dosages over long periods. Should not be taken with other psychoactive medications.
Valerian *(Valeriana officinalis)*	Used to treat nervousness and insomnia. Produces restful sleep without morning "hangover." The root may be used to make a tea, or capsules are available in a variety of dosages. Mechanism of action is similar to benzodi-azepines, but without addicting properties. Daily dosage range: 100–1000 mg.	Generally recognized as safe when taken at rec-ommended dosages. Side effects may include mild headache or upset stomach. Taking doses higher than rec-ommended may result in severe headache, nausea, morning grog-giness, blurry vision. Should not be taken concurrently with CNS depressants or during pregnancy.

Sources: Adapted from Holt, G.A., & Kouzi, S. (2002*). Herbs through the ages.* In M.A. Bright (Ed.), *Holistic health and healing.* Philadelphia: F.A. Davis; Thomson Healthcare. (2007). *PDR for Herbal Medicines* (4th ed.). Montvale, NJ: Author; Pranthikanti, S. Ayurvedic treatments. In J.H. Lake & D. Spiegel (Eds.), *Complementary and alternative treatments in mental health care.* (2007). Washington, DC: American Psychiatric Publishing; Sadock, B.J., Sadock, V.A., & Ruiz, P. (2015). *Synopsis of psychiatry: Behavioral sciences/clinical psychiatry* (11th ed.). Philadelphia: Lippincott Williams & Wilkins; Mayo Clinic. (2019). *Drugs and supplements.* Retrieved from https://www.mayoclinic.org/drugs-supplements/

obstructions in the flow of healing energy and to restore the body to a healthier functioning. In acupuncture, hair-thin, sterile, disposable, stainless-steel needles are inserted into acupoints to dissolve the obstructions along the meridians. The needles may be left in place for a specified length of time, they may be rotated, or a mild electric current may be applied.

The Western medical philosophy regarding acupressure and acupuncture is that they stimulate the body's own painkilling chemicals—the morphine-like substances known as *endorphins*. Some studies have found that several factors, including expectation and beliefs, may account for the effectiveness of these procedures for treating pain conditions (National Center for Complementary and Integrative Health [NCCIH], 2017b). Acupuncture has a wealth of research behind it, and there is evidence that indicates effectiveness in treating pain conditions, but the benefits in treating other conditions remain uncertain (NCCIH, 2017b). Acupuncture is gaining wide acceptance in the United States by both patients and physicians. This treatment can be administered at the same time other techniques are being used, including conventional Western techniques, although it is essential that all health-care providers have knowledge of all treatments being received. One recent study found evidence that acupuncture, when combined with nimodipine to treat mild cognitive impairment following a cerebral infarction, enhanced the effectiveness of the medication to a greater extent than either treatment used alone (Wang et al, 2016). Ongoing research may reveal additional benefits of combination therapies. Acupuncture should be administered by a physician or an acupuncturist who is licensed by the state in which the service is provided. Typical training for licensed acupuncturists, doctors of oriental medicine, and acupuncture physicians is a 3- or 4-year program of 2,500 to 3,500 hours.

Diet and Nutrition

The value of nutrition in the healing process has long been underrated. Mazur and Litch (2019) state:

> Nutritional changes are essential to prevent medical conditions and diseases caused by nutrient deficiencies, such as iron-deficiency anemia. Excessive body weight is clearly related to heart disease, stroke, type 2 diabetes mellitus, some cancers, joint diseases, and some fertility disorders. The difficulty lies in motivating people to change behavior today for possible benefits in the future (p. 3).

Individuals select the foods they eat based on a number of factors, not the least of which is enjoyment. Eating must serve social and cultural, as well as nutritional, needs. The U.S. Departments of Agriculture (USDA) and Health and Human Services (USDHHS) have collaborated on a set of guidelines to help individuals understand what types of foods to eat and the healthy lifestyle they need to pursue in order to promote health and prevent disease. Following is a list of key recommendations from these guidelines (USDA/USDHHS, 2015): The eighth edition of *Dietary Guidelines for Americans 2015–2020* shifts the focus from food groups to developing healthy eating patterns. The key guidelines are stated as follows:

1. Follow a healthy eating pattern across the life span. All food and beverage choices matter. Choose a healthy eating pattern at an appropriate calorie level to help achieve and maintain a healthy body weight, support nutrient adequacy, and reduce the risk of chronic disease.

2. Focus on variety, nutrient density, and amount. To meet nutrient needs within calorie limits, choose a variety of nutrient-dense foods across and within all food groups in recommended amounts.

3. Limit calories from added sugars and saturated fats and reduce sodium intake. Consume an eating pattern low in added sugars, saturated fats, and sodium. Cut back on foods and beverages higher in these components to amounts that fit within healthy eating patterns.

4. Shift to healthier food and beverage choices. Choose nutrient-dense foods and beverages across and within all food groups in place of less healthy choices. Consider cultural and personal preferences to make these shifts easier to accomplish and maintain.

5. Support healthy eating patterns for all. Everyone has a role in helping to create and support healthy eating patterns in multiple settings nationwide, from home to school to work to communities (p. xii).

Foods and Food Components to Reduce

The following key recommendations are taken from the *Dietary Guidelines for Americans 2015*.

- Reduce daily sodium intake to less than 2,300 milligrams (mg) and further reduce intake to 1,500 mg among persons who are 51 and older and those of any age who are African American or have hypertension, diabetes, or chronic kidney disease. The 1,500 mg recommendation applies to about half of the U.S. population, including children and the majority of adults.
- Consume less than 10% of calories from saturated fatty acids by replacing them with monounsaturated and polyunsaturated fatty acids.
- Consume less than 300 mg per day of dietary cholesterol.
- Keep *trans*-fatty acid consumption as low as possible by limiting foods that contain synthetic sources of *trans*-fats, such as partially hydrogenated oils, and by limiting other solid fats.
- Reduce the intake of calories from solid fats and added sugars.

- Limit the consumption of foods that contain refined grains, especially refined grain foods that contain solid fats, added sugars, and sodium.
- If alcohol is consumed, it should be consumed in moderation—up to one drink per day for women and two drinks per day for men—and only by adults of legal drinking age.
  One drink is defined as:
- 12 ounces of regular beer (150 calories)
- 5 ounces of wine (100 calories)
- 1.5 ounces of 80-proof distilled spirits (100 calories)

The guidelines advise that alcohol should be avoided by individuals who are unable to restrict their intake; women who are pregnant (no safe level of alcohol intake during pregnancy has been established), may become pregnant, or are breastfeeding; and individuals who are taking medications that may interact with alcohol or who have specific medical conditions (USDA/USDHHS, 2015).

Foods and Nutrients to Increase

Individuals should meet the following recommendations as part of a healthy eating pattern while staying within their calorie needs:

- Increase vegetable and fruit intake.
- Eat a variety of vegetables, especially dark-green, red, and orange vegetables and beans and peas.
- Consume at least half of all grains as whole grains. Increase whole-grain intake by replacing refined grains with whole grains.
- Increase intake of fat-free or low-fat milk and milk products, such as milk, yogurt, cheese, or fortified soy beverages.
- Choose a variety of protein foods that includes seafood, lean meat and poultry, eggs, beans and peas, soy products, and unsalted nuts and seeds.
- Increase the amount and variety of seafood consumed by choosing seafood in place of some meat and poultry.
- Replace protein foods that are higher in solid fats with choices that are lower in solid fats and calories and/or are sources of oils.
- Use oils to replace solid fats when possible.
- Choose foods that provide more potassium, dietary fiber, calcium, and vitamin D, which are nutrients of concern in American diets. These foods include vegetables, fruits, whole grains, and milk and milk products.
- Meet recommended intakes within energy needs by adopting a balanced eating pattern, such as the USDA Food Guide (Table 20–2). Table 20–3 provides a summary of information about essential vitamins and minerals (USDA/USDHHS, 2015).

TABLE 20–2 **Sample USDA Food Guide at the 2,000-Calorie Level**

Food Groups and Subgroups	USDA Food Guide Daily Amount	Examples/Equivalent Amounts
Fruit Group	2 cups (4 servings)	½-cup equivalent is: • ½ cup fresh, frozen, or canned fruit • 1 medium fruit • ¼ cup dried fruit • ½ cup fruit juice
Vegetable Group	2.5 cups (5 servings) • Dark green vegetables: 1.5 cups/wk • Red and orange vegetables: 5.5 cups/wk • Legumes (dry beans/peas): 1.5 cups/wk • Starchy vegetables: 5 cups/wk • Other vegetables: 4 cups/wk	½-cup equivalent is: • ½ cup cut-up raw or cooked vegetable • 1 cup raw leafy vegetable • ½ cup vegetable juice
Grain Group	6 oz equivalents • Whole grains: 3 oz equivalents • Other grains: 3 oz equivalents	1 oz equivalent is: • 1 slice bread • 1 cup dry cereal • ½ cup cooked rice, pasta, cereal
Protein Foods	5.5 oz equivalents • Seafood: 8 oz equivalent/wk • Meat, poultry, eggs: 26 oz equivalent/wk • Nuts, seeds, soy products: 5 oz equivalent/wk	1 oz equivalent is: • 1 oz cooked lean meat, poultry, or fish • 1 egg • ¼ cup cooked dry beans or tofu • 1 tbsp peanut butter • ½ oz nuts or seeds
Dairy	3 cups	1-cup equivalent is: • 1 cup low-fat/fat-free milk • 1 cup low-fat/fat-free yogurt • 1.5 oz low-fat/fat-free natural cheese • 2 oz low-fat/fat-free processed cheese

(Continued)

TABLE 20–2	Sample USDA Food Guide at the 2,000-Calorie Level—cont'd	
Food Groups and Subgroups	USDA Food Guide Daily Amount	Examples/Equivalent Amounts
Oils	27 grams	1 tsp equivalent is: • 1 tbsp low-fat mayonnaise • 2 tbsp light salad dressing • 1 tsp vegetable oil • 1 tsp soft margarine with zero *trans*-fat
Discretionary Calorie Allowance	270 calories Example of distribution: • Solid fats, 18 grams (e.g., saturated and trans fats) • Added sugars, 8 tsp (e.g., sweetened cereals)	1 added sugar equivalent is: • ½ oz jelly beans • 8 oz lemonade Examples of solid fats: • Fat in whole milk or ice cream • Fatty meats Essential oils (above) are not considered part of the discretionary calories.

Source: U.S. Department of Agriculture & U.S. Department of Health and Human Services (2015). *Dietary guidelines for Americans 2015–2020* (8th ed.). Washington, DC: Office of Disease Prevention and Health Promotion. Retrieved from https://health.gov/dietaryguidelines/2015/resources/2015-2020_Dietary_Guidelines.pdf

Building Healthy Eating Patterns

• Select an eating pattern that meets nutrient needs over time at an appropriate calorie level.
• Account for all foods and beverages consumed and assess how they fit within a total healthy eating pattern.
• Follow food safety recommendations when preparing and eating foods to reduce the risk of food-borne illnesses (USDA/USDHHS, 2010, p. 43).

Chiropractic Medicine

Chiropractic medicine is probably the most widely used form of alternative healing in the United States. It was developed in the late 1800s by a self-taught healer named David Palmer and was later reorganized and expanded by his son Joshua, a trained practitioner. Palmer's objective was to find a cure for disease and illness that did not use drugs but instead relied on more natural methods of healing. Palmer's theory behind chiropractic medicine was that energy flows from the brain to all parts of the body

(Text continued on page 381)

TABLE 20-3	Essential Vitamins and Minerals			
Vitamin/Mineral	Function	DRI (UL)*	Food Sources	Comments
Vitamin A	Prevention of night blindness; calcification of growing bones; resistance to infection	Men: 900 mcg (3,000 mcg) Women: 700 mcg (3,000 mcg) **900 mcg of retinol activity equivalents (RAE)	Liver, butter, cheese, whole milk, egg yolk, fish, green leafy vegetables, carrots, pumpkin, sweet potatoes	May be of benefit in prevention of cancer because of its antioxidant properties, which are associated with control of free radicals that damage DNA and cell membranes.†
Vitamin D	Promotes absorption of calcium and phosphorus in the small intestine; prevention of rickets	Men and women: 15 mcg (100 mcg) Men and women >70 years of age: 20 mcg (100 mcg) ** 20 mcg	Fortified milk and dairy products, egg yolk, fish liver oils, liver, oysters; formed in the skin by exposure to sunlight	Without vitamin D, very little dietary calcium can be absorbed.
Vitamin E	An antioxidant that prevents cell membrane destruction	Men and women: 15 mg (1,000 mg) **15 mg α-Tocopherol	Vegetable oils, wheat germ, whole grain or fortified cereals, green leafy vegetables, nuts	As an antioxidant, may have implications in the prevention of Alzheimer's disease, heart disease, breast cancer.†
Vitamin K	Synthesis of prothrombin and other clotting factors; normal blood coagulation	Men: 120 mcg (not determined [ND]) Women: 90 mcg (ND)	Green vegetables (collards, spinach, lettuce, kale, broccoli, Brussels sprouts, cabbage), plant oils, and margarine	Individuals on anticoagulant therapy should monitor vitamin K intake.

(Continued)

TABLE 20-3 Essential Vitamins and Minerals—cont'd

Vitamin/Mineral	Function	DRI (UL)*	Food Sources	Comments
Vitamin C	Formation of collagen in connective tissues; a powerful antioxidant; facilitates iron absorption; aids in the release of epinephrine from the adrenal glands during stress	Men: 90 mg (2,000 mg) Women: 75 mg (2,000 mg)	Citrus fruits, tomatoes, potatoes, green leafy vegetables, strawberries	As an antioxidant, may have implications in the prevention of cancer, cataracts, heart disease. It may stimulate the immune system to fight various types of infection.†
Vitamin B₁ (thiamine)	Essential for normal functioning of nervous tissue; coenzyme in carbohydrate metabolism	Men: 1.2 mg (ND) Women: 1.1 mg (ND)	Whole grains, legumes, nuts, egg yolk, meat, green leafy vegetables	Large doses may improve mental performance in people with Alzheimer's disease.
Vitamin B₂ (riboflavin)	Coenzyme in the metabolism of protein and carbohydrate for energy	Men: 1.3 mg (ND) Women: 1.1 mg (ND)	Meat, dairy products, whole or enriched grains, legumes, nuts	May help in the prevention of cataracts; high-dose therapy may be effective in migraine prophylaxis and in the treatment of Parkinson's disease (Marashly & Bohlega, 2017).

Vitamin B₃ (niacin)	Coenzyme in the metabolism of protein and carbohydrates for energy	Men: 16 mg (35 mg) Women: 14 mg (35 mg) **16 mg niacin equivalents (NE)	Milk, eggs, meats, legumes, whole grain and enriched cereals, nuts	High doses of niacin have been successful in decreasing levels of cholesterol in some individuals.
Vitamin B₆ (pyridoxine)	Coenzyme in the synthesis and catabolism of amino acids; essential for metabolism of tryptophan to niacin	Men and women: 1.3 mg (100 mg) After age 50: Men: 1.7 mg Women: 1.5 mg	Meat, fish, grains, legumes, bananas, nuts, white and sweet potatoes	May decrease depression in some individuals by increasing levels of serotonin; deficiencies may contribute to memory problems; also used in the treatment of migraines and premenstrual discomfort.
Vitamin B₁₂	Necessary in the formation of DNA and the production of red blood cells; associated with folic acid metabolism	Men and women: 2.4 mcg (ND)	Found in animal products (e.g., meats, eggs, dairy products)	Deficiency may contribute to memory problems. Vegetarians can get this vitamin from fortified foods. Intrinsic factor must be present in the stomach for absorption of vitamin B₁₂.

(Continued)

TABLE 20-3 Essential Vitamins and Minerals—cont'd

Vitamin/Mineral	Function	DRI (UL)*	Food Sources	Comments
Folic acid (folate)	Necessary in the formation of DNA and the production of red blood cells	Men and women: 400 mcg (1000 mcg) Pregnant women: 600 mcg ** 400 mcg dietary folate equivalents (DFE)	Meat; green leafy vegetables; beans; peas; fortified cereals, breads, rice, and pasta	Important in women of childbearing age to prevent fetal neural tube defects; may contribute to prevention of heart disease and colon cancer.
Calcium	Necessary in the formation of bones and teeth; neuron and muscle functioning; blood clotting	Men and women: 1000 mg (2,500 mg) After age 50: Men and women: 1200 mg	Dairy products, kale, broccoli, spinach, sardines, oysters, salmon	Calcium has been associated with preventing headaches, muscle cramps, osteoporosis, and premenstrual problems. Requires vitamin D for absorption.
Phosphorus	Necessary in the formation of bones and teeth; a component of DNA, RNA, adenosine diphosphate, and adenosine-5′-triphosphate; helps control acid-base balance in the blood	Men and women: 700 mg (4,000 mg)	Milk, cheese, fish, meat, yogurt, ice cream, peas, eggs	

Nutrient	Function	Amount	Sources	Comments
Magnesium	Protein synthesis and carbohydrate metabolism; muscular relaxation following contraction; bone formation	Men: Age 19-30: 410 mg Age 31 and older: 420 mg (350 mg)‡ Women: Age 19-30: 310 mg Age 31 and older: 320 mg (350 mg)‡	Green vegetables, legumes, seafood, milk, nuts, meat	May aid in prevention of asthmatic attacks and migraine headaches. Deficiencies may contribute to insomnia, premenstrual problems.
Iron	Synthesis of hemoglobin and myoglobin; cellular oxidation	Men: 8 mg (45 mg) Women: (45 mg, all adult women) Childbearing age: 18 mg Over 50: 8 mg Pregnant: 27 mg Breastfeeding: 9 mg	Meat, fish, poultry, eggs, nuts, dark green leafy vegetables, dried fruit, enriched pasta and bread	Iron deficiencies can result in headaches and feeling chronically fatigued.
Iodine	Aids in the synthesis of T_3 and T_4	Men and women: 150 mcg (1100 mcg)	Iodized salt, seafood	Exerts strong controlling influence on overall body metabolism.
Selenium	Works with vitamin E to protect cellular compounds from oxidation	Men and women: 55 mcg (400 mcg)	Seafood, low-fat meats, dairy products, liver	As an antioxidant combined with vitamin E, may have some anticancer effect.† Deficiency has also been associated with depressed mood.

(Continued)

TABLE 20–3	Essential Vitamins and Minerals—cont'd			
Vitamin/Mineral	Function	DRI (UL)*	Food Sources	Comments
Zinc	Involved in synthesis of DNA and RNA; energy metabolism and protein synthesis; wound healing; increased immune functioning; necessary for normal smell and taste sensation.	Men: 11 mg (40 mg) Women: 8 mg (40 mg)	Meat, seafood, fortified cereals, poultry, eggs, milk	An important source for the prevention of infection and improvement in wound healing.

*Dietary Reference Intakes (UL), the most recent set of dietary recommendations for adults established by the National Academies of Sciences, Engineering, and Medicine (2018). UL is the upper limit of intake considered to be safe for use by adults (includes total intake from food, water, and supplements). In addition to the UL, DRIs are composed of the Recommended Dietary Allowance (RDA, the amount considered sufficient to meet the requirements of 97% to 98% of all healthy individuals) and the Adequate Intake (AI, the amount considered sufficient where no RDA has been established).

** In 2019, the FDA recommended converting units of measure on nutrition labels for Vitamins A, D, E, niacin, and folate based on recommendations for the National Academy of Medicine (U.S. Food and Drug Administration [FDA], 2019).

† The health benefits of antioxidants continue to be investigated.

‡ UL for magnesium applies only to intakes from dietary supplements, excluding intakes from food and water.

Source: Adapted from National Academies of Science, Engineering, and Medicine (2018). *Dietary reference intakes (DRIs) tables. Food and Nutrition Board, Institute of Medicine.* Retrieved from www.nationalacademies.org/hmd/Activities/Nutrition/SummaryDRIs/DRI-Tables.aspx; and Sadock, B.J., Sadock, V.A., & Ruiz, P. (2015). *Synopsis of psychiatry: Behavioral sciences/clinical psychiatry* (11th ed.). Philadelphia: Lippincott Williams & Wilkins.

through the spinal cord and spinal nerves. When vertebrae of the spinal column become displaced, they may press on a nerve and interfere with the normal nerve transmission. Palmer named the displacement of these vertebrae *subluxation*, and he alleged that the way to restore normal function was to manipulate the vertebrae back into their normal positions. These manipulations are called *adjustments*.

Adjustments are usually performed by hand, although some chiropractors have special treatment tables equipped to facilitate these manipulations. Other processes used to facilitate the outcome of the spinal adjustment by providing muscle relaxation include massage tables, application of heat or cold, and ultrasound treatments.

The chiropractor takes a medical history and performs a clinical examination, which usually includes x-ray films of the spine. Today's chiropractors may practice "straight" therapy, meaning subluxation adjustments are the only procedure provided. *Mixer* is a term applied to a chiropractor who combines adjustments with adjunct therapies, such as exercise, heat treatments, or massage.

Individuals seek treatment from chiropractors for many types of ailments and illnesses, most commonly back pain. In addition, chiropractors treat patients with headaches, neck injuries, scoliosis, carpal tunnel syndrome, respiratory and gastrointestinal disorders, menstrual difficulties, allergies, sinusitis, and certain sports injuries. Some chiropractors are employed by professional sports teams as their team physicians. In 2017, the American College of Physicians updated practice guidelines to recommend nondrug treatments, such as spinal manipulation, as first-line treatments for acute low back pain (Qaseem et al, 2017). The epidemic numbers of individuals now addicted to prescription opiate medications will no doubt continue to fuel research into and acceptance of alternative medical treatments for pain.

Chiropractors are licensed to practice in all 50 states, and treatment costs are covered by government and most private insurance plans. There are over 70,000 licensed chiropractors who collectively treat more than 35 million people in the United States annually (American Chiropractic Association, 2019).

Therapeutic Touch and Massage

Therapeutic Touch

The technique of therapeutic touch was developed in the 1970s by Dolores Krieger, a nurse associated with the New York University School of Nursing. This therapy is based on the philosophy that the human body projects a field of energy around it. When this field of energy becomes blocked, pain or illness occurs. Practitioners of therapeutic touch use this technique to correct these blockages, thereby relieving the discomfort and improving health.

The premise that the energy field extends beyond the surface of the body means the practitioner need not actually touch the patient's skin. Instead, the therapist's hands are passed over the patient's body, remaining 2 to 4 inches from the skin. The goal is to repattern the energy field by performing slow, rhythmic, sweeping hand motions over the entire body. Heat should be felt where the energy is blocked. The therapist "massages" the energy field in that area, smoothing it out and thus correcting the obstruction. Therapeutic touch is thought to reduce pain and anxiety and promote relaxation and health maintenance. It has been useful in the treatment of chronic health conditions.

Massage

Massage is the technique of manipulating the muscles and soft tissues of the body. Chinese physicians prescribed massage for the treatment of disease more than 5,000 years ago. The Eastern style focuses on balancing the body's vital energy (qi) as it flows through pathways (meridians), as described earlier in the discussion of acupressure and acupuncture. The Western style of massage focuses on muscles, connective tissues (e.g., tendons and ligaments), and the cardiovascular system. Its benefits are believed to include improved blood circulation, lymph flow, and muscle tone as well as tranquilizing effects (Sadock, Sadock, & Ruiz, 2015). Swedish massage, which is probably the best-known Western style, uses a variety of gliding and kneading strokes along with deep circular movements and vibrations to relax the muscles, improve circulation, and increase mobility.

Massage has been shown to be beneficial in reducing anxiety and pain perception, particularly pain associated with joint disease (Sadock et al, 2015). However, it is contraindicated in certain conditions, including high blood pressure, acute infection, osteoporosis, phlebitis, skin conditions, and varicose veins. It also should not be performed over the site of a recent injury, bruise, or burn. Massage therapists require specialized training in a program accredited by the American Massage Therapy Association and must pass the National Certification Examination for Therapeutic Massage and Bodywork. Laws related to licensure requirements vary from state to state.

It should be noted that some spas offer relaxation massages conducted by nonlicensed personnel and training, if any, is highly variable. States that require licensing may specify that these individuals are not permitted identify their massage as "clinical" or "medical" massage.

Yoga

Yoga is thought to have developed in India some 5,000 years ago and is attributed to an Indian physician and Sanskrit scholar named Patanjali. The objective of yoga is to integrate the physical, mental, and spiritual energies that enhance health and well-being.

Yoga has been found to be especially helpful in relieving stress and improving overall physical and psychological wellness. Proper breathing is a major component of yoga. It is believed that yoga breathing—a deep, diaphragmatic breathing—increases oxygen to brain and body tissues, thereby easing stress and fatigue and boosting energy.

Another component of yoga is meditation. Individuals who practice the meditation and deep breathing associated with yoga find that they are able to achieve a profound feeling of relaxation. The most familiar type of yoga practiced in Western countries is hatha yoga. Hatha yoga uses body postures, along with the meditation and breathing exercises, to achieve a balanced, disciplined workout that releases muscle tension, tones the internal organs, and energizes the mind, body, and spirit to allow natural healing to occur. The complete routine of poses is designed to work all parts of the body—stretching and toning muscles and keeping joints flexible. Studies have shown that yoga benefits some individuals with back pain, stress, migraine, insomnia, high blood pressure, rapid heart rates, and limited mobility (Sadock et al, 2015).

Mindfulness Meditation

Mindfulness meditation has its roots in Buddhist traditions and was popularized in America by Jon Kabat-Zinn (2012). The practice focuses on becoming more aware of the present moment through meditations that focus on breathing awareness, relaxation, and nonjudgmental self-awareness. This kind of meditation has become a fundamental complement to various forms of psychotherapy, including cognitive behavior therapy, dialectical behavior therapy, and acceptance and commitment therapy. In addition to relaxation, mindfulness meditation is believed to be beneficial in helping patients learn how to stay focused on the present (rather than ruminating about the past or worrying about the future), which facilitates problem-solving and behavior change.

Pet Therapy

The therapeutic value of pets is no longer just theory. Evidence has shown that animals can directly influence a person's mental and physical well-being. Many pet therapy programs have been established across the country, and the numbers are increasing regularly. Several studies have provided information about the positive results of human interaction with pets. Some of these include the following:

1. Petting a dog or cat has been shown to lower blood pressure. In one study, volunteers experienced a 7.1 mm Hg drop in systolic and an 8.1 mm Hg decrease in diastolic blood pressure when they talked to and petted their dogs, compared

with blood pressure when reading aloud or resting quietly (Whitaker, 2000).

2. Bringing a pet into a nursing home or other institution for the elderly has been shown in numerous studies to enhance a patient's mood and social interaction (Banks & Banks, 2002; Godenne, 2001; Marx et al, 2010; Moretti et al, 2011).

3. One study of 96 patients who had been admitted to a coronary care unit for heart attack or angina revealed that in the year following hospitalization, the mortality among those who did not own pets was 22% higher than among pet owners (Whitaker, 2000).

4. Multiple studies have demonstrated the efficacy of pet therapy in reducing symptoms of depression (Siegel et al, 1999; Souter & Miller, 2007).

5. Animal-assisted therapy with patients in acute care centers has been shown to decrease anxiety, reduce blood pressure, lower stress hormone release, increase feelings of safety, and improve cooperation and participation in the patient's own recovery (Ernst, 2012).

6. The American Heart Association released a statement based on a survey of research studies stating that "there is a substantial body of data that suggests that pet ownership is associated with a reduction in CVD risk factors and increased survival in individuals with established CVD" (Levine et al, 2013, p. 7).

7. Lundqvist and associates (2017) conducted a systematic review of the literature on the benefits of dog-assisted interventions and found that dog-assisted therapy had the greatest potential in treatment of psychiatric disorders among both young and adult patients where other health outcome measures (such as physiological parameters) did not show significant improvement. Dog-assisted activities had some positive effects on health, well-being, depression, and quality of life for patients with severe cognitive disorders. Dog-assisted support had positive effects on stress and mood.

Some researchers believe that animals actually may retard the aging process among those who live alone. Loneliness often results in premature death, and having a pet mitigates the effects of loneliness and isolation.

Whitaker (2000) suggests:

Though owning a pet doesn't make you immune to illness, pet owners are on the whole healthier than those who don't own pets. Study after study shows that people with pets have fewer minor health problems, require fewer visits to the doctor and less medication, and have fewer risk factors for heart disease, such as high blood pressure or cholesterol levels. (p. 7)

It may never be known precisely why animals affect humans the way they do, but for those who have pets to love, the therapeutic benefits come as no surprise. Pets provide unconditional, nonjudgmental love and affection, which can be the perfect antidote for a depressed mood or a stressful situation. The role of animals in the human healing process still requires more research, but its validity is now widely accepted in both the medical and lay communities.

■ SUMMARY

Complementary therapies help the practitioner view the patient in a holistic manner. Most complementary therapies consider the mind and body connection and strive to enhance the body's own natural healing powers.

Some commonly practiced complementary and alternative practices include herbal medicine, acupressure, acupuncture, diet and nutrition, chiropractic medicine, therapeutic touch, massage, yoga, mindfulness meditation, and pet therapy. Nurses must be familiar with these therapies, existing evidence supporting their benefits, and potential adverse reactions associated with their use as consumers continue to seek alternatives or complements to traditional medical interventions.

INTERNET REFERENCES

Additional information related to complementary therapies may be located at the following Web sites:
- http://abc.herbalgram.org/site/PageServer
- http://nutritiondata.self.com
- https://www.nutrition.gov
- www.chiropractic.org
- www.shanti.org
- https://www.therapydogs.com
- www.holisticmed.com/www/acupuncture.html

CHAPTER 21

Loss and Bereavement

■ BACKGROUND ASSESSMENT DATA

Loss is the experience of separation from something of personal importance. Loss is anything that is perceived as such by the individual. The separation from loved ones or the giving up of treasured possessions, for whatever reason; the experience of failure, either real or perceived; or life events that create change in a familiar pattern of existence—all can be experienced as loss, and all can trigger behaviors associated with the grieving process. Loss and bereavement are universal events encountered by all beings that experience emotions. Following are examples of some notable forms of loss:

1. A significant other (person or pet) through death, divorce, or separation for any reason.
2. Illness or debilitating conditions. Examples include (but are not limited to) diabetes, stroke, cancer, rheumatoid arthritis, multiple sclerosis, Alzheimer's disease, hearing or vision loss, and spinal cord or head injuries. Some of these conditions not only incur a loss of physical and/or emotional wellness but also may result in the loss of personal independence.
3. Developmental/maturational changes or situations, such as menopause, andropause, infertility, "empty nest" syndrome, aging, impotence, or hysterectomy.
4. A decrease in self-esteem due to inability to meet self-expectations or the expectations of others (even if these expectations are only perceived by the individual as unfulfilled). This includes a loss of potential hopes and dreams.
5. Personal possessions that symbolize familiarity and security in a person's life. Separation from these familiar and personally valued external objects represents a loss of material extensions of the self.

Some texts differentiate the terms *mourning* and *grief* by describing mourning as the psychological process (or stages) through which the individual passes on the way to successful adaptation to the loss of a valued object. Grief may be viewed as the subjective states that accompany mourning, or the emotional work involved in the mourning process. For purposes of this text, grief work and the process of mourning are collectively referred to as the *grief response*.

Theoretical Perspectives on Loss and Bereavement (Symptomatology)

Stages of Grief

Behavior patterns associated with the grief response include many individual variations. However, sufficient similarities have been observed to warrant characterization of grief as a syndrome that has a predictable course with an expected resolution. Early theorists, including Elisabeth Kübler-Ross (1969), John Bowlby (1961), and George Engel (1964), described behavioral stages through which individuals advance in their progression toward resolution. A number of variables influence one's progression through the grief process. Some individuals may reach acceptance, only to revert back to an earlier stage; some may never complete the sequence; and some may never progress beyond the initial stage.

A more contemporary grief specialist, J. William Worden (2009), offers a set of tasks that must be processed in order to complete the grief response. He suggests that it is possible for a person to accomplish some of these tasks and not others, resulting in an incomplete bereavement and thus impairing further growth and development.

Elisabeth Kübler-Ross

These well-known stages of the grief process were identified by Kübler-Ross in her extensive work with dying patients. Behaviors associated with each of these stages can be observed in individuals experiencing the loss of any concept of personal value.

- **Stage I: Denial.** The individual does not acknowledge that the loss has occurred. He or she may say, "No, it can't be true!" or "It's just not possible." This stage may protect the individual against the psychological pain of reality.
- **Stage II: Anger.** This is the stage when reality sets in. Feelings associated with this stage include sadness, guilt, shame, helplessness, and hopelessness. Self-blame or blaming of others may lead to feelings of anger toward the self and others. The anxiety level may be elevated, and the individual may experience confusion and a decreased ability to function independently. He or she may be preoccupied with an idealized image of what has been lost. Numerous somatic complaints are common.
- **Stage III: Bargaining.** The individual attempts to strike a bargain with God for a second chance or for more time. The person acknowledges the loss, or impending loss, but holds out hope for additional alternatives, as evidenced by such statements as, "If only I could . . ." or "If only I had. . . ."
- **Stage IV: Depression.** The individual mourns for that which has been or will be lost. This is a very painful stage during which the individual must confront feelings associated with having lost someone or something of value (called *reactive*

depression). An example might be the individual who is mourning a change in body image. Feelings associated with an impending loss (called *preparatory* depression) are also confronted. Examples include permanent lifestyle changes related to the altered body image or even an impending loss of life itself. Regression, withdrawal, and social isolation may be observed behaviors with this stage. Therapeutic intervention should be available, but not imposed, and with guidelines for implementation based on patient readiness.

- **Stage V: Acceptance.** The individual has worked through the behaviors associated with the other stages and either accepts or is resigned to the loss. Anxiety decreases, and methods for coping with the loss have been established. The patient is less preoccupied with what has been lost and increasingly interested in other aspects of the environment. If this is an impending death of self, the individual is ready to die. The person may become very quiet and withdrawn, seemingly devoid of feelings. These behaviors are an attempt to facilitate the passage by slowly disengaging from the environment.

Recently Davis Kessler (2019), who collaborated with Kübler-Ross in exploring the grief response, advanced the concept that there is a sixth stage of the grief response. Kessler contends that, when moving beyond the original five stages, one must find meaning in the loss to return to a state of peace and hopefulness.

John Bowlby

John Bowlby hypothesized four stages in the grief process. He implied that these behaviors can be observed in all individuals who have experienced the loss of something or someone of value, even in infants as young as 6 months of age.

- **Stage I: Numbness or Protest.** This stage is characterized by a feeling of shock and disbelief that the loss has occurred. Reality of the loss is not acknowledged.
- **Stage II: Disequilibrium.** During this stage, the individual has a profound urge to recover what has been lost. Behaviors associated with this stage include a preoccupation with the loss, intense weeping and expressions of anger toward the self and others, and feelings of ambivalence and guilt associated with the loss.
- **Stage III: Disorganization and Despair.** Feelings of despair occur in response to the realization that the loss has occurred. Activities of daily living become increasingly disorganized, and behavior is characterized by restlessness and aimlessness. Efforts to regain productive patterns of behavior are ineffective, and the individual experiences fear, helplessness, and hopelessness. Somatic complaints are common. Perceptions of visualizing or being in the presence of that

which has been lost may occur. Social isolation is common, and the individual may feel a great deal of loneliness.
- **Stage IV: Reorganization.** The individual accepts or becomes resigned to the loss. New goals and patterns of organization are established. The individual begins a reinvestment in new relationships and indicates a readiness to move forward within the environment. Grief subsides and recedes into valued remembrances.

George Engel

- **Stage I: Shock and Disbelief.** The initial reaction to a loss is a stunned, numb feeling and refusal by the individual to acknowledge the reality of the loss. Engel states that this stage is an attempt by the individual to protect the self "against the effects of the overwhelming stress by raising the threshold against its recognition or against the painful feelings evoked thereby" (Engel, 1964).
- **Stage II: Developing Awareness.** This stage begins within minutes to hours of the loss. Behaviors associated with this stage include excessive crying and regression to a state of helplessness and a childlike manner. Awareness of the loss creates feelings of emptiness, frustration, anguish, and despair. Anger may be directed toward the self or toward others in the environment who are held accountable for the loss.
- **Stage III: Restitution.** The various rituals associated with loss within a culture are performed. Examples include funerals, wakes, special attire, a gathering of friends and family, and religious practices customary to the spiritual beliefs of the bereaved. Participation in these rituals is thought to assist the individual to accept the reality of the loss and to facilitate the recovery process.
- **Stage IV: Resolution of the Loss.** This stage is characterized by a preoccupation with the loss. The concept of the loss is idealized, and the individual may even imitate admired qualities of the lost entity. Preoccupation with the loss gradually decreases over a year or more, and the individual eventually begins to reinvest feelings in others.
- **Stage V: Recovery.** Obsession with the loss has ended, and the individual is able to go on with his or her life.

J. William Worden

Worden views the bereaved person as active and self-determining rather than a passive participant in the grief process. He proposes that bereavement includes a set of tasks that must be reconciled in order to complete the grief process. Worden's four tasks of mourning include the following:
- **Task I: Accepting the Reality of the Loss.** When something of value is lost, it is common for individuals to refuse

to believe that the loss has occurred. Behaviors include misidentifying individuals in the environment for their lost loved one, retaining possessions of the lost loved one as though he or she has not died, and removing all reminders of the lost loved one so as not to have to face the reality of the loss. Worden (2009) states:

> Coming to an acceptance of the reality of the loss takes time since it involves not only an intellectual acceptance but also an emotional one. The bereaved person may be intellectually aware of the finality of the loss long before the emotions allow full acceptance of the information as true. (p. 42)

Belief and denial are intermittent when grappling with this task. It is thought that traditional rituals such as the funeral help some individuals move toward acceptance of the loss.

- **Task II: Processing the Pain of Grief.** Pain associated with a loss includes both physical pain and emotional pain. This pain must be acknowledged and worked through. To avoid or suppress it serves only to delay or prolong the grieving process. People accomplish this by refusing to allow themselves to think painful thoughts, by idealizing or avoiding reminders of the lost entity, and by using alcohol or drugs. The intensity of the pain and the manner in which it is experienced are different for all individuals. But the commonality is that it *must* be experienced. Failure to do so generally results in some form of depression that commonly requires therapy, which then focuses on working through the pain of grief that the individual failed to work through at the time of the loss. In this very difficult Task II, individuals must "allow themselves to process the pain—to feel it and to know that one day it will pass" (p. 45).

- **Task III: Adjusting to a World Without the Lost Entity.** It usually takes a number of months for a bereaved person to realize what his or her world will be like without the lost entity. In the case of a lost loved one, how the environment changes will depend on the types of roles that person fulfilled in life. In the case of a changed lifestyle, the individual will be required to make adaptations to his or her environment in terms of the changes as they are presented in daily life. In addition, those individuals who had defined their identity through the lost entity will require an adjustment to their own sense of self. Worden states:

> The coping strategy of redefining the loss in such a way that it can redound to the benefit of the survivor is often part of the successful completion of Task III. (p. 47)

If the bereaved person experiences failures in his or her attempt to adjust in an environment without the lost entity, feelings of low self-esteem may result. Regressed behaviors and feelings of helplessness and inadequacy are not uncommon. Worden states:

> [Another] area of adjustment may be to one's sense of the world. Loss through death can challenge one's fundamental life values and philosophical beliefs—beliefs that are influenced by our families, peers, education, and religion as well as life experiences. The bereaved person searches for meaning in the loss and its attendant life changes in order to make sense of it and to regain some control of his or her life. (pp. 48–49)

To be successful in Task III, bereaved individuals must develop new skills to cope with and adapt to their new environment without the lost entity. Successful achievement of this task determines the outcome of the mourning process—that of continued growth or a state of arrested development.

- **Task IV: Finding an Enduring Connection With the Lost Entity in the Midst of Embarking on a New Life.** This task allows for the bereaved person to identify a special place for the lost entity. Individuals need not purge from their history or find a replacement for that which has been lost. Instead, there is a kind of continued presence of the lost entity that only becomes *relocated* in the life of the bereaved. Successful completion of Task IV involves letting go of past attachments and forming new ones. However, there is also the recognition that although the relationship between the bereaved and what has been lost is changed, it is nonetheless still a relationship. Worden suggests that one never loses memories of a significant relationship. He states:

> For many people Task IV is the most difficult one to accomplish. They get stuck at this point in their grieving and later realize that their life in some way stopped at the point the loss occurred. (p. 52)

Worden relates the story of a teenaged girl who had a difficult time adjusting to the death of her father. After 2 years, when she began to finally fulfill some of the tasks associated with successful grieving, she wrote these words that express rather clearly what bereaved people in Task IV struggle to understand: "There are other people to be loved, and it doesn't mean that I love Dad any less" (p. 52).

Length of the Grief Process

Stages of grief allow bereaved persons an orderly approach to the resolution of mourning. Each stage presents tasks that must be overcome through a painful experiential process. Engel (1964) stated that successful resolution of the grief response is thought to have occurred when a bereaved individual is able "to remember comfortably and realistically both the pleasures and disappointments of [what has been lost]." The duration of the grief process depends on the individual and can last for a number of years without being maladaptive. The acute phase of normal grieving usually lasts 6 to 8 weeks—longer in older adults—but complete resolution of the grief response may take much longer. Sadock, Sadock, and Ruiz (2015) state:

> Ample evidence suggests that the bereavement process does not end within a prescribed interval; certain aspects persist indefinitely for many otherwise high-functioning, normal individuals. . . . Other common manifestations of protracted grief occur intermittently. . . . Most grief does not fully resolve or permanently disappear; rather grief becomes circumscribed and submerged only to reemerge in response to certain triggers. (p. 1355)

A number of factors influence the eventual outcome of the grief response. The grief response can be more difficult if:

- The bereaved person was strongly dependent on or perceived the lost entity as an important means of physical and/or emotional support.
- The relationship with the lost entity was highly ambivalent. A love-hate relationship may instill feelings of guilt that can interfere with the grief work.
- The individual has experienced a number of recent losses. Grief tends to be cumulative, and if previous losses have not been resolved, each succeeding grief response becomes more difficult.
- The loss is that of a young person. Grief over loss of a child is often more intense than it is over the loss of an elderly person. Traumatic death in general increases the likelihood of abnormal grief, but when a child dies a sudden or violent death evidence supports an increased incidence of posttraumatic stress disorder (PTSD) in parents (Kearns, 2014). One study found PTSD symptoms in more than 25% of the mothers up to 5 years after the death (Parris, 2011).
- The state of the person's physical or psychological health is unstable at the time of the loss.
- The bereaved person perceives (whether real or imagined) some responsibility for the loss.
- The loss is secondary to suicide.
- The loss is a traumatic death such as murder.

The grief response may be facilitated if:

- The individual has the support of significant others to assist him or her through the mourning process.
- The individual has the opportunity to prepare for the loss. Grief work is more intense when the loss is sudden and unexpected. The experience of *anticipatory grieving* is thought to facilitate the grief response that occurs at the time of the actual loss.

Worden (2009) states:

> There is a sense in which mourning can be finished, when people regain an interest in life, feel more hopeful, experience gratification again, and adapt to new roles. There is also a sense in which mourning is never finished. [People must understand] that mourning is a long-term process, and that the culmination [very likely] will not be to a pre-grief state. (p. 77)

Anticipatory Grief

Anticipatory grieving is the experiencing of the feelings and emotions associated with the normal grief response before the loss actually occurs. One dissimilar aspect relates to the fact that conventional grief tends to diminish in intensity with the passage of time. Anticipatory grief can become more intense as the expected loss becomes imminent.

Although anticipatory grief is thought to facilitate the actual mourning process following the loss, there may be some problems. In the case of a dying person, difficulties can arise when the family members complete the process of anticipatory grief and detachment from the dying person occurs prematurely. The person who is dying experiences feelings of loneliness and isolation as the psychological pain of imminent death is faced without family support. Another example of difficulty associated with premature completion of the grief response is one that can occur on the return of persons long absent and presumed dead (e.g., soldiers missing in action or prisoners of war). In this instance, resumption of the previous relationship may be difficult for the bereaved person.

Anticipatory grieving may serve as a defense for some individuals to ease the burden of loss when it actually occurs. It may prove to be less functional for others who, because of interpersonal, psychological, or sociocultural variables, are unable in advance of the actual loss to express the intense feelings that accompany the grief response.

One qualitative study examined the unique process of grief for family caregivers of a relative who has dementia. One common theme was that in addition to anticipatory grief related to the final loss, these family members were, at the same time, grieving actual losses throughout the journey of their family member's illness (Peacock, Hammond-Collins, & Ford, 2014). These included grieving the loss of the ill person's personality, companionship, social self, and cognition as the disease progressed. The grief reactions of these active caregivers were similar to those of bereaved caregivers although their family member was still alive. This study highlights the multiplicity of factors that can influence the grieving process.

Maladaptive Responses to Loss

When, then, is the grieving response considered to be maladaptive (sometimes referred to as complicated grief)? Three types of complicated grief reactions have been described. These include delayed or inhibited grief, an exaggerated or distorted grief response, and chronic or prolonged grief.

Delayed or Inhibited Grief

Delayed or inhibited grief refers to the absence of evidence of grief when it ordinarily would be expected. Many times, cultural influences, such as the expectation to keep a "stiff upper lip," cause the delayed response.

Delayed or inhibited grief is potentially pathological because the person is simply not dealing with the reality of the loss. He or she remains fixed in the denial stage of the grief process, sometimes for many years. When this occurs, the grief response may be triggered, sometimes many years later, when the individual experiences a subsequent loss. Sometimes the grief process is triggered spontaneously or in response to a seemingly insignificant event. Overreaction to another person's loss may be one manifestation of delayed grief.

The recognition of delayed grief is critical because, depending on the profoundness of the loss, the failure of the mourning process may prevent assimilation of the loss and thereby delay a return to satisfying living. Delayed grieving most commonly occurs because of ambivalent feelings toward the lost entity, outside pressure to resume normal function, or perceived lack of internal and external resources to cope with a profound loss.

Distorted (Exaggerated) Grief Response

In the distorted grief reaction, all of the symptoms associated with normal grieving are exaggerated. Feelings of sadness, helplessness, hopelessness, powerlessness, anger, and guilt, as well as numerous somatic complaints, render the individual dysfunctional in terms of management of daily living. Morrow (2019) describes this as a state of feeling "trapped" in one's grief during which the grief response either stays the same or intensifies over a prolonged period.

When the exaggerated reaction occurs, the individual remains fixed in the anger stage of the grief response. This anger may be directed toward others in the environment to whom the individual may be attributing the loss. However, many times the anger is turned inward on the self. When this occurs, depression is the result. Depressive mood disorder is a type of exaggerated grief reaction. This should be distinguished, though, from the depression that is considered part of the normal grieving process. (See Table 21–1.)

Chronic or Prolonged Grieving

Some authors have discussed a chronic or prolonged grief response as a type of maladaptive grief response. Care must be taken in making this determination because, as was stated previously, length of the grief response depends on the individual. An adaptive response may take years for some people. A prolonged process may be considered maladaptive when certain behaviors are exhibited.

Although Morrow (2019) identifies that it is difficult to establish a time frame signaling the difference between normal and maladaptive grieving, several symptoms are red flags of complicated grief. These include:

- Episodes of rage or prolonged, unresolved anger
- Inability to focus on anything but the loss
- Intense focus or avoidance of any reminders of the lost entity
- Prolonged difficulty accepting the reality of the loss
- Self destructive behaviors, including alcohol and drug abuse
- Suicidal thoughts and actions

TABLE 21–1 Normal Grief Reactions Versus Symptoms of Clinical Depression

Normal Grief	Clinical Depression
Self-esteem intact	Self-esteem is disturbed
May openly express anger	Usually does not directly express anger
Experiences a mixture of "good and bad days"	Persistent state of dysphoria
Able to experience moments of pleasure	Anhedonia is prevalent
Accepts comfort and support from others	Does not respond to social interaction and support from others
Maintains feeling of hope	Feelings of hopelessness prevail
May express guilt feelings over some aspect of the loss	Has generalized feelings of guilt
Relates feelings of depression to specific loss experienced	Does not relate feelings to a particular experience
May experience transient physical symptoms	Expresses chronic physical complaints

Sources: Corr, C.A., & Corr, D.M. (2013). *Death & dying: Life & living* (7th ed.). Belmont, CA: Wadsworth; Pies, R.W. (2013). Grief and depression: The sages knew the difference. *Psychiatric Times, 30*(6); and Sadock, B.J., Sadock, V.A., & Ruiz, P. (2015). *Synopsis of psychiatry: Behavioral sciences/clinical psychiatry* (11th ed.). Philadelphia: Lippincott Williams & Wilkins.

Normal versus Maladaptive Grieving

Several authors have identified a crucial difference between normal and maladaptive grieving: the loss of self-esteem. Marked feelings of worthlessness are indicative of a depressive disorder rather than uncomplicated bereavement. Corr and Corr (2013) state, "Normal grief reactions do not include the loss of self-esteem commonly found in most clinical depression" (p. 215). Pies (2013) affirmed:

> Unlike the person with [major depressive disorder] MDD, most recently bereaved individuals are usually not preoccupied with feelings of worthlessness, hopelessness, or unremitting gloom; rather, self-esteem is usually preserved; the bereaved person can envision a "better day"; and positive thoughts and feelings are often interspersed with negative ones.

Hensley and Clayton (2013) add that when clinically depressed inpatients were compared to individuals experiencing depression associated with bereavement, four symptoms were absent in the bereavement population: suicidal thoughts, feeling like they were a burden to others, feeling like they would rather be dead, and psychomotor retardation. These may be considered associated symptoms of low self-esteem and feelings of worthlessness. The presence of suicidal ideation automatically indicates an abnormal grief reaction and requires careful assessment and immediate intervention to prevent the risk for completed suicide.

It is thought that this major difference between normal grieving and maladaptive grieving (the feeling of worthlessness or low self-esteem) ultimately precipitates depression, which can be a progressive process for some individuals.

Concepts of Death–Developmental Issues
Children

- **Birth to Age 2:** Infants are unable to recognize and understand death, but they can experience the feelings of loss and separation. Infants who are separated from their mothers may become quiet, lose weight, and sleep less. Children at this age will likely sense changes in the atmosphere of the home in which a death has occurred. They often react to the emotions of adults by becoming more irritable and crying more.
- **Ages 3 to 5:** Preschoolers and kindergartners have some understanding about death but often have difficulty distinguishing between fantasy and reality. They believe death is reversible, and their thoughts about death may include magical thinking. For example, they may believe that their thoughts or behaviors caused a person to become sick or to die.

  Children of this age are capable of understanding at least some of what they see and hear from adult conversations or media reports. They become frightened if they feel a threat to themselves or to their loved ones. They are concerned with safety issues and require a great deal of personal reassurance that they will be protected. Regressive behaviors, such as loss of bladder or bowel control, thumb-sucking, and temper tantrums, are not uncommon. Changes in eating and sleeping patterns may also occur.

- **Ages 6 to 9:** Children at this age begin to understand the finality of death. They are able to understand a more detailed explanation of why or how the person died, although the concept of death is often associated with old age or with accidents. They may believe that death is contagious and avoid association with individuals who have experienced a loss by death. Death is often personified in the form of a "bogey man" or a monster—someone who takes people away or someone they can avoid if they try hard enough. It is difficult for them to perceive their own death. Normal grief reactions at this age include regressive and aggressive behaviors, withdrawal, school phobias, somatic symptoms, and clinging behaviors.
- **Ages 10 to 12:** Preadolescent children are able to understand that death is final and eventually affects everyone, including themselves. They are interested in the physical aspects of dying and the final disposition of the body. They may ask questions about how the death will affect them personally. Feelings of anger, guilt, and depression are common. Peer relationships and school performance may be disrupted. There may be a preoccupation with the loss and a withdrawal into the self. They will require support, flexibility in management of anger responses, and reassurance of their own safety and self-worth.

Adolescents

Adolescents are usually able to view death on an adult level. They understand death to be universal and inevitable; however, they have difficulty tolerating the intense feelings associated with the death of a loved one. They may or may not cry. They may withdraw into themselves or attempt to go about usual activities in an effort to avoid dealing with the pain of the loss. Some teens exhibit acting-out behaviors, such as aggression and defiance. It is often easier for adolescents to discuss their feelings with peers than with their parents or other adults. Some adolescents may show regressive behaviors whereas others react by trying to take care of their loved ones who are also grieving. In general, individuals of this age group have an attitude of immortality. Although they understand that their own death is inevitable, the concept is so far-reaching as to be imperceptible.

Adults

The adult's concept of death is influenced by cultural and religious backgrounds. Behaviors associated with grieving in the adult were discussed in the section "Theoretical Perspectives on Loss and Bereavement (Symptomatology)."

Older Adults

Philosophers and poets have described late adulthood as the "season of loss." By the time individuals reach their 60s and 70s, they have experienced numerous losses, and mourning has become a life-long process. Those who are most successful at adapting to losses earlier in life will similarly cope better with the losses and grief inherent in aging. Unfortunately, with the aging process comes a convergence of losses, the timing of which makes it impossible for the aging individual to complete the grief process in response to one loss before another occurs. Because grief is cumulative, this can result in *bereavement overload;* the person is less able to adapt and reintegrate, and mental and physical health is jeopardized. Bereavement overload has been implicated as a predisposing factor in the development of depressive disorder in older adults.

Some believe that bereavement among elderly couples is also associated with increased risk for mortality. While many variables influence mortality in this population, evidence suggests that, in cases where the loss is anticipated, there is not an increased risk for mortality, but when the loss was unexpected there was indeed an increased risk (King et al, 2013; Shah et al, 2013). This research highlights the need for additional assessment and support during the bereavement period when loss, particularly of a spouse, is unexpected.

Common Nursing Diagnoses and Interventions for the Individual Who Is Grieving

■ RISK FOR COMPLICATED GRIEVING

Definition: Susceptible to a disorder that occurs after the death of a significant other [or any other loss of significance to the individual], in which the experience of distress accompanying bereavement fails to follow normative expectations and manifests in functional impairment, which may compromise health (NANDA International [NANDA-I], 2018, p. 341)

Risk Factors ("related to")

[Actual or perceived object loss (e.g., people, pets, possessions, job, status, home, ideals, parts and process of the body)]
[Denial of loss]
[Interference with life functioning]
[Reliving of past experiences with little or no reduction (diminishment) of intensity of the grief]
Lack of social support
Emotional instability

Goals/Objectives

Short-term Goals

1. The patient will acknowledge awareness of the loss.
2. The patient will express feelings about the loss.
3. The patient will verbalize own position in the grief process.

Long-term Goal

The patient will progress through the grief process in a healthful manner toward resolution.

Interventions With *Selected Rationales*

1. Assess the patient's stage and adaptation in the grief process. Assess for bereavement risk factors. *Accurate baseline data are required to provide appropriate assistance. Several tools have been developed to assess the risk for maladaptive grief responses. They are framed to identify multiple risk factors commonly associated with complicated grief reactions that may require additional resources and intervention. Some factors that may increase risk for maladaptive grief include:*
   Additional financial problems posed by the loss
   Lack of coping skills or lack of experience in responding to loss
   Emotional or physical dependence on the lost person or item
   History of mental illness or substance abuse
   History of trauma, including abuse
   Multiple losses within a short time frame

2. Develop trust. Show empathy, concern, and unconditional positive regard. *Developing trust provides the basis for a therapeutic relationship.*

3. Help the patient actualize the loss by talking about it—"When did it happen?," "How did it happen?," and so forth. *Reviewing the events of the loss can help the patient come to full awareness of the loss.*

4. Help the patient identify and express feelings. *Until the patient can recognize and accept personal feelings regarding the loss, grief work cannot progress.* Some common troubling feelings include:
   a. **Anger:** The anger may be directed at the deceased, at God, displaced on others, or retroflected inward on the self. Encourage the patient to examine this anger and validate the appropriateness of this feeling. *Many people will not admit to angry feelings, believing it is inappropriate and unjustified. Expression of this emotion is necessary to prevent fixation in this stage of grief.*
   b. **Guilt:** The patient may feel that he or she did not do enough to prevent the loss. Help the patient by reviewing the circumstances of the loss and assisting the patient to gain insight about those things over which they have control and those they do not. Validate that guilt is a common reaction as people struggle with the reality of loss. *Patients may express "If only I had done . . ." as a way struggling toward the recognition that some things are beyond their control. Unexamined feelings of guilt prolong resolution of the grief process.*
   c. **Anxiety and Helplessness:** Help the patient to recognize the way that life was managed before the loss. Help the

patient to put the feelings of helplessness into perspective by pointing out ways that he or she managed situations effectively without help from others. Role-play life events and assist with decision-making situations. *The patient may have fears that he or she will not be able to carry on alone.*

5. Identify normal behaviors associated with grieving and provide the patient with adequate time to grieve. *Understanding of the grief process will help the patient understand the groundswell of uncomfortable emotions that often accompany grief (e.g., anger, guilt, sadness) and the fact that these feelings may leave and return at different points in the grieving process. Individuals need adequate time to adjust to the loss and all its ramifications. This involves getting past birthdays and anniversaries of which the deceased was a part.*

6. Provide continuing support. If this is not possible by the nurse, then offer referrals to support groups. Support groups of individuals going through the same experiences can be very helpful for the grieving individual. *The availability of emotional support systems facilitates the grief process.*

7. Identify pathological defenses that the patient may be using (e.g., drug/alcohol use, somatic complaints, social isolation). Assist the patient in understanding why these are not healthy defenses and how they delay the process of grieving. *The bereavement process is impaired by behaviors that mask the pain of the loss.*

8. Encourage the patient to make an honest review of the relationship with the lost entity. Journal-keeping is a facilitative tool with this intervention. *When the patient is able to see both positive and negative aspects related to the loss the grieving process is facilitated.*

Outcome Criteria

1. The patient is able to express feelings about the loss.
2. The patient verbalizes stages of the grief process and behaviors associated with each.
3. The patient acknowledges own position in the grief process and recognizes the appropriateness of the associated feelings and behaviors.

■ RISK FOR SPIRITUAL DISTRESS

Definition: Susceptible to an impaired ability to experience and integrate meaning and purpose in life through connectedness within self, others, literature, nature, and/or a power greater than oneself, which may compromise health (NANDA-I, 2018, p. 377)

Risk Factors ("related to")

Loss [of any concept of value to the individual]
Low self-esteem

Natural disasters
Physical illness
Depression; anxiety; stress
Separated from support systems
Life changes

Goals/Objectives

Short-term Goal

The patient will identify meaning and purpose in life, moving forward with hope for the future.

Long-term Goal

The patient will express achievement of support and personal satisfaction from spiritual practices.

Interventions With *Selected Rationales*

1. Assess the patient's perspective about spiritual needs. *Encouraging the patient to discuss spirituality informs the patient that the nurse is open to addressing the patient's spiritual needs and sets the foundation for patient-centered care.*
2. Be accepting and nonjudgmental when the patient expresses anger and bitterness toward God. Stay with the patient. *The nurse's presence and nonjudgmental attitude increase the patient's feelings of self-worth and promote trust in the relationship.*
3. Encourage the patient to ventilate feelings related to meaning of own existence in the face of current loss. *The patient may believe he or she cannot go on living without the lost entity. Catharsis can provide relief and put life back into realistic perspective.*
4. Encourage the patient as part of grief work to reach out to previously used spiritual support systems and practices. Encourage the patient to discuss these practices and how they provided support in the past. *The patient may find comfort in spiritual practices and support systems with which he or she is familiar.*
5. Ensure the patient that he or she is not alone when feeling inadequate in the search for life's answers. *Validation of the patient's feelings and assurance that they are shared by others offer encouragement and an affirmation of acceptability.*
6. Contact spiritual leader of the patient's choice, if he or she requests. *These individuals serve to provide relief from spiritual distress and often can do so when other support persons cannot.*

Outcome Criteria

1. The patient verbalizes increased sense of self-concept and hope for the future.
2. The patient verbalizes meaning and purpose in life that reinforces hope, peace, and contentment.

3. The patient expresses personal satisfaction and support from spiritual practices.

@ INTERNET REFERENCES

Additional references related to bereavement may be located at the following Web sites:

- www.journeyofhearts.org
- https://www.nhpco.org
- www.hospicefoundation.org
- www.livingwithloss.com
- www.caringinfo.org
- www.aahpm.org

CHAPTER 22

Military Families

■ BACKGROUND ASSESSMENT DATA

There are currently almost 1.3 million individuals on active duty in the U.S. Armed Forces in more than 150 countries around the world and another 809,000 serving in the National Guard and Reserves forces (Department of Defense [DoD], 2017). In 2017, the number of women in the military reached an all-time high of 16% among enlisted personnel and 21% among officers. Veterans currently number more than 20 million, about 9% of whom are women (U.S. Census Bureau, 2016).

Because of U.S. involvement in conflicts around the world, perhaps at no time in modern history has so much attention been given to what individuals and families experience as a result of their lives in the military. There is an ongoing effort by organizations that provide services for active-duty military personnel and veterans of military combat to keep up with the growing demand, and resources for these services will be required for many years to come. The need for mental health-care practitioners will rise as the increasing number of veterans and their family members struggle to cope with the effects of military deployment.

The Military Family

The military lifestyle offers both positive and negative aspects to those who choose this way of life. Hall (2012) summarizes a number of pros and cons about what is sometimes called the Warrior Society. Some advantages include:

- Early retirement compared to civilian counterparts
- A vast resource system to meet family needs
- Job security with a guaranteed paycheck
- Health-care benefits
- Opportunities to see different areas of the world
- Educational opportunities

Some disadvantages include:

- Frequent familial separations and reunions
- Regular household relocations

- Living life under the maxim of "the mission must always come first"
- A pattern of rigidity, regimentation, and conformity in family life
- Feelings of detachment from nonmilitary community
- The social effects of "rank"
- The lack of control over pay, promotion, and other benefits

Mary Wertsch (1996), who conducted a vast amount of research on the culture of the military family, stated, "The great paradox of the military is that its members, the self-appointed frontline guardians of our cherished American democratic values, do not live in democracy themselves" (p. 15). The military is maintained by a rigid authoritarian structure, and these characteristics often extend into the structure of the home.

Isolation and alienation are common facets of military life. To compensate for the extreme mobility, the focus of this lifestyle turns inward to the military world rather than outward to the local community. Children of military families almost always report that no matter what school they attend, they feel "different" from the other students (Wertsch, 1996). These descriptions apply principally to career military families. There is another type of military family that has become a familiar part of the American culture in recent years. The military campaigns of Operation Enduring Freedom (OEF) and Operation Iraqi Freedom (OIF) together make up the longest sustained U.S. military operation since the Vietnam War, and they are the first extended conflicts to depend on an all-volunteer military (Institute of Medicine [IOM], 2013). There has been heavy dependence on the National Guard and Reserves and an escalation in the pace, duration, and number of deployments and redeployments experienced by these individuals. Many had joined the National Guard or Reserves as a second job for financial reasons or for the educational opportunities available to them. Little thought had been given to the possibility of actually fighting in a war.

Military Spouses and Children

A military spouse inherently knows and lives with the concept of "mission first." Devries and colleagues (2012) state, "While the military works hard to value the family lives of service members and their welfare, the nature of the job is that the mission trumps all other concerns" (p. 11). However, times have changed from the days when life in the military was viewed as a two-person career in which a woman was expected to "create the right family setting so that her husband's work reflected his life at home, by staying positive, being interested in his duty, and being flexible and adaptable" (Hall, 2012, p. 148). Many of today's military spouses have their own careers or are pursuing higher levels of education. They do not view the military as a joint career with their service member spouse.

The lives of military spouses and children are clearly affected when the active-duty assignments of the service member require frequent family moves. Wakefield (2007) has stated, "The many short-term relationships, complications of spousal employment, university transfer issues, escalated misbehavior of the children, day-care arrangements, spousal loneliness, and increased financial obligations are just some of the issues military personnel face that can lead to frustration." In most instances, when the service member receives orders for a new geographical assignment, the spouse's education, career, or both are put on hold, and the entire family is relocated. Other occasions may arise when the family is unable to immediately follow the service member to the new location. In certain instances, such as when a student may be about to complete a semester or is about to graduate, the service member may proceed to the new assignment without the family. This is difficult for the military spouse who is left alone to care for the children, as well as to deal with all aspects of the move. Among active-duty members, 59 percent have children (DoD, 2017).

Military children face unique challenges. They primarily attend civilian public schools in which they form a unique subculture among staff and peers who often do not understand their life experiences. Children who grow up in a career military family learn to adapt to changing situations very quickly and to hide a certain level of fear associated with the nomadic lifestyle.

The Impact of Deployment

Not since the Vietnam War have so many U.S. military families been affected by deployment-related family separation, combat injury, and death. Many service members have been deployed multiple times. Those who are deployed most frequently describe their greatest fear as having to leave their spouse and children. Lengthy separations pose many challenges to all members of the family. Spouses undertake all the challenges of managing the household, in addition to assuming the role of the single parent. The pressure and stress are intense as the spouse attempts to maintain an atmosphere of strength for the children while experiencing the fears and anxiety associated with the life-threatening conditions facing his or her service member partner.

Approximately 2 million children have experienced the deployment of a parent to Iraq or Afghanistan, and thousands have either lost a parent or have a parent who was wounded in these conflicts. Children often have difficulty understanding and accepting the changes in appearance, personality, or behavior of parents upon their return from the combat experience. The following behaviors have been reported in children in response to the deployment of a parent (American Academy of Child & Adolescent Psychiatry, 2016):

- Infants (birth to 12 months): May respond to disruptions in their schedule with decreased appetite, weight loss, irritability, and apathy.
- Toddlers (1 to 3 years): May become sullen, tearful, throw temper tantrums, or develop sleep problems.
- Preschoolers (3 to 6 years): May regress in areas such as toilet training, sleep, separation fears, physical complaints, or thumb sucking. May assume blame for the parent's departure.
- School-aged children (6 to 12 years): Are more aware of potential dangers to the parent. May exhibit irritable behavior, aggression, or whininess. May become more regressed and fearful about the parent's safety.
- Adolescents (13 to 18 years): May be rebellious, irritable, or more challenging of authority. Parents need to be alert to high-risk behaviors, such as problems with the law, sexual acting out, and drug or alcohol abuse.

Women in the Military

Women make up approximately 16% of the U.S. military and 19% of National Guard and Reserve members (DoD, 2017). Women have been serving in the military since the time of the Civil War, mostly as nurses, spies, and support persons. In recent years, the Pentagon has relaxed its ban on women serving in combat roles, and "women began to fly combat aircraft, staff missile placements, drive convoys in the desert, and participate in other roles that involved potential combat exposure" (Mathewson, 2011, p. 217). Early in 2013, the Secretary of Defense lifted the ban on combat jobs to women, gradually opening direct combat units to female troops. Currently, certain specialty positions continue to remain off limits, although the plan is to eventually integrate women into these positions. Flexibility in the new law exists for exemptions to occur if further assessment reveals that some jobs are inappropriate for women.

Special Concerns of Women in the Military

- **Sexual Harassment:** Sexual harassment includes "unwelcome sexual advances, requests for sexual favors, and other verbal or physical harassment of a sexual nature" (U.S. Equal Employment Opportunity Commission [EEOC], n.d.). In addition to overt sexual behavior, sexual harassment includes making offensive comments about a person's gender, statements such as "You look nice this morning" or "Hey, you smell good" as well as blatant suggestions or requests for sexual interactions. Wolfe and associates (1998), in a study of women on active duty during the Persian Gulf War, found that both physical and sexual harassment were higher than typically found in peacetime military samples. Reports by military therapists convey that these women who were sexually harassed when in the military had higher than average rates of a range of problems following discharge, including poor self-image, relationship issues, drug use, depression, and posttraumatic stress disorder (PTSD).

- **Sexual Assault:** The DoD defines "sexual assault" as referring to a range of crimes, including rape, sexual assault, forcible sodomy, aggravated sexual contact, abusive sexual contact, and attempts to commit offenses. The DoD (2019) reported 20,500 incidents (6.2%) of active service member sexual assaults in 2018. This number increased from 4.3% in the year prior to the survey. The incidents of sexual assault on males remained consistent (around 7,500) but the incidents of sexual assault on women increased to around 13,000. It is estimated that only about 33% of sexual assaults in the military are reported. Reasons for not reporting include being afraid of causing trouble in their unit, fear that their commanders and fellow soldiers would turn against them, that they would be passed over for well-deserved promotions, or be transferred and removed from duty altogether (Vlahos, 2012). In 2000, following incidents of military sexual assaults that were made public, the Veteran's Health Administration mandated universal health screening for sexual trauma among military personnel. But despite the efforts within the Department of Defense to identify and correct this problem, incidents continue, suggesting that sexual assault remains a part of military culture. The DoD (2019) reports having taken disciplinary action in 65% of reported incidents.

- **Differential Treatment and Conditions:** Although their numbers have increased, women still constitute a minority in the military. Because of the small number of women in any given unit, officers and enlisted personnel are often housed together. Officers report missing being with other officers to discuss work and to be able to spend time with their peers, and enlisted women often report feeling uncomfortable with an officer in their presence. Burgess and associates (2013) add that when sexual trauma occurs among military personnel, it is occurring in the workplace, and as such, the victim often has ongoing contact with the perpetrator and may also be in a dependent position if the perpetrator was in a supervisory role.

   Women's military careers are often limited by their exclusions from occupational specialties. These sanctions often preclude female officers and enlisted personnel from the most prestigious units and occupations in the military, their participation in which is essential to ascending in the ranks should they choose to make the military a career. Although many bans have been lifted and occupations are now open to women that, historically, have been off limits, the manner in which military culture will respond to those changes remains to be seen.

- **Parenting Issues:** Women's feelings associated with leaving their children often differ from those of men. Women seem to struggle more with guilt feelings for "abandoning" their children, whereas men have stronger emotions tied to a sense of doing their duty. Although men also experience regret at leaving their children, they often rely on the assurance that the children have their mothers to care for them.

Veterans

Most veterans returning from a combat zone undergo a period of adjustment. A recent study of young veterans (Pedersen, Marshall, & Kurz, 2016) identified that 70% screened as positive for behavioral health problems, less than a third of whom received adequate psychotherapy or psychotropic treatment. Many veterans suffer from migraine headaches and experience cognitive difficulties, such as memory loss. Hypervigilance, insomnia, and jitteriness are common. The Substance Abuse and Mental Health Services Administration (Pemberton et al, 2016) reported that, particularly in the 18 to 25 age group of veterans, there is a higher incidence of nonmedical use of pain relievers, amphetamine use, and alcohol abuse or dependence than nonveterans and higher incidence of mental illness, including major depressive episodes and severe mental illnesses. Plach and Sells (2013) identified in a study of veterans that over 50% screened positive for problem drinking, and over 90% had engaged in hazardous drinking (Cogan, 2014). In addition, SAMSHA (2017) reports that veterans make up about 10% of the homeless population, and among this group, 75% have mental and/or substance use disorders.

Traumatic Brain Injury

The Departments of Veterans Affairs and Defense (DVA/DoD, 2016, p. 6) offer the following definition of traumatic brain injury (TBI):

A traumatically induced structural injury and/or physiological disruption of brain function as a result of an external force that is indicated by new onset or worsening of at least one of the following clinical signs, immediately following the event:
- Any period of loss of or a decreased level of consciousness
- Any loss of memory for events immediately before or after the injury (posttraumatic amnesia)
- Any alteration in mental state at the time of the injury (confusion, disorientation, slowed thinking, etc.) (Alteration of consciousness/mental state)

- Neurological deficits (weakness, loss of balance, change in vision, praxis, paresis/plegia, sensory loss, aphasia, etc.) that may or may not be transient
- Intracranial lesion

Symptoms may be classified as mild, moderate, or severe. Blasts from explosive devices are the leading cause of TBI for active-duty military personnel in combat. TBI also results from penetrating wounds, severe blows to the head with shrapnel or debris, and falls or bodily collisions with objects following a blast.

Posttraumatic Stress Disorder

PTSD is the most common mental disorder among veterans returning from military combat. The disorder can occur when an individual is exposed to an accident or violence in which death or serious injury to others or oneself occurs or is threatened. Symptoms of PTSD include:

- Reliving the trauma through flashbacks, nightmares, and intrusive thoughts
- Intensive efforts to avoid activities, people, places, situations, or objects that arouse recollections of the trauma
- Chronic negative emotional state and diminished interest or participation in significant activities
- Aggressive, reckless, or self-destructive behavior
- Hypervigilance and exaggerated startle response
- Angry outbursts, problems with concentration, and sleep disturbances

Symptoms of PTSD may be delayed, in some instances for years. When emotions regarding the trauma are constricted, they may suddenly appear at some time in the future following a major life event, stressor, or an accumulation of stressors with time that challenge the person's defenses. Co-occurring disorders are common in individuals with PTSD, including major depressive disorder, substance use disorders, and anxiety disorders. Individuals with TBI also may develop PTSD, depending on the degree of amnesia experienced immediately following the cerebral trauma.

Depression and Suicide

Reports by the DoD and VA indicate that the number of suicides among veterans and active-duty military has risen dramatically since 2001, the year that detailed record-keeping began. This number reached an all-time high in 2012 with a rate of 22.7 suicides per 100,000 population (319) of active-duty military personnel. While that number declined somewhat in 2013 to 18.7 per 100,000 (259), the number of suicides among reservists and National Guard members remained alarmingly high at 23.4 to 28.9 per 100,000 respectively (Kime, 2015). In 2018, the year for which the most recent data are available, the suicide rate was again at a high of 22.9 per 100,000, and the rate among active-duty members rose significantly to 24.8 per 100,000 (DoD, 2018). The DoD reports that when statistics are adjusted for age and sex, these numbers approximate the suicide rates in the general population (with the exception of the National Guard, which had the highest suicide rate at 30.6 suicides per 100,000 members). In any scenario, the rates of suicide are alarmingly high and underscore the need for intensive and ongoing suicide prevention initiatives.

When suicides among veterans are added to the numbers, the incidence is even higher. In 2017, the U.S. Department of Veterans Affairs released a report that examined suicide rates among veterans from 1979 to 2014. One significant finding was that the incidence of suicide among veterans is 22% higher than the general population and that 65% of all military personnel who die by suicide are veterans aged 50 or older. For female veterans, the highest suicide rate is among those aged 18 to 29. Whereas the use of firearms as a method for suicide has declined in the civilian population, it remains high among veterans and has increased among female veterans. The U.S. Department of Veteran Affairs (2017) concludes "these results strongly suggest that firearms safety initiatives are likely an important component of an effective suicide prevention strategy for male and female veterans" (p. 47). A common theme among investigations of suicide attempts and completed suicides by military service members is marital/relationship distress. Devries and associates (2012) stated:

> From 2005 to 2009, relationship problems were a factor in over 50 percent of the suicides in the Army. The health of our military fighting force is directly related to the health of our military marriages. What we see in the military is a common drama of relationship problems played out in an environment of uncommon stressors. (p. 7)

A study by Jakupcak and associates (2010) concluded that veterans who are unmarried or those who report lower satisfaction with their social support networks are also at increased risk for suicide.

In 2015 President Obama signed into law the Clayton Hunt SAV (suicide prevention for American veterans) Act which intends to, among other things, expand peer support for troubled veterans, streamline transitions for exiting servicemen, and mandate annual surveying of VA mental health and suicide prevention programs, among other initiatives (National Alliance on Mental Illness, 2015). Clayton Hunt was a decorated Marine who struggled with PTSD and depression after returning home from active duty and took his own life in 2011.

Substance Use Disorder

In addition to rising suicide rates, substance use disorder has also been on the rise in the military. The Army Suicide Prevention

Task Force reported that 29% of active-duty military suicides between 2005 and 2009 involved alcohol or drugs, and in 2009 about one-third of these involved prescription drugs (National Institute on Drug Abuse [NIDA], 2013). Substance use disorder is a common co-occurring condition with PTSD. Other studies found that around 22% of all service members report heavy alcohol use (Braneu et al, 2011; Herberman et al, 2016). Among veterans who sought treatment for substance use disorder, 65% (almost double that of the nonveteran population) identified alcohol as their primary substance of abuse; 10% identified heroin as their primary drug; and 6.2% primarily used cocaine (SAMHSA, 2015). As with U.S. civilians, opioid pain medication use and abuse among military personnel has been on the rise. NIDA (2019) reported that from 2005 to 2009, prescriptions for pain medications prescribed by military physicians quadrupled. Crosby (2015) reports that smoking tobacco among military personnel is also higher (24%) than that in the general population. The IOM report (2013) on readjustment needs of veterans identified that as many as 39% of veterans are struggling with substance use issues. Their recommendations included supporting research to identify evidence-based treatments for substance use disorders as well as reevaluating policies about access to abused substances within the military.

■ SYMPTOMATOLOGY (SUBJECTIVE AND OBJECTIVE DATA)

Posttraumatic Stress Disorder

1. Rage reactions
2. Aggression; irritability
3. Substance abuse
4. Flashbacks; nightmares; startle reaction
5. Depression; anxiety; suicidal ideation
6. Feelings of hopelessness
7. Guilt
8. Emotional numbness
9. Panic attacks
10. Confusion, fear, and anxiety among family members

Traumatic Brain Injury

1. Impaired mobility; limited range of motion
2. Decreased muscle strength
3. Perceptual or cognitive impairment
4. Seizures
5. Memory deficits
6. Distractibility; altered attention span or concentration
7. Impaired ability to make decisions, solve problems, reason, or conceptualize

8. Personality changes
9. Inability to perform activities of daily living
10. Confusion, fear, and anxiety among family members

Family Members' Issues

1. Children
   a. Regressive behaviors
   b. Loss of appetite
   c. Temper tantrums
   d. Clinging behaviors
   e. Guilt and self-blame
   f. Sleep problems
   g. Irritability
   h. Aggression
2. Adolescents
   a. Rebelliousness
   b. Irritability
   c. Acting-out behaviors
   d. Promiscuity
   e. Substance abuse
3. Spouse/Partner
   a. Depression
   b. Anxiety
   c. Loneliness
   d. Fear
   e. Feeling overwhelmed and powerless
   f. Anger
4. Spouse/Partner Caregiver
   a. Anger
   b. Anxiety; frustration
   c. Ineffective coping
   d. Sleep deprivation
   e. Somatic symptoms
   f. Fatigue

Common Nursing Diagnoses and Interventions for Military Service Members, Veterans, and Their Families

■ POSTTRAUMA SYNDROME

Definition: Sustained maladaptive response to a traumatic, overwhelming event (NANDA International [NANDA-I], 2018, p. 316)

Possible Contributing Factors ("related to")

War
Witnessing violent death

Witnessing mutilation
Serious threat or injury to self [or others]
Events outside the range of usual human experience

Defining Characteristics ("evidenced by")

Anger; aggression
Depression
Difficulty concentrating
Flashbacks; nightmares; intrusive dreams
Exaggerated startle response
Panic attacks
Hypervigilance
Substance abuse

Goals/Objectives

Short-term Goals

1. The patient will begin a healthy grief resolution, initiating the process of psychological healing (within time frame specific to individual).
2. The patient will demonstrate ability to deal with emotional reactions in an individually appropriate manner.

Long-term Goal

The patient will integrate the traumatic experience into his or her persona, renew significant relationships, and establish meaningful goals for the future.

Interventions With *Selected Rationales*

1. Stay with the patient during periods of flashbacks and nightmares. Offer reassurance of safety and security and that these symptoms are not uncommon following a trauma of the magnitude he or she has experienced. *The presence of a trusted individual may help to calm fears for personal safety and reassure the anxious patient that he or she is not "going crazy."*
2. Encourage the patient to talk about the trauma at his or her own pace. Provide a nonthreatening, private environment, and include a significant other if the patient wishes. Acknowledge and validate the patient's feelings as they are expressed. *This debriefing process is the first step in the progression toward resolution.*
3. Discuss coping strategies used in response to the trauma. Determine those that have been most helpful, including available support systems and religious and cultural influences. Identify maladaptive coping strategies being used, such as substance abuse or psychosomatic responses, and discuss more adaptive coping strategies. *Resolution of the*

posttrauma response is largely dependent on the effectiveness of the coping strategies employed.

4. Help the patient understand that *use of substances merely numbs feelings and delays healing.* Refer for treatment of substance use disorder if need is determined.

5. Discuss the use of stress-management techniques, such as deep breathing, meditation, relaxation techniques, and physical exercise. *These interventions help to maintain anxiety at a manageable level and prevent escalation to panic.*

6. Administer medications as prescribed, and provide medication education. *A number of medications have been used for patients with PTSD. Some of these include the selective serotonin reuptake inhibitors, trazodone, amitriptyline, imipramine, and phenelzine. Benzodiazepines are sometimes prescribed for their antipanic effects, although their addictive properties make them less desirable. Propranolol and clonidine have been successful in alleviating symptoms such as nightmares, intrusive recollections, hypervigilance, insomnia, startle responses, and angry outbursts.*

7. Explore available resources for ongoing support, particularly support groups for veterans. *Support groups for individuals with shared military and combat experiences provide a powerful network for mutual understanding and healing.*

Outcome Criteria

1. The patient is able to discuss the traumatic experience with trusted nurse/therapist.

2. The patient recognizes own position in grief process and demonstrates the initiation of psychological healing.

3. The patient has established meaningful, realistic goals and expresses hope for a positive future.

■ RISK FOR SUICIDE

Definition: Susceptible to self-inflicted, life-threatening injury (NANDA International [NANDA-I], 2018, p. 422)

Risk Factors ("related to")

[Depression]
[Perception of lack of social support]
[Physical disabilities from combat injuries]
[Feelings of hopelessness]
Substance abuse
Poor support systems
States desire to die

Goals/Objectives

Short-term Goals

1. The patient will seek out staff member when suicidal feelings occur or intensify.
2. The patient will verbalize adaptive coping strategies for use when suicidal feelings occur.

Long-term Goals

1. The patient will demonstrate adaptive coping strategies for use when suicidal feelings occur.
2. The patient will not harm self.

Interventions With *Selected Rationales*

1. Assess degree of risk according to seriousness of threat, existence of a plan, and availability and lethality of the means. Ask directly if the person is thinking of acting on thoughts or feelings. *The risk of suicide is greatly increased if the patient has developed a plan and particularly if means exist for the patient to execute the plan. It is important to get the subject out in the open. This places some of the responsibility for his or her safety with the patient.*
2. Ascertain presence of significant others for support. *The presence of a strong support system decreases the risk of suicide.*
3. Determine whether substance abuse is a factor. *The abuse of substances increases the risk of suicide.*
4. Encourage expression of feelings, including appropriate expression of anger. *It is vital that the patient express angry feelings, because suicide and other self-destructive behaviors are often viewed as the result of anger turned inward on the self.*
5. Ensure that the environment is safe. Remove all dangerous objects from the patient's environment (e.g., sharp items, belts, ties, straps, breakable items, smoking materials). *Patient safety is a nursing priority.*
6. Collaborate with the patient to establish a comprehensive safety plan and offer hope for the future. *In the patient's current state of mind, he or she may not be able to see any hope for positive life change. Discussion with a trusted individual may help the patient identify options that provide for safety, encouragement, and hope for improvement.*
7. Involve family/significant others in the planning. *This problem affects all members of the family. Outcomes are more successful when all persons involved are allowed input into the plan for intervention.*

Outcome Criteria

1. The patient is able to discuss feelings about current situation with nurse or therapist.

2. The patient expresses commitment to a plan for safety and hope for the future.
3. The patient has not harmed self.

■ DISTURBED THOUGHT PROCESSES

Definition: Disruption in cognitive operations and activities (Note: This diagnosis has been retired by NANDA-I but is retained in this text because of its appropriateness in describing these specific behaviors.)

Possible Contributing Factors ("related to")

[Response to having experienced a trauma outside the range of usual human experience]
[Physical trauma to the brain]

Defining Characteristics ("evidenced by")

[Memory deficits]
[Distractibility]
[Altered attention span or concentration]
[Impaired ability to make decisions, solve problems, reason, or conceptualize]
[Personality changes]

Goals/Objectives

Short-term Goal

The patient will perform self-care activities with assistance as required.

Long-term Goal

The patient will regain cognitive ability to execute mental functions realistic with the extent of the condition or injury.

Interventions With *Selected Rationales*

1. Evaluate mental status. *An accurate assessment of the patient's strengths and limitations is essential to providing appropriate care and fulfilling the patient's needs. Consideration should be given to the following issues and concerns:*
   • Extent of impairment in thinking ability
   • Remote and recent memory
   • Orientation to person, place, time, and situation
   • Insight and judgment
   • Changes in personality
   • Attention span, distractibility, and ability to make decisions or solve problems
   • Ability to communicate appropriately

- Anxiety level
- Evidence of psychotic behavior

2. Report to the physician any cognitive changes that become obvious. *This is important to ensure that any reversible condition is addressed and that patient safety is assured.*
3. Note behavior indicative of potential for violence and take appropriate action *to prevent harm to the patient and others.*
4. Provide safety measures as required. Institute seizure precautions if indicated. Assist with limited mobility issues. Monitor medication regimen. *Patient safety is a nursing priority.*
5. Refer to appropriate rehabilitation providers. *Individuals with TBI will require assistance from multidisciplinary providers in an effort to achieve his or her highest level of self-care ability.*

Outcome Criteria

1. The patient is able to assist with aspects of self-care.
2. The patient has not experienced injury as a result of cognitive limitations.
3. The patient participates in decision-making situations that relate to life situations.

■ INTERRUPTED FAMILY PROCESSES

Definition: Break in the continuity of family functioning which fails to support the well-being of its members (NANDA-I, 2018, p. 293)

Possible Contributing Factors ("related to")

Situational transition or crisis precipitated by:
    [Family member returns from combat with PTSD]
    [Family member returns from combat with TBI]
    [Family member experiences repeated deployments]

Defining Characteristics ("evidenced by")

[Confusion, fear, and anxiety among family members]
[Inability to adapt to changes associated with veteran member's condition/injury]
[Difficulty accepting/receiving help]
[Inability to express or to accept each other's feelings]

Goals/Objectives

Short-term Goal

Family members will accept assistance from multidisciplinary services in an effort to restore adaptive family functioning.

Long-term Goal

Family will verbalize understanding of trauma-related illness, demonstrate ability to maintain anxiety at a manageable level, and make appropriate decisions to stabilize family functioning.

Interventions With *Selected Rationales*

1. Encourage continuous, open dialogue between family members. *This promotes understanding and assists family members to maintain clear communication and resolve problems effectively.*
2. Assist the family to identify and use previously successful coping strategies. *Most people have developed effective coping skills that when identified can be useful in current situation.*
3. Encourage family participation in multidisciplinary team conference or group therapy. *Participation in family and group therapy for an extended period increases likelihood of success as interactional issues (e.g., marital conflict, scapegoating) can be addressed and dealt with.*
4. Involve family in social support and community activities of their interest and choice. *Involvement with others can help family members to experience new ways of interacting and gain insight into their behavior, providing opportunity for change.*
5. Assist the family to identify situations that may lead to fear or anxiety. Encourage the use of stress-management techniques. *A high level of anxiety and stress interferes with the ability to cope and solve problems effectively.*
6. Make necessary referrals (e.g., Parent Effectiveness, specific disease or disability support groups, self-help groups, clergy, psychological counseling, or family therapy). *Multidisciplinary specialties may be required to effect positive change and enhance conflict resolution. If substance abuse is a problem, all family members should be encouraged to seek support and assistance in dealing with the situation to promote a healthy outcome.*
7. Involve the family in mutual setting of goals to plan for the future. *When all members of the family are involved, commitment to goals and continuation of the plan are more likely to be maintained.*
8. Identify community agencies from which family may seek assistance (e.g., Meals on Wheels, visiting nurse, trauma support group, American Cancer Society, Veterans Administration). *These agencies may provide both immediate and long-term support to individual members and to the family as a group.*

Outcome Criteria

1. Family members verbalize understanding of illness/trauma, treatment regimen, and prognosis.

2. Family members demonstrate ability to express feelings openly and communicate with each other in an appropriate and healthy manner.
3. Family members seek out and accept assistance from community agencies.

■ RISK FOR COMPLICATED GRIEVING

Definition: Susceptible to a disorder that occurs after the death of a significant other [or any loss or perceived loss of significance to the individual], in which the experience of distress accompanying bereavement fails to follow normative expectations and manifests in functional impairment, which may compromise health (NANDA-I, 2018, p. 341)

Risk Factors ("related to")

[Military deployment of the individual's spouse/partner, resulting in:
    Depression
    Anxiety
    Loneliness
    Fear
    Feeling overwhelmed
    Powerlessness
    Anger]

Goals/Objectives

Short-term Goal

The patient will acknowledge feelings of anger and powerlessness associated with spouse's/partner's extended absence.

Long-term Goal

The patient will work through stages of grief, achieve a healthy acceptance, and express a sense of control over the present situation and future outcome.

Interventions With *Selected Rationales*

1. Help family members to realize that all of the feelings they are having are a normal part of the grieving process. Validate their feelings of anger, loneliness, fear, powerlessness, dysphoria, and distress at separation from their loved one. *Understanding of the grief process will help prevent feelings of guilt generated by these responses. Individuals need adequate time to accommodate to the loss and all its ramifications.*
2. Help the parent to understand that children's and adolescents' problematic behaviors are symptoms of grieving and that they should not be deemed unacceptable and result in punishment

but rather be recognized as having their basis in grief. *Children and adolescents exhibit grief differently than adults, and they must be allowed to grieve in their own way. Caring support and assistance is required when the behaviors become problematic or maladaptive.*

3. Children should be allowed an appropriate amount of time to grieve. *Some experts believe children need at least 4 weeks to adjust to a parent's deployment* (Gabany & Shellenbarger, 2010). Refer for professional help if improvement is not observed in a reasonable period of time.

4. Assess if maladaptive coping strategies, such as substance abuse, are being used. Assist the patient to understand why these are not healthy defenses. *Behaviors that mask the pain of loss delay the process of adaptation.*

5. Suggest caution against spending too much time alone. Encourage resuming involvement in usual activities, and employ previously used successful coping strategies. *Most people have developed effective coping skills that can be useful in the current situation. Keeping busy and receiving support from others eases the burden of loneliness.*

6. Suggest keeping a journal of experiences and feelings. *Journaling can be therapeutic because it helps to get in touch with emotions that are sometimes difficult to express verbally. Writing down thoughts and feelings helps to sort through problems and come to a deeper understanding of oneself or the issues in one's life.*

7. Refer to other resources as needed, such as psychotherapy, family counseling, religious references or pastor, or grief support group. *The individual may require ongoing support to work through the feelings of loss associated with long-term separation issues.*

Outcome Criteria

1. The patient recognizes and verbalizes own position in grief process.

2. The patient keeps a journal of feelings and emotions.

3. Grieving behaviors of children and adolescents are recognized and accepted. Caring assistance is provided.

4. Family demonstrates ability to adapt to the life change associated with the absence of the service member and to accept assistance and support from others.

■ CAREGIVER ROLE STRAIN

Definition: Difficulty in fulfilling care responsibilities, expectations, and/or behaviors for family or significant others (NANDA-I, 2018, pp. 278–282)

Possible Contributing Factors ("related to")

24-hour care responsibilities
Severity, chronicity, and unpredictability of illness/[injury] course

Increasing care needs [of care receiver]

Cognitive or psychological problems [of care receiver]

Defining Characteristics ("evidenced by")

Anger

Stress; anxiety

Frustration

Ineffective coping

Sleep deprivation

Somatization

Goals/Objectives

Short-term Goal

The patient will identify resources within self and from others to assist with and manage caregiving responsibilities.

Long-term Goal

Caregiver will demonstrate effective problem-solving skills and develop adaptive coping mechanisms to regain equilibrium.

Interventions With *Selected Rationales*

1. Assess the spouse's/caregiver's ability to anticipate and fulfill the injured service member's unmet needs. Note the caregiver's physical and emotional health, developmental level and abilities, and additional responsibilities of the caregiver (e.g., job, raising family). *It is important to ensure that the caregiver has realistic self-expectations. Failure in the caregiver role is likely to occur in a situation in which the caregiver is overburdened and undersupported.*

2. Ensure that the caregiver encourages the injured service member to be as independent as possible. *Not only does this relieve the caregiver of some of the responsibilities, it provides the care receiver with increased feelings of capability, personal control, and self-esteem.*

3. Encourage the caregiver to express feelings and to participate in a support group. *Having others with whom to share concerns and fears is therapeutic. Support group members provide ideas for different ways to manage problems, helping caregivers deal more effectively with the situation.*

4. Provide information or demonstrate techniques for dealing with acting-out, violent, or disoriented behavior by the injured service member. *The presence of cognitive impairment necessitates learning these techniques or skills to enhance safety of the caregiver and receiver.*

5. Encourage attention to own needs (e.g., eating and sleeping regularly, setting realistic goals, talking with trusted friend, periodic respite from caregiving), accepting own feelings,

acknowledging frustrations and limitations, and being realistic about loved one's condition. *This supports and enhances the caregiver's general well-being and coping ability.*

6. Discuss and demonstrate stress management techniques and importance of self-nurturing (e.g., pursuing self-development interests, hobbies, social activities, spiritual enrichment). *Being involved in activities such as these can prevent caregiver burnout.*

Outcome Criteria

1. Caregiver is able to solve problems effectively regarding care of their loved one.
2. Caregiver demonstrates adaptive coping strategies for dealing with stress of the caregiver role.
3. Caregiver openly expresses feelings.
4. Caregiver expresses desire to join a support group of other caregivers.

@ INTERNET REFERENCES

The following Web sites provide information for and about military service members, their families, and veterans:

- https://www.va.gov
- www.dvnf.org
- https://nvf.org
- https://www.ptsd.va.gov
- https://www.ptsd.va.gov/professional/assessment/overview/index.asp
- www.mayoclinic.org/diseases-conditions/post-traumatic-stress-disorder/symptoms-causes/dxc-20308550
- https://www.cdc.gov/traumaticbraininjury
- https://www.ninds.nih.gov/Disorders/All-Disorders/Traumatic-Brain-Injury-Information-Page
- www.militaryfamily.org
- https://www.woundedwarriorproject.org

Movie Connections

The Best Years of Our Lives (1946) • *The Deer Hunter* (1978) • *Jarhead* (2005) • *In the Valley of Elah* (2007) • *The Lucky Ones* (2008) • *A Walk in My Shoes* (2010) • *The Invisible War* (2012) • *Of Men and War* (2014) • *Fort Bliss* (2014) • *Disorder* (2015) • *Thank-You for Your Service* (2017)

PSYCHOTROPIC MEDICATIONS

CHAPTER **23**

Antianxiety Agents

■ ANTIHISTAMINES

Examples

Generic Name	Trade Name	Half-life	Available Forms (mg)
Hydroxyzine	Vistaril	20 hr	**CAPS:** 25, 50, 100 **ORAL SUSP:** 25/5 mL **SYRUP:** 10/5 mL **INJ:** 25/mL, 50/mL
	Atarax		**TABS:** 10, 25, 50

Indications

- Anxiety disorders
- Temporary relief of anxiety symptoms
- Allergic reactions producing pruritic conditions
- Antiemetic
- Reduction of narcotic requirement, alleviation of anxiety, and control of emesis in preoperative/postoperative patients (parenteral only)

Action

- Exerts central nervous system (CNS) depressant activity at the subcortical level of the CNS
- Has anticholinergic, antihistaminic, and antiemetic properties
- Blocks histamine 1 receptors

Contraindications and Precautions

Contraindicated in: • Hypersensitivity • Pregnancy and lactation

Use Cautiously in: • Elderly or debilitated patients (dosage reduction recommended) • Hepatic or renal dysfunction • Concomitant use of other CNS depressants

Adverse Reactions and Side Effects

- Dry mouth
- Drowsiness
- Pain at intramuscular site

Interactions

- Additive CNS depression with other **CNS depressants** (e.g., **alcohol, other anxiolytics, opioid analgesics**, and **sedative/ hypnotics**) and with **herbal depressants** (e.g., **kava, valerian**).
- Additive anticholinergic effects with other **drugs possessing anticholinergic properties** (e.g., **antihistamines, antidepressants, atropine, haloperidol, phenothiazines**) and **herbal products** such as **angel's trumpet, jimson weed,** and **scopolia.**
- Can antagonize the vasopressor effects of **epinephrine.**

Route and Dosage

INTRAMUSCULAR

- **Anxiety**
  Adults: 50 to 100 mg 4 times/day
- **Pruritus**
  Adults: 25 mg 3 or 4 times/day
- **Pre- and postoperative sedative**
  Adults: 50 to 100 mg
  Children: 0.6 mg/kg
- **Antiemetic/adjunctive therapy to analgesia**
  Adults: 25 to 100 mg q 4 to 6 hours as needed
  Children: 0.5 to 1 mg/kg q 4 to 6 hours as needed

ORAL

- **Anxiety**
  Adults: 25 to 100 mg 4 times/day
  Children (≥6 yr): 50 to 100 mg/day in divided doses
  Children (<6 yr): 50 mg/day or 2 mg/kg/day in divided doses
- **Pruritus**
  Adults: 25 mg 3 or 4 times/day
  Children (≥6 yr): 50 to 100 mg/day in divided doses
  Children (<6 yr): 50 mg/day in divided doses

- **Pre- and postoperative sedative**
  Adults: 50 to 100 mg
  Children: 0.6 mg/kg

■ BENZODIAZEPINES
Examples

Generic (Trade) Name	Half-life (hr)	Indications	Available Forms (mg)
Alprazolam (Xanax)	6.3–26.9 10.7–15.8 (ER)	• Anxiety disorders • Anxiety symptoms • Anxiety associated with depression • Panic disorder **Unlabeled uses:** • Premenstrual dysphoric disorder • Irritable bowel syndrome and other somatic symptoms associated with anxiety	TABS: 0.25, 0.5, 1.0, 2.0 TABS ER: 0.5, 1.0, 2.0, 3.0 TABS (ORALLY DISINTEGRATING): 0.25, 0.5, 1.0, 2.0 ORAL SOLU: 1/mL
Chlordiazepoxide (Librium)	5–30	• Anxiety disorders • Anxiety symptoms • Acute alcohol withdrawal • Preoperative sedation	CAPS: 5, 10, 25
Clonazepam (Klonopin)	18–50	• Petit mal, akinetic, and myoclonic seizures • Panic disorder **Unlabeled uses:** • Acute manic episodes • Neuralgias • Restless leg syndrome • Adjunct therapy in schizophrenia • Tic disorders	TABS: 0.5, 1.0, 2.0 TABS (ORALLY DISINTEGRATING): 0.125, 0.25, 0.5, 1.0, 2.0
Clorazepate (Tranxene-T)	48	• Anxiety disorders • Anxiety symptoms • Acute alcohol withdrawal • Partial seizures	TABS: 3.75, 7.5, 15
Diazepam (Valium)	20–100	• Anxiety disorders • Anxiety symptoms • Skeletal muscle relaxant • Acute alcohol withdrawal • Adjunct therapy in convulsive disorders • Status epilepticus • Preoperative sedation	TABS: 2, 5, 10 ORAL SOLU: 5/5 mL, 5/mL INJ: 5/mL RECTAL GEL: 2.5, 10, 20

(Continued)

Generic (Trade) Name	Half-life (hr)	Indications	Available Forms (mg)
Lorazepam (Ativan)	10–20	• Anxiety disorders • Anxiety symptoms • Status epilepticus • Preoperative sedation **Unlabeled uses:** • Acute alcohol withdrawal • Insomnia • Chemotherapy-induced nausea and vomiting	TABS: 0.5, 1.0, 2.0 ORAL SOLU: 2/mL INJ: 2/mL, 4/mL
Oxazepam	5.7–10.9	• Anxiety disorders • Anxiety symptoms • Acute alcohol withdrawal	CAPS: 10, 15, 30

Action

• Benzodiazepines are thought to potentiate the effects of gamma-aminobutyric acid (GABA), a powerful inhibitory neurotransmitter, thereby producing a calmative effect. The activity may involve the spinal cord, brain stem, cerebellum, limbic system, and cortical areas.

Contraindications and Precautions

Contraindicated in: • Hypersensitivity • Psychoses • Acute narrow-angle glaucoma • Preexisting CNS depression • Pregnancy and lactation • Shock • Coma

Use Cautiously in: • Elderly or debilitated patients (reduced dosage recommended) • Hepatic/renal/pulmonary impairment • History of drug abuse/dependence • Depressed/suicidal patients • Children

Adverse Reactions and Side Effects

• Drowsiness; dizziness, lethargy
• Nausea and vomiting
• Ataxia
• Dry mouth
• Blurred vision
• Rash
• Hypotension
• Tolerance
• Physical and psychological addiction
• Paradoxical excitation

Interactions

• Additive CNS depression with other **CNS depressants** (e.g., **alcohol, other anxiolytics, opioid analgesics,** and **sedative/hypnotics**) and with **herbal depressants** (e.g., **kava, valerian**).
• The FDA (2016a) added a **boxed warning** (its strongest warning) related to the serious risks and possible death associated

with combining **benzodiazepines with opioid pain or cough medicines.**

- **Cimetidine, oral contraceptives, disulfiram, fluoxetine, isoniazid, ketoconazole, metoprolol, propoxyphene, propranolol,** or **valproic acid** may enhance effects of benzodiazepines.
- Benzodiazepines may decrease the efficacy of **levodopa.**
- Sedative effects of benzodiazepines may be decreased by **theophylline.**
- **Rifampin** and **St. John's wort** may decrease the efficacy of benzodiazepines.
- Serum concentration of **digoxin** may be increased (and subsequent toxicity can occur) with concurrent benzodiazepine therapy.

Route and Dosage

ALPRAZOLAM (Xanax)

Anxiety disorders and anxiety symptoms: **PO** *(Adults):* 0.25 to 0.5 mg 3 times/day. Maximum daily dose 4 mg in divided doses.

> *In elderly or debilitated patients:* **PO:** 0.25 mg 2 or 3 times/day. Gradually increase if needed and tolerated. Total daily dosages of greater than 2 mg should not be used.

Panic disorder: **PO** *(Adults):* Initial dose: 0.5 mg 3 times/day. Increase dose at intervals of 3 to 4 days in increments of no more than 1 mg/day.

> *Extended-release tablets:* **PO** *(Adults):* 0.5 to 1 mg once daily. May increase the dose at intervals of 3 to 4 days in increments of no more than 1 mg/day until desired effect has been achieved. Total daily dose range: 3 to 6 mg.

CHLORDIAZEPOXIDE (Librium)

Mild to moderate anxiety: **PO** *(Adults):* 5 or 10 mg 3 or 4 times/day.

> *Children (≥6 yr):* 5 mg 2 to 4 times/day. May be increased to 10 mg 2 or 3 times/day if needed.

Severe anxiety: **PO** *(Adults):* 20 or 25 mg 3 or 4 times/day.

> *Elderly or debilitated patients:* **PO:** 5 mg 2 times/day. Increase gradually as needed and tolerated.

Preoperative sedation: **PO** *(Adults):* 5 to 10 mg 3 or 4 times/day.

Acute alcohol withdrawal: **PO** *(Adults):* 50 to 100 mg; repeat as needed up to 300 mg/day.

CLONAZEPAM (Klonopin)

Seizures: Adults: **PO:** 0.5 mg 3 times/day. May increase by 0.5 to 1 mg every 3 days. Total daily maintenance dose not to exceed 20 mg.

> *Children (<10 yr or 30 kg):* **PO:** Initial daily dose 0.01 to 0.03 mg/kg/day (not to exceed 0.05 mg/kg/day) given in 2 to 3 equally divided doses; increase by not more

than 0.25 to 0.5 mg every third day until a daily maintenance dose of 0.1 to 0.2 mg/kg has been reached.

Therapeutic serum concentrations of clonazepam are 20 to 80 mg/ml.

Panic disorder: **PO** *(Adults):* Initial dose: 0.25 mg 2 times/day. Increase after 3 days toward target dose of 1 mg/day. Some patients may require up to 4 mg/day, in which case the dose may be increased in increments of 0.125 to 0.25 mg twice daily every 3 days until symptoms are controlled.

Acute manic episode: **PO** *(Adults):* 2 to 16 mg/day.

Tic disorders: **PO** *(Adults and children):* 0.5 to 12 mg/day.

Restless leg syndrome: **PO** *(Adults):* 0.5 to 2 mg 30 minutes before bedtime.

CLORAZEPATE (Tranxene-T)

Anxiety disorders/anxiety symptoms: **PO** *(Adults):* 7.5 to 15 mg 2 to 4 times/day. Adjust gradually to dose within range of 15 to 60 mg/day. May also be given in a single daily dose at bedtime. The recommended initial dose is 15 mg. Adjust subsequent dosages according to patient response.

Geriatric or debilitated patients: **PO:** 7.5 to 15 mg/day.

Acute alcohol withdrawal: **PO** *(Adults):* Day 1: 30 mg initially, followed by 15 mg 2 to 4 times/day.

Day 2: 45 to 90 mg in divided doses.

Day 3: 22.5 to 45 mg in divided doses.

Day 4: 15 to 30 mg in divided doses.

Thereafter, gradually reduce the daily dose to 7.5 to 15 mg. Discontinue drug as soon as patient's condition is stable.

Partial seizures: *Adults and children >12 years:* **PO:** 7.5 mg 3 times/day. Can increase by no more than 7.5 mg/day at weekly intervals (daily dose not to exceed 90 mg).

Children (9 to 12 yr): **PO:** 7.5 mg 2 times/day initially; may increase by 7.5 mg/week (not to exceed 60 mg/day).

DIAZEPAM (Valium)

Antianxiety/adjunct anticonvulsant: **PO** *(Adults):* 2 to 10 mg 2 to 4 times/day.

Antianxiety: **PO** *(Children ≥6 months):* 1 to 2.5 mg 3 to 4 times/day.

Moderate to severe anxiety: **IM** or **IV** *(Adults):* 2 to 10 mg. Repeat in 3 to 4 hours if necessary.

Skeletal muscle relaxant: **PO** *(Adults):* 2 to 10 mg 3 or 4 times/day.

Children (≥6 mo): **PO:** 0.12 to 0.8 mg/kg/day divided into 3 to 4 equal doses.

Geriatric or debilitated patients: **PO:** 2 to 2.5 mg 1 to 2 times daily initially. Increase gradually as needed and tolerated.

Acute alcohol withdrawal: **PO** *(Adults):* 10 mg 3 to 4 times/day in first 24 hours; decrease to 5 mg 3 or 4 times/day as needed. **IM** or **IV** *(Adults):* 10 mg initially, then 5 to 10 mg in 3 to 4 hours, if necessary.

Status epilepticus/acute seizure activity: **IV** *(Adults)* (IM route may be used if IV route is unavailable): 5 to 10 mg; may repeat every 10 to 15 minutes to a total of 30 mg; may repeat regimen again in 2 to 4 hours.

> *Children (≥5 yr):* **IM** or **IV:** 0.05 to 0.3 mg/kg/dose given over 3 to 5 minutes every 15 to 30 minutes to a total dose of 10 mg; repeat every 2 to 4 hours.

> *Children (1 mo to 5 yr):* **IM** or **IV:** 0.05 to 0.3 mg/kg/dose given over 3 to 5 minutes every 15 to 30 minutes to a maximum dose of 5 mg; repeat in 2 to 4 hours if needed.

Preoperative sedation: **IM** *(Adults):* 10 mg.

LORAZEPAM (Ativan)

Anxiety disorders/anxiety symptoms: **PO** *(Adults):* 2 to 6 mg/day (varies from 1 to 10 mg/day) given in divided doses; take the largest dose before bedtime.

> *Geriatric or debilitated patient:* **PO:** 0.5 to 2 mg/day in divided doses; adjust as needed and tolerated.

> *Children:* **PO:** 0.05 mg/kg/dose every 4 to 8 hours. Maximum dose: 2 mg/dose.

Insomnia: **PO** *(Adults):* 2 to 4 mg at bedtime.

> *Geriatric or debilitated patient:* **PO:** 0.25 to 1 mg at bedtime.

Preoperative sedation: **IM** *(Adults):* 0.05 mg/kg (maximum 4 mg) 2 hours before surgery; **IV** *(Adults):* Initial dose is 2 mg or 0.044 mg/kg, whichever is smaller, given 15 to 20 minutes before the procedure.

Status epilepticus: **IV** *(Adults):* 4 mg given slowly (2 mg/min). May be repeated after 10 to 15 minutes if seizures continue or recur.

> *Neonates and children <18 years:* **IV:** 0.05 to 0.1 mg/kg given over 2 to 5 minutes. If needed, a dosage of 0.05 mg/kg may be repeated in 10 to 15 minutes. Maximum dose: 4 mg.

Antiemetic: **IV** *(Adults):* 2 mg 30 minutes prior to chemotherapy; may be repeated every 4 hours as needed

OXAZEPAM

Mild to moderate anxiety: **PO** *(Adults and children >12 yr):* 10 to 15 mg 3 or 4 times/day.

Severe anxiety states: **PO** *(Adults and children >12 yr):* 15 to 30 mg 3 or 4 times/day.

> *Geriatric patients:* **PO:** Initial dosage: 10 mg 3 times/day. If necessary, increase cautiously to 15 mg 3 or 4 times/day.

Acute alcohol withdrawal: **PO** *(Adults):* 15 to 30 mg 3 or 4 times/day.

■ CARBAMATE DERIVATIVES
Examples

Generic Name	Half-life (hr)	Available Forms (mg)
Meprobamate	6–16	TABS: 200, 400

Indications
- Anxiety disorders
- Temporary relief of anxiety symptoms

Action
- Depresses multiple sites in the CNS, including the thalamus and limbic system
- May act by blocking the reuptake of adenosine

Contraindications and Precautions

Contraindicated in: • Hypersensitivity to the drug • Combination with other CNS depressants • Children under age 6 • Pregnancy and lactation • Acute intermittent porphyria

Use Cautiously in: • Elderly or debilitated patients • Hepatic or renal dysfunction • Individuals with a history of drug abuse/addiction • Patients with a history of seizure disorders • Depressed/suicidal patients

Adverse Reactions and Side Effects
- Palpitations, tachycardia
- Drowsiness, dizziness, ataxia
- Nausea, vomiting, diarrhea
- Tolerance
- Physical and psychological addiction

Interactions
- Additive CNS depression with other **CNS depressants** (e.g., **alcohol, other anxiolytics, opioid analgesics,** and **sedative-hypnotics**) and with **herbal depressants** (e.g., **kava, valerian**).

Route and Dosage
Anxiety disorders/anxiety symptoms: **PO** *(Adults and children >12 yr):* 1200 to 1600 mg/day in 3 or 4 divided doses.
Children (6 to 12 yr): **PO:** 100 to 200 mg 2 or 3 times/day.

■ AZAPIRONES

Examples

Generic Name	Half-life (hr)	Available Forms (mg)
Buspirone HCI	2–3	TABS: 5, 7.5, 10, 15, 30

Indications
- Anxiety disorders
- Anxiety symptoms

Unlabeled uses:
- Symptomatic management of premenstrual syndrome

Actions
- Unknown
- May produce desired effects through interactions with serotonin, dopamine, and other neurotransmitter receptors
- Delayed onset (a lag time of 7 to 10 days between onset of therapy and subsiding of anxiety symptoms)
- Cannot be used on a prn basis

Contraindications and Precautions

Contraindicated in: • Hypersensitivity to the drug • Severe hepatic or renal impairment • Concurrent use with MAO inhibitors

Use Cautiously in: • Elderly or debilitated patients • Pregnancy and lactation • Children • Buspirone will not block the withdrawal syndrome in patients with a history of chronic benzodiazepine or other sedative/hypnotic use. Patients should be withdrawn gradually from these medications before beginning therapy with buspirone.

Adverse Reactions and Side Effects
- Drowsiness, dizziness
- Excitement, nervousness
- Fatigue, headache
- Nausea, dry mouth
- Incoordination, numbness
- Palpitations, tachycardia

Interactions
- Increased effects of buspirone with **cimetidine, erythromycin, itraconazole, nefazodone, ketoconazole, clarithromycin, diltiazem, verapamil, fluvoxamine,** and **ritonavir.**

- Decreased effects of buspirone with **rifampin, rifabutin, phenytoin, phenobarbital, carbamazepine, fluoxetine,** and **dexamethasone.**
- Increased serum concentrations of **haloperidol** when used concomitantly with buspirone.
- Use of buspirone with an **MAO inhibitor** may result in elevated blood pressure.
- Increased risk of hepatic effects when used concomitantly with **nefazodone.**
- Additive effects when used with certain **herbal products** (e.g., **kava, valerian**).
- **Grapefruit juice** increases the absorption in the bloodstream and increases the risk for unwanted side effects.

Route and Dosage

Anxiety: **PO** (*Adults*): Initial dosage 7.5 mg 2 times/day. Increase by 5 mg/day every 2 to 3 days as needed. Maximum daily dosage: 60 mg.

The FDA has approved SSRIs paroxetine (Paxil), escitalopram (Lexapro), and SSNRIs duloxetine (Cymbalta), and extended release venlafaxine (Effexor XR) in the treatment of GAD. Atypical antidepressants such as nefazodone (Serzone) and mirtazapine (Remeron), although not FDA approved for anxiety disorder treatment, have also been identified as beneficial (Bhatt, 2018). These medications are discussed in more detail in Chapter 24, Antidepressants.

■ NURSING DIAGNOSES RELATED TO ALL ANTIANXIETY AGENTS

1. Risk for injury related to seizures, panic anxiety, acute agitation from alcohol withdrawal (indications); abrupt withdrawal from the medication after long-term use; effects of medication intoxication or overdose.
2. Anxiety (specify) related to threat to physical integrity or self-concept.
3. Risk for activity intolerance related to medication side effects of sedation, confusion, and lethargy.
4. Disturbed sleep pattern related to situational crises, physical condition, severe level of anxiety.
5. Deficient knowledge related to medication regimen.
6. Risk for acute confusion related to action of the medication on the CNS.

■ NURSING IMPLICATIONS FOR ANTIANXIETY AGENTS

1. Instruct the patient not to drive or operate dangerous machinery when taking the medication.

2. Advise the patient receiving long-term therapy not to quit taking the drug abruptly. Abrupt withdrawal can be life threatening (with the exception of buspirone). Symptoms include depression, insomnia, increased anxiety, abdominal and muscle cramps, tremors, vomiting, sweating, convulsions, and delirium.

3. Instruct the patient not to drink alcohol or take other medications that depress the CNS while taking this medication.

4. Assess mood daily. *May aggravate symptoms in depressed persons.* Take necessary precautions for potential suicide.

5. Monitor lying and standing blood pressure and pulse every shift. Instruct the patient to arise slowly from a lying or sitting position.

6. Withhold drug and notify the physician should paradoxical excitement occur.

7. Have the patient take frequent sips of water, ice chips, suck on hard candy, or chew sugarless gum to relieve dry mouth.

8. Have the patient take drug with food or milk to prevent nausea and vomiting.

9. Symptoms of sore throat, fever, malaise, easy bruising, or unusual bleeding should be reported to the physician immediately. They may be indications of blood dyscrasias.

10. Ensure that the patient taking buspirone understands there is a lag time of 7 to 10 days between onset of therapy and subsiding of anxiety symptoms. The patient should continue to take the medication during this time. (Note: This medication is not recommended for prn administration because of this delayed therapeutic onset. There is no evidence that buspirone creates tolerance or physical dependence as do the CNS depressant anxiolytics.)

■ PATIENT/FAMILY EDUCATION RELATED TO ALL ANTIANXIETY AGENTS

- Do not drive or operate dangerous machinery. Drowsiness and dizziness can occur.
- Do not stop taking the drug abruptly. Can produce serious withdrawal symptoms, such as depression, insomnia, anxiety, abdominal and muscle cramps, tremors, vomiting, sweating, convulsions, and delirium.
- *(With buspirone only):* Be aware of lag time between start of therapy and subsiding of symptoms. Relief is usually evident within 7 to 10 days. Take the medication regularly, as ordered, so that it has sufficient time to take effect. Grapefruit juice interacts with buspirone to increase the absorption of buspirone into the bloodstream and increases the risk for side effects.
- Do not consume other CNS depressants (including alcohol).
- Do not take nonprescription medication without approval from physician.

- Rise slowly from the sitting or lying position to prevent a sudden drop in blood pressure.
- Report to physician immediately symptoms of sore throat, fever, malaise, easy bruising, unusual bleeding, or motor restlessness.
- Be aware of risks of taking these drugs during pregnancy. (Congenital malformations have been associated with use during the first trimester). If pregnancy is suspected or planned, the patient should notify the physician of the desirability to discontinue the drug.
- Be aware of possible side effects. Refer to written materials furnished by health-care providers regarding the correct method of self-administration.
- Carry card or piece of paper at all times stating names of medications being taken.

@ INTERNET REFERENCES

- www.mentalhealth.com
- https://www.nimh.nih.gov/index.shtml
- https://www.nimh.nih.gov/health/topics/mental-health-medications/index.shtml
- https://medlineplus.gov/druginformation.html
- https://www.drugguide.com/ddo (Davis's Drug Guide)
- http://centerwatch.com

CHAPTER 24

Antidepressants

■ TRICYCLICS AND RELATED (NONSELECTIVE REUPTAKE INHIBITORS)

Examples

Generic (Trade) Name	Half-life (hr)	Indications	Therapeutic Plasma Level Range (ng/mL)	Available Forms (mg)
Tricyclics				
Amitriptyline	10–50	• Depression **Unlabeled uses:** • Migraine prevention • Chronic headache prevention • Fibromyalgia • Postherpetic neuralgia	80–200	**TABS:** 10, 25, 50, 75, 100, 150
Clomipramine (Anafranil)	19–37	• Obsessive-compulsive disorder (OCD) **Unlabeled uses:** • Premenstrual symptoms • Panic disorder	70–200	**CAPS:** 25, 50, 75
Desipramine (Norpramin)	15–24	• Depression **Unlabeled uses:** • Alcoholism • Attention-deficit/hyperactivity disorder (ADHD) • Bulimia nervosa • Diabetic neuropathy • Postherpetic neuralgia • Irritable bowel syndrome	150–250	**TABS:** 10, 25, 50, 75, 100, 150

(Continued)

Generic (Trade) Name	Half-life (hr)	Indications	Therapeutic Plasma Level Range (ng/mL)	Available Forms (mg)
Doxepin (Sinequan)	8–25	• Depression or anxiety • Depression or anxiety associated with alcoholism • Depression or anxiety associated with organic disease • Psychotic depressive disorders with anxiety **Unlabeled uses:** • Migraine prevention	50–100	CAPS: 10, 25, 50, 75, 100, 150
Imipramine (Tofranil)	8–16	• Depression • Nocturnal enuresis **Unlabeled uses:** • Alcoholism • ADHD • Bulimia nervosa • Migraine prevention • Urinary incontinence	175–300	HCL TABS: 10, 25, 50 PAMOATE CAPS: 75, 100, 125, 150
Nortriptyline (Aventyl; Pamelor)	18–28	• Depression **Unlabeled uses:** • ADHD • Postherpetic neuralgia • Irritable bowel syndrome	50–150	CAPS: 10, 25, 50, 75 ORAL SOLUTION: 10/5 mL
Protriptyline (Vivactil)	67–89	• Depression **Unlabeled uses:** • Migraine prevention	50–170	TABS: 5, 10
Trimipramine (Surmontil)	7–30	• Depression	50–300	CAPS: 25, 50, 100
Amoxapine	8	• Depression • Depression with anxiety	200–400	TABS: 25, 50, 100, 150
Tetracyclics Maprotiline (no longer available in the United States)	21–25	• Depression • Depression with anxiety **Unlabeled uses:** • Postherpetic neuralgia	180–300	TABS: 25, 50, 75

Generic (Trade) Name	Half-life (hr)	Indications	Therapeutic Plasma Level Range (ng/mL)	Available Forms (mg)
Mirtazapine (Remeron)	20–40	• Depression **Unlabeled uses:** • Chronic urticaria • Insomnia associated with depression	4.0–40.0 (expected steady state concentration at recommended daily doses)	TABS: 7.5, 15, 30, 45 TABS (ORALLY DISINTEGRATING): 15, 30, 45

Action

• Inhibit reuptake of norepinephrine or serotonin at the presynaptic neuron

Contraindications and Precautions

Contraindicated in: • Hypersensitivity to any tricyclic or related drug • Concomitant use with monoamine oxidase inhibitors (MAOIs) • Acute recovery period following myocardial infarction • Narrow angle glaucoma • Pregnancy and lactation (safety not established) • Known or suspected seizure disorder (maprotiline)

Use Cautiously in: • Patients with history of seizures (maprotiline contraindicated) • Patients with tendency to have urinary retention • Benign prostatic hypertrophy • Cardiovascular disorders • Hepatic or renal insufficiency • Psychotic patients • Elderly or debilitated patients

Adverse Reactions and Side Effects

• Drowsiness; fatigue
• Dry mouth
• Blurred vision
• Orthostatic hypotension
• Tachycardia; arrhythmias
• Constipation
• Urinary retention
• Blood dyscrasias
• Nausea and vomiting
• Photosensitivity
• Possible QT prolongation (maprotiline)
• Increased risk of suicidality in children and adolescents (**black-box warning**)

Interactions

• Increased effects of tricyclic antidepressants with **bupropion, cimetidine, haloperidol, selective serotonin reuptake inhibitors (SSRIs),** and **valproic acid.**
• Decreased effects of tricyclic antidepressants with **carbamazepine, barbiturates,** and **rifamycins.**

- Hyperpyretic crisis, convulsions, and death can occur with **MAOIs.**
- Coadministration with **clonidine** may produce hypertensive crisis.
- Decreased effects of **levodopa** and **guanethidine** with tricyclic antidepressants.
- Potentiation of pressor response with direct-acting **sympathomimetics.**
- Increased anti-coagulation effects may occur with **dicumarol.**
- Increased serum levels of **carbamazepine** occur with concomitant use of tricyclics.
- Increased risk of seizures with concomitant use of maprotiline and **phenothiazines.**
- Potential for cardiovascular toxicity of maprotiline when given concomitantly with **thyroid hormones** (e.g., **levothyroxine**).
- Impairment of motor skills is increased with concomitant use of mirtazapine and **central nervous system (CNS) depressants** (e.g., **benzodiazepines**).
- Concomitant use of maprotiline and **other drugs that prolong QT interval** may result in life-threatening cardiac arrhythmia because of possible additive effects.
- Increased effects of mirtazapine with concomitant use of **SSRIs.**

Route and Dosage

AMITRIPTYLINE

Depression: **PO** *(Adults):* 75 mg/day in divided doses. May gradually increase to 150 mg/day. Alternative dosing: May initiate at 50 to 100 mg at bedtime; increase by 25 to 50 mg as necessary, to a total of 150 mg/day.
  Hospitalized patients: May require up to 300 mg/day.
  Adolescent and elderly patients: 10 mg 3 times/day and 20 mg at bedtime.
Migraine prevention: **PO** *(Adults):* Common dosage: 50 to 100 mg/day in divided doses. Range: 10 to 300 mg/day.
Prevention of chronic headache: **PO** *(Adults):* 20 to 100 mg/day.
Fibromyalgia: **PO** *(Adults):* 10 to 50 mg at bedtime.
Postherpetic neuralgia: **PO** *(Adults):* 65 to 100 mg/day for at least 3 weeks.

CLOMIPRAMINE (Anafranil)

Obsessive-compulsive disorder: **PO** *(Adults):* 25 mg/day. Gradually increase to 100 mg/day during first 2 weeks, given in divided doses. May increase gradually over several weeks to maximum of 250 mg/day.
  Children and adolescents: 25 mg/day. Gradually increase during first 2 weeks to daily dose of 3 mg/kg or 100 mg, whichever is smaller. Maximum daily dose: 3 mg/kg or 200 mg, whichever is smaller.

Premenstrual symptoms: **PO** *(Adults):* 25 to 75 mg/day for irritability and dysphoria.

Panic disorder: **PO** *(Adults):* Initial dosage: 10 mg. Increase to a maximum dose of 150 mg given as multiple daily doses.

DESIPRAMINE (Norpramin)

Depression: **PO** *(Adults):* 100 to 200 mg/day in divided doses or as a single daily dose. May increase to maximum dose of 300 mg/day.

> *Elderly and adolescents:* 25 to 100 mg/day in divided doses or as a single daily dose. Maximum dose: 150 mg/day.

Alcoholism: **PO** *(Adults):* 200 to 275 mg/day.

Attention-deficit/hyperactivity disorder (ADHD): **PO** *(Adults):* 100 to 200 mg/day.

> *Children and adolescents:* Has been studied at dosages of 75 mg/day and 4.6 mg/kg/day. Should be initiated at the lowest dose and then increased according to tolerability and clinical response.

Bulimia nervosa: **PO** *(Adults):* Initial dose: 25 mg 3 times a day. Titrate dosage up to 200 to 300 mg/day, depending on response and adverse effects.

Diabetic neuropathy: **PO** *(Adults):* 50 to 250 mg/day.

Postherpetic neuralgia: **PO** *(Adults):* 94 to 167 mg/day for at least 6 weeks.

Irritable bowel syndrome: **PO** *(Adults):* 10 to 50 mg/day. May titrate dosage based on response to therapy up to 100 to 200 mg/day.

DOXEPIN (Sinequan)

Depression and/or anxiety: **PO** *(Adults and children ≥12 years):* (Mild to moderate illness) 75 mg/day. May increase to maximum dose of 150 mg/day.

> (Mild symptoms associated with organic illness): 25 to 50 mg/day.
>
> (Severe symptoms): 50 mg 3 times/day; may gradually increase to 300 mg/day.

Migraine prevention: **PO** *(Adults):* 75 to 150 mg/day. Occasionally dosages up to 300 mg/day may be required.

IMIPRAMINE (Tofranil)

Depression: **PO** *(Adults):* 75 mg/day. May increase to maximum of 200 mg/day. Hospitalized patients may require up to 300 mg/day.

> *Adolescent and geriatric patients:* 30 to 40 mg/day. May increase to maximum of 100 mg/day.

Nocturnal enuresis: **PO** *(Children ≥6 years of age):* 25 mg/day 1 hour before bedtime. May increase after 1 week to 50 mg/night if <12 years of age; up to 75 mg/night if >12 years of age. Maximum dose: 2.5 mg/kg/day.

Alcoholism: **PO** *(Adults):* 50 mg/day titrated by 50 mg every 3 to 5 days to a maximum daily dose of 300 mg.

ADHD: **PO** *(Children and adolescents):* 1 mg/kg/day titrated to a maximum dose of 4 mg/kg/day or 200 mg/day, whichever is smaller.

Bulimia nervosa: **PO** *(Adults):* 50 mg/day titrated to 100 mg 2 times a day.

Migraine prevention: **PO** *(Adults):* 10 to 25 mg 3 times a day.

Urinary incontinence: **PO** *(Adults):* 25 mg 2 to 3 times a day.

NORTRIPTYLINE (Aventyl; Pamelor)

Depression: **PO** *(Adults):* 25 mg 3 or 4 times a day. The total daily dose may be given at bedtime.

> *Elderly and adolescent patients:* 30 to 50 mg daily in divided doses or total daily dose may be given once/day.

ADHD: **PO** *(Adults):* 25 mg 3 to 4 times/day.

> *Children and adolescents:* 0.5 mg/kg/day, titrated to a maximum dose of 2 mg/kg/day or 100 mg, whichever is less.

Postherpetic neuralgia: **PO** *(Adults):* Dosage range: 58 to 89 mg/day for at least 5 weeks.

Irritable bowel syndrome: **PO** *(Adults):* 10 to 50 mg/day. May titrate dosage based on response to therapy up to 100 to 200 mg/day.

PROTRIPTYLINE (Vivactil)

Depression: **PO** *(Adults):* 15 to 40 mg/day divided into 3 or 4 doses. Maximum daily dose: 60 mg.

> *Adolescent and elderly patients:* 5 mg 3 times/day.

TRIMIPRAMINE (Surmontil)

Depression: **PO** *(Adults):* 75 mg/day. Increase gradually to 150 to 200 mg/day. Hospitalized patients may require up to 300 mg/day.

> *Adolescent and elderly patients:* Initially, 50 mg/day, with gradual increments up to 100 mg/day.

AMOXAPINE (Asendin)

Depression/depression with anxiety: **PO** *(Adults):* 50 mg 2 or 3 times daily. May increase to 100 mg 2 or 3 times daily by end of first week. Maintenance dosage is the lowest dose that will maintain remission.

> *Elderly patients:* 25 mg 2 or 3 times a day. May increase by end of first week to 50 mg 2 or 3 times a day.

MAPROTILINE (Generic Only)

Depression/depression with anxiety: **PO** *(Adults):* Initial dosage: 75 mg/day. After 2 weeks, may increase gradually in 25 mg increments. Maximum daily dose: 150 mg.

> *Hospitalized patients with severe depression:* **PO** *(Adults):* Initial dosage: 100 to 150 mg/day. May increase

gradually and as tolerated to a maximum dosage of 225 mg/day.

Elderly patients: **PO:** Initiate dosage at 25 mg/day; 50 to 75 mg/day may be sufficient for maintenance therapy in elderly patients.

Postherpetic neuralgia: **PO** *(Adults):* 100 mg/day for 5 weeks.

MIRTAZAPINE (Remeron)

Depression: **PO** *(Adults):* Initial dosage: 15 mg/day as a single dose, preferably in the evening before bedtime. The effective dose range is generally 15 to 45 mg/day.

Chronic urticaria: **PO** *(Adults):* 15 to 30 mg/day.

Insomnia associated with depression: **PO** *(Adults):* 15 to 45 mg orally once daily before bedtime.

■ SELECTIVE SEROTONIN REUPTAKE INHIBITORS (SSRIs)

Examples

Generic (Trade) Name	Half-life	Indications	Available Forms (mg)
Citalopram (Celexa)	~35 hr	• Treatment of depression **Unlabeled uses:** • Alcoholism • Binge-eating disorder • Generalized anxiety disorder (GAD) • OCD • Premenstrual dysphoric disorder (PMDD)	**TABS:** 10, 20, 40 **ORAL SOLUTION:** 10/5 mL
Escitalopram (Lexapro)	27–32 hr	• Major depressive disorder • GAD **Unlabeled uses:** • Posttraumatic stress disorder (PTSD)	**TABS:** 5, 10, 20 **ORAL SOLUTION:** 1/mL
Fluoxetine (Prozac; Sarafem; Selfemra)	1 to 6 days	• Depression • Depressive episodes associated with bipolar I disorder and treatment-resistant depression (in combination with olanzapine) • OCD • Bulimia nervosa • Panic disorder • PMDD (Sarafem; Selfemra only) **Unlabeled uses:** • Alcoholism • Borderline Personality Disorder • Fibromyalgia	**TABS:** 10, 15, 20, 60 **CAPS:** 10, 20, 40 **CAPS, DELAYED-RELEASE:** 90 **ORAL SOLUTION:** 20/5 mL

(Continued)

Generic (Trade) Name	Half-life	Indications	Available Forms (mg)
		• Hot flashes • PTSD • Migraine prevention • Raynaud phenomenon • Irritable bowel syndrome	
Fluvoxamine (Luvox)	13.6–15.6 hr	• OCD • Social anxiety disorder **Unlabeled uses:** • Panic disorder • PTSD • Bulimia nervosa • Depression and anxiety in children and adolescents	**TABS:** 25, 50, 100 **CAPS (ER):** 100, 150
Paroxetine (Paxil)	21 hr (CR: 15–20 hr)	• Major depressive disorder • Panic disorder • OCD • Social anxiety disorder • GAD • PTSD • PMDD **Unlabeled uses:** • Hot flashes • Diabetic neuropathy • Irritable bowel syndrome	**TABS:** 10, 20, 30, 40 **ORAL SUSPENSION:** 10/5 mL **TABS (CR):** 12.5, 25, 37.5
Sertraline (Zoloft)	24	• Major depressive disorder • OCD • Panic disorder • PTSD • PMDD • Social anxiety disorder	**TABS:** 25, 50, 100 **ORAL CONCENTRATE:** 20/mL
Vilazodone (Viibryd)	25 hr	• Major depressive disorder	**TABS:** 10, 20, 40
Vortioxetine (Trintellix)	66 hr	• Major depressive disorder	**TABS:** 5, 10, 15, 20

Action

- Selectively inhibit the central nervous system neuronal uptake of serotonin (5-hydroxytryptamine [5-HT]). Vilazodone (Viibryd) is also a partial agonist at serotonergic 5-HT$_{1A}$ receptors. Vortioxetine (Trintellix) also exhibits agonist activity for 5-HT$_{1A}$ receptors, as well as antagonism for 5-HT$_3$ receptors.

Contraindications and Precautions

Contraindicated in: • Hypersensitivity to SSRIs • Concomitant use of SSRIs with, or within 14 days' use of, MAOIs • Concomitant use of SSRIs with pimozide • *Fluoxetine:* concomitant use with thioridazine • *Fluvoxamine:* concomitant use with alosetron, astemizole, cisapride, terfenadine, thioridazine, or tizanidine • *Paroxetine:* concomitant use with thioridazine • *Sertraline:* coadministration of oral solution with disulfiram because of alcohol content • *Citalopram:* in patients with congenital long QT syndrome

Use Cautiously in: • Patients with history of seizures • Underweight or anorexic patients • Hepatic or renal insufficiency • Elderly or debilitated patients • Suicidal patients • Patients taking anticoagulants • Pregnancy and lactation

Adverse Reactions and Side Effects

- Headache
- Insomnia
- Nausea
- Anorexia
- Diarrhea
- Constipation
- Sexual dysfunction
- Somnolence
- Dry mouth
- Increased risk of suicidality in children and adolescents (**black-box warning**)
- Serotonin syndrome. Can occur if taken concurrently with other medications that increase levels of serotonin (e.g., MAOIs, tryptophan, amphetamines, other antidepressants, buspirone, lithium, dopamine agonists, or serotonin 5-HT$_1$ receptor agonists [agents for migraine]). Symptoms of serotonin syndrome include diarrhea, cramping, tachycardia, labile blood pressure, diaphoresis, fever, tremor, shivering, restlessness, confusion, disorientation, mania, myoclonus, hyperreflexia, ataxia, seizures, cardiovascular shock, and death.

Interactions

- Toxic, sometimes fatal, reactions have occurred with concomitant use of **MAOIs.**
- Increased effects of SSRIs with **cimetidine, L-tryptophan, lithium, linezolid,** and **St. John's wort.**
- Serotonin syndrome may occur with concomitant use of SSRIs and **metoclopramide, sibutramine, tramadol, serotonin 5-HT1 receptor agonists** (agents for migraine), or any drug that increases levels of serotonin.
- Concomitant use of SSRIs may increase effects of **hydantoins, tricyclic antidepressants, cyclosporine, benzodiazepines, beta blockers, methadone, carbamazepine, clozapine, olanzapine, pimozide, haloperidol, mexiletine, phenothiazines, St. John's wort, sumatriptan, trazodone, sympathomimetics, theophylline, procyclidine, propafenone, risperidone, ropivacaine, warfarin,** and **zolpidem.**

- Concomitant use of SSRIs may decrease effects of **buspirone** and **digoxin**.
- **Lithium** levels may be increased with concomitant use of SSRIs (these drugs interact synergistically).
- Decreased effects of SSRIs with concomitant use of **carba-mazepine** and **cyproheptadine**.
- Increased effects of vortioxetine with concomitant use of **bupropion, fluoxetine, paroxetine,** or **quinidine**.
- Decreased effects of vortioxetine with concomitant use of **CYP inducers** (e.g., **rifampicin, carbamazepine, phenytoin**).

Route and Dosage

CITALOPRAM (Celexa)

Depression: **PO** *(Adults):* Initial dosage: 20 mg/day as a single daily dose. May increase in increments of 20 mg at intervals of no less than 1 week. Maximum dose: 40 mg/day.
   Elderly patients: 20 mg/day.

Alcoholism: **PO** *(Adults):* 20 to 40 mg/day.

Binge-eating disorder: **PO** *(Adults):* 20 to 60 mg/day.

GAD: **PO** *(Adults):* 10 mg/day, titrated up to 40 mg/day.

OCD: **PO** *(Adults):* Initial dosage: 20 mg/day. Titrate to a target dosage of 40 to 60 mg/day. Maximum dosage: 80 mg/day.

PMDD: **PO** *(Adults):* 5 mg initiated on estimated day of ovulation. Increase on subsequent days by 5 mg/day to the maximum dose of 30 mg. On the first day of menses, decrease dose to 20 mg and then to 10 mg on second day of menses. Discontinue medication on day 3 of menses. Repeat medication regimen beginning on following initial day of ovulation.

ESCITALOPRAM (Lexapro)

Depression: **PO** *(Adults):* Initial dosage: 10 mg/day as a single daily dose. May increase to 20 mg/day after 1 week.
   Elderly patients: **PO:** 10 mg/day.
   Children 12 to 17 years: **PO:** Initial dosage: 10 mg/day as a single daily dose. May increase gradually to 20 mg after a minimum of 3 weeks.

GAD: **PO** *(Adults):* Initial dosage: 10 mg/day as a single daily dose. May increase to 20 mg/day after 1 week.

PTSD: **PO** *(Adults):* Initial dose: 10 mg/day as a single daily dose. Increase to 20 mg once daily after 4 weeks.

FLUOXETINE (Prozac; Sarafem; Selfemra)

Depression: **PO** *(Adults):* Initial dosage: 20 mg/day in the morning. May increase dosage after several weeks if sufficient clinical improvement is not observed. Maximum dose: 80 mg/day.
   Children ≥8 years: **PO:** Initial dosage: 10 mg/day. May increase after 1 week to 20 mg/day.

OCD: **PO** *(Adults):* Initial dosage: 20 mg/day in the morning. May increase dosage after several weeks if sufficient clinical improvement is not observed. Maximum dose: 80 mg/day.

> *Children 7 to 17 years:* **PO** *Adolescents and higher-weight children:* 10 mg/day. May be increased after 2 weeks to 20 mg/day; additional increases may be made after several more weeks (range 20 to 60 mg/day). **PO** *Lower-weight children:* 10 mg/day initially. Dosage may be increased after several more weeks (range 20 to 30 mg/day).

Depressive episodes associated with bipolar I disorder and treatment-resistant depression (in combination with olanzapine): **PO** *(Adults):* Fluoxetine 20 mg and olanzapine 5 mg are administered once daily in the evening without regard to meals. Dosage adjustments, if indicated, should be made with the individual components according to efficacy and tolerability (dosage range fluoxetine 20 to 50 mg and oral olanzapine 5 to 20 mg).

Bulimia nervosa: **PO** *(Adults):* 60 mg/day administered in the morning. May need to titrate up to this target dose in some patients.

Panic disorder: **PO** *(Adults):* Initial dose: 10 mg/day. After 1 week, increase dose to 20 mg/day. If no improvement is seen after several weeks, may consider dose increases up to 60 mg/day.

PMDD (Sarafem and Selfemra only): **PO** *(Adults):* Initial dose: 20 mg/day. Maximum: 80 mg/day. May be given continuously throughout the cycle or intermittently (only during the 14 days prior to anticipated onset of menses).

Alcoholism: **PO** *(Adults):* Initial dosage: 20 mg/day. Titrate to 40 mg/day after 2 weeks, if needed.

Borderline personality disorder: **PO** *(Adults):* 20 to 80 mg/day.

Fibromyalgia: **PO** *(Adults):* 20 mg/day (in the morning) for up to 6 weeks.

Hot flashes: **PO** *(Adults):* 20 mg/day for 4 weeks.

PTSD: **PO** *(Adults):* Initial dosage 10 to 20 mg/day. Average target dose: 20 to 50 mg/day in adults and 20 mg in older adults. Highest target dosage: 80 mg/day. Duration of therapy is 6 to 12 months for acute PTSD and 12 to 24 months for chronic PTSD. Dose tapering over 2 to 4 weeks is recommended to avoid withdrawal symptoms.

> *Children and adolescents:* Average target dose: 10 to 20 mg/day. Duration and tapering of therapy is the same as for adults.

Migraine prevention: **PO** *(Adults):* 10 to 40 mg/day.

Raynaud phenomenon: **PO** *(Adults):* 20 to 60 mg/day.

Irritable bowel syndrome: **PO** *(Adults):* 10 to 20 mg/day.

FLUVOXAMINE (Luvox)

> *OCD:* **PO** *(Adults):* Initial dose: 50 mg (immediate release tabs) or 100 mg (extended-release caps) at bedtime. May increase dose in 50 mg increments every week until therapeutic benefit

is achieved. Maximum dose: 300 mg. Administer daily doses of immediate release tabs >100 mg in 2 divided doses. If unequal, give larger dose at bedtime.

> *Children 8 to 17 years*: Initial dose: 25 mg single dose at bedtime. May increase the dose in 25 mg increments every 4 to 7 days to a maximum dose of 200 mg/day. Some adolescents may require up to a maximum dose of 300 mg/day to achieve a therapeutic benefit. Divide daily doses >50 mg into 2 doses. If unequal, give larger dose at bedtime.

Social anxiety disorder: **PO** *(Adults):* (extended release capsules): Initial dose: 100 mg/day as a single daily dose at bedtime. Increase in 50 mg increments every week, as tolerated, until maximum therapeutic benefit is achieved. Maximum dose: 300 mg/day.

Panic disorder: **PO** *(Adults):* Initial dosage: 50 mg/day. Gradually increase after several days to 150 mg/day. For patients who fail to respond after several weeks of treatment, further increases up to 300 mg/day may be considered.

Bulimia nervosa: **PO** *(Adults):* 50 mg/day, titrated up based on therapeutic response to 200 mg/day for up to 12 weeks.

PTSD: **PO** *(Adults):* Initial dosage: 50 mg/day. Increase gradually to target dose of 100 to 250 mg/day in adults, and 100 mg/day in older adults. Maximum recommended dosage: 300 mg/day. Duration of therapy is 6 to 12 months for acute PTSD and 12 to 24 months for chronic PTSD. Dose tapering over 2 to 4 weeks is recommended to avoid withdrawal symptoms.

> *Children and adolescents:* Target dose: 50 mg/day. Duration and tapering of therapy is the same as for adults.

Depression or anxiety disorder in children and adolescents: **PO** *(≥12 years):* Initial dosage: 25 to 50 mg at bedtime. Maintenance dosage: 150 to 300 mg/day. **PO** *(<12 years):* Initial dosage: 25 mg at bedtime. Maintenance dosage: 100 to 200 mg/day.

PAROXETINE (Paxil)

Depression: **PO** *(Adults):* 20 mg/day in the morning. May increase dose in 10 mg increments at intervals of at least 1 week to a maximum of 50 mg/day.

> *Controlled release*: Initial dose: 25 mg/day in the morning. May increase dose in 12.5 mg increments at intervals of at least 1 week to a maximum of 62.5 mg/day.

Panic disorder: **PO** *(Adults):* 10 mg/day in the morning. May increase dose in 10 mg/day increments at intervals of at least 1 week to a target dose of 40 mg/day. Maximum dose: 60 mg/day.

> *Controlled release:* Initial dose: 12.5 mg/day. May increase dose in 12.5 mg/day increments at intervals of at least 1 week to a maximum dose of 75 mg/day.

OCD: **PO** *(Adults):* 20 mg/day. May increase dose in 10 mg/day increments at intervals of at least 1week. Recommended dose: 40 mg/day. Maximum dose: 60 mg/day.

> *Children and adolescents (7 to 17 years):* **PO:** Initial dosage: 10 mg/day. If needed, may increase dosage by 10 mg/day no more frequently than every 7 days, to a maximum dosage of 50 mg/day.

Social anxiety disorder: **PO** *(Adults):* 20 mg/day. Usual range is 20 to 60 mg/day.

> *Controlled release:* 12.5 mg/day. May increase dosage at intervals of at least 1 week, in increments of 12.5 mg/day to a maximum of 37.5 mg/day.

> *Children and adolescents (8 to 17 years):* **PO:** Initial dosage: 10 mg/day. If needed, may increase dose by 10 mg/day no more frequently than every 7 days, to a maximum dosage of 50 mg/day.

GAD and PTSD: **PO** *(Adults)*: Initial dose: 20 mg/day. Usual range is 20 to 50 mg/day. Doses may be increased in increments of 10 mg/day at intervals of at least 1 week.

PMDD: **PO** *(Adults): Controlled release:* Initial dose: 12.5 mg/day. Usual range: 12.5 to 25 mg/day. Dosage increases may be made at intervals of at least 1 week. May be administered daily throughout the menstrual cycle or limited to luteal phase of menstrual cycle.

Hot flashes: **PO** *(Adults):* 10 to 20 mg/day. *Controlled release:* 12.5 to 25 mg/day.

Diabetic neuropathy: **PO** *(Adults):* Initial dose: 10 mg/day. Titrate to 20 to 60 mg/day.

Irritable bowel syndrome: **PO** *(Adults):* 20 to 40 mg/day. *Controlled release:* 12.5 to 50 mg/day.

Elderly or debilitated patients: **PO:** Initial dose 10 mg/day. Maximum dose: 40 mg/day. *Controlled release:* Initial dose: 12.5 mg/day. Maximum dose: 50 mg/day.

SERTRALINE (Zoloft)

Depression and OCD: **PO** *(Adults):* 50 mg/day (either morning or evening). May increase dosage at 1 week intervals to a maximum of 200 mg/day.

> *Children and adolescents:* **PO** *(≥13 years):* 50 mg/day. May increase by 50 mg at weekly intervals to maximum dosage of 200 mg/day. **PO** *(6 to 12 years):* 25 mg/day. May increase by 25 mg at weekly intervals to maximum dosage of 200 mg/day.

Panic disorder and PTSD: **PO** *(Adults):* Initial dose: 25 mg/day. After 1 week, increase dose to 50 mg/day. If needed, may increase dosage at 1 week intervals to a maximum of 200 mg/day.

PMDD: **PO** *(Adults):* 50 mg/day given on each day of the menstrual cycle or only during each day of the luteal phase of the menstrual cycle. For patients not responding, may increase dosage in 50 mg increments per menstrual cycle up to 150 mg/day when dosing throughout the cycle, or 100 mg/day when dosing only during the luteal phase. If 100 mg/day has been established with luteal phase dosing, titrate at 50 mg/day for first 3 days of each luteal phase dosing period.

Social anxiety disorder: **PO** *(Adults):* Initial dose: 25 mg/day. After 1 week, increase dose to 50 mg/day. May be increased at weekly intervals up to 200 mg/day.

VILAZODONE (Viibryd)

Major depressive disorder: **PO** *(Adults):* Initial dosage: 10 mg once daily. After 1 week, increase dosage to 20 mg once daily. After the second week, increase the dosage to 40 mg once daily. Should be taken with food.

VORTIOXETINE (Trintellix)

Major depressive disorder: **PO** *(Adults):* Initial dosage: 10 mg once daily. Dosage may be titrated to 20 mg/day, and may be administered without regard to meals.

■ NOREPINEPHRINE-DOPAMINE REUPTAKE INHIBITORS (NDRIs)

Examples

Generic (Trade) Name	Half-life (hr)	Indications	Available Forms (mg)
Bupropion (Wellbutrin; Wellbutrin SR; Wellbutrin XL; Budeprion SR; Budeprion XL; Aplenzin; Zyban)	8–24	• Depression (all except Zyban) • Seasonal affective disorder (Wellbutrin XL; Aplenzin) • Smoking cessation (Zyban) **Unlabeled uses:** • ADHD (Wellbutrin; Wellbutrin SR; Wellbutrin XL)	**TABS:** 75, 100 **TABS (SR):** 100, 150, 200 **TABS (XL):** 150, 300, 450 **TABS (ER) (APLENZIN):** 174, 348, 522

SR = 12-hour tablets; XL and ER = 24-hour tablets

Action

• Action is unclear. Thought to inhibit the reuptake of norepinephrine and dopamine into presynaptic neurons.

Contraindications and Precautions

Contraindicated in: • Hypersensitivity to the drug • Concomitant use with, or within 2 weeks use of, MAOIs • Known or suspected seizure disorder • Alcohol or benzodiazepine (or other sedatives) withdrawal • Current or prior diagnosis of bulimia or anorexia nervosa • Concomitant use with more than one bupropion product • Lactation

Use Cautiously in: • Patients with urinary retention • Patients with hepatic or renal function impairment • Patients with suicidal ideation • Patients with recent history of myocardial infarction or unstable heart disease • Pregnancy (safety not established) • Elderly and debilitated patients

Adverse Reactions and Side Effects
- Dry mouth
- Blurred vision
- Agitation; aggression
- Insomnia
- Tremor
- Sedation; dizziness
- Tachycardia
- Excessive sweating
- Headache
- Nausea/vomiting
- Anorexia; weight loss
- Seizures
- Constipation
- Neuropsychiatric symptoms (e.g., delusions, hallucinations, suicidal ideation)
- Increased risk of suicidality in children and adolescents (**black-box warning**)

Interactions
- Increased effects of bupropion with **amantadine, levodopa, clopidogrel, CYP2B6 inhibitors** (e.g., **cimetidine, ticlopidine, clopidogrel**), **guanfacine,** and **linezolid.**
- Increased risk of acute toxicity with **MAOIs.** Coadministration is contraindicated.
- Coadministration with a **nicotine replacement agent** may cause hypertension.
- Concomitant use with **alcohol** may produce adverse neuropsychiatric events (alcohol tolerance is reduced).
- Decreased effects of bupropion with **carbamazepine, ritonavir,** and **CYP2B6 inducers** (e.g., **efavirenz, phenobarbital, phenytoin, rifampin**).
- Increased anticoagulant effect of **warfarin** with bupropion.
- Increased effects of drugs metabolized by CYP2D6 isoenzyme (e.g., **nortriptyline, imipramine, desipramine, paroxetine, fluoxetine, sertraline, haloperidol, risperidone, thioridazine, metoprolol, propafenone,** and **flecainide**).
- Increased risk of seizures when bupropion is coadministered with drugs that lower the seizure threshold (e.g., **antidepressants, antipsychotics, systemic steroids, theophylline, tramadol**).

Route and Dosage

BUPROPION (Wellbutrin; Budeprion; Aplenzin; Zyban)

Depression (Wellbutrin; Budeprion): **PO** *(Adults): (immediate release tabs):* 100 mg 2 times/day. May increase after 3 days to 100 mg given 3 times/day. For patients who do not show improvement after several weeks of dosing at 300 mg/day, an increase in dosage up to 450 mg/day may be considered. No single dose of bupropion should exceed 150 mg. To prevent the risk of seizures, administer with 4 to 6 hours between doses.

Sustained release tabs (Wellbutrin SR; Budeprion SR): Give as a single 150 mg dose in the morning. May increase to twice a day (total 300 mg), with at least 8 hours between doses. Maximum dose: 400 mg, administered as 200 mg twice a day, with at least 8 hours between doses.

Extended release tabs (Wellbutrin XL; Budeprion XL): Begin dosing at 150 mg/day, given as a single daily dose in the morning. May increase after 3 days to 300 mg/day, given as a single daily dose in the morning. Maximum dose: 450 mg administered as a single daily dose in the morning.

Aplenzin: Initial dose: 174 mg once daily. After 4 days, may increase the dose to 348 mg once daily.

Seasonal affective disorder (Wellbutrin XL): **PO** *(Adults):* 150 mg administered each morning beginning in the autumn prior to the onset of depressive symptoms. Dose may be up titrated to the target dose of 300 mg/day after 1 week. Therapy should continue through the winter season before being tapered to 150 mg/day for 2 weeks prior to discontinuation in early spring.

Aplenzin: **PO** *(Adults):* 174 mg once daily beginning in the autumn prior to the onset of seasonal depressive symptoms. After 1 week, may increase the dose to 348 mg once daily. Continue treatment through the winter season.

Smoking cessation (Zyban): **PO** *(Adults):* Begin dosing at 150 mg given once a day in the morning for 3 days. If tolerated well, increase to target dose of 300 mg/day given in doses of 150 mg twice daily with an interval of 8 hours between doses. Continue treatment for 7 to 12 weeks. Some patients may need treatment for as long as 6 months.

ADHD (Wellbutrin; Wellbutrin SR; Wellbutrin XL): **PO** *(Adults):* 150 to 450 mg/day. Initiate therapy with 150 mg/day and titrate based on tolerability and efficacy. Doses can be given as divided doses or in SR or XL formulations.

Children and adolescents (Wellbutrin; Wellbutrin SR; Wellbutrin XL): Up to 3 mg/kg/day or 150 mg/day initially, titrated to a maximum dosage of up to 6 mg/kg/day or 300 mg/day. Single dose should not exceed 150 mg. Usually given in divided doses for safety and effectiveness: twice daily for children and 3 times daily for adolescents.

■ SEROTONIN-NOREPINEPHRINE REUPTAKE INHIBITORS (SNRIs)

Examples

Generic (Trade) Name	Half-life (hr)	Indications	Available Forms (mg)
Desvenlafaxine (Pristiq)	11–14	• Depression	TABS ER: 50, 100
Duloxetine (Cymbalta)	8–17	• Depression • Chronic musculoskeletal pain • Diabetic peripheral neuropathic pain • Fibromyalgia • GAD; new indication: GAD in children 7–17 yr **Unlabeled uses:** • Stress urinary incontinence	CAPS: 20, 30, 60
Venlafaxine (Effexor)	5–11 (incl. metabolite)	• Depression • GAD (extended release [ER only]) • Social anxiety disorder (ER) • Panic disorder (ER) **Unlabeled uses:** • Hot flashes • PMDD • Diabetic neuropathy • Anxiety and depression in children and adolescents	TABS: 25, 37.5, 50, 75, 100 CAPS XR: 37.5, 75, 150 TABS XR: 37.5, 75, 150, 225
Levomilnacipran (Fetzima)	12	• Major depressive disorder	CAPS: 20, 40, 80, 120

Action
• SNRIs are potent inhibitors of neuronal serotonin and norepinephrine reuptake; weak inhibitors of dopamine reuptake

Contraindications and Precautions

Contraindicated in: • Hypersensitivity to the drug • Children (safety not established) • Concomitant (or within 14 days) use with MAOIs • Severe renal or hepatic impairment • Pregnancy and lactation (safety not established) • Uncontrolled narrow-angle glaucoma

Use Cautiously in: • Hepatic and renal insufficiency • Elderly and debilitated patients • Patients with history of drug abuse • Patients with suicidal ideation • Patients with history of or existing cardiovascular disease • Patients with history of mania • Patients with history of seizures • Children (Venlafaxine has been used off label with children and adolescents.)

Adverse Reactions and Side Effects
• Headache
• Dry mouth

- Nausea
- Somnolence
- Dizziness
- Insomnia
- Asthenia
- Constipation
- Diarrhea
- Tachycardia; palpitations
- Activation of mania/hypomania
- Abnormal bleeding
- Hypertension
- Mydriasis (venlafaxine)
- Increased risk of suicidality in children and adolescents (**black-box warning**)
- Discontinuation syndrome. Abrupt withdrawal may result in symptoms such as nausea, vomiting, nervousness, dizziness, headache, insomnia, nightmares, paresthesias, agitation, irritability, sensory disturbances, and tinnitus. A gradual reduction in dosage is recommended.

Interactions

- Concomitant use of SNRIs with **MAOIs** results in serious, sometimes fatal, effects resembling neuroleptic malignant syndrome. Coadministration is contraindicated.
- Serotonin syndrome may occur when SNRIs are used concomitantly with **St. John's wort, 5-HT$_1$ receptor agonists (triptans), sibutramine, trazodone,** or other drugs that increase levels of serotonin.
- Increased effects of **haloperidol, clozapine,** and **tricyclic antidepressants** when used concomitantly with venlafaxine.
- Increased effects of venlafaxine with **cimetidine, terbinafine,** and **azole antifungals.**
- Decreased effects of venlafaxine with **cyproheptadine.**
- Decreased effects of **indinavir** and **metoprolol** with venlafaxine.
- Increased effects of **warfarin and other drugs with anticoagulant effects** with all SNRIs.
- Increased effects of duloxetine with **CYP1A2 inhibitors** (e.g., cimetidine, fluvoxamine, quinolone antibiotics) and **CYP2D6 inhibitors** (e.g., fluoxetine, quinidine, paroxetine).
- Increased risk of liver injury with concomitant use of **alcohol** and duloxetine.
- Increased risk of toxicity or adverse effects from drugs extensively metabolized by CYP2D6 (e.g., **flecainide, phenothiazines, propafenone, tricyclic antidepressants, thioridazine**) when used concomitantly with duloxetine.
- Increased effects of **tricyclic antidepressants** with desvenlafaxine.
- Decreased effects of **midazolam** with desvenlafaxine.

- Increased effects of desvenlafaxine and levomilnacipran with concomitant use of potent **CYP3A4 inhibitors** (e.g., ketoconazole).

Route and Dosage

DESVENLAFAXINE (Pristiq)

Depression: **PO** *(Adults):* 50 mg once daily, with or without food.

DULOXETINE (Cymbalta)

Depression: **PO** *(Adults):* 40 mg/day (given as 20 mg twice a day) to 60 mg/day (given either once a day or as 30 mg twice daily) without regard to meals.

Diabetic peripheral neuropathic pain: **PO** *(Adults):* 60 mg/day given once daily without regard to meals.

Fibromyalgia: **PO** *(Adults):* 30 mg once daily for 1 week and then increase to 60 mg once daily, if needed.

GAD: **PO** *(Adults):* 60 mg once daily. For some patients, it may be desirable to start at 30 mg once daily for 1 week to allow the patient to adjust to the medication before increasing to 60 mg once daily. If desired results are not achieved on 60 mg/day, may increase in daily increments of 30 mg to a maximum dosage of 120 mg/day.

Chronic musculoskeletal pain: **PO** *(Adults):* Initial dosage: 30 mg/day for 1 week, then increase to 60 mg/day.

Stress urinary incontinence: **PO** *(Adults):* 80 mg/day in a single dose or two divided doses (range 20 to 120 mg) for 12 weeks.

VENLAFAXINE (Effexor)

Depression: **PO** *(Adults): Immediate-release tabs:* Initial dosage: 75 mg/day in 2 or 3 divided doses, taken with food. May increase in increments up to 75 mg/day at intervals of at least 4 days up to 225 mg/day (not to exceed 375 mg/day in 3 divided doses).

Depression and GAD: **PO** *(Adults): Extended-release caps:* Initial dosage: 75 mg/day, administered in a single dose. May increase dose in increments of up to 75 mg/day at intervals of at least 4 days to a maximum of 225 mg/day.

Social anxiety disorder: **PO** *(Adults): Extended-release caps:* 75 mg/day as a single dose.

Panic disorder: **PO** *(Adults): Extended-release caps:* Initial dosage: 37.5 mg/day for 7 days. After 7 days, increase dosage to 75 mg/day. May increase dose in increments of up to 75 mg/day at intervals of at least 7 days to a maximum of 225 mg/day.

Hot flashes: **PO** *(Adults): Immediate-release forms:* 12.5 mg 2 times a day for 4 weeks.

   Extended-release forms: 37.5 to 150 mg once a day for up to 3 months. Titrate doses.

Premenstrual dysphoric disorder: **PO** *(Adults):* 37.5 to 200 mg/day, starting with either 37.5 mg once daily or 25 mg twice daily during the first menstrual cycle, then decreasing the dose as necessary at the start of subsequent menstrual cycles. Alternatively, intermittent dosing may be used by starting 14 days prior to the start of menses with either 37.5 or 75 mg daily for 2 days, then increasing to either 75 or 112.5 mg daily for 12 days or until the start of menses, followed by 37.5 or 75 mg daily for 2 days.

***Diabetic neuropathy:* PO** *(Adults):* Initial dosage: 37.5 mg once or twice daily. May increase by 75 mg each week to a maximum dosage of 225 mg/day.

***Anxiety and depression in children and adolescents:* PO** *(Adolescents):* Initial dosage: 37.5 to 75 mg/day. Maintenance dosage: 150 to 300 mg/day. **PO** *(Children):* Initial dosage 37.5 mg/day. Maintenance dosage: 75 to 150 mg/day.

LEVOMILNACIPRAN (Fetzima)

***Major depressive disorder:* PO** *(Adults):* Initial dosage: 20 mg once daily for 2 days, and then increase to 40 mg once daily. May increase dosage in increments of 40 mg at intervals of at least 2 days to the maximum dose of 120 mg once daily.

■ OTHER ATYPICAL ANTIDEPRESSANTS: SEROTONIN-5HT₂ ANTAGONISTS/REUPTAKE INHIBITORS (SARIs)

Examples

Generic (Trade) Name	Half-life	Indications	Therapeutic Plasma Level Range (ng/mL)	Available Forms (mg)
Nefazodone*	2–4 hr	• Depression	100–4000	**TABS:** 50, 100, 150, 200, 250
Trazodone (Oleptro [ER])	5–9 hr	• Depression **Unlabeled uses:** • Aggressive behavior • Insomnia • Migraine prevention • Depression in children and adolescents	800–1600	**TABS:** 50, 100, 150, 300 **TABS (ER):** 150, 300

* Bristol-Myers Squibb voluntarily removed its brand of nefazodone (Serzone) from the market in 2004. The generic equivalent is currently available through various other manufacturers.

Action

• Trazodone inhibits neuronal reuptake of serotonin; nefazodone inhibits neuronal reuptake of serotonin and norepinephrine, and both act as antagonists at central 5-HT₂ receptors

Contraindications and Precautions

Contraindicated in: • Hypersensitivity • Coadministration with terfenadine, astemizole, cisapride, pimozide, carbamazepine, or triazolam (nefazodone) • Patients with liver disease or baseline increases in serum transaminases (nefazodone) • Concomitant use with, or within 2 weeks of use of, MAOIs • Acute phase of myocardial infarction

Use Cautiously in: • Pregnancy and lactation (safety not established) • Children (safety not established) • Patients with suicidal ideation • Hepatic, renal, or cardiovascular disease • Elderly and debilitated patients

Adverse Reactions and Side Effects

- Drowsiness; dizziness
- Fatigue
- Orthostatic hypotension
- Headache
- Nervousness; insomnia
- Dry mouth
- Nausea
- Somnolence
- Constipation
- Blurred vision
- Priapism *(trazodone)*
- Erectile dysfunction
- Increased risk of suicidality in children and adolescents (**black-box warning**)
- Risk of hepatic failure *(nefazodone)* (**black-box warning**)

Interactions

- Increased effects of **CNS depressants, carbamazepine, digoxin,** and **phenytoin** with trazodone.
- Increased effects of trazodone with **phenothiazines, delavirdine, ginkgo biloba, clarithromycin, azole antifungals,** and **protease inhibitors.**
- Risk of serotonin syndrome with concomitant use of trazodone and **SSRIs** or **SNRIs.**
- Decreased effects of trazodone and nefazodone with **carbamazepine.**
- Increases or decreases in prothrombin time with concurrent use of trazodone and **warfarin.**
- Symptoms of serotonin syndrome and those resembling neuroleptic malignant syndrome may occur with concomitant use of **MAOIs.** Should not be used concurrently or within 2 weeks of use of MAOIs. Nefazodone and trazodone should be discontinued at least 14 days before starting MAOI therapy.
- Risk of serotonin syndrome with concomitant use of trazodone or nefazodone and **sibutramine, triptans, or other drugs that increase serotonin.**
- Increased effects of both drugs with concomitant use of **buspirone** and nefazodone.

- Increased effects of **benzodiazepines, carbamazepine, cisapride, cyclosporine, digoxin,** and **St. John's wort** with nefazodone.
- Risk of rhabdomyolysis with concomitant use of nefazodone and **HMG-CoA reductase inhibitors** (e.g., **simvastatin, atorvastatin, lovastatin**).

Route and Dosage

NEFAZODONE

Depression: **PO** *(Adults):* Initial dosage: 100 mg twice daily. May increase in increments of 100 to 200 mg/day, again on a twice-daily schedule, at intervals of no less than 1 week. Maintenance dosage: 300 to 600 mg/day.

> *Elderly and debilitated patients:* **PO:** 50 mg twice daily.

TRAZODONE

Depression: **PO:** *Adults: Immediate-release tablets:* Initial dosage: 150 mg/day in divided doses. May increase gradually by 50 mg/day every 3 to 4 days. Maximum dose: *Inpatients:* 600 mg/day in divided doses. *Outpatients:* 400 mg/day in divided doses.

> *Extended-release tablets:* Initial dosage: 150 mg once daily. May increase by 75 mg/day every 3 days to maximum dose of 375 mg/day.

> *Children and adolescents (≥6 years):* 1.5 to 2 mg/kg/day in 2 or 3 divided doses. Gradually increase every 3 to 4 days to maximum dose of 6 mg/kg/day in 3 divided doses.

Aggressive behavior: **PO** *(Adults):* 50 mg twice daily. Titrate dose over 1 to 6 weeks based on response and tolerability. Maintenance dosage: 75 to 400 mg/day in 2 to 4 divided dosages.

> *Children:* **PO:** 50 mg once daily at bedtime, titrated up as tolerated and based on response over approximately 1 week. Maintenance dosage: 150 to 200 mg/day in 3 divided doses.

Insomnia: **PO** *(Adults):* 50 to 100 mg at bedtime.

Migraine prevention: **PO** *(Adults):* 100 mg/day.

■ MONOAMINE OXIDASE INHIBITORS (MAOIs)

Examples

Generic (Trade) Name	Half-life	Indications	Available Forms (mg)
Isocarboxazid (Marplan)	Not established	Depression	**TABS:** 10
Phenelzine (Nardil)	11.6	Depression	**TABS:** 15
Tranylcypromine (Parnate)	2.4–2.8 hr	Depression	**TABS:** 10
Selegiline Transdermal System (Emsam)	18–25 hr (including metabolites)	Depression	**TRANSDERMAL PATCHES:** 6, 9, 12

Action

- Inhibition of the enzyme monoamine oxidase, which is responsible for the decomposition of the biogenic amines, epinephrine, norepinephrine, dopamine, and serotonin. This action results in an increase in the concentration of these endogenous amines.

Contraindications and Precautions

Contraindicated in: • Hypersensitivity • Pheochromocytoma • Hepatic or renal insufficiency • History of or existing cardiovascular disease • Hypertension • History of severe or frequent headaches • Concomitant use with other MAOIs, tricyclic antidepressants, carbamazepine, cyclobenzaprine, bupropion, SSRIs, SARIs, buspirone, sympathomimetics, meperidine, dextromethorphan, anesthetic agents, CNS depressants, antihypertensives, caffeine, and food with high tyramine content • Children younger than 16 years of age • Pregnancy and lactation (safety not established)

Use Cautiously in: • Patients with a history of seizures • Diabetes mellitus • Patients with suicidal ideation • Agitated or hypomanic patients • History of angina pectoris or hyperthyroidism

Adverse Reactions and Side Effects

- Dizziness
- Headache
- Orthostatic hypotension
- Constipation or diarrhea
- Nausea
- Disturbances in cardiac rate and rhythm
- Blurred vision
- Dry mouth
- Weight gain
- Hypomania
- Site reactions (itching, irritation) (with selegiline transdermal system)
- Increased risk of suicidality in children and adolescents (**black-box warning**)

Interactions

- Serious, potentially fatal adverse reactions may occur with concurrent use of other **antidepressants, carbamazepine, cyclobenzaprine, bupropion, SSRIs, SARIs, buspirone, sympathomimetics, L-tryptophan, dextromethorphan, anesthetic agents, CNS depressants,** and **amphetamines.** Avoid using within 2 weeks of each other (5 weeks after therapy with **fluoxetine**). (See contraindications.)

- Hypertensive crisis may occur with **amphetamines, methyldopa, levodopa, dopamine, epinephrine, norepinephrine, guanethidine, methylphenidate, guanadrel, reserpine,** or **vasoconstrictors.**
- Hypertension or hypotension, coma, convulsions, and death may occur with **opioids** (avoid use of **meperidine** within 14 to 21 days of MAOI therapy).
- Additive hypotension may occur with **antihypertensives, thiazide diuretics,** or **spinal anesthesia.**
- MAOIs may inhibit the hypotensive effects of **guanethidine.**
- Additive hypoglycemia may occur with **insulins** or **oral hypoglycemic agents.**
- **Doxapram** may increase pressor response.
- Serotonin syndrome may occur with concomitant use of **St. John's wort.**
- Hypertensive crisis may occur with ingestion of foods or other products containing high concentrations of **tyramine** (see Nursing Implications).
- Consumption of foods or beverages with high **caffeine** content increases the risk of hypertension and arrhythmias.
- Bradycardia may occur with concurrent use of MAOIs and **beta blockers.**
- There is a risk of toxicity from the **5-HT₁ receptor agonists** (e.g., **triptans**) with concurrent use of MAOIs.

Route and Dosage

ISOCARBOXAZID (Marplan)

> *Depression:* **PO** *(Adults):* Initial dose: 10 mg twice daily. May increase dosage by 10 mg every 2 to 4 days to 40 mg by end of first week. If needed, may continue to increase dosage by increments of up to 20 mg/week. Maximum dosage: 60 mg/day divided into 2 to 4 doses. Gradually reduce to smallest effective dose.

PHENELZINE (Nardil)

> *Depression:* **PO** *(Adults):* Initial dose: 15 mg 3 times/day. Increase to 60 to 90 mg/day in divided doses until therapeutic response is achieved. Then gradually reduce to smallest effective dose (15 mg/day or every other day).

TRANYLCYPROMINE (Parnate)

> *Depression:* **PO** *(Adults):* 30 mg/day in divided doses. After 2 weeks, may increase by 10 mg/day, at 1 to 3 week intervals, up to a maximum dose of 60 mg/day.

SELEGILINE TRANSDERMAL SYSTEM (Emsam)

> *Depression:* **Transdermal patch** *(Adults):* Initial dose: 6 mg/24 hr. If necessary, dosage may be increased in increments

of 3 mg/24 hr at intervals of no less than 2 weeks up to a maximum dose of 12 mg/24 hr.
Elderly patients: The daily recommended dosage is 6 mg/24 hr.

■ NMDA ANTAGONIST

Generic (Trade) Name	Half-life (hr)	Indications	Available Forms (mg)
Esketamine nasal spray (Spravato)	Rapid decline in initial 4 Mean terminal: 8	• Treatment-resistant depression	28

Action

Esketamine is a nonselective, noncompetitive antagonist of the N-methyl-D-aspartate (NMDA) receptor which is a glutamate receptor. Its mechanism of action in exerting antidepressant effects is unknown.

Contraindications and Precautions

Contraindicated in: • Hypersensitivity • Aneurysmal vascular disease • Arterial venous malformations • History of intracerebral hemorrhage

Use Cautiously in: • Because of the possibility of prolonged or delayed sedation and dissociation, patients should be monitored by a healthcare provider for at least 2 hours at each treatment and determined to be clinically stable before releasing the patient • Esketamine is a Schedule III controlled substance and may be subject to abuse and diversion • Esketamine is only available through certified healthcare settings where patients are enrolled in a **Risk Evaluation and Mitigation Strategy (REMS) program** • History of hypertension • History of hallucinations

Adverse Reactions and Side Effects

• Sedation
• Dissociation
• Increase in Blood Pressure
• Cognitive Impairment
• Impaired Ability to Drive and Operate Machinery
• Ulcerative or Interstitial Cystitis
• Embryo-fetal Toxicity

Interactions

• Combining with **CNS depressants** (e.g., **benzodiazepines, opioids, alcohol**) may increase sedation.
• Combining with **psychostimulants** (e.g., **amphetamines, methylphenidate, modafinil, armodafinil**) may increase blood pressure.

- Combining with **monoamine oxidase inhibitors (MAOIs)** may increase blood pressure

Route and Dosage

Adults: Initial dosage: 56 mg intranasal (one spray in each nostril); weeks 1 to 4: administer twice a week at 56 or 84 mg; weeks 5 to 8: administer once a week at 56 or 84 mg; weeks 9 and thereafter: administer once every two weeks or once a week at 56 or 84 mg. (Dosage frequency is individualized based on response and remission of symptoms.)

■ PSYCHOTHERAPEUTIC COMBINATIONS*

Examples

Generic (Trade) Name	Indications	Available Forms (mg)
Olanzapine/fluoxetine (Symbyax)	• For the acute treatment of depressive episodes associated with bipolar I disorder in adults • Treatment-resistant depression	CAPS: olanzapine 3/fluoxetine 25; olanzapine 6/fluoxetine 25; olanzapine 6/fluoxetine 50; olanzapine 12/fluoxetine 25; olanzapine 12/fluoxetine 50
Chlordiazepoxide/ amitriptyline (Limbitrol)	• For the treatment of moderate to severe depression associated with moderate to severe anxiety	TABS: chlordiazepoxide 5/amitriptyline 12.5; chlordiazepoxide 10/ amitriptyline 25
Perphenazine/ amitriptyline HCl (Etrafon)	• For the treatment of moderate to severe anxiety or agitation and depressed mood • For the treatment of patients with schizophrenia who have associated symptoms of depression	TABS: perphenazine 2/ amitriptyline 10; perphenazine 2/ amitriptyline 25; perphenazine 4/amitriptyline 10; perphenazine 4/amitriptyline 25; perphenazine 4/amitriptyline 50

* These medications are presented for general information only. For detailed information, the reader is directed to the chapters that deal with each of the specific drugs that make up these combinations.

Route and Dosage

OLANZAPINE/FLUOXETINE (Symbyax)

> ***Depression associated with bipolar I disorder and treatment-resistant depression:*** **PO** *(Adults):* Initial dosage: olanzapine 6 mg/fluoxetine 25 mg once daily in the evening. Dosage adjustments, if indicated, can be made according to efficacy and tolerability.
>
> *Elderly:* **PO:** Initial dosage: olanzapine 3 to 6 mg/fluoxetine 25 mg once daily in the evening. Dosage adjustments should be made with caution.

CHLORDIAZEPOXIDE/AMITRIPTYLINE (Limbitrol)

Moderate to severe depression associated with moderate to severe anxiety: **PO** *(Adults):* Initial dose: chlordiazepoxide 10 mg/amitriptyline 25 mg given 3 or 4 times a day in divided doses. May increase to 6 times a day, as required. Some patients respond to smaller doses and can be maintained on 2 tablets daily.

PERPHENAZINE/AMITRIPTYLINE HCL (Etrafon)

Anxiety/agitation/depression: **PO** *(Adults):* Initial dose: perphenazine 2 to 4 mg/amitriptyline 10 to 25 mg administered 3 or 4 times a day, or perphenazine 4 mg/amitriptyline 50 mg administered 2 times a day. Once a satisfactory response is achieved, reduce to smallest amount necessary to obtain relief.

■ NURSING DIAGNOSES RELATED TO ALL ANTIDEPRESSANTS

1. Risk for suicide related to depressed mood.
2. Risk for injury related to possible side effects of sedation, lowered seizure threshold, orthostatic hypotension, priapism, photosensitivity, arrhythmias, hypertensive crisis, or serotonin syndrome.
3. Social isolation related to depressed mood.
4. Risk for constipation or diarrhea related to possible side effects of the medication.
5. Insomnia related to depressed mood and elevated level of anxiety.
6. Knowledge deficit related to insufficient information.

■ NURSING IMPLICATIONS FOR ANTIDEPRESSANTS

The plan of care should include monitoring for the following side effects from antidepressant medications. Nursing implications are designated by an asterisk (*).

1. **May occur with all chemical classes:**
   a. **Dry mouth**
      * Offer the patient sugarless candy, ice, frequent sips of water.
      * Strict oral hygiene is very important.
   b. **Sedation**
      * Request an order from the physician for the drug to be given at bedtime.
      * Request that the physician decrease the dosage or perhaps order a less sedating drug.
      * Instruct the patient not to drive or use dangerous equipment when experiencing sedation.

c. **Nausea**
   * Medication may be taken with food to minimize GI distress.

d. **Discontinuation syndrome**
   * All classes of antidepressants have varying potentials to cause discontinuation syndromes. Abrupt withdrawal following long-term therapy with SSRIs and SNRIs may result in dizziness, lethargy, headache, and nausea. Fluoxetine is less likely to result in withdrawal symptoms because of its long half-life. Abrupt withdrawal from tricyclics may produce hypomania, akathisia, cardiac arrhythmias, gastrointestinal upset, and panic attacks. The discontinuation syndrome associated with MAOIs includes flulike symptoms, confusion, hypomania, and worsening of depressive symptoms. All antidepressant medication should be tapered gradually to prevent withdrawal symptoms.

2. **Most commonly occur with tricyclics and related medications and others, such as the SARIs and bupropion:**
   a. **Blurred vision**
      * Offer reassurance that this symptom should subside after a few weeks.
      * Instruct the patient not to drive until vision is clear.
      * Clear small items from routine pathway to prevent falls.
   b. **Constipation**
      * Order foods high in fiber; increase fluid intake if not contraindicated; and encourage the patient to increase physical exercise, if possible.
   c. **Urinary retention**
      * Instruct the patient to report hesitancy or inability to urinate.
      * Monitor intake and output.
      * Try various methods to stimulate urination, such as running water in the bathroom or pouring water over the perineal area.
   d. **Orthostatic hypotension**
      * Instruct the patient to rise slowly from a lying or sitting position.
      * Monitor blood pressure (lying and standing) frequently, and document and report significant changes.
      * Avoid long hot showers or tub baths.
   e. **Reduction of seizure threshold**
      * Observe patients with history of seizures closely.
      * Institute seizure precautions as specified in hospital procedure manual.
      * Bupropion (Wellbutrin) should be administered in doses of no more than 150 mg and should be given at least 4 hours apart. Bupropion has been associated with a relatively high incidence of seizure activity in anorexic and cachectic patients.

f. **Tachycardia; arrhythmias**
  * Carefully monitor blood pressure and pulse rate and rhythm, and report any significant change to the physician.
g. **Photosensitivity**
  * Ensure that the patient wears sunblock lotion, protective clothing, and sunglasses when outdoors.
h. **Weight gain**
  * Provide instructions for reduced-calorie diet.
  * Encourage increased level of activity, if appropriate.
3. **Most commonly occur with SSRIs and SNRIs:**
a. **Insomnia; agitation**
  * Administer or instruct the patient to take dose early in the day.
  * Instruct the patient to avoid caffeinated food and drinks.
  * Teach relaxation techniques to use before bedtime.
b. **Headache**
  * Administer analgesics, as prescribed.
  * If relief is not achieved, physician may order another antidepressant.
c. **Weight loss** (may occur early in therapy)
  * Ensure that the patient is provided with caloric intake sufficient to maintain desired weight.
  * Caution should be taken in prescribing these drugs for patients with *anorexia nervosa*.
  * Weigh the patient daily or every other day, at the same time and on the same scale if possible.
  * After prolonged use, some patients may gain weight on these drugs.
d. **Sexual dysfunction**
  * Men may report abnormal ejaculation or impotence.
  * Women may experience delayed or loss of orgasm.
  * If side effect becomes intolerable, a switch to another antidepressant may be necessary.
e. **Serotonin syndrome** (may occur when two drugs that potentiate serotonergic neurotransmission are used concurrently [see "Interactions"]).
  * Most frequent symptoms include changes in mental status, restlessness, myoclonus, hyperreflexia, tachycardia, labile blood pressure, diaphoresis, shivering, and tremors.
  * Discontinue offending agent immediately.
  * The physician may prescribe medications to block serotonin receptors, relieve hyperthermia and muscle rigidity, and prevent seizures. In severe cases, artificial ventilation may be required. The histamine-1 receptor antagonist cyproheptadine is commonly used to treat the symptoms of serotonin syndrome.

* Supportive nursing measures include monitoring vital signs, providing safety measures to prevent injury when muscle rigidity and changes in mental status are present, cooling blankets and tepid baths to assist with temperature regulation, and monitoring intake and output (Cooper & Sejnowski, 2013).

* The condition will usually resolve on its own once the offending medication has been discontinued. However, if left untreated, the condition may progress to life-threatening complications such as seizures, coma, hypotension, ventricular arrhythmias, disseminated intravascular coagulation, rhabdomyolysis, metabolic acidosis, and renal failure (Cooper & Sejnowski, 2013).

f. Risk for hyponatremia is increased with SSRIs, especially in the elderly. Monitor electrolytes.

4. **Most commonly occur with MAOIs:**

  a. **Hypertensive crisis**

   * Hypertensive crisis occurs if the individual consumes foods or other substances containing tyramine when receiving MAOI therapy. Foods that should be avoided include aged cheeses, raisins, fava beans, red wines, smoked and processed meats, caviar, pickled herring, soy sauce, monosodium glutamate (MSG), beer, chocolate, yogurt, and bananas. Drugs that should be avoided include other antidepressants, sympathomimetics (including over-the-counter cough and cold preparations), stimulants (including over-the-counter diet drugs), antihypertensives, meperidine and other opioid narcotics, and antiparkinsonian agents, such as levodopa.

   * Symptoms of hypertensive crisis include severe occipital headache, palpitations, nausea and vomiting, nuchal rigidity, fever, sweating, marked increase in blood pressure, chest pain, and coma.

   * Treatment of hypertensive crisis: Discontinue drug immediately; monitor vital signs; administer short-acting antihypertensive medication, as ordered by physician; use external cooling measures to control hyperpyrexia.

   * *Note:* Hypertensive crisis has not shown to be a problem with selegiline transdermal system at the 6 mg/24 hr dosage, and dietary restrictions at this dose are not recommended. Dietary modifications are recommended, however, at the 9 mg/24 hr and 12 mg/24 hr dosages.

  b. **Application site reactions** (with selegiline transdermal system [Emsam])

   * The most common reactions include rash, itching, erythema, redness, irritation, swelling, or urticarial lesions. Most reactions resolve spontaneously, requiring no treatment. However, if reaction becomes problematic, it should

be reported to the physician. Topical corticosteroids have been used in treatment.
5. **Miscellaneous side effects:**
   a. **Priapism (with trazodone)**
      * Priapism is a rare side effect, but it has occurred in some men taking trazodone.
      * If prolonged or inappropriate penile erection occurs, the medication should be withheld and the physician notified immediately.
      * Priapism can become very problematic, requiring surgical intervention, and, if not treated successfully, can result in impotence.
   b. **Hepatic failure (with nefazodone)**
      * Cases of life-threatening hepatic failure have been reported in patients treated with nefazodone.
      * Advise patients to be alert for signs or symptoms suggestive of liver dysfunction (e.g., jaundice, anorexia, GI complaints, or malaise) and to report them to the physician immediately.

■ PATIENT/FAMILY EDUCATION RELATED TO ALL ANTIDEPRESSANTS

* Continue to take the medication even though the symptoms have not subsided. Optimum effects may not be seen for as long as 4 to 6 weeks. If after this length of time no improvement is noted, the physician may prescribe a different medication.
* Use caution when driving or operating dangerous machinery. Drowsiness and dizziness can occur. If these side effects become persistent or interfere with activities of daily living, the patient should report them to the physician. Dosage adjustment may be necessary.
* Do not stop taking the drug abruptly. To do so might produce withdrawal symptoms, such as nausea, vertigo, insomnia, headache, malaise, nightmares, and return of symptoms for which the medication was prescribed.
* Use sunblock lotion and wear protective clothing when spending time outdoors. The skin may be sensitive to sunburn.
* Report occurrence of any of the following symptoms to the physician immediately: sore throat, fever, malaise, yellowish skin, unusual bleeding, easy bruising, persistent nausea and vomiting, severe headache, rapid heart rate, difficulty urinating, anorexia or weight loss, seizure activity, stiff or sore neck, and chest pain.
* Rise slowly from a sitting or lying position to prevent a sudden drop in blood pressure.
* Take frequent sips of water, chew sugarless gum, or suck on hard candy if dry mouth is a problem. Good oral care (frequent brushing, flossing) is very important.

- Do not consume the following foods or medications when taking MAOIs: aged cheese, wine (especially Chianti), beer, chocolate, colas, coffee, tea, sour cream, smoked and processed meats, chicken or beef liver, soy sauce, pickled herring, yogurt, raisins, caviar, broad beans, cold remedies, diet pills. To do so could cause a life-threatening hypertensive crisis.
- Follow the correct procedure for applying the selegiline transdermal patch:
  - Apply to dry, intact skin on upper torso, upper thigh, or outer surface of upper arm.
  - Apply approximately same time each day to new spot on skin, after removing and discarding old patch.
  - Wash hands thoroughly after applying the patch.
  - Avoid exposing application site to direct heat (e.g., heating pads, electric blankets, heat lamps, hot tub, or prolonged direct sunlight).
  - If patch falls off, apply new patch to a new site and resume previous schedule.
- Avoid smoking when receiving tricyclic therapy. Smoking increases the metabolism of tricyclics, requiring an adjustment in dosage to achieve the therapeutic effect.
- Do not drink alcohol when taking antidepressant therapy. These drugs potentiate the effects of each other.
- Avoid the use of other medications (including over-the-counter medications) without the physician's approval when receiving antidepressant therapy. Many medications contain substances that, in combination with antidepressant medication, could precipitate a life-threatening hypertensive crisis.
- Notify the physician immediately if inappropriate or prolonged penile erections occur when taking trazodone. If the erection persists longer than 4 hours, seek emergency department treatment. This condition is rare but has occurred in some men who have taken trazodone. If measures are not instituted immediately, impotence can result.
- Do not "double up" on medication if a dose of bupropion (Wellbutrin) is missed unless advised to do so by the physician. Taking bupropion in divided doses will decrease the risk of seizures and other adverse effects.
- Be aware of possible risks of taking antidepressants during pregnancy. Safe use during pregnancy and lactation has not been fully established. These drugs are believed to readily cross the placental barrier; if so, the fetus could experience adverse effects of the drug. Inform the physician immediately if pregnancy occurs, is suspected, or is planned.
- Be aware of the side effects of antidepressants. Refer to written materials furnished by health-care providers for safe self-administration.

- Carry a card or other identification at all times describing the medications being taken.
- *Specifically for esketamine:* Do not eat or drink for 2 hours prior to treatment. If taking nasal decongestants or intranasal corticosteroids they should be taken at least 1 hour prior to treatment. The patient will need someone to drive him or her home after the treatment. Report immediately any experience of dizziness; fainting; anxiety; feeling disconnected from one's body, thoughts, or emotions; shortness of breath; chest pain; uncontrollable shaking; vision changes; sudden, severe headache; seizures; or suicidal thoughts.

 INTERNET REFERENCES

- www.mentalhealth.com
- https://www.nimh.nih.gov/index.shtml
- https://www.nimh.nih.gov/health/publications/mental-health-medications/index.shtml
- https://medlineplus.gov/druginformation.html
- http://www.dbsalliance.org

CHAPTER 25

Mood-Stabilizing Agents

■ ANTIMANIC

Examples

Generic (Trade) Name	Half-life	Indications	Therapeutic Plasma Level Range	Available Forms (mg)
Lithium Carbonate (Lithobid) Lithium Citrate	20–27 hr	• Manic episodes associated with bipolar disorder • Maintenance therapy to prevent or diminish intensity of subsequent manic episodes **Unlabeled uses:** • Borderline personality disorder • Neutropenia • Cluster headaches (prophylaxis) • Alcohol dependence • Bulimia • Postpartum affective psychosis • Corticosteroid-induced psychosis	Acute mania: 1.0–1.5 mEq/L Maintenance: 0.6–1.2 mEq/L	**CAPS:** 150, 300, 600 **TABS:** 300 **TABS (ER):** 300, 450 **SYRUP:** 8 mEq lithium (as citrate equivalent to 300 mg lithium carbonate)/5 mL

Action

• Not fully understood, but lithium may have an influence on the reuptake of norepinephrine and serotonin. Effects on other neurotransmitters have also been noted. Lithium also alters sodium transport in nerve and muscle cells. The subsiding of manic symptoms with lithium may take 1 to 3 weeks.

Contraindications and Precautions

Contraindicated in: • Hypersensitivity • Severe cardiovascular or renal disease • Dehydrated or debilitated patients • Sodium depletion • Pregnancy and lactation

Use Cautiously in: • Elderly patients • Any degree of cardiac, renal, or thyroid disease • Diabetes mellitus • Urinary retention • Children under the age of 12 years (safety not established)

Adverse Reactions and Side Effects
• Drowsiness, dizziness, headache
• Seizures
• Dry mouth, thirst
• Indigestion, nausea, anorexia
• Fine hand tremors
• Hypotension, arrhythmias, ECG changes
• Polyuria, glycosuria
• Weight gain
• Hypothyroidism
• Dehydration
• Leukocytosis

Interactions
• The effects of lithium (and potential for toxicity) are increased with concurrent use of **carbamazepine, fluoxetine, haloperidol, loop diuretics, methyldopa, NSAIDs,** and **thiazide diuretics.**
• The effects of lithium are decreased with concurrent use of **acetazolamide, osmotic diuretics, theophylline,** and **urinary alkalinizers.**
• Increased effects of **neuromuscular blocking agents** and **tricyclic antidepressants** with concurrent use of lithium.
• Decreased pressor sensitivity of **sympathomimetics** with lithium.
• Neurotoxicity may occur with concurrent use of lithium and **phenothiazines** or **calcium channel blockers.**

Route and Dosage
> *Acute mania and maintenance:* **PO** *(Adults and children* ≥*12 years): Immediate-release tabs and caps:* Initial dosage: 300 to 600 mg 3 times daily. Usual maintenance dose is 300 mg 3 to 4 times daily. *Extended-release (ER) tabs:* 450 to 900 mg twice daily or 300 to 600 mg 3 times daily. Usual maintenance dose is 450 mg twice daily or 300 mg 3 times daily.
>> *Children* <*12 years:* **PO:** Initial dosage: 15 to 20 mg/kg/day in 2 to 3 divided doses. Dosage may be adjusted weekly until therapeutic level has been achieved.
>> Serum lithium levels should be taken twice weekly at the initiation of therapy and until therapeutic level has been achieved.

■ ANTICONVULSANT MOOD STABILIZERS
Examples

Generic (Trade) Name	Half-life (hr)	Indications	Therapeutic Plasma Level Range	Available Forms (mg)
Carbamazepine* (Tegretol, Epitol, Carbatrol, Equetro, Teril, Tegretol-XR)	25–65 (initial) 12–17 (repeated doses)	• Epilepsy (except *Equetro*) • Trigeminal neuralgia (except *Equetro*) • Bipolar disorder (FDA approved: *Equetro* only) **Unlabeled uses:** • Borderline personality disorder • Management of alcohol withdrawal • Restless legs syndrome • Postherpetic neuralgia	4–12 mcg/mL	**TABS:** 100, 200 **TABS XR:** 100, 200, 400 **CAPS XR:** 100, 200, 300 **ORAL SUSPENSION:** 100/5 mL
Clonazepam (C-IV) (Klonopin)	18–60	• Petit mal, akinetic, and myoclonic seizures • Panic disorder **Unlabeled uses:** • Acute manic episodes • Restless leg syndrome • Tic disorders	20–80 ng/mL	**TABS:** 0.5, 1, 2 **TABS (DISINTEGRATING ORAL):** 0.125, 0.25, 0.5, 1, 2
Valproic acid* (Depakene; Depakote; Stavzor; Depacon)	5–20	• Epilepsy • Manic episodes (FDA approved: *Stavzor* only) • Migraine prophylaxis (FDA approved: *Stavzor* only) **Unlabeled uses:** • Borderline personality disorder	50–150 mcg/mL	**CAPS:** 250 **CAPS (DR):** 125, 250, 500 **SYRUP:** 250/5 mL **TABS (DR):** 125, 250, 500 **TABS (ER):** 250, 500 **CAPS (SPRINKLE):** 125 **INJECTION:** 100/mL in 5 mL vial
Lamotrigine* (Lamictal)	~33	• Epilepsy • Bipolar disorder	Not established	**TABS:** 25, 50, 100, 150, 200, 250 **TABS (CHEWABLE, DISPERSIBLE):** 2, 5, 25

Generic (Trade) Name	Half-life (hr)	Indications	Therapeutic Plasma Level Range	Available Forms (mg)
				TABS (DISINTEGRATING ORAL): 25, 50, 100, 200 TABS (ER): 25, 50, 100, 200, 250, 300
Topiramate* (Topamax)	21	• Epilepsy • Migraine prophylaxis **Unlabeled uses:** • Bipolar disorder • Bulimia nervosa	Not established	TABS: 25, 50, 100, 200 CAPS (SPRINKLE): 15, 25
Oxcarbazepine* (Trileptal)	2 (metabolite 9 hr)	• Epilepsy **Unlabeled uses:** • Alcohol withdrawal • Bipolar disorder • Diabetic neuropathy	Not established	TABS: 150, 300, 600 ORAL SUSP: 60/mL

*The FDA has issued a warning indicating reports of suicidal behavior or ideation associated with the use of these drugs (and other antiepileptic medications). The FDA now requires that all manufacturers of drugs in this class include a warning in their labeling to this effect. Results of a study published in the December 2009 issue of *Archives of General Psychiatry* indicate that antiepileptic medications "do not increase risk of suicide attempts in patients with bipolar disorder" (Gibbons et al., 2009).

Action
• Action in the treatment of bipolar disorder is unclear.

Contraindications and Precautions
Carbamazepine

Contraindicated in: • Hypersensitivity • With monoamine oxidase inhibitors (MAOIs) • Lactation • History of previous bone marrow depression

Use Cautiously in: • Elderly • Liver/renal/cardiac disease • Pregnancy

Clonazepam

Contraindicated in: • Hypersensitivity to clonazepam or other benzodiazepines • Acute narrow-angle glaucoma • Liver disease • Pregnancy and lactation

Use Cautiously in: • Elderly • Liver/renal disease

Valproic Acid

Contraindicated in: • Hypersensitivity • Liver disease

Use Cautiously in: • Elderly • Renal/cardiac diseases • Pregnancy and lactation • Patients with bleeding disorders or bone marrow depression

Lamotrigine

Contraindicated in: • Hypersensitivity • Lactation

Use Cautiously in: • Renal/hepatic/cardiac insufficiency • Pregnancy

Topiramate

Contraindicated in: • Hypersensitivity • Lactation

Use Cautiously in: • Renal and hepatic impairment • Pregnancy • Children and the elderly

Oxcarbazepine

Contraindicated in: • Hypersensitivity (cross sensitivity with carbamazepine may occur) • Lactation

Use Cautiously in: • Renal impairment • Pregnancy • Children under the age of 4 years

Adverse Reactions and Side Effects

Carbamazepine

- Drowsiness, ataxia
- Nausea, vomiting
- Blood dyscrasias

Clonazepam

- Drowsiness, ataxia
- Dependence, tolerance
- Blood dyscrasias

Valproic Acid

- Drowsiness, dizziness
- Nausea, vomiting
- Prolonged bleeding time
- Tremor

Lamotrigine

- Ataxia, dizziness, headache
- Nausea, vomiting
- Risk of severe rash (Stevens-Johnson syndrome)
- Photosensitivity

Topiramate

- Drowsiness, dizziness, fatigue, ataxia
- Impaired concentration, nervousness
- Vision changes

- Nausea, weight loss
- Decreased efficacy with oral contraceptives

Oxcarbazepine

- Dizziness, drowsiness
- Headache
- Nausea and vomiting
- Abnormal vision, diplopia, nystagmus
- Ataxia
- Tremor

Interactions

The effects of:	Are increased by:	Are decreased by:	Concurrent use may result in:
Carbamazepine	Verapamil, diltiazem, erythromycin, clarithromycin, selective serotonin reuptake inhibitors (SSRIs), tricyclic antidepressants, cimetidine, isoniazid, danazol, lamotrigine, niacin, acetazolamide, dalfopristin, valproate, nefazodone	Cisplatin, doxorubicin, felbamate, rifampin, barbiturates, hydantoins, primidone, theophylline	Decreased levels of corticosteroids, doxycycline, felbamate, quinidine, warfarin, estrogen-containing contraceptives, cyclosporine, benzodiazepines, theophylline, lamotrigine, valproic acid, bupropion, haloperidol, olanzapine, tiagabine, topiramate, voriconazole, ziprasidone, levothyroxine, antidepressants. Increased levels of lithium; life-threatening hypertensive reaction with MAOIs.
Clonazepam	Central nervous system (CNS) depressants, cimetidine, hormonal contraceptives, disulfiram, fluoxetine, isoniazid, ketoconazole, metoprolol, propranolol, valproic acid, or probenecid	Rifampin, theophylline (↓ sedative effects), phenytoin	Increased phenytoin levels. Decreased efficacy of levodopa.
Valproic acid	Chlorpromazine, cimetidine, erythromycin, felbamate, salicylates	Rifampin, carbamazepine, cholestyramine, lamotrigine, phenobarbital, ethosuximide, hydantoins	Increased effects of tricyclic antidepressants, carbamazepine, CNS depressants, ethosuximide, lamotrigine, phenobarbital, warfarin, zidovudine, hydantoins.

(Continued)

The effects of:	Are increased by:	Are decreased by:	Concurrent use may result in:
Lamotrigine	Valproic acid	Primidone, phenobarbital, phenytoin, rifamycin, succinimides, oral contraceptives, oxcarbazepine, carbamazepine, acetaminophen	Decreased levels of valproic acid. Increased levels of carbamazepine and topiramate.
Topiramate	Metformin; hydrochlorothiazide	Phenytoin, carbamazepine, valproic acid, lamotrigine	Increased risk of CNS depression with alcohol or other CNS depressants. Increased risk of kidney stones with carbonic anhydrase inhibitors. Increased effects of phenytoin, metformin, amitriptyline; decreased effects of oral contraceptives, digoxin, lithium, risperidone, and valproic acid.
Oxcarbazepine		Carbamazepine, phenobarbital, phenytoin, valproic acid, verapamil	Increased concentrations of phenobarbital and phenytoin. Decreased effects of oral contraceptives, felodipine, and lamotrigine.

Route and Dosage

CARBAMAZEPINE (Tegretol)

> *Seizure disorders:* **PO** *(Adults and children >12 years):* 200 mg 2 times a day (tablets) or 100 mg 4 times a day (suspension). Increase by 200 mg/day every 7 days until therapeutic levels are achieved (range is 600 to 1200 mg/day in divided doses every 6 to 8 hours). Extended-release products are given twice daily. Maximum dose: 1000 mg/day in children 12 to 15 yr; 1200 mg/day in patients >15 yr.
>
> > *Children 6 to 12 yr:* **PO:** 100 mg 2 times a day (tablets) or 50 mg 4 times/day (suspension). Increase by 100 mg weekly until therapeutic levels are obtained. (Usual range: 400 to 800 mg/day). Maximum daily dose: 1000 mg. Extended-release products are given twice daily.
> >
> > *Children <6 yr:* **PO:** 10 to 20 mg/kg/day in 2 to 3 divided doses. May increase weekly until optimal response and therapeutic levels are achieved. Usual maintenance dose is 250 to 350 mg/day. Maximum daily dose: 35 mg/kg/day.

Trigeminal neuralgia: **PO** *(Adults):* Initial dose 100 mg 2 times a day (tablets) or 50 mg 4 times a day (suspension). May increase by up to 200 mg/day until pain is relieved, then maintenance dose of 200 to 1200 mg/day in divided doses (usual range, 400 to 800 mg/day).

Bipolar disorder, mania: (Equetro only) **PO** *(Adults):* Initial dose: 200 mg 2 times a day. Dosage may be adjusted in 200 mg daily increments to achieve optimal clinical response. Doses higher than 1600 mg/day have not been studied.

Borderline personality disorder: **PO** *(Adults):* 400 mg/day in 2 divided doses. May increase dose in increments of 200 mg/day depending on response, tolerability, and plasma concentrations. Maximum dosage: 1600 mg/day.

Management of alcohol withdrawal: **PO** *(Adults):* Dosage on day 1: 600 to 1200 mg. Dosage is then tapered over 5 to 10 days to 0 mg.

Restless leg syndrome: **PO** *(Adults):* 100 to 600 mg daily for up to 5 weeks.

Postherpetic neuralgia: **PO** *(Adults):* 100 to 200 mg/day, slowly increased to a maximum of 1200 mg/day.

CLONAZEPAM (Klonopin)

Seizures: **PO** *(Adults and children >10 years or more than 30 kg):* 0.5 mg 3 times a day; may increase by 0.5 to 1 mg every 3 days until seizures are adequately controlled. Maximum daily dose: 20 mg.

> *Children <10 years or 30 kg:* **PO:** Initial daily dose 0.01 to 0.03 mg/kg/day (not to exceed 0.05 mg/kg/day) given in 2 or 3 divided doses; increase by no more than 0.25 to 0.5 mg every third day until a daily maintenance dose of 0.1 to 0.2 mg/kg (in 3 divided doses) has been reached, unless seizures are controlled or side effects preclude further increase.

Panic disorder: **PO** *(Adults):* Initial dose: 0.25 mg 2 times a day. May increase in increments of 0.125 to 0.25 mg twice daily every 3 days until symptoms are controlled or until side effects preclude further increase. Usual dose: 1 mg/day. Maximum dose: 4 mg/day.

Bipolar disorder, mania: **PO** *(Adults):* 2 to 16 mg/day.

Restless leg syndrome: **PO** *(Adults):* 0.5 to 2 mg administered 30 minutes before bedtime.

Tic disorders: **PO** *(Adults and children):* 0.5 to 12 mg (after dose titration).

VALPROIC ACID (Depakene; Depakote)

Epilepsy: **PO:** *(Adults and children ≥10 years):* Initial dose: 5 to 15 mg/kg/day. Increase by 5 to 10 mg/kg/week until therapeutic levels are reached. Maximum recommended dosage:

60 mg/kg/day. When daily dosage exceeds 250 mg, give in 2 divided doses.

Manic episodes: **PO** *(Adults):* Initial dose: 750 mg in divided doses. Titrate rapidly to achieve the lowest therapeutic dose that produces the desired response or trough plasma levels of 50 to 125 mcg/mL. Maximum recommended dose: 60/mg/kg/day.

Migraine prophylaxis: **PO** *(Adults and children ≥16 years):* 250 mg twice daily. Some patients may require up to 1000 mg/day.

Borderline personality disorder: **PO** *(Adults):* 750 mg/day in divided doses. Titrate to maintain a therapeutic plasma level of 50 to 100 mcg/mL.

LAMOTRIGINE (Lamictal)

Epilepsy: **PO** *(Adults and children >12 years):*

For patients not taking carbamazepine, valproate, phenobarbital, phenytoin, or primidone: Weeks 1 and 2: 25 mg/day; weeks 3 and 4: 50 mg/day; week 5 onward to maintenance: Increase by 50 mg/day every 1 to 2 weeks; usual maintenance dosage: 225 to 375 mg/day in 2 divided doses.

For patients taking valproate: Weeks 1 and 2: 25 mg every other day; weeks 3 and 4: 25 mg/day; week 5 onward to maintenance: increase by 25 to 50 mg/day every 1 to 2 weeks; usual maintenance dosage: 100 to 400 mg/day in 1 or 2 divided doses (maintenance dose of 100 to 200 mg/day if receiving valproate alone).

For patients taking carbamazepine, phenobarbital, phenytoin, or primidone, but not valproate: Weeks 1 and 2: 50 mg/day; weeks 3 and 4: 100 mg/day in 2 divided doses; week 5 onward to maintenance: increase by 100 mg/day every 1 to 2 weeks; usual maintenance dosage: 300 to 500 mg/day in 2 divided doses.

Children 2 to 12 years: Refer to manufacturer's dosing recommendations.

Bipolar disorder (escalation regimen):

For patients not taking carbamazepine, valproate, phenobarbital, phenytoin, or primidone: **PO** *(Adults):* Weeks 1 and 2: 25 mg/day; weeks 3 and 4: 50 mg/day; week 5: 100 mg/day; then 200 mg/day.

For patients taking valproate: **PO** *(Adults):* Weeks 1 and 2: 25 mg every other day; weeks 3 and 4: 25 mg/day; week 5: 50 mg/day; then 100 mg/day.

For patients taking carbamazepine, phenobarbital, phenytoin, or primidone, but not valproate: **PO** *(Adults):* Weeks 1 and 2: 50 mg/day; weeks 3 and 4: 100 mg/day in divided doses; week 5: 200 mg/day in divided doses; week 6: 300 mg/day in divided doses; then up to 400 mg/day in divided doses.

TOPIRAMATE (Topamax)

Epilepsy (monotherapy): Adults and children ≥10 years: **PO:** 25 mg twice daily initially, gradually increasing at weekly intervals to 200 mg twice daily over a 6-week period.

> *Children 2 to <10 years and ≤11 kg:* **PO:** 25 mg daily in the evening initially, gradually increasing at weekly intervals to 75 mg twice daily over a 5 to 7 week period; if needed, may continue to titrate dose on a weekly basis up to 150 mg twice daily.

> *Children 2 to <10 years and 12 to 22 kg:* **PO:** 25 mg daily in the evening initially, gradually increasing at weekly intervals to 100 mg twice daily over a 5 to 7 week period; if needed may continue to titrate dose on a weekly basis up to 150 mg twice daily.

> *Children 2 to <10 years and 23 to 31 kg:* **PO:** 25 mg daily in the evening initially, gradually increasing at weekly intervals to 100 mg twice daily over a 5 to 7 week period; if needed may continue to titrate dose on a weekly basis up to 175 mg twice daily.

> *Children 2 to <10 years and 32 to 38 kg:* **PO:** 25 mg daily in the evening initially, gradually increasing at weekly intervals to 125 mg twice daily over a 5 to 7 week period; if needed may continue to titrate dose on a weekly basis up to 175 mg twice daily.

> *Children 2 to <10 and >38 kg:* **PO:** 25 mg daily in the evening initially, gradually increasing at weekly intervals to 125 mg twice daily over a 5 to 7 week period; if needed may continue to titrate dose on a weekly basis up to 200 mg twice daily.

Epilepsy (adjunctive therapy): **PO** *(Adults and children ≥17 years):* 25 to 50 mg/day increasing by 25 to 50 mg/day at weekly intervals up to 200 to 400 mg/day in 2 divided doses (200 to 400 mg day in 2 divided doses for partial seizures and 400 mg/day in 2 divided doses for primary generalized tonic-clonic seizures). Maximum dose: 1600 mg/day.

Bipolar disorder: **PO** *(Adults):* Initial dose: 25 to 50 mg/day. Increase to target range of 100 to 200 mg/day in divided doses. Maximum dosage: 400 mg/day.

Bulimia nervosa: **PO** *(Adults):* 25 mg/day for the first week, then titrated by 25 to 50 mg/week to the minimal effective dosage or a maximum dosage of 400 mg/day.

OXCARBAZEPINE (Trileptal)

Epilepsy: **PO** *(Adults): Adjunctive therapy:* 300 mg twice daily, may be increased by up to 600 mg/day at weekly intervals up to 1200 mg/day (up to 2400 mg/day may be needed).

> *Conversion to monotherapy:* 300 mg twice daily; may be increased by 600 mg/day at weekly intervals, whereas

other antiepileptic drugs are tapered over 3 to 6 weeks; dose of oxcarbazepine should be increased up to 2400 mg/day over a period of 2 to 4 weeks.

Initiation of monotherapy: 300 mg twice daily, increase by 300 mg/day every third day, up to 1200 mg/day. Maximum maintenance dose should be achieved over 2 to 4 weeks.

Children 2 to 16 years: **PO:** *Adjunctive therapy:* 4 to 5 mg/kg twice daily (up to 600 mg/day), increased over 2 weeks to achieve 900 mg/day in patients 20 to 29 kg, 1200 mg/day in patients 29.1 to 39 kg, and 1800 mg/day in patients >39 kg (range 6 to 51 mg/kg/day). In patients <20 kg, initial dose of 16 to 20 mg/kg/day may be used, not to exceed 60 mg/kg/day.

Conversion to monotherapy: 8 to 10 mg/kg/day given twice daily; may be increased by 10 mg/kg/day at weekly intervals, whereas other antiepileptic drugs are tapered over 3 to 6 weeks; dose of oxcarbazepine should be increased up to 600 to 900 mg/day in patients ≤20 kg, 900 to 1200 mg/day in patients 25 to 30 kg, 900 to 1500 mg/day in patients 35 to 40 kg, 1200 to 1500 mg/day in patients 45 kg, 1200 to 1800 mg/day in patients 50 to 55 kg, 1200 to 2100 mg/day in patients 60 to 65 kg, and 1500 to 2100 mg/day in patients 70 kg. Maximum maintenance dose should be achieved over 2 to 4 weeks.

Alcohol withdrawal: **PO** *(Adults):* 600 to 1800 mg in divided doses for 6 weeks to 6 months.

Bipolar disorder: **PO** *(Adults):* Initial dose: 300 mg/day. Titrate to a maximum dose of 900 to 2400 mg/day.

Diabetic neuropathy: **PO** *(Adults):* Initial dose: 150 to 300 mg/day. Titrate to recommended dose of 900 to 1200 mg/day. Maximum dose: 1800 mg/day.

■ ANTIPSYCHOTICS
Examples

Generic (Trade) Name	Half-life (hr)	Indications	Available Forms (mg)
Olanzapine (Zyprexa)	21–54	• Schizophrenia • Bipolar disorder • Agitation associated with schizophrenia and mania (IM)	**TABS:** 2.5, 5, 7.5, 10, 15, 20 **TABS (ORALLY DISINTEGRATING):** 5, 10, 15, 20 **POWDER FOR INJECTION (IM):** 10 mg/vial **POWDER FOR SUSPENSION, ER (PER VIAL):** 210, 300, 405
Olanzapine and fluoxetine (Symbyax)*		Symbyax: • For the treatment of depressive episodes associated with bipolar disorder	Symbyax: **CAPS:** 3 olanzapine/25 fluoxetine, 6 olanzapine/25 fluoxetine

Generic (Trade) Name	Half-life (hr)	Indications	Available Forms (mg)
		• Treatment-resistant depression	6 olanzapine/50 fluoxetine, 12 olanzapine/25 fluoxetine, 12 olanzapine/50 fluoxetine
Aripiprazole (Abilify)	75–94 (including metabolite)	• Bipolar mania • Schizophrenia • Irritability associated with autistic disorder • Major depressive disorder (adjunctive treatment)	**TABS:** 2, 5, 10, 15, 20, 30 **TABS (ORALLY DISINTEGRATING):** 10, 15 **ORAL SOLUTION:** 1/mL **INJECTION:** 7.5/mL
Quetiapine (Seroquel)	6	• Schizophrenia • Acute manic episodes • Major depression (adjunctive therapy) • Obsessive-compulsive disorder (OCD)	**TABS:** 25, 50, 100, 200, 300, 400 **TABS (XR):** 50, 150, 200, 300, 400
Risperidone (Risperdal)	3–20 (including metabolite)	• Bipolar mania • Schizophrenia • Irritability associated with autistic disorder **Unlabeled uses:** • OCD	**TABS:** 0.25, 0.5, 1, 2, 3, 4 **TABS (ORALLY DISINTEGRATING):** 0.5, 1, 2, 3, 4 **ORAL SOLUTION:** 1/mL **POWDER FOR INJECTION:** 12.5/vial, 25/vial, 37.5/vial, 50/vial
Ziprasidone (Geodon)	7 (oral); 2–5 (IM)	• Bipolar mania • Schizophrenia • Acute agitation in schizophrenia (IM)	**CAPS:** 20, 40, 60, 80 **POWDER FOR INJECTION:** 20/vial
Asenapine (Saphris)	24	• Schizophrenia • Bipolar disorder	**TABS (SUBLINGUAL):** 5, 10
Cariprazine (Vraylar)	2–4 days; didesmethyl-cariprazine *(DDCAR)*— 1–3 weeks	• Schizophrenia • Acute treatment of mania/mixed episodes in bipolar I disorder	**CAPSULES:** 1.5, 3, 4.5, 6

*For information related to action, contraindications/precautions, adverse reactions and side effects, and interactions, refer to the monographs for olanzapine (Chapters 25 and 26) and fluoxetine (Chapter 24).

Action

- Efficacy in schizophrenia is achieved through a combination of dopamine and serotonin type 2 ($5HT_2$) antagonism.
- Mechanism of action in the treatment of acute manic episodes is unknown.

- Cariprazine: Acts as a partial agonist at dopamine D_3/D_2 receptors in the CNS with preferential binding to dopamine D_3, and partial agonist at serotonin 5-HT_{1A}; also acts as an antagonist at 5-HT_{2A} receptors.

Contraindications and Precautions

Olanzapine

Contraindicated in: • Hypersensitivity • Lactation • *Orally disintegrating tablets only:* Phenylketonuria (orally disintegrating tablets contain aspartame)

Use Cautiously in: • Hepatic insufficiency • Elderly patients (reduce dosage) • Pregnancy and children (safety not established) • Cardiovascular or cerebrovascular disease • History of glaucoma • History of seizures • History of attempted suicide • Prostatic hypertrophy • Diabetes or risk factors for diabetes • Narrow-angle glaucoma • History of paralytic ileus • Patients with preexisting low white blood cell count and/or history of drug-induced leukopenia/neutropenia • Elderly patients with psychosis related to neurocognitive disorder (NCD) (black-box warning).

Aripiprazole

Contraindicated in: • Hypersensitivity • Lactation

Use Cautiously in: • Cardiovascular or cerebrovascular disease • Conditions that cause hypotension (dehydration, treatment with antihypertensives or diuretics) • Elderly patients • Pregnancy, children, and adolescents (safety not established) • Patients with diabetes or seizure disorders • Elderly patients with NCD-related psychosis (black-box warning)

Quetiapine

Contraindicated in: • Hypersensitivity • Lactation • Concurrent use with drugs that prolong the QT interval • Patients with history of arrhythmias, including bradycardia

Use Cautiously in: • Cardiovascular or cerebrovascular disease • Dehydration or hypovolemia (increased risk of hypotension) • Elderly patients • Hepatic impairment • Hypothyroidism • History of suicide attempt • Patients with diabetes or a history of seizures • Pregnancy or children (safety not established) • Elderly patients with NCD-related psychosis (black-box warning)

Risperidone

Contraindicated in: • Hypersensitivity • Lactation

Use Cautiously in: • Elderly or debilitated patients • Renal or hepatic impairment • Cardiovascular disease • History of seizures • History of suicide attempt or drug abuse • Diabetes or risk factors for diabetes • Pregnancy or children (safety not established) • Elderly patients with NCD-related psychosis (black-box warning)

Ziprasidone

Contraindicated in: • Hypersensitivity • History of QT prolongation, arrhythmias, recent myocardial infarction, or uncompensated heart failure • Concurrent use of other drugs known to prolong QT interval • Hypokalemia or hypomagnesemia • Lactation

Use Cautiously in: • Concurrent diuretic therapy or diarrhea (may increase the risk of hypotension, hypokalemia, or hypomagnesemia) • Hepatic impairment • Cardiovascular or cerebrovascular disease • Hypotension, concurrent antihypertensive therapy, dehydration, or hypovolemia (may increase risk of orthostatic hypotension) • Elderly patients • Patients at risk for aspiration pneumonia • History of suicide attempt • Pregnancy and children (safety not established) • Patients with preexisting low white blood cell count and/or history of drug-induced leukopenia/neutropenia • Elderly patients with NCD-related psychosis (black-box warning)

Asenapine

Contraindicated in: • Hypersensitivity • Lactation • History of QT prolongation or arrhythmias • Concurrent use of other drugs known to prolong QT interval

Use Cautiously in: • Patients with hepatic, renal, or cardiovascular insufficiency • Diabetes or risk factors for diabetes • History of seizures • History of suicide attempt • Patients at risk for aspiration pneumonia • Elderly patients • Pregnancy and children (safety not established) • Elderly patients with NCD-related psychosis (black-box warning)

Cariprazine

Contraindicated in: • Hypersensitivity • Concurrent use of strong CYP3A4 inhibitors • Concurrent use of strong CYP3A4 inducers

Use Cautiously in: • Known cerebrovascular/cardiovascular disease, dehydration, concurrent use of diuretics/antihypertensives or syncope (↑ risk of orthostatic hypotension) • Preexisting ↓ WBC or ANC or history of drug-induced leukopenia/neutropenia • Elderly patients with dementia-related psychosis (↑ risk of adverse cardiovascular effects and death)—consider age-related ↓ in renal/hepatic/cardiovascular function, concurrent disease states and medications (↓ initial dose recommended) • Patients at risk of aspiration • Neonates exposed in the third trimester may experience extrapyramidal symptoms/withdrawal • Lactation—consider maternal and fetal benefits against possible adverse effects in infant.

Adverse Reactions and Side Effects
Olanzapine

- Drowsiness, dizziness, weakness
- Dry mouth, constipation, increased appetite

- Nausea
- Weight gain or loss
- Orthostatic hypotension, tachycardia
- Restlessness
- Rhinitis
- Tremor
- Headache

Aripiprazole

- Drowsiness, light-headedness
- Headache
- Insomnia, restlessness
- Constipation
- Nausea
- Weight loss

Quetiapine

- Drowsiness, dizziness
- Hypotension, tachycardia
- Headache
- Constipation
- Dry mouth
- Nausea
- Weight gain

Risperidone

- Agitation, anxiety
- Drowsiness, dizziness
- Extrapyramidal symptoms
- Headache
- Insomnia
- Constipation
- Nausea/vomiting
- Weight gain
- Rhinitis
- Sexual dysfunction
- Diarrhea
- Dry mouth

Ziprasidone

- Drowsiness, dizziness
- Restlessness
- Headache
- Constipation
- Diarrhea
- Dry mouth
- Nausea

- Weight gain
- Prolonged QT interval
- Sexual dysfunction

Asenapine

- Constipation
- Dry mouth
- Nausea and vomiting
- Weight gain
- Restlessness
- QTc interval prolongation
- Tachycardia
- Extrapyramidal symptoms
- Drowsiness, dizziness
- Insomnia
- Headache

Cariprazine

- Drowsiness
- Extreme tiredness
- Restlessness
- Anxiety
- Agitation
- Difficulty falling asleep or staying asleep
- Dizziness
- Weight gain
- Constipation
- Indigestion
- Increased saliva or drooling
- Blurred vision

Interactions

The effects of:	Are increased by:	Are decreased by:	Concurrent use may result in:
Olanzapine	Fluvoxamine and other CYP1A2 inhibitors, fluoxetine	Carbamazepine and other CYP1A2 inducers, omeprazole, rifampin	Decreased effects of levodopa and dopamine agonists. Increased hypotension with antihypertensives. Increased CNS depression with alcohol or other CNS depressants.
Aripiprazole	Ketoconazole and other CYP3A4 inhibitors; quinidine, fluoxetine, paroxetine, or other potential CYP2D6 inhibitors	Carbamazepine, famotidine, valproate	Increased CNS depression with alcohol or other CNS depressants. Increased hypotension with antihypertensives.

(Continued)

The effects of:	Are increased by:	Are decreased by:	Concurrent use may result in:
Quetiapine	Cimetidine; ketoconazole, itraconazole, fluconazole, erythromycin, or other CYP3A4 inhibitors	Phenytoin; thioridazine	Decreased effects of levodopa and dopamine agonists. Increased CNS depression with alcohol or other CNS depressants. Increased hypotension with antihypertensives.
Risperidone	Clozapine, fluoxetine, paroxetine, or ritonavir	Carbamazepine	Decreased effects of levodopa and dopamine agonists. Increased effects of clozapine and valproate. Increased CNS depression with alcohol or other CNS depressants. Increased hypotension with antihypertensives.
Ziprasidone	Ketoconazole and other CYP3A4 inhibitors	Carbamazepine	Life-threatening prolongation of QT interval with quinidine, dofetilide, other class Ia and III antiarrhythmics, pimozide, sotalol, thioridazine, chlorpromazine, pentamidine, arsenic trioxide, mefloquine, dolasetron, tacrolimus, droperidol, gatifloxacin, or moxifloxacin. Decreased effects of levodopa and dopamine agonists. Increased CNS depression with alcohol or other CNS depressants. Increased hypotension with antihypertensives.
Asenapine	Fluvoxamine; imipramine; valproate	Carbamazepine; cimetidine; paroxetine	Increased effects of paroxetine and dextromethorphan. Increased CNS depression with alcohol or other CNS depressants. Increased hypotension with antihypertensives; additive effect of QT interval prolongation with quinidine, dofetilide, other class Ia and III antiarrhythmics, pimozide, sotalol, thioridazine, chlorpromazine, pentamidine, arsenic trioxide, mefloquine, dolasetron, tacrolimus, droperidol, gatifloxacin, or moxifloxacin.

The effects of:	Are increased by:	Are decreased by:	Concurrent use may result in:
Cariprazine			Blood levels, effects and risk of toxicity ↑ by concurrent use of **strong CYP3A4 inhibitors,** including **itraconazole** and **ketoconazole;** concurrent use not recommended. Blood levels and effectiveness may be ↓ by concurrent use of **strong CYP3A4 inducers,** including **carbamazepine** and **rifampin;** concurrent use not recommended. Concurrent use of **diuretics/ antihypertensives** (↑ risk of orthostatic hypotension/ syncope).

Route and Dosage

OLANZAPINE (Zyprexa)

> *Bipolar disorder:* **PO** *(Adults):* 10 to 15 mg once daily initially; may increase every 24 hours by 5 mg/day (not to exceed 20 mg/day).
>> *Children ≥13 years:* **PO:** Initial dosage: 2.5 or 5 mg once daily. May increase in increments of 2.5 or 5 mg. Recommended maintenance dosage: 10 mg/day.
> *Schizophrenia:* **PO** *(Adults):* 5 to 10 mg/day initially; may increase at weekly intervals by 5 mg/day (not to exceed 20 mg/day).
>> *Children ≥13 years:* **PO:** Initial dosage: 2.5 or 5 mg once daily. May increase in increments of 2.5 or 5 mg. Recommended maintenance dosage 10 mg/day.
> *Agitation associated with schizophrenia or mania:* **IM** *(Adults):* 10 mg, administered slowly, deep into muscle mass. May repeat in 2 to 4 hours, as needed. Maximum dose: 30 mg/day IM. (Dosage for elderly or debilitated patients: 2.5 to 5 mg.)

OLANZAPINE AND FLUOXETINE (Symbyax)

> *Depressive episodes associated with bipolar disorder:* **PO** *(Adults):* Initial dosage: 6/25 given once daily in the evening. Adjust dosage according to efficacy and tolerability to within a range of 6 to 12 olanzapine/25 to 50 fluoxetine.

ARIPIPRAZOLE (Abilify)

> *Bipolar mania:* **PO** *(Adults):* Usual starting dose: 15 mg once daily as monotherapy, or 10 to 15 mg as adjunctive therapy with lithium or valproate given once daily. Dosage may be increased to 30 mg/day based on clinical response.

The safety of dosages higher than 30 mg have not been evaluated.

> *Children 10 to 17 years:* **PO:** Initial dosage: 2 mg/day. Titrate to 5 mg/day after 2 days and to the target dosage of 10 mg/day after 2 additional days. Subsequent dosage increases should be administered in 5 mg/day increments. Usual dosage: 10 mg/day as monotherapy, or as adjunctive therapy with lithium or valproate.

Major depressive disorder (adjunctive treatment): **PO** *(Adults):* Initial dosage: 2 to 5 mg/day for patients already taking another antidepressant. May increase dosage by up to 5 mg/day at intervals of at least a week. Maintenance dosage range: 2 to 15 mg/day.

Schizophrenia: **PO** *(Adults):* Initial dosage: 10 or 15 mg/day as a single dose. Doses up to 30 mg have been used. Dosage increases should not be made before 2 weeks, the time required to achieve steady state.

> *Children 13 to 17 years:* **PO:** Initial dosage: 2 mg/day. Titrate to 5 mg after 2 days and to the target dose of 10 mg after 2 additional days. Subsequent dose increases should be administered in 5 mg increments. Maintenance dosage: 10 to 30 mg/day.

Irritability associated with autistic disorder: **PO** *(Children 6 to 17 years):* Initial dosage: 2 mg/day. The dosage should be increased to 5 mg/day, with subsequent increases to 10 or 15 mg/day if needed. Dosage adjustments of up to 5 mg/day should occur gradually, at intervals of no less than 1 week. Usual dosage: 5 to 15 mg/day.

CARIPRAZINE

Schizophrenia: **PO** *(Adults):* 1.5 mg/day initially; may be increased on second day to 3 mg; further increments of 1.5 mg or 3 mg may be made depending on response/tolerance up to maintenance dose of 1.5 to 6 mg/day.

Bipolar mania: **PO** *(Adults):* 1.5 mg/day initially; may be increased on second day to 3 mg; further increments of 1.5 mg or 3 mg may be made depending on response/tolerance up to maintenance dose of 1.5 to 6 mg/day titrated up to 3 to 6 mg/day. *Concurrent use of strong CYP3A4 inhibitors*—decrease dose by 50%.

QUETIAPINE (Seroquel)

Schizophrenia: **PO** *(Adults): Immediate-release:* 25 mg twice daily initially, increased by 25 to 50 mg 2 to 3 times daily over 3 days, up to 300 to 400 mg/day in 2 to 3 divided doses by the fourth day (not to exceed 800 mg/day). *Extended-release:* 300 mg once daily. Increase by 300 mg/day (not to exceed 800 mg/day).

Children 13 to 17 years: **PO:** *Immediate-release:* 25 mg twice daily on Day 1; increase to 50 mg twice daily on Day 2; then increase to 100 mg twice daily on Day 3; then increase to 150 mg twice daily on Day 4; then increase to 200 mg twice daily on Day 5. May then increase by no more than 100 mg/day (not to exceed 800 mg/day).

Bipolar mania: PO *(Adults): Immediate-release:* 50 mg twice daily on Day 1; then increase to 100 mg twice daily on Day 2; then increase to 150 mg twice daily on Day 3; then increase to 200 mg twice daily on Day 4. May then increase by no more than 200 mg/day up to 400 mg twice daily on Day 6, if needed. *Extended-release:* 300 mg once daily on Day 1; then 600 mg once daily on Day 2; then 400 to 800 mg once daily starting on Day 3.

Children 10 to 17 years: **PO:** *Immediate release:* 25 mg twice daily on Day 1; then increase to 50 mg twice daily on Day 2; then increase to 100 mg twice daily on Day 3; then increase to 150 mg twice daily on Day 4; then increase to 200 mg twice daily on Day 5. May then increase by no more than 100 mg/day (not to exceed 600 mg/day).

Major depression (adjunctive therapy): PO *(Adults): Extended-release:* Initial dosage: 50 mg once daily in the evening. On Day 3, the dose may be increased to 150 mg once daily in the evening. Usual dosage: 150 to 300 mg/day.

Obsessive-compulsive disorder: PO *(Adults):* Initial dosage: 50 mg/day and increased based on therapeutic effect and tolerance. Dosage range: 25 to 400 mg/day.

RISPERIDONE (Risperdal)

Bipolar mania: PO *(Adults):* 2 to 3 mg/day as a single daily dose; dose may be increased at 24-hour intervals by 1 mg (range 1 to 6 mg/day). **IM** *(Adults):* 25 mg every 2 weeks; some patients may require larger dose of 37.5 or 50 mg every 2 weeks.

Children 10 to 17 years: **PO:** Initial dosage: 0.5 mg once daily in either morning or evening. May be increased at intervals of at least 24 hours in increments of 0.5 or 1 mg/day, to a recommended dosage of 2.5 mg/day.

Schizophrenia: PO *(Adults):* Initial dosage: 2 mg/day administered as a single dose or in two divided doses. May increase dose at 24-hour intervals in increments of 1 to 2 mg/day to a recommended dose of 4 to 8 mg/day. **IM** *(Adults):* 25 mg every 2 weeks; some patients may require larger dose of 37.5 or 50 mg every 2 weeks.

Adolescents (13 to 17 years): **PO:** Initial dosage: 0.5 mg once daily, increased by 0.5 to 1.0 mg no more frequently than every 24 hours to 3 mg daily. May administer half the daily dose twice daily if drowsiness persists.

Irritability associated with autistic disorder: **PO** *(Children and adolescents 5 to 16 years weighing <20 kg):* 0.25 mg/day initially. After at least 4 days of therapy, may increase to 0.5 mg/day. Dose increases in increments of 0.25 mg/day may be considered at 2-week or longer intervals. May be given as a single dose or in divided doses.

Children and adolescents 5 to 16 years weighing ≥20 kg: **PO:** 0.5 mg/day initially. After at least 4 days of therapy, may increase to 1.0 mg/day. Dose increases in increments of 0.5 mg/day may be considered at 2-week or longer intervals. May be given as a single dose or in divided doses.

Obsessive-compulsive disorder: **PO** *(Adults):* Initial dosage: 0.5 or 1 mg/day. May be increased by 0.5 or 1 mg weekly based on therapeutic effect and tolerance. Dosage range: 0.5 to 4 mg/day.

ZIPRASIDONE (Geodon)

Bipolar mania: **PO** *(Adults):* Initial dosage: 40 mg twice daily. Increase dose to 60 or 80 mg twice/day on the second day of treatment. Adjust dose on the basis of toleration and efficacy within the range of 40 to 80 mg twice/day.

Schizophrenia: **PO** *(Adults):* Initial dose: 20 mg twice daily. Dose increments may be made at 2-day intervals up to 80 mg twice daily.

Acute agitation in schizophrenia: **IM** *(Adults):* 10 to 20 mg as needed up to 40 mg/day. May be given as 10 mg every 2 hours or 20 mg every 4 hours. Maximum dosage: 40 mg/day.

ASENAPINE (Saphris)

Schizophrenia: **PO** *(Adults):* Usual dosage: 5 mg twice daily. May increase up to 10 mg twice daily after 1 week based on tolerability.

Bipolar disorder: **PO** *(Adults):* Usual dose: 10 mg twice daily. Decrease to 5 mg twice daily if there are adverse effects or based on individual tolerability. *As adjunctive therapy with lithium or valproate:* Initial dosage: 5 mg twice daily. Increase to 10 mg twice daily depending on the clinical response and tolerability.

■ NURSING DIAGNOSES RELATED TO ALL MOOD-STABILIZING AGENTS

1. Risk for injury related to manic hyperactivity.
2. Risk for self-directed or other-directed violence related to unresolved anger turned inward on the self or outward on the environment.
3. Risk for injury related to lithium toxicity.
4. Risk for injury related to adverse effects of mood-stabilizing drugs.
5. Risk for activity intolerance related to side effects of drowsiness and dizziness.

■ NURSING IMPLICATIONS FOR MOOD-STABILIZING AGENTS

The plan of care should include monitoring for the following side effects from mood-stabilizing drugs. Nursing implications are designated by an asterisk (*).

1. **May occur with lithium:**
   a. **Drowsiness, dizziness, headache**
      * Ensure that the patient does not participate in activities that require alertness or operate dangerous machinery.
   b. **Dry mouth; thirst**
      * Provide sugarless candy, ice, frequent sips of water. Ensure that strict oral hygiene is maintained.
   c. **GI upset; nausea/vomiting**
      * Administer medications with meals to minimize GI upset.
   d. **Fine hand tremors**
      * Report to physician, who may decrease dosage. Some physicians prescribe a small dose of beta-blocker propranolol to counteract this effect.
   e. **Hypotension; arrhythmias; pulse irregularities**
      * Monitor vital signs two or three times a day. Physician may decrease dose of medication.
   f. **Polyuria; dehydration**
      * May subside after initial week or two. Monitor daily intake and output and weight. Monitor skin turgor daily.
   g. **Weight gain**
      * Provide instructions for reduced calorie diet. Emphasize importance of maintaining adequate intake of sodium.

2. **May occur with anticonvulsants:**
   a. **Nausea/vomiting**
      * May give with food or milk to minimize GI upset.
   b. **Drowsiness; dizziness**
      * Ensure that the patient does not operate dangerous machinery or participate in activities that require alertness.
   c. **Blood dyscrasias**
      * Ensure that the patient understands the importance of regular blood tests while receiving anticonvulsant therapy.
   d. **Prolonged bleeding time (with valproic acid)**
      * Ensure that platelet counts and bleeding time are determined before initiation of therapy with valproic acid. Monitor for spontaneous bleeding or bruising.
   e. **Risk of severe rash (with lamotrigine)**
      * Ensure that the patient is informed that he or she must report evidence of skin rash to physician immediately.
   f. **Decreased efficacy of oral contraceptives (with topiramate)**
      * Ensure that the patient is aware of decreased efficacy of oral contraceptives with concomitant use.

g. **Risk of suicide with all antiepileptic drugs** (warning by FDA, December 2008)
  * Monitor for worsening of depression, suicidal thoughts or behavior, or any unusual changes in mood or behavior.

3. **May occur with antipsychotics:**
  a. **Drowsiness; dizziness**
    * Ensure that the patient does not operate dangerous machinery or participate in activities that require alertness.
  b. **Dry mouth; constipation**
    * Provide sugarless candy or gum, ice, and frequent sips of water. Provide foods high in fiber; encourage physical activity and fluid if not contraindicated.
  c. **Increased appetite; weight gain**
    * Provide calorie-controlled diet; provide opportunity for physical exercise; provide diet and exercise instruction.
  d. **ECG changes**
    * Monitor vital signs. Observe for symptoms of dizziness, palpitations, syncope, or weakness.
  e. **Extrapyramidal symptoms**
    * Monitor for symptoms. Administer prn medication at first sign.
  f. **Hyperglycemia and diabetes**
    * Monitor blood glucose regularly. Observe for the appearance of symptoms of polydipsia, polyuria, polyphagia, and weakness at any time during therapy.

■ PATIENT/FAMILY EDUCATION RELATED TO MOOD-STABILIZING AGENTS

* Do not drive or operate dangerous machinery. Drowsiness or dizziness can occur.
* Do not stop taking the drug abruptly. Can produce serious withdrawal symptoms. The physician will administer orders for tapering the drug when therapy is to be discontinued.
* Report the following symptoms to the physician immediately:
  * *Patient taking anticonvulsant:* Unusual bleeding, spontaneous bruising, sore throat, fever, malaise, skin rash, dark urine, and yellow skin or eyes.
  * *Patient taking lithium:* Ataxia, blurred vision, severe diarrhea, persistent nausea and vomiting, tinnitus, excessive urine output, increasing tremors, or mental confusion.
  * *Patient taking antipsychotic:* Sore throat, fever, malaise, unusual bleeding, easy bruising, persistent nausea and vomiting, severe headache, rapid heart rate, difficulty urinating, muscle twitching, tremors, darkly colored urine, excessive urination, excessive thirst, excessive hunger, weakness, pale stools, yellow skin or eyes, muscular incoordination, or skin rash.

- For the patient on lithium: Ensure that the diet contains adequate sodium. Drink 6 to 8 glasses of water each day. Avoid drinks that contain caffeine (that have a diuretic effect). Have serum lithium level checked every 1 to 2 months, or as advised by physician.
- For the patient on asenapine: Place the tablet *under* the tongue and allow to dissolve completely. Do not chew or swallow tablet. Do not eat or drink for 10 minutes.
- Avoid consuming alcoholic beverages and nonprescription medications without approval from physician.
- Carry card at all times identifying the name of medications being taken.

@ INTERNET REFERENCES

- www.mentalhealth.com
- https://www.nimh.nih.gov/index.shtml
- https://www.nimh.nih.gov/health/publications/mental-health-medications/index.shtml
- https://www.nlm.nih.gov/medlineplus/druginformation.html
- www.dbsalliance.org/site/PageServer?pagename=home
- https://www.drugguide.com/ddo (Davis's Drug Guide)
- www.centerwatch.com

CHAPTER 26

Antipsychotic Agents

CONVENTIONAL (First Generation) ANTIPSYCHOTIC AGENTS

■ PHENOTHIAZINES

Examples

Generic (Trade) Name	Half-life (hr)	Indications	Available Forms (mg)
Chlorpromazine	24	• Schizophrenia • Bipolar mania • Emesis/hiccoughs • Acute intermittent porphyria • Hyperexcitable, combative behavior in children • Preoperative apprehension	**TABS:** 10, 25, 50, 100, 200 **INJ:** 25/mL
Fluphenazine	HCl: 18 Decanoate: 6.8–9.6 days	• Psychotic disorders	**TABS:** 1, 2.5, 5, 10 **ELIXIR:** 0.5/mL **CONC:** 5/mL **INJ:** 2.5/mL **INJ (DECANOATE):** 25/mL
Perphenazine	9–12	• Schizophrenia • Nausea and vomiting	**TABS:** 2, 4, 8, 16
Prochlorperazine	3–5 (oral) 6.9 (IV)	• Schizophrenia • Nonpsychotic anxiety • Nausea and vomiting	**TABS:** 5, 10 **SUPP:** 25 **INJ:** 5/mL
Thioridazine	24	• Management of schizophrenia in patients who do not have an acceptable response to other antipsychotic therapy	**TABS:** 10, 25, 50, 100
Trifluoperazine	18	• Schizophrenia • Nonpsychotic anxiety	**TABS:** 1, 2, 5, 10

Action

- These drugs are thought to work by blocking postsynaptic dopamine receptors in the basal ganglia, hypothalamus, limbic system, brainstem, and medulla.
- They also demonstrate varying affinity for cholinergic, alpha$_1$-adrenergic, and histaminic receptors.
- Antipsychotic effects may also be related to inhibition of dopamine-mediated transmission of neural impulses at the synapses.

Contraindications and Precautions

Contraindicated in: • Hypersensitivity (cross-sensitivity may exist among phenothiazines) • Comatose or severely CNS-depressed patients • Poorly controlled seizure disorders • Patients with blood dyscrasias • Narrow-angle glaucoma • Patients with liver, renal, or cardiac insufficiency • Bone marrow depression • Concurrent pimozide use • Coadministration with other drugs that prolong QT interval or in patients with long QT syndrome or history of cardiac arrhythmias

Use Cautiously in: • Elderly and debilitated patients • Children with acute illnesses, infections, gastroenteritis, or dehydration (increased risk of extrapyramidal reactions) • Diabetes • Respiratory disease • Prostatic hypertrophy • Central nervous system (CNS) tumors • Epilepsy • Intestinal obstruction • Pregnancy or lactation (safety not established) • Elderly patients with psychosis related to neurocognitive disorder (NCD) (**black-box warning**). Antipsychotics are not approved for the treatment of dementia-related psychosis • Opioids should be prescribed only with benzodiazepines or other CNS depressants when other treatments are deemed inadequate (**black-box warning**)

Adverse Reactions and Side Effects

- Dry mouth
- Blurred vision
- Constipation
- Urinary retention
- Nausea
- Skin rash
- Sedation
- Orthostatic hypotension
- Photosensitivity
- Decreased libido
- Amenorrhea
- Retrograde ejaculation
- Gynecomastia
- Weight gain
- Reduction of seizure threshold

- Agranulocytosis
- Extrapyramidal symptoms
- Tardive dyskinesia
- Neuroleptic malignant syndrome
- Prolongation of QT interval **(thioridazine)**

Interactions

- Coadministration of phenothiazines and **beta blockers** may increase effects from either or both drugs.
- Increased effects of phenothiazines with **paroxetine.**
- Concurrent administration with **meperidine** may produce excessive sedation and hypotension.
- Therapeutic effects of phenothiazines may be decreased by **centrally acting anticholinergics.** Anticholinergic effects are increased.
- Concurrent use may result in decreased hypotensive effect of **guanethidine.**
- Phenothiazines may reduce effectiveness of **oral anticoagulants.**
- Concurrent use with phenothiazines may increase or decrease **phenytoin** levels.
- Increased orthostatic hypotension with **thiazide diuretics.**
- Increased CNS depression with **alcohol** or other **CNS depressants.**
- Increased hypotension with **antihypertensives.**
- Concurrent use with **epinephrine** or **dopamine** may result in severe hypotension.

Route and Dosage

CHLORPROMAZINE

Psychotic disorders: **PO** *(Adults and children ≥12 years):* 10 to 25 mg 2 to 4 times/day. May increase by 20 to 50 mg every 3 to 4 days until effective dose is reached, usually 200 to 400 mg/day (up to 1000 mg/day). **IM** *(Adults and children ≥12 years):* Initial dose: 25 to 50 mg. May give additional 25 to 50 mg in 1 hour. Increase gradually over several days (up to 400 mg every 3 to 12 hours in severe cases—maximum of 1000 mg/day).

Pediatric behavioral disorders: **PO** *(Children 6 months to 12 years):* 0.55 mg/kg every 4 to 6 hours as needed. **IM** *(Outpatients):* 0.55 mg/kg every 6 to 8 hours, as needed. *(Hospitalized patients):* Start with low dosage and increase gradually. In severe behavior disorders, 50 to 100 mg/day, or in older children, 200 mg/day or more may be necessary. Maximum dosage: 40 mg/day in children 6 months to 4 years (or weighing 22.7 kg) or 75 mg/day in children 5 to 12 years (or weighing 22.7 to 45.5 kg).

Nausea and vomiting: **PO** *(Adults and children ≥12 years):* 10 to 25 mg every 4 to 6 hr. **IM** *(Adults and children ≥12 years):* 25 mg initially, may repeat 25 to 50 mg every 3 to 4 hours, as needed, until vomiting stops.

Children >6 mo: **PO:** 0.55 mg/kg every 4 to 6 hours. **IM:** 0.55 mg/kg every 6 to 8 hours, not to exceed 40 mg/day in children up to 5 years (or weighing 22.7 kg) or 75 mg/day in children 5 to 12 years (or weighing 22.7 to 45.5 kg).

Intractable hiccoughs: **PO** *(Adults and children ≥12 years):* 25 to 50 mg 3 or 4 times daily. If symptoms persist for 2 to 3 days, give 25 to 50 mg **IM.**

Preoperative sedation: **PO** *(Adults and children ≥12 years):* 25 to 50 mg 2 to 3 hours before surgery, or **IM:** 12.5 to 25 mg 1 to 2 hours before surgery.

Children >6 mo: **PO:** 0.55 mg/kg 2 to 3 hours before surgery, or **IM:** 0.5 mg/kg 1 to 2 hours before surgery.

Acute intermittent porphyria: **PO** *(Adults):* 25 to 50 mg 3 or 4 times/day, or **IM** *(Adults):* 25 mg 3 or 4 times/day until patient can take **PO.**

FLUPHENAZINE

Psychotic disorders: **PO** *(Adults):* Initial dose: 2.5 to 10 mg/day in divided doses every 6 to 8 hours. Maintenance dose: 1 to 5 mg/day. **IM** *(Adults):* Initial dose: 1.25 mg. Usual dosage range: 2.5 to 10 mg/day in divided doses at 6 to 8 hour intervals.

Elderly or debilitated patients: **PO:** 1 to 2.5 mg/day initially. Adjust dosage according to response.

Decanoate formulation: **IM, SC** *(Adults):* Initial dose: 12.5 to 25 mg. May be repeated every 3 to 4 weeks. Dosage may be slowly increased in 12.5 mg increments as needed (not to exceed 100 mg/dose).

PERPHENAZINE

Schizophrenia: **PO** *(Adults and children ≥12 years): Outpatients:* 4 to 8 mg 3 times/day initially. Reduce as soon as possible to minimum effective dose. *Hospitalized patients:* 8 to 16 mg 2 to 4 times a day, not to exceed 64 mg/day.

Nausea and vomiting: **PO** *(Adults):* 8 to 16 mg daily in divided doses, up to 24 mg, if necessary.

PROCHLORPERAZINE

Schizophrenia: **PO** *(Adults) Mild conditions:* 5 or 10 mg 3 or 4 times a day. *Moderate conditions:* 10 mg 3 or 4 times/day. Gradually increase dosage by small increments over 2 or 3 days to 50 to 75 mg/day. *Severe conditions:* 100 to 150 mg/day. **IM** *(Adults):* 10 to 20 mg every 2 to 4 hours for up to 4 doses, then 10 to 20 mg every 4 to 6 hours, if needed. When control is achieved, switch to oral dosage.

Children ≥12 years: **PO:** 5 to 10 mg 3 to 4 times/day.

Children 2 to 12 years: **PO:** 2.5 mg 2 to 3 times/day. Maximum dose: 20 mg/day.

Nonpsychotic anxiety: **PO** *(Adults):* 5 mg 3 to 4 times/day, not to exceed 20 mg/day or longer than 12 weeks.

Nausea and vomiting: **PO** *(Adults):* 5 to 10 mg 3 or 4 times a day. **Rectal** *(Adults):* 25 mg twice daily. **IM:** 5 to 10 mg. May repeat every 3 or 4 hours, not to exceed 40 mg/day.

> *Children 9.1 to 13.2 kg:* **PO:** 2.5 mg 1 or 2 times a day, not to exceed 7.5 mg/day.
> *Children 13.6 to 17.7 kg:* **PO:** 2.5 mg 2 or 3 times a day, not to exceed 10 mg/day.
> *Children 18.2 to 38.6 kg:* **PO:** 2.5 mg 3 times a day or 5 mg twice daily, not to exceed 15 mg/day.
> *Children 2 years and older and at least 9.1 kg:* **IM:** 0.132 mg/kg. Usually only 1 dose is required.

THIORIDAZINE

Schizophrenia (intractable to other antipsychotics): **PO** *(Adults):* Initial dose: 50 to 100 mg 3 times a day. May increase gradually to maximum dosage of 800 mg/day. Once effective response has been achieved, may reduce gradually to determine the minimum maintenance dose. Usual daily dosage range: 200 to 800 mg, divided into 2 to 4 doses.

> *Children:* **PO:** Initial dose: 0.5 mg/kg/day given in divided doses. Increase gradually until therapeutic effect has been achieved or maximum dose of 3 mg/kg/day has been reached.

TRIFLUOPERAZINE

Schizophrenia: **PO** *(Adults and children ≥12 years):* 2 to 5 mg twice daily. Usual optimum dosage range: 15 to 20 mg/day, although a few may require 40 mg/day or more.

> *Children 6 to 12 years:* **PO:** Initial dose: 1 mg once or twice daily. May increase dose gradually to a maximum of 15 mg/day.

Nonpsychotic anxiety: **PO** *(Adults):* 1 or 2 mg twice daily. Do not administer more than 6 mg/day or for longer than 12 weeks.

■ THIOXANTHENES

Examples

Generic (Trade) Name	Half-life (hr)	Indications	Available Forms (mg)
Thiothixene (Navane)	34	• Schizophrenia	CAPS: 1, 2, 5, 10

Action

- Blocks postsynaptic dopamine receptors in the basal ganglia, hypothalamus, limbic system, brainstem, and medulla.
- Demonstrates varying affinity for cholinergic, alpha$_1$-adrenergic, and histaminic receptors.

Contraindications and Precautions

Contraindicated in: • Hypersensitivity • Comatose or severely CNS-depressed patients • Bone marrow depression or blood dyscrasias • Parkinson's disease • Severe hypotension or hypertension • Circulatory collapse • Children under age 12 • Pregnancy and lactation (safety not established)

Use Cautiously in: • Patients with history of seizures • Respiratory, renal, hepatic, thyroid, or cardiovascular disorders • Elderly or debilitated patients • Patients exposed to extreme environmental heat • Patients taking atropine or atropine-like drugs • Elderly patients with NCD-related psychosis (**black-box warning**). Antipsychotics are not approved for the treatment of dementia-related psychosis • Opioids should be prescribed only with benzodiazepines or other CNS depressants when other treatments are deemed inadequate (**black-box warning**)

Adverse Reactions and Side Effects
• Refer to this section under Phenothiazines.

Interactions
• Additive CNS depression with **alcohol** and other **CNS depressants.**
• Additive anticholinergic effects with other drugs that have anticholinergic properties.
• Possible additive hypotension with **antihypertensive agents.**
• Concurrent use with **epinephrine** or **dopamine** may result in severe hypotension.

ROUTE AND DOSAGE

Schizophrenia: **PO** *(Adults and children ≥12 years): Mild conditions:* Initial dosage: 2 mg 3 times/day. May increase to 15 mg/day. *Severe conditions:* Initial dosage: 5 mg twice daily. Optimal dose is 20 to 30 mg/day. If needed, may increase gradually, not to exceed 60 mg/day.

■ BUTYROPHENONE AND DIPHENYLBUTYLPIPERIDINE
Examples

Generic (Trade) Name	Half-life (hr)	Indications	Available Forms (mg)
Haloperidol (Haldol) [butyrophenone]	~18 hr (oral); ~3 wk (IM decanoate)	• Psychotic disorders • Tourette's disorder • Pediatric behavior problems and hyperactivity	**TABS:** 0.5, 1, 2, 5, 10, 20 **CONC:** 2/mL **INJ (LACTATE):** 5/mL **INJ (DECANOATE):** 50/mL; 100/mL
Pimozide (Orap) [diphenylbutylpiperidine]	~55 hr	• Tourette's disorder • Second line treatment after failure with atypical antipsychotics	**TABS:** 1, 2

Action

• Blocks postsynaptic dopamine receptors in the hypothalamus, limbic system, and reticular formation.
• Demonstrates varying affinity for cholinergic, alpha$_1$-adrenergic, and histaminic receptors.

Contraindications and Precautions

Contraindicated in: • Hypersensitivity to the drug • Coadministration with other drugs that prolong the QT interval • Coadministration with drugs that inhibit CYP3A enzymes **(pimozide)** • Treatment of tics other than those associated with Tourette's disorder **(pimozide)** • Coadministration with other drugs that may cause tics (e.g., pemoline, methylphenidate, amphetamines) until it has been determined whether the tics are caused by the medications or Tourette's disorder **(pimozide)** • Parkinson disease **(haloperidol)** • In comatose or severely CNS-depressed patients • Patients with blood dyscrasias or bone marrow depression • Narrow-angle glaucoma • Patients with liver, renal, or cardiac insufficiency • Pregnancy and lactation (safety not established)

Use Cautiously in: • Elderly and debilitated patients • Diabetic patients • Depressed patients • Patients with history of seizures • Patients with respiratory insufficiency • Prostatic hypertrophy • Children • Elderly patients with NCD-related psychosis **(black-box warning)**. Antipsychotics are not approved for the treatment of dementia-related psychosis • Opioids should be prescribed only with benzodiazepines or other CNS depressants when other treatments are deemed inadequate **(black-box warning)**

Adverse Reactions and Side Effects

• Dry mouth
• Blurred vision
• Constipation
• Urinary retention
• Nausea
• Skin rash
• Sedation
• Orthostatic hypotension
• Photosensitivity
• Decreased libido
• Amenorrhea
• Retrograde ejaculation
• Gynecomastia
• Weight gain
• Reduction of seizure threshold
• Agranulocytosis
• Extrapyramidal symptoms
• Tardive dyskinesia

- Neuroleptic malignant syndrome
- Prolongation of QT interval

Interactions

- Decreased serum concentrations of haloperidol, worsening schizophrenic symptoms, and tardive dyskinesia with concomitant use of **anticholinergic agents.**
- Increased plasma concentrations when administered with drugs that inhibit CYP3A enzymes **(azole antifungal agents; macrolide antibiotics)** and CYP1A2 enzymes **(fluoxetine; fluvoxamine).**
- Decreased therapeutic effects of haloperidol with **carbamazepine;** increased effects of **carbamazepine.**
- Additive hypotension with **antihypertensives.**
- Additive CNS depression with **alcohol** or other **CNS depressants.**
- Coadministration of haloperidol and **lithium** may result in alterations in consciousness, encephalopathy, extrapyramidal effects, fever, leukocytosis, and increased serum enzymes.
- Decreased therapeutic effects of haloperidol with **rifamycins.**
- Concurrent use with **epinephrine** or **dopamine** may result in severe hypotension.
- Additive effects with other drugs that prolong QT interval (e.g., **phenothiazines, tricyclic antidepressants, antiarrhythmic agents**).

Route and Dosage

HALOPERIDOL (Haldol)

Psychotic disorders: **PO** *(Adults and children ≥12 years): Moderate symptoms or geriatric or debilitated patients:* 0.5 to 2 mg 2 or 3 times a day. *Severe symptoms or chronic or resistant patients:* 3 to 5 mg 2 or 3 times a day. Some patients may require dosages up to 100 mg/day.

> *Children (3 to 12 years; weight range 15 to 40 kg):* Initial dose: 0.5 mg/day. May increase in 0.5 mg increments at 5- to 7-day intervals up to 0.15 mg/kg/day or until therapeutic effect is obtained. Administer in 2 or 3 divided doses.

Control of acutely agitated schizophrenic patient: **IM (lactate)** *(Adults):* 2 to 5 mg. May be repeated every 1 to 8 hours, not to exceed 100 mg/day.

Chronic psychosis requiring prolonged antipsychotic therapy: **IM (decanoate)** *(Adults):* 10 to 15 times the previous daily oral dose, not to exceed 100 mg initially. Repeat every 4 weeks, or adjust interval to patient response. For maintenance, titrate dosage upward or downward based on therapeutic response.

Tourette's disorder: **PO** *(Adults and children ≥12 years):* Initial dosage: 0.5 to 2 mg given 2 or 3 times/day.

> *Children (3 to 12 years; 15 to 40 kg):* **PO:** 0.25 to 0.5 mg/day given in 2 to 3 divided doses; may increase by 0.25 to 0.5 mg every 5 to 7 days; maximum dose: 0.15 mg/kg/day.

Behavioral disorders/hyperactivity: **PO** *(Children 3 to 12 years; 15 to 40 kg):* 0.25 to 0.5 mg/day given in 2 to 3 divided doses; may increase by 0.25 to 0.5 mg every 5 to 7 days; maximum dose: 0.15 mg/kg/day.

PIMOZIDE (Orap)

Tourette's disorder: **PO** *(Adults): Initial dose:* 1 to 2 mg/day in divided doses. Thereafter, increase dose every other day. *Maintenance dose:* Less than 0.2 mg/kg/day or 10 mg/day, whichever is less. Doses greater than 0.2 mg/kg/day or 10 mg/day are not recommended.

> *Children (12 years and older):* **PO:** Initial dose: 0.05 mg/kg, preferably taken once at bedtime. The dose may be increased every third day to a maximum of 0.2 mg/kg, not to exceed 10 mg/day.

ATYPICAL (Second Generation) ANTIPSYCHOTIC AGENTS
■ DIBENZAPINE DERIVATIVES
Examples

Generic (Trade) Name	Half-life (hr)	Indications	Available Forms (mg)
Asenapine (Saphris)	24	• Schizophrenia • Bipolar disorder	**TABS (SUBLINGUAL):** 5, 10
Clozapine (Clozaril)	8 (single dose); 12 (at steady state)	• Treatment-resistant schizophrenia • Recurrent suicidal behavior	**TABS:** 12.5, 25, 50, 100, 200 **TABS (ORALLY DISINTEGRATING):** 12.5, 25, 100, 150, 200
Loxapine	8	• Schizophrenia	**CAPS:** 5, 10, 25, 50
Olanzapine (Zyprexa)	21–54	• Schizophrenia • Bipolar disorder • Acute agitation associated with schizophrenia and mania (IM)	**TABS:** 2.5, 5, 7.5, 10, 15, 20 **TABS (ORALLY DISINTEGRATING [ZYDIS]):** 5, 10, 15, 20 **POWDER FOR INJECTION (IM):** 10/vial **POWDER FOR SUSPENSION, ER (PER VIAL):** 210, 300, 405
Quetiapine (Seroquel)	6	• Schizophrenia • Acute manic episodes • Major depression (adjunctive therapy) • Obsessive-compulsive disorder	**TABS:** 25, 50, 100, 200, 300, 400 **TABS (XR):** 50, 150, 200, 300, 400

Action
Asenapine

• Efficacy in schizophrenia is achieved through a combination of dopamine and serotonin type 2 ($5\text{-}HT_2$) antagonism.

- Mechanism of action in the treatment of acute manic episodes is unknown.

Clozapine

- Exerts an antagonistic effect on dopamine receptors, with a particularly high affinity for the D_4 receptor.
- It appears to be more active at limbic than at striatal dopamine receptors.
- Also acts as an antagonist at adrenergic, cholinergic, histaminergic, and serotonergic receptors.

Loxapine

- Mechanism of action has not been fully established.
- Exerts strong antagonistic effects on dopamine D_2, histamine H_1, alpha-adrenergic, and muscarinic M_1 receptors.

Olanzapine

- Efficacy in schizophrenia is mediated through a combination of dopamine and 5-HT_2 antagonism.
- Also shows antagonism for muscarinic, histaminic, and adrenergic receptors.
- The mechanism of action of olanzapine in the treatment of bipolar mania is unknown.

Quetiapine

- Antipsychotic activity is thought to be mediated through a combination of dopamine and serotonin receptor antagonism. Other effects may be due to antagonism of histamine H_1 receptors and alpha-adrenergic receptors.

Contraindications and Precautions

Asenapine

Contraindicated in: • Hypersensitivity • Lactation • History of QT prolongation or arrhythmias • Concurrent use of other drugs known to prolong QT interval

Use Cautiously in: • Patients with hepatic, renal, or cardiovascular insufficiency • Diabetes or risk factors for diabetes • History of seizures • History of suicide attempt • Patients at risk for aspiration pneumonia • Elderly patients • Pregnancy and children (safety not established) • Elderly patients with NCD-related psychosis (**black-box warning**)

Clozapine

Contraindicated in: • Hypersensitivity • Myeloproliferative disorders • History of clozapine-induced agranulocytosis or severe granulocytopenia • Concomitant use with other drugs that have the potential to suppress bone marrow function • Severe CNS depression or comatose states • Uncontrolled epilepsy • Lactation • Children (safety not established)

Use Cautiously in: • Patients with hepatic, renal, respiratory, or cardiac insufficiency • Patients with QT syndrome or risk factors for QT interval prolongation or ventricular arrhythmias • Diabetes mellitus or risk factors for diabetes • Prostatic enlargement • Narrow-angle glaucoma • Pregnancy • Elderly patients with NCD-related psychosis (**black-box warning**)

Loxapine

Contraindicated in: • Hypersensitivity • Comatose or severe drug-induced depressed states • Patients with blood dyscrasias • Hepatic, renal, or cardiac insufficiency • Severe hypotension or hypertension • Children, pregnancy, and lactation (safety not established)

Use Cautiously in: • Patients with epilepsy or history of seizures • Glaucoma • Urinary retention • Respiratory insufficiency • Prostatic hypertrophy • Elderly patients with NCD-related psychosis (**black-box warning**)

Olanzapine

Contraindicated in: • Hypersensitivity • Lactation • *Orally disintegrating tablets only:* Phenylketonuria (orally disintegrating tablets contain aspartame)

Use Cautiously in: • Hepatic insufficiency • Elderly patients (reduce dosage) • Pregnancy and children (safety not established) • Cardiovascular or cerebrovascular disease • History of glaucoma • History of seizures • History of attempted suicide • Prostatic hypertrophy • Diabetes or risk factors for diabetes • Narrow-angle glaucoma • History of paralytic ileus • Patients with preexisting low white blood cell count and/or history of drug-induced leukopenia/neutropenia • Elderly patients with NCD-related psychosis (**black-box warning**)

Quetiapine

Contraindicated in: • Hypersensitivity • Lactation • Concurrent use with drugs that prolong the QT interval • Patients with history of arrhythmias, including bradycardia

Use Cautiously in: • Cardiovascular or cerebrovascular disease • Dehydration or hypovolemia (increased risk of hypotension) • Hepatic impairment • Hypothyroidism • History of suicide attempt • Pregnancy or children (safety not established) • Patients with diabetes or risk factors for diabetes • History of seizures • Elderly patients with NCD-related psychosis (**black-box warning**)

Adverse Reactions and Side Effects

Asenapine

- Drowsiness, light-headedness
- Fatigue, irritability
- Headache

- Insomnia, restlessness
- Constipation
- Nausea
- Weight gain
- Neuroleptic malignant syndrome
- QT Interval prolongation
- Hyperprolactinemia

Clozapine

- Drowsiness, dizziness, sedation
- Nausea and vomiting
- Dry mouth; blurred vision
- Neutropenia (must monitor absolute neutrophil count [ANC] during treatment)
- Agranulocytosis
- Seizures (appear to be dose related)
- Salivation
- Myocarditis; cardiomyopathy
- Tachycardia
- Constipation
- Fever
- Weight gain
- Orthostatic hypotension
- Neuroleptic malignant syndrome
- Hyperglycemia

Loxapine

- Drowsiness, dizziness
- Anticholinergic effects (dry mouth, blurred vision, urinary retention, constipation, paralytic ileus)
- Nausea and vomiting
- Extrapyramidal symptoms
- Seizures
- Hypotension; hypertension; tachycardia
- Blood dyscrasias
- Neuroleptic malignant syndrome

Olanzapine

- Drowsiness, dizziness, weakness
- Dry mouth, constipation, increased appetite
- Nausea; weight gain
- Orthostatic hypotension, tachycardia
- Restlessness; insomnia
- Rhinitis
- Tremor
- Headache
- Hyperglycemia
- DRESS (drug reaction with eosinophilia and systemic symptoms)

Quetiapine
- Drowsiness, dizziness
- Hypotension, tachycardia
- Headache
- Nausea, dry mouth, constipation
- Weight gain
- Hyperglycemia

Interactions

The effects of:	Are increased by:	Are decreased by:	Concurrent use may result in:
Asenapine	Fluvoxamine; imipramine; valproate	Carbamazepine; cimetidine; paroxetine	Increased effects of paroxetine and dextromethorphan. Increased CNS depression with alcohol or other CNS depressants. Increased hypotension with antihypertensives. Additive effects on QT interval prolongation with quinidine, dofetilide, other class Ia and III antiarrhythmics, pimozide, sotalol, thioridazine, chlorpromazine, pentamidine, arsenic trioxide, mefloquine, dolasetron, tacrolimus, droperidol, gatifloxacin, or moxifloxacin.
Clozapine	Caffeine, citalopram, cimetidine, fluoxetine, fluvoxamine, sertraline, CYP3A4-inhibiting drugs (e.g., ketoconazole), risperidone, ritonavir	CYP1A2 inducers (e.g., carbamazepine, omeprazole, rifampin), phenobarbital, phenytoin, nicotine	Additive CNS depression with alcohol or other CNS depressants. Increased hypotension with antihypertensive agents. Additive anticholinergic effects with anticholinergic agents. Concomitant use with benzodiazepines may result in respiratory depression, stupor, hypotension, and/or respiratory or cardiac arrest. Increased effects of risperidone with chronic coadministration.
Loxapine			Additive CNS depression with alcohol or other CNS depressants. Increased hypotension with antihypertensive agents. Additive anticholinergic effects with anticholinergic agents.

The effects of:	Are increased by:	Are decreased by:	Concurrent use may result in:
			Concomitant use with lorazepam (and possibly other benzodiazepines) may result in respiratory depression, stupor, hypotension, and/or respiratory or cardiac arrest.
Olanzapine	Fluvoxamine and other CYP1A2 inhibitors, fluoxetine	Carbamazepine and other CYP1A2 inducers, omeprazole, rifampin	Decreased effects of levodopa and dopamine agonists. Increased hypotension with antihypertensives. Increased CNS depression with alcohol or other CNS depressants. Increased anticholinergic effects with anticholinergic agents.
Quetiapine	Cimetidine; ketoconazole, itraconazole, fluconazole, erythromycin, or other CYP3A4 inhibitors	Phenytoin, thioridazine	Decreased effects of levodopa and dopamine agonists. Increased CNS depression with alcohol or other CNS depressants. Increased hypotension with antihypertensives. Additive anticholinergic effects with anticholinergic agents.

Opioids should be prescribed only with benzodiazepines or other CNS depressants when other treatments are deemed inadequate (**black box warning**).

Route and Dosage

ASENAPINE (Saphris)

Schizophrenia: **PO** *(Adults):* Usual starting and target dose: 5 mg twice daily. The safety of doses above 10 mg twice daily has not been evaluated in clinical trials.

Bipolar disorder: **PO** *(Adults):* Recommended initial dose: 10 mg twice daily. The dose can be decreased to 5 mg twice daily if there are adverse effects. The safety of doses above 10 mg twice daily has not been evaluated in clinical trials.

CLOZAPINE (Clozaril)

Schizophrenia and recurrent suicidal behavior: **PO** *(Adults):* Initial dose: 12.5 mg once or twice daily. May increase dosage by 25 to 50 mg/day over a period of 2 weeks to a target dose of 300 to 450 mg/day. If required, make additional increases in increments of 100 mg not more than once or twice weekly to a maximum dosage of 900 mg/day. Titrate dosage slowly to observe for possible seizures and agranulocytosis. Dosage should be maintained at the lowest level effective for controlling symptoms.

NOTE: A baseline ANC must be taken, with a baseline ANC count of at least 1,500 µL before initiation of treatment with clozapine and done weekly for the first 6 months of treatment. Because of the risk of severe neutropenia, clozapine is available only in a 1-week supply through the *Clozapine Risk Evaluation and Mitigation Strategy (REMS)* program, which combines ANC testing, patient monitoring, and controlled distribution through certified pharmacies. Prescribers must also be certified at www.clozapinerems.com. Treatments will be based on the new protocols established and based on ANC monitoring and counts. Prescribers should familiarize themselves with these new protocols that can be found on the clozapine REMS Web site (prescribing information).

LOXAPINE

Schizophrenia: **PO** *(Adults):* Initial dosage: 10 mg twice daily, although some severely disturbed patients may require up to 50 mg/day. Increase dosage fairly rapidly over the first 7 to 10 days until symptoms are controlled. The usual therapeutic and maintenance dosage range is 60 to 100 mg/day. Doses higher than 250 mg/day are not recommended. Dosage should be maintained at the lowest level effective for controlling symptoms.

OLANZAPINE (Zyprexa)

Schizophrenia: **PO** *(Adults—most patients):* 5 to 10 mg/day initially; may ↑ at weekly intervals by 5 mg/day (target dose = 10 mg/day; not to exceed 20 mg/day).

    PO *(Adults—debilitated or nonsmoking female patients ≥65 yr):* Initiate therapy at 5 mg/day.

    PO *(Children 13 to 17 years):* 2.5 to 5 mg/day initially; may ↑ at weekly intervals by 2.5 to 5 mg/day (target dose = 10 mg/day; not to exceed 20 mg/day).

    IM *(Adults): Oral olanzapine dose = 10 mg/day*—210 mg every 2 weeks or 410 mg every 4 weeks for the first 8 weeks, then 150 mg every 2 weeks or 300 mg every 4 weeks as maintenance therapy. *Oral olanzapine dose = 15 mg/day*—300 mg every 2 weeks for the first 8 weeks, then 210 mg every 2 weeks or 405 mg every 4 weeks as maintenance therapy. *Oral olanzapine dose = 20 mg/day*—300 mg every 2 weeks for the first 8 weeks, then 300 mg every 2 weeks as maintenance therapy.

    IM *(Adults—debilitated or nonsmoking female patients ≥65 yr):* Initiate therapy at 150 mg every 4 weeks.

Acute manic or mixed episodes associated with bipolar I disorder: **PO** *(Adults):* 10 to 15 mg/day initially (use 10 mg/day when used with lithium or valproate); may ↑ every 24 hours by 5 mg/day (not to exceed 20 mg/day).

PO *(Children 13 to 17 years):* 2.5 to 5 mg/day initially; may ↑ by 2.5 to 5 mg/day (target dose = 10 mg/day; not to exceed 20 mg/day).

Maintenance treatment of bipolar I disorder: **PO** *(Adults):* Continue at the dose required to maintain symptom remission (usual dose: 5 to 20 mg/day).

PO *(Children 13 to 17 years):* Continue at the lowest dose required to maintain symptom remission.

Acute agitation due to schizophrenia or bipolar I mania: **IM** *(Adults):* 10 mg, may repeat in 2 hours, then 4 hours later. **IM** *(Adults >65 yr):* Initiate therapy with 5 mg.

Depressive episodes associated with bipolar I disorder: **PO** *(Adults):* 5 mg/day with fluoxetine 20 mg/day (both given in evening); may ↑ fluoxetine dose up to 50 mg/day and olanzapine dose up to 12.5 mg/day.

PO *(Children 10 to 17 years):* 20 mg/day with olanzapine 2.5 mg/day (both given in evening); may ↑ fluoxetine dose up to 50 mg/day and olanzapine dose up to 12 mg/day.

Treatment-resistant depression: **PO** *(Adults):* 5 mg/day with fluoxetine 20 mg/day (both given in evening); may ↑ fluoxetine dose up to 50 mg/day and olanzapine dose up to 20 mg/day.

QUETIAPINE (Seroquel)

Schizophrenia: **PO** *(Adults): Immediate-release:* 25 mg twice daily initially, increased by 25 to 50 mg 2 to 3 times daily over 3 days, up to 300 to 400 mg/day in 2 to 3 divided doses by the fourth day (not to exceed 800 mg/day). *Extended-release:* 300 mg once daily. Increase by 300 mg/day (not to exceed 800 mg/day).

Children 13 to 17 years: **PO:** *Immediate-release:* 25 mg twice daily on Day 1; increase to 50 mg twice daily on Day 2; then increase to 100 mg twice daily on Day 3; then increase to 150 mg twice daily on Day 4; then increase to 200 mg twice daily on Day 5. May then increase by no more than 100 mg/day (not to exceed 800 mg/day).

Acute manic episodes: **PO** *(Adults): Immediate-release:* 50 mg twice daily on Day 1; then increase to 100 mg twice daily on Day 2; then increase to 150 mg twice daily on Day 3; then increase to 200 mg twice daily on Day 4. May then increase by no more than 200 mg/day up to 400 mg twice daily on Day 6, if needed. *Extended-release:* 300 mg once daily on Day 1; then 600 mg once daily on Day 2; then 400 to 800 mg once daily starting on Day 3.

Children 10 to 17 years: **PO:** *Immediate release:* 25 mg twice daily on Day 1; then increase to 50 mg twice daily on Day 2; then increase to 100 mg twice daily on Day 3; then increase to 150 mg twice daily on Day 4; then increase to 200 mg twice daily on Day 5. May then increase by no more than 100 mg/day (not to exceed 600 mg/day).

Major depression (adjunctive therapy): **PO** *(Adults): Extended-release:* Initial dosage: 50 mg once daily in the evening. On Day 3, the dose may be increased to 150 mg once daily in the evening. Usual dosage: 150 to 300 mg/day.

Obsessive-compulsive disorder: **PO** *(Adults):* Initial dosage: 50 mg/day and increased based on therapeutic effect and tolerance. Dosage range: 25 to 400 mg/day.

■ BENZISOXAZOLE DERIVATIVES
Example

Generic (Trade) Name	Half-life	Indications	Available Forms (mg)
Risperidone (Risperdal)	3–20 hr (including metabolite)	• Bipolar mania • Schizophrenia • Irritability associated with autistic disorder **Unlabeled uses:** • Obsessive-compulsive disorder	TABS: 0.25, 0.5, 1, 2, 3, 4 TABS (ORALLY DISINTE-GRATING): 0.5, 1, 2, 3, 4 ORAL SOLUTION: 1/mL POWDER FOR INJECTION: 12.5/vial, 25/vial, 37.5/vial, 50/vial
Paliperidone (Invega)	23 hr (oral) 25–49 days (IM Sustenna) 84–139 days (IM Trinza)	• Schizophrenia • Schizoaffective disorder	TABS (ER): 1.5, 3, 6, 9 INJ: EXTENDED-RELEASE IM (INVEGA SUSTENNA): 39, 78, 117, 156, 234 EXTENDED-RELEASE IM (INVEGA TRINZA): 273, 410, 546, 819
Iloperidone (Fanapt)	18–33 hr	• Schizophrenia	TABS: 1, 2, 4, 6, 8, 10, 12
Ziprasidone (Geodon)	7 hr (oral) 2–5 hr (IM)	• Schizophrenia • Bipolar mania • Acute agitation in schizophrenia (IM)	CAPS: 20, 40, 60, 80 POWDER FOR INJECTION: 20/vial

Action
• Exerts antagonistic effects on dopamine, serotonin, alpha adrenergic, and histaminergic receptors

Contraindications and Precautions
Contraindicated in: • Known hypersensitivity • Comatose or severely depressed patients • Bradycardia, recent myocardial

infarction, or uncompensated heart failure • Lactation • Patients with history of QT prolongation or cardiac arrhythmias • Concurrent use with drugs known to cause QT prolongation

Use Cautiously in: • Patients with hepatic or renal impairment • Patients with history of seizures • Patients with diabetes or risk factors for diabetes • Patients exposed to temperature extremes • Elderly or debilitated patients • Patients with history of suicide attempt • Pregnancy and children (safety not established) • Elderly patients with NCD-related psychosis (**black-box warning**). Antipsychotics are not approved for the treatment of dementia-related psychosis • Opioids should only be prescribed with benzodiazepines or other CNS depressants when other treatments are deemed inadequate (**black-box warning**) • Conditions that increase risk of hypotension (e.g., dehydration [including from diuretic therapy or diarrhea], hypovolemia, concurrent antihypertensive therapy)

Adverse Reactions and Side Effects

- Anxiety
- Agitation
- Dry mouth
- Weight gain
- Orthostatic hypotension
- Insomnia
- Sedation
- Extrapyramidal symptoms
- Dizziness
- Headache
- Constipation
- Diarrhea
- Nausea
- Rhinitis
- Rash
- Tachycardia
- Hyperglycemia
- Prolonged QT interval

Interactions

- Increased effects of risperidone with **clozapine** or **ritonavir.**
- Increased effects of iloperidone, paliperidone, and risperidone with concomitant use of **CYP2D6 inhibitors** (e.g., **fluoxetine, paroxetine**).
- Decreased effects of **levodopa** and **other dopamine agonists** with risperidone, paliperidone, and ziprasidone.
- Decreased effectiveness of risperidone, paliperidone, and ziprasidone with **carbamazepine.**

- Additive CNS depression with **CNS depressants,** such as **alcohol, antihistamines, sedative/hypnotics,** or **opioid analgesics.**
- Increased effects of **clozapine** and **valproate** with risperidone.
- Additive hypotension with **antihypertensive agents.**
- Additive orthostatic hypotension with coadministration of other drugs that result in this adverse reaction.
- Additive anticholinergic effects with **anticholinergic agents.**
- Serious life-threatening arrhythmias with drugs known to prolong QT interval (e.g., **antiarrhythmics** [such as **quinidine, procainamide, amiodarone, sotalol], chlorpromazine, thioridazine, gatifloxacin, moxifloxacin, pentamidine, levomethadyl**).
- Increased risk of life-threatening arrhythmias with concurrent use of paliperidone and **chloroquine.**
- Increased effects of iloperidone and ziprasidone with concomitant use of **CYP3A4 inhibitors** (e.g., **ketoconazole**).
- Increased risk of seizures with coadministration of ziprasidone and **tramadol.**

Route and Dosage

RISPERIDONE (Risperdal)

Bipolar mania: **PO** *(Adults):* 2 to 3 mg/day as a single daily dose; dose may be increased at 24-hour intervals by 1 mg (range 1 to 6 mg/day). **IM** *(Adults):* 25 mg every 2 weeks; some patients may require larger dose of 37.5 or 50 mg every 2 weeks.

    Children 10 to 17 years: **PO:** Initial dosage: 0.5 mg once daily in either morning or evening. May be increased at intervals of at least 24 hours in increments of 0.5 or 1 mg/day, to a recommended dosage of 2.5 mg/day.

Schizophrenia: **PO** *(Adults):* Initial dosage: 2 mg/day administered as a single dose or in two divided doses. May increase dose at 24-hour intervals in increments of 1 to 2 mg/day to a recommended dose of 4 to 8 mg/day. **IM** *(Adults):* 25 mg every 2 weeks; some patients may require larger dose of 37.5 or 50 mg every 2 weeks.

    Adolescents (13 to 17 years): **PO:** Initial dosage: 0.5 mg once daily, increased by 0.5 to 1.0 mg no more frequently than every 24 hours to 3 mg daily. May administer half the daily dose twice daily if drowsiness persists.

Irritability associated with autistic disorder: **PO** *(Children and adolescents 5 to 16 years weighing <20 kg):* 0.25 mg/day initially. After at least 4 days of therapy, may increase to 0.5 mg/day. Dose increases in increments of 0.25 mg/day may be considered at 2-week or longer intervals. May be given as a single dose or in divided doses.

Children and adolescents 5 to 16 years weighing ≥20 kg: **PO:** 0.5 mg/day initially. After at least 4 days of therapy, may increase to 1.0 mg/day. Dose increases in increments of 0.5 mg/day may be considered at 2-week or longer intervals. May be given as a single dose or in divided doses.

Obsessive-compulsive disorder: **PO** *(Adults):* Initial dosage: 0.5 or 1 mg/day. May be increased by 0.5 or 1 mg weekly based on therapeutic effect and tolerance. Dosage range: 0.5 to 4 mg/day.

PALIPERIDONE (Invega)

Schizophrenia: **PO** *(Adults):* 6 mg once daily; may titrate by 3 mg/day at intervals of at least 5 days (range 3 to 12 mg/day).

PO *(Children 12 to 17 years):* 3 mg once daily; may titrate by 3 mg/day at intervals of at least 5 days (not to exceed 6 mg if <51 kg or 12 mg if ≥51 kg).

IM *(Adults): Invega Sustenna*—234 mg initially, then 156 mg 1 week later; continue with monthly maintenance dose of 117 mg (range of 39 to 234 mg based on efficacy and/or tolerability). *Invega Trinza*—dose should be based on dose of previous 1-month injection dose of Invega Sustenna. If last dose of Invega Sustenna was 78 mg, administer 273 mg of Invega Trinza; if last dose of Invega Sustenna was 117 mg, administer 410 mg of Invega Trinza; if last dose of Invega Sustenna was 156 mg, administer 546 mg of Invega Trinza; if last dose of Invega Sustenna was 234 mg, administer 819 mg of Invega Trinza. Administer dose q 3 months; may adjust dose based on efficacy and/or tolerability (range: 273 to 819 mg).

Schizoaffective Disorder: **PO** *(Adults):* 6 mg/day; may titrate by 3 mg/day at intervals of at least 4 days (range 3 to 12 mg/day).

ILOPERIDONE (Fanapt)

Schizophrenia: **PO** *(Adults):* Initiate treatment with 1 mg twice daily on the first day, then 2 mg twice daily the second day, then increase by 2 mg/day every day until a target dose of 12 to 24 mg/day given in two divided doses is reached.

ZIPRASIDONE (Geodon)

Bipolar mania: **PO** *(Adults):* Initial dosage: 40 mg twice daily. Increase dose to 60 or 80 mg twice/day on the second day of treatment. Adjust dose on the basis of toleration and efficacy within the range of 40 to 80 mg twice/day.

Schizophrenia: **PO** *(Adults):* Initial dose: 20 mg twice daily. Dose increments may be made at 2-day intervals up to 80 mg twice daily.

Acute agitation in schizophrenia: **IM** *(Adults):* 10 to 20 mg as needed up to 40 mg/day. May be given as 10 mg every 2 hours or 20 mg every 4 hours. Maximum dosage: 40 mg/day.

■ QUINOLINONES; UNDETERMINED (CARIPRAZINE AND BREXIPIPRAZOLE)

Example

Generic (Trade) Name	Half-life (hr)	Indications	Available Forms (mg)
Aripiprazole (Abilify)	75 (aripiprazole); 94 (metabolite)	• Bipolar mania • Schizophrenia • Schizophrenia relapse: Abilify Maintena) • Irritability associated with autistic disorder • Major depressive disorder (adjunctive treatment)	**TABS:** 2, 5, 10, 15, 20, 30 **TABS (ORALLY DISINTE-GRATING):** 10, 15 **ORAL SOLUTION:** 1/mL **INJ:** 5.25/0.7 mL, 9.75/1.3 mL, 15/2 mL **ER INJ (MAINTENA):** 400/vial: 1.9 mL sterile water for injection 300/vial: 1.5 mL sterile water for injection **ER INJECTABLE SUSPEN-SION (ARISTADA):** 441/1.6 mL, 662/2.4 mL, 882/3.2 mL
Brexipiprazole (Rexulti)	91	• Schizophrenia • Major depressive disorder (adjunctive treatment)	**TABS:** 0.25, 0.5, 1, 2, 3, 4
Cariprazine (Vraylar)	2–4 days; *didesmethyl-cariprazine (DDCAR)*—1–3 weeks	• Schizophrenia • Acute treatment of mania/mixed episodes in bipolar I disorder	**CAPS:** 1.5, 3, 4.5, 6

Action

• Aripiprazole: The efficacy of aripiprazole is thought to occur through a combination of partial agonist activity at D_2 and 5-HT_{1A} receptors and antagonist activity at 5-HT_{2A} receptors.
• Also exhibits antagonist activity at adrenergic α_1 receptors.
  Brexipiprazole: Psychotropic activity may be due to partial agonist activity at dopamine D_2 and serotonin 5-HT_{1A} receptors and antagonist activity at the 5-HT_{2A} receptor.
  Cariprazine: Acts as a partial agonist at dopamine D_3/D_2 receptors in the CNS with preferential binding to dopamine D_3, and partial agonist at serotonin 5–HT_{1A}; also acts an antagonist at 5-HT_{2A} receptors.

Contraindications and Precautions

Aripiprazole

Contraindicated in: • Hypersensitivity • Lactation

Use Cautiously in: • History of seizures • Hepatic or renal impairment • Known cardiovascular or cerebrovascular disease • Conditions that cause hypotension (dehydration, hypovolemia, treatment with antihypertensive medication) • Conditions that increase the core body temperature (excessive exercise, exposure to extreme heat, dehydration) • Patients with diabetes or risk factors for diabetes • Pregnancy (weigh benefits of the drug to potential risk to fetus) • Children and adolescents (safety and effectiveness not established) • Elderly patients with NCD-related psychosis (**black-box warning**)

Brexpiprazole

Contraindicated in: • Hypersensitivity

Use Cautiously in: • History of seizures, concurrent use of medications that may ↓ seizure threshold • Preexisting cardiovascular disease, dehydration, hypotension, concurrent antihypertensives, diuretics, electrolyte imbalance (↑ risk of orthostatic hypotension, correct deficits before treatment) • Preexisting low WBC (may ↑ risk of leukopenia/neutropenia) • History of diabetes, metabolic syndrome or dyslipidemia (may exacerbate) • Patients <24 years (may ↑ suicidal ideation/behaviors, monitor carefully) • Elderly patients with dementia-induced psychoses (↑ risk of serious adverse cardiovascular reactions and death), consider age, concurrent medical conditions and medications, renal/hepatic/cardiac function (**black-box warning**) • Poor CYP2D6 metabolizers (PM), dose ↓ required • Safe use in pregnancy has not been established; use during third trimester may result in extrapyramidal/withdrawal symptoms in infant • Lactation, consider health benefits against risk of adverse effects in infant • Safe and effective use in children has not been established (may ↑ suicidal ideation/behaviors)

Cariprazine

Contraindicated in: • Hypersensitivity • Concurrent use of strong CYP3A4 inhibitors • Concurrent use of strong CYP3A4 inducers

Use Cautiously in: • Known cerebrovascular/cardiovascular disease, dehydration, concurrent use of diuretics/antihypertensives or syncope (↑ risk of orthostatic hypotension) • Preexisting ↓ WBC or ANC or history of drug-induced leukopenia/neutropenia • Elderly patients with dementia-related psychosis (↑ risk of adverse cardiovascular effects and death) (**black-box warning**) • Antipsychotics are not approved for the treatment of dementia-related psychosis • Opioids should be prescribed only with benzodiazepines or other CNS depressants when other treatments are deemed inadequate (**black-box warning**), consider age-related ↓ in renal/hepatic/cardiovascular function, concurrent disease states and medications (↓ initial dose recommended) • Patients at risk of aspiration

• Neonates exposed in the third trimester may experience extrapyramidal symptoms/withdrawal • Lactation, consider maternal and fetal benefits against possible adverse effects in infant • Safe and effective use in children has not been established

Adverse Reactions and Side Effects

• Headache
• Nausea and vomiting
• Dyspepsia, dysphagia
• Constipation, diarrhea
• Anxiety, restlessness
• Akathisia
• Insomnia
• Light-headedness
• Drowsiness, sedation, somnolence
• Weight gain
• Blurred vision
• Increased salivation
• Extrapyramidal symptoms
• Hyperglycemia
• Disruption in the body's ability to reduce core body temperature
• Compulsive behaviors/uncontrollable urges (shopping, gambling) (Aripiprazole)

Interactions

Aripiprazole

• Decreased plasma levels of aripiprazole with **carbamazepine** and other **CYP3A4 inducers.**
• Increased plasma levels and potential for aripiprazole toxicity with **CYP2D6 inhibitors,** such as **quinidine, fluoxetine,** and **paroxetine.**
• Decreased metabolism and increased effects of aripiprazole with **ketoconazole** or **other CYP3A4 inhibitors.**
• Additive hypotensive effects with **antihypertensive drugs.**
• Additive CNS effects with **alcohol** and other **CNS depressants.**

Brexpiprazole

• Concurrent use with strong CYP3A4 inhibitors including **clarithromycin, itraconazole,** or **ketoconazole** ↑ blood levels, effects, and risk of adverse reactions; ↓ dose of brexpiprazole required.
• Concurrent use with strong CYP2D6 inhibitors including **fluoxetine, paroxetine,** or **quinidine** ↑ blood levels, effects, and risk of adverse reactions; ↓ dose of brexpiprazole required.
• Combined use of **strong or moderate CYP3A4 inhibitors with strong or moderate CYP2D6 inhibitors** in addition to brexpiprazole, including combinations of **itraconazole + quinidine, fluconazole + paroxetine, itraconazole + duloxetine,** or **fluconazole + duloxetine,** ↑ blood levels, effects, and risk of toxicity; ↓ dose of brexpiprazole required.

- Concurrent use of **strong inducers of CYP3A4** including **rifampin** ↓ blood levels and effectiveness; ↑ dose of brexipiprazole required.
- Concurrent use of **antihypertensives** or **diuretics** (↑ risk of hypotension).
- Concurrent use of **medications that may ↓ seizure threshold** (↑ risk of seizures).

HerbalProducts

Concurrent use of **St. John's wort** ↓ blood levels and effectiveness; ↑ dose of brexipiprazole required.

Cariprazine

- Blood levels, effects, and risk of toxicity ↑ by concurrent use of **strong CYP3A4 inhibitors** including **itraconazole** and **ketoconazole;** concurrent use not recommended.
- Blood levels and effectiveness may be ↓ by concurrent use of **strong CYP3A4 inducers,** including **carbamazepine** and **rifampin;** concurrent use not recommended.
- Concurrent use of **diuretics/antihypertensives** (↑ risk of orthostatic hypotension/syncope).

Route and Dosage
ARIPIPRAZOLE (Abilify)

Bipolar mania: **PO** *(Adults):* Usual starting dose: 15 mg once daily as monotherapy, or 10 to 15 mg as adjunctive therapy with lithium or valproate given once daily. Dosage may be increased to 30 mg/day based on clinical response. The safety of dosages higher than 30 mg has not been evaluated.

> *Children 10 to 17 years:* **PO:** Initial dosage: 2 mg/day. Titrate to 5 mg/day after 2 days and to the target dosage of 10 mg/day after 2 additional days. Subsequent dosage increases should be administered in 5 mg/day increments. Usual dosage: 10 mg/day as monotherapy or as adjunctive therapy with lithium or valproate.

Major depressive disorder (adjunctive treatment): **PO** *(Adults):* Initial dosage: 2 to 5 mg/day for patients already taking another antidepressant. May increase dosage by up to 5 mg/day at intervals of at least a week. Maintenance dosage range: 2 to 15 mg/day.

Schizophrenia: **PO** *(Adults):* Initial dosage: 10 or 15 mg/day as a single dose. Doses up to 30 mg have been used. Dosage increases should not be made before 2 weeks, the time required to achieve steady state.

> *Children 13 to 17 years:* **PO:** Initial dosage: 2 mg/day. Titrate to 5 mg after 2 days and to the target dose of 10 mg after 2 additional days. Subsequent dose increases should be

administered in 5 mg increments. Maintenance dosage: 10 to 30 mg/day.

IM *(Adults):* 400 mg every month; after first injection, continue treatment with oral aripiprazole (10 to 20 mg/day) for 14 days; if no adverse reactions to 400 mg/month dose, may ↓ dose to 300 mg every month.

Irritability associated with autistic disorder: **PO** *(Children 6 to 17 years):* Initial dosage: 2 mg/day. The dosage should be increased to 5 mg/day, with subsequent increases to 10 or 15 mg/day if needed. Dosage adjustments of up to 5 mg/day should occur gradually, at intervals of no less than 1 week. Usual dosage: 5 to 15 mg/day.

Brexpiprazole (Rexulti)

Schizophrenia: **PO** *(Adults):* 1 mg daily initially, may be increased to 2 to 4 mg daily (not to exceed 4 mg daily).

Major depressive disorder: **PO** *(Adults):* 0.5 or 1 mg daily initially, may be increased to 2 mg daily (not to exceed 3 mg daily).

Cariprazine (Vraylar)

Schizophrenia: **PO** *(Adults):* 1.5 mg/day initially, may be increased on second day to 3 mg; further increments of 1.5 mg or 3 mg may be made depending on response/tolerance up to maintenance dose of 1.5–6 mg/day.

Bipolar mania: **PO** *(Adults):* 1.5 mg/day initially, may be increased on second day to 3 mg; further increments of 1.5 mg or 3 mg may be made depending on response/tolerance up to maintenance dose of 1.5 to 6 mg/day titrated up to 3 to 6 mg/day. *Concurrent use of strong CYP3A4 inhibitors*—decrease dose by 50%.

■ BENZOTHIAZOL DERIVATIVE

Example

Generic (Trade) Name	Half-life (hr)	Indications	Available Forms (mg)
Lurasidone (Latuda)	18	• Schizophrenia • Depressive episodes associated with bipolar I disorder	**TABS:** 20, 40, 60, 80, 120

Action

• The efficacy of lurasidone in schizophrenia is thought to be mediated through a combination of central dopamine type 2 (D_2) and serotonin Type 2 (5-HT_{2A}) receptor antagonism.

Contraindications and Precautions

Contraindicated in: • Hypersensitivity • Children (safety not established)

Use Cautiously in: • Renal or hepatic impairment • History of suicide attempt • Diabetes mellitus • Overheating/dehydration • History of leukopenia or previous drug-induced leukopenia • Elderly or debilitated patients • Pregnancy • Elderly patients with NCD-related psychosis (**black-box warning**). Antipsychotics are not approved for the treatment of dementia-related psychosis • Opioids should be prescribed only with benzodiazepines or other CNS depressants when other treatments are deemed inadequate (**black-box warning**)

Adverse Reactions and Side Effects

- Akathisia
- Drowsiness
- Parkinsonism
- Agitation
- Dizziness
- Nausea
- Neuroleptic malignant syndrome
- Seizures
- Agranulocytosis

Interactions

- Decreased effects of lurasidone with **CYP3A4 inducers** (e.g., **carbamazepine, dexamethasone, phenobarbital, phenytoin, rifampin**).
- Increased effects of lurasidone with **CYP3A4 inhibitors** (e.g., **ketoconazole**).
- Increased effects of **digoxin** and **midazolam** with concomitant use of lurasidone.
- Coadministration of lurasidone and **lithium** may result in alterations in consciousness, encephalopathy, extrapyramidal effects, fever, leukocytosis, and increased serum enzymes.
- Increased sedation may occur with other **CNS depressants,** including **alcohol, sedative/hypnotics, opioids,** some **antidepressants,** and **antihistamines.**

Route and Dosage

LURASIDONE (Latuda)

*Schizophrenia: **PO** (Adults):* Initial dosage: 40 mg once daily. Usual dosage range: 40 to 80 mg/day. Maximum dose: 160 mg/day.

*Depressive episodes associated with bipolar I disorder: **PO** (Adults):* Initial dosage: 20 mg once daily as monotherapy or as adjunctive therapy with lithium or valproate. Usual dosage range: 20 to 120 mg/day. Maximum dose: 120 mg/day.

NOTE: *Lurasidone (Latuda) should be taken with food (at least 350 calories).* Administration with food substantially increases the absorption of this medication.

■ NURSING DIAGNOSES RELATED TO ALL ANTIPSYCHOTIC AGENTS

1. Risk for other-directed violence related to panic anxiety and mistrust of others.
2. Risk for injury related to medication side effects of sedation, photosensitivity, reduction of seizure threshold, agranulocytosis, extrapyramidal symptoms, tardive dyskinesia, neuroleptic malignant syndrome, and/or QT prolongation.
3. Risk for activity intolerance related to medication side effects of sedation, blurred vision, and/or weakness.
4. Nonadherence with medication regimen related to suspiciousness and mistrust of others.

■ NURSING IMPLICATIONS FOR ANTIPSYCHOTIC AGENTS

The plan of care should include monitoring for the following side effects from antipsychotic medications. Nursing implications related to each side effect are designated by an asterisk (*).

1. Anticholinergic effects
   a. Dry mouth
      * Provide the patient with sugarless candy or gum, ice, and frequent sips of water.
      * Ensure that the patient practices strict oral hygiene.
   b. Blurred vision
      * Explain that this symptom will most likely subside after a few weeks.
      * Advise the patient not to drive a car until vision clears.
      * Clear small items from pathway to prevent falls.
   c. Constipation
      * Order foods high in fiber; encourage increase in physical activity and fluid intake if not contraindicated.
   d. Urinary retention
      * Instruct the patient to report any difficulty urinating; monitor intake and output.
2. Nausea; gastrointestinal (GI) upset (may occur with all classifications)
      * Tablets or capsules may be administered with food to minimize GI upset.
      * Concentrates may be diluted and administered with fruit juice or other liquid; they should be mixed immediately before administration.
3. Skin rash (may occur with all classifications)
      * Report appearance of any rash on skin to physician.
      * Avoid spilling any of the liquid concentrate on skin; contact dermatitis can occur.

4. Sedation
   * Discuss with physician possibility of administering drug at bedtime.
   * Discuss with physician possible decrease in dosage or order for less-sedating drug.
   * Instruct the patient not to drive or operate dangerous equipment when experiencing sedation.
5. Orthostatic hypotension
   * Instruct the patient to rise slowly from a lying or sitting position.
   * Monitor blood pressure (lying and standing) each shift; document and report significant changes.
6. Photosensitivity (may occur with all classifications)
   * Ensure that the patient wears protective sunblock lotion, clothing, and sunglasses when spending time outdoors.
7. Hormonal effects (may occur with all classifications, but more common with typical antipsychotics)
   a. Decreased libido, retrograde ejaculation, gynecomastia (men)
      * Provide explanation of the effects and reassurance of reversibility. If necessary, discuss with physician possibility of ordering alternate medication.
   b. Amenorrhea (women)
      * Offer reassurance of reversibility; instruct patient to continue use of contraception, because amenorrhea does not indicate cessation of ovulation.
   c. Weight gain (may occur with all classifications; has been problematic with the atypical antipsychotics)
      * Weigh patient every other day; order calorie-controlled diet; provide opportunity for physical exercise; provide diet and exercise instruction.
8. ECG changes. ECG changes, including prolongation of the QT interval, are possible with most of the antipsychotics. This is particularly true with ziprasidone, thioridazine, pimozide, haloperidol, paliperidone, iloperidone, asenapine, and clozapine. Caution is advised in prescribing this medication to individuals with history of arrhythmias. Conditions that produce hypokalemia and/or hypomagnesemia, such as diuretic therapy or diarrhea, should be taken into consideration when prescribing. Routine ECG should be taken before initiation of therapy and periodically during therapy. Clozapine has also been associated with other cardiac events, such as ischemic changes, arrhythmias, congestive heart failure, myocarditis, and cardiomyopathy.
   * Monitor vital signs every shift.
   * Observe for symptoms of dizziness, palpitations, syncope, weakness, dyspnea, and peripheral edema.

9. Reduction of seizure threshold (more common with the typical than the atypical antipsychotics, with the exception of clozapine)
   * Closely observe patients with history of seizures.
   * **NOTE:** This is particularly important with patients taking clozapine (Clozaril), with which seizures have been frequently associated. Dose appears to be an important predictor, with a greater likelihood of seizures occurring at higher doses. Extreme caution is advised in prescribing clozapine for patients with history of seizures.
10. Agranulocytosis (more common with the typical than the atypical antipsychotics, with the exception of clozapine)
    * Agranulocytosis usually occurs within the first 3 months of treatment. Observe for symptoms of sore throat, fever, malaise. A complete blood count should be monitored if these symptoms appear.
    * **EXCEPTION:** There is a significant risk of agranulocytosis with clozapine (Clozaril). In May 2016, a new set of protocols was established to monitor for severe neutropenia (ANC of less than 500/μL). There is now a single shared system for providers and pharmacies for monitoring patients receiving clozapine. Both providers and pharmacies must now be certified at www.clozapinerems.com. This is the Clozapine REMS program and Web site. Protocols are provided for initiating clozapine, for continuation based on ANC levels, as well as interrupting or discontinuing treatment.
11. Hypersalivation (most common with clozapine)
    * A significant number of patients receiving clozapine (Clozaril) therapy experience extreme salivation. Offer support to the patient because this may be an embarrassing situation. It may even be a safety issue (e.g., risk of aspiration) if the problem is very severe. Management has included the use of sugar-free gum to increase the swallowing rate, as well as the prescription of medications such as an anticholinergic (e.g., scopolamine patch) or alpha$_2$-adrenoceptor agonist (e.g., clonidine).
12. Extrapyramidal symptoms (EPS)
    * Observe for symptoms and report; administer antiparkinsonian drugs, as ordered (see Chapter 27)
    a. Pseudoparkinsonism (tremor, shuffling gait, drooling, rigidity)
       * Symptoms may appear 1 to 5 days following initiation of antipsychotic medication; occurs most often in women, the elderly, and dehydrated patients.

b. Akinesia (muscular weakness)
    * Same as pseudoparkinsonism.
c. Akathisia (continuous restlessness and fidgeting)
    * This occurs most frequently in women; symptoms may occur 50 to 60 days following initiation of therapy.
d. Dystonia (involuntary muscular movements [spasms] of face, arms, legs, and neck)
    * This occurs most often in men and in people younger than 25 years of age.
e. Oculogyric crisis (uncontrolled rolling back of the eyes)
    * This may appear as part of the syndrome described as dystonia. It may be mistaken for seizure activity. Dystonia and oculogyric crisis should be treated as an emergency situation. The physician should be contacted, and intravenous benztropine mesylate (Cogentin) is commonly administered. Stay with the patient and offer reassurance and support during this frightening time.
13. Tardive dyskinesia (bizarre facial and tongue movements, stiff neck, and difficulty swallowing) (may occur with all classifications, but more common with typical antipsychotics)
    * All patients receiving long-term (months or years) antipsychotic therapy are at risk.
    * The symptoms are potentially irreversible.
    * The drug should be withdrawn at first sign, which is usually vermiform movements of the tongue; prompt action may prevent irreversibility.
    * The Abnormal Involuntary Movement Scale (AIMS) is a rating scale that was developed in the 1970s by the National Institute of Mental Health to measure involuntary movements associated with tardive dyskinesia. The AIMS aids in early detection of movement disorders and provides a means for ongoing surveillance. The AIMS assessment tool, examination procedure, and interpretation of scoring are presented in Appendix P.
14. Neuroleptic malignant syndrome (NMS) (more common with the typical than the atypical antipsychotics)
    * This is a relatively rare, but potentially fatal, complication of treatment with antipsychotic drugs. Routine assessments should include temperature and observation for parkinsonian symptoms.
    * Onset can occur within hours or even years after drug initiation, and progression is rapid over the following 24 to 72 hours.
    * Symptoms include severe parkinsonian muscle rigidity, very high fever, tachycardia, tachypnea, fluctuations in blood pressure, diaphoresis, and rapid deterioration of mental status to stupor and coma.

* Discontinue neuroleptic medication immediately.
* Monitor vital signs, degree of muscle rigidity, intake and output, level of consciousness.
* The physician may order bromocriptine (Parlodel) or dantrolene (Dantrium) to counteract the effects of NMS.

15. Hyperglycemia and diabetes (more common with atypical antipsychotics). Studies have suggested an increased risk of treatment-emergent, hyperglycemia-related adverse events in patients using atypical antipsychotics (e.g., risperidone, clozapine, olanzapine, quetiapine, ziprasidone, paliperidone, iloperidone, asenapine, lurasidone, and aripiprazole). The U.S. Food and Drug Administration recommends that patients with diabetes starting on atypical antipsychotic drugs be monitored regularly for worsening of glucose control. Patients with risk factors for diabetes should undergo fasting blood glucose testing at the beginning of treatment and periodically thereafter. All patients taking these medications should be monitored for symptoms of hyperglycemia (polydipsia, polyuria, polyphagia, and weakness). If these symptoms appear during treatment, the patient should undergo fasting blood glucose testing.

16. Increased risk of mortality in elderly patients with psychosis related to NCD. Studies have indicated that elderly patients with NCD-related psychosis who are treated with antipsychotic drugs are at increased risk of death, compared with placebo. Causes of death are most commonly related to infections or cardiovascular problems. All antipsychotic drugs now carry black-box warnings to this effect. They are not approved for treatment of elderly patients with NCD-related psychosis.

■ PATIENT/FAMILY EDUCATION RELATED TO ALL ANTIPSYCHOTICS

* Use caution when driving or operating dangerous machinery. Drowsiness and dizziness can occur.
* Do not stop taking the drug abruptly after long-term use. To do so might produce withdrawal symptoms, such as nausea, vomiting, dizziness, gastritis, headache, tachycardia, insomnia, and tremulousness.
* Use sunblock lotion and wear protective clothing when spending time outdoors. Skin is more susceptible to sunburn, which can occur in as little as 30 minutes.
* Report weekly (if receiving clozapine therapy) to have blood levels drawn and to obtain a weekly supply of the drug.
* Report occurrence of any of the following symptoms to the physician immediately: sore throat, fever, malaise, unusual bleeding, easy bruising, persistent nausea and vomiting, severe headache, rapid heart rate, fainting, difficulty urinating, muscle

twitching, tremors, darkly colored urine, excessive urination, excessive thirst, excessive hunger, weakness, pale stools, yellow skin or eyes, muscular incoordination, or skin rash.

- Rise slowly from a sitting or lying position to prevent a sudden drop in blood pressure.
- Take frequent sips of water, chew sugarless gum, or suck on hard candy if experiencing a problem with dry mouth. Good oral care (frequent brushing, flossing) is very important.
- Consult the physician regarding smoking when taking this medication. Smoking increases the metabolism of some antipsychotics, possibly requiring adjustment in dosage to achieve therapeutic effect.
- Dress warmly in cold weather and avoid extended exposure to very high or low temperatures. Body temperature is harder to maintain with this medication. Avoid drinking alcohol when on antipsychotic therapy. These drugs potentiate each other's effects.
- Do not consume other medications (including over-the-counter products) without physician's approval. Many medications contain substances that interact with antipsychotics in a way that may be harmful. Opiates and benzodiazepines can be particularly dangerous in combination with antipsychotics and should not be taken unless first discussed with the physician.
- Be aware of possible risks of taking antipsychotic medication during pregnancy. Safe use during pregnancy and lactation has not been established. Antipsychotics are thought to readily cross the placental barrier; if so, a fetus could experience adverse effects of the drug. Inform the physician immediately if pregnancy occurs, is suspected, or is planned.
- Be aware of side effects of antipsychotic drugs. Refer to written materials furnished by health-care providers for safe self-administration.
- Continue to take medication, even if feeling well and as though it is not needed. Symptoms may return if medication is discontinued.
- Carry card or other identification at all times describing medications being taken.

@ INTERNET REFERENCES

- www.mentalhealth.com
- https://www.nimh.nih.gov/index.shtml
- https://www.nimh.nih.gov/health/topics/mental-health-medications/index.shtml
- https://medlineplus.gov/druginformation.html
- www.schizophrenia.com
- https://drugguide.com (Davis's Drug Guide)
- http://centerwatch.com

CHAPTER 27

Antiparkinsonian and Tardive Dyskinesia Agents*

■ ANTICHOLINERGICS
Examples

Generic (Trade) Name	Half-life (hr)	Indications	Available Forms (mg)
Benztropine (Cogentin)	Unknown	• Parkinsonism • Drug-induced extrapyramidal symptoms (EPS)	TABS: 0.5, 1, 2 INJ: 1/mL
Biperiden (Akineton)	18.4–24.3	• Parkinsonism • Drug-induced EPS	TABS: 2
Trihexyphenidyl (Artane)	5.6–10.2	• Parkinsonism • Drug-induced EPS	TABS: 2, 5 ELIXIR: 2/5 mL
Diphenhydramine (Benadryl)	4–15	• Parkinsonism • Drug-induced EPS • Motion sickness • Allergy reactions • Insomnia • Cough suppressant	TABS & CAPS: 25, 50 TABS, CHEWABLE: 12.5 STRIPS (ORALLY DISINTEGRATING): 12.5, 25 ELIXIR/SYRUP/ORAL SOLU: 12.5/5 mL ORAL SUSPENSION: 25/5 mL INJ: 50/mL

*This chapter includes only those antiparkinsonian agents indicated for treatment of antipsychotic-induced extrapyramidal symptoms or neuroleptic malignant syndrome (bromocriptine).

Action

- Blocks acetylcholine receptors to diminish excess cholinergic effects. May also inhibit the reuptake and storage of dopamine at central dopamine receptors, thereby prolonging the action of dopamine.
- Diphenhydramine also blocks histamine release by competing with histamine for H_1 receptor sites. Decreased allergic response and somnolence are affected by diminished histamine activity.

Contraindications and Precautions

Contraindicated in: • Hypersensitivity • Angle-closure glaucoma • Pyloric or duodenal obstruction • Peptic ulcers • Prostatic hypertrophy • Bladder neck obstructions • Megaesophagus • Megacolon • Myasthenia gravis • Lactation • Children (*except* diphenhydramine)

Use Cautiously in: • Tachycardia • Cardiac arrhythmias • Hypertension • Hypotension • Tendency toward urinary retention • Patients exposed to high environmental temperatures • Pregnancy

Adverse Reactions and Side Effects

- Dry mouth
- Blurred vision
- Constipation
- Paralytic ileus
- Urinary retention
- Tachycardia
- Agitation, nervousness
- Decreased sweating
- Elevated temperature
- Nausea/vomiting
- Sedation
- Dizziness
- Exacerbation of psychoses
- Orthostatic hypotension

Interactions

- *(Diphenhydramine):* Additive sedative effects with **central nervous system (CNS) depressants.**
- Increased effects of **beta blockers** with diphenhydramine.
- Additive anticholinergic effects with other drugs that have anticholinergic properties.
- Anticholinergic drugs counteract the cholinergic effects of **bethanechol.**

- Possible increased **digoxin** levels with anticholinergics.
- Concomitant use of anticholinergics with **haloperidol** may result in worsening of psychotic symptoms, decreased haloperidol serum levels, and development of tardive dyskinesia.
- Possible decreased efficacy of **phenothiazines** and increased incidence of anticholinergic side effects with concomitant use.
- Decreased effects of **levodopa** with concomitant use.

Route and Dosage

BENZTROPINE (Cogentin)

Parkinsonism: **PO** *(Adults):* 0.5 to 2 mg/day in 1 or 2 divided doses (range 0.5 to 6 mg/day).

Drug-induced EPS: **PO, IM, IV** *(Adults):* 1 to 4 mg given once or twice daily.

Acute dystonic reactions: **IM, IV** *(Adults):* 1 to 2 mg, then 1 to 2 mg PO twice daily.

BIPERIDEN (Akineton)

Parkinsonism: **PO** *(Adults):* 2 mg 3 or 4 times/day, not to exceed 16 mg/24 hr.

Drug-induced EPS: **PO** *(Adults):* 2 mg 1 to 3 times/day.

TRIHEXYPHENIDYL (Artane)

Parkinsonism: **PO** *(Adults):* Initial dose: 1 mg the first day; increase by 2 mg increments at 3 to 5 day intervals, up to a daily dose of 6 to 10 mg in 3 divided doses taken at mealtimes.

Drug-induced EPS: **PO** *(Adults):* Initial dosage: 1 mg. Repeat dosage every few hours until symptoms are controlled. Maintenance or prophylactic use: 5 to 15 mg/day.

DIPHENHYDRAMINE (Benadryl)

Parkinsonism and drug-induced EPS/Motion sickness/Allergy reactions: **PO** *(Adults and children ≥12 years):* 25 to 50 mg every 4 to 6 hours. Maximum dosage: 300 mg/day. **IM/IV** *(Adults):* 10 to 50 mg IV or 100 mg IM. Maximum daily dose: 400 mg.

    Children 6 to 12 years: **PO:** 12.5 to 25 mg every 4 to 6 hours, not to exceed 150 mg/day.

Insomnia: **PO** *(Adults and children ≥12 years):* 50 mg at bedtime.

Cough suppressant: *(Adults and children ≥12 years):* **PO Liquid:** 25 to 50 mg every 4 hours, not to exceed 300 mg/day. **PO Syrup:** 25 mg every 4 hours, not to exceed 150 mg/day.

    Children 6 to 12 yr: **PO Liquid:** 12.5 to 25 mg every 4 hours, not to exceed 150 mg/day. **PO Syrup:** 12.5 mg every 4 hours, not to exceed 75 mg/day.

    Children 2 to 6 yr: **PO Syrup:** 6.25 mg every 4 hours, not to exceed 25 mg/day.

■ DOPAMINERGIC AGONISTS
Examples

Generic (Trade) Name	Half-life (hr)	Indications	Available Forms (mg)
Amantadine (Osmolex ER)	10–25	• Parkinsonism • Drug-induced EPS • Prophylaxis and treatment of influenza A viral infection	TABS, CAPS: 100 SYRUP: 50/5 mL ER: 129, 193, 258
Bromocriptine (Parlodel)	8–20	• Parkinsonism • Hyperprolactinemia • Acromegaly • Neuroleptic malignant syndrome	TABS: 2.5 CAPS: 5

Action
- Amantadine increases dopamine at the receptor either by releasing intact striatal dopamine stores or by blocking neuronal dopamine reuptake. It also inhibits the replication of influenza A virus isolates from each of the subtypes.
- Bromocriptine increases dopamine by direct stimulation of dopamine receptors.

Contraindications and Precautions
Contraindicated in:

AMANTADINE: • Hypersensitivity to the drug • Pregnancy, lactation, and in children under 1 year (safety not established) • Angle-closure glaucoma

BROMOCRIPTINE: • Hypersensitivity to this drug, other ergot alkaloids, or sulfites (contained in some preparations) • Uncontrolled hypertension • Pregnancy, lactation, and children (has been used in children ages 11 to 16 years in the treatment of prolactin-secreting adenomas)

Use Cautiously in: • Hepatic or renal impairment • Uncontrolled psychiatric disturbances • History of congestive heart failure, myocardial infarction, or ventricular arrhythmia • Elderly or debilitated patients • Orthostatic hypotension

AMANTADINE: • Patients with a history of seizures • Concurrent use of CNS stimulants

BROMOCRIPTINE: • Patients with history of peptic ulcer or gastrointestinal bleeding

Adverse Reactions and Side Effects
Amantadine
- Nausea
- Dizziness

- Insomnia; somnolence
- Depression; anxiety
- Hallucinations
- Arrhythmia; tachycardia
- Dry mouth
- Blurred vision

Bromocriptine

- Nausea and vomiting
- Headache; dizziness; drowsiness
- Orthostatic hypotension
- Confusion
- Constipation; diarrhea
- Skin mottling
- Exacerbation of Raynaud's syndrome
- Ataxia

Interactions

The effects of:	Are increased by:	Are decreased by:	Concurrent use may result in:
Amantadine	Quinidine, quinine, triamterene, thiazide diuretics, trimethoprim/ sulfamethoxazole, thioridazine		Potentiation of anticholinergic side effects with anticholinergic agents; increased effects of CNS stimulants with concurrent use.
Bromocriptine	Erythromycin, protease inhibitors, isometheptene, phenylpropanolamine (and other sympathomimetics)	Phenothiazines (and other antipsychotics), metoclopramide	Additive vasoconstriction with triptans; increased plasma levels of probenecid, methyldopa, salicylates, and sulfonamides

Route and Dosage

AMANTADINE

Parkinsonism: **PO** *(Adults):* 100 mg 1 to 2 times/day (up to 400 mg/day).

Drug-induced EPS: **PO** *(Adults):* 100 mg twice daily (up to 300 mg/day in divided doses). Extended release (Osmolex ER), 129 mg daily, maximum daily dose 322 mg.

Influenza A viral infection: **PO** *(Adults and children >12 yr):* 200 mg/day as a single dose or 100 mg twice daily.
　　Children 9 to 12 years: **PO:** 100 mg twice daily.
　　Children 1 to 9 years: **PO:** 4.4 to 8.8 mg/kg/day, not to exceed 150 mg/day.

BROMOCRIPTINE (Parlodel)

Parkinsonism: **PO** *(Adults):* Initial dose: 1.25 mg twice daily with meals. May increase dosage every 2 to 4 weeks by 2.5 mg/day with meals. Assessments are advised at 2-week intervals to ensure that the lowest dosage producing an optimal therapeutic response is not exceeded.

Hyperprolactinemia: **PO** *(Adults and children ≥16 years):* Initial dose: 1.25 to 2.5 mg/day with meals. May increase by 2.5 mg every 2 to 7 days. Usual therapeutic dosage range: 2.5 to 15 mg/day.

> *Children 11 to 15 years:* **PO:** Initial dosage: 1.25 to 2.5 mg/day. Dosage may be increased as tolerated until a therapeutic response is achieved. Therapeutic dosage range: 2.5 to 10 mg/day.

Acromegaly: **PO** *(Adults):* Initial dosage: 1.25 to 2.5 mg for 3 days (with food) at bedtime. May increase by 1.25 to 2.5 mg/day every 3 to 7 days. Usual therapeutic dosage range: 20 to 30 mg/day. Maximum dosage: 100 mg/day.

Neuroleptic malignant syndrome: **PO** *(Adults):* 5 mg every 4 hours.

■ ANTIDOPAMINERGIC AGENTS

Generic (Trade) Name	Half-life (hr)	Indications	Available Forms (mg)
Valbenazine (Ingrezza) (FDA approved 2017)	15–22	• Adults with tardive dyskinesia	CAPS: 40, 80
Deutetrabenazine (Austedo) (FDA approved 2017)	9–10	• Adults with tardive dyskinesia or Huntington's chorea	TABS: 6,9, and 12

Action

• The mechanism of action is unknown, but valbenazine is known to cause reversible reduction of dopamine release by selectively inhibiting presynaptic human vesicular monoamine transporter type 2 (VMAT2), a transporter that regulates monoamine uptake from the cytoplasm to the synaptic vesicle for storage and release. The precise mechanism by which deutetrabenazine exerts its effects in the treatment of tardive dyskinesia and chorea in patients with Huntington's disease is unknown but is believed to be related to its effect as a reversible depletor of monoamines (such as dopamine, serotonin, norepinephrine, and histamine) from nerve terminals. The major circulating metabolites (a-dihydrotetrabenazine [HTBZ] and b-HTBZ) of deutetrabenazine, are reversible inhibitors of VMAT2.

Contraindications and Precautions

Contraindicated in: Deutetrabenazine is contraindicated when taking reserpine, MAOIs, tetrabenazine or valbenazine, in patients with hepatic impairment, and in patients with Huntington's disease who are suicidal.

Use Cautiously in: • Valbenazine and deutetrabenazine should be avoided in patients with congenital long QT syndrome or with arrhythmias associated with a prolonged QT interval. For patients at increased risk of a prolonged QT interval, assess the QT interval before increasing the dosage. Not recommended for patients with severe renal impairment. Advise not to breastfeed.

Adverse Reactions and Side Effects
• Somnolence
• QT prolongation

Interactions
Dose adjustments due to drug interactions:

Factors	Dose adjustments for valbenazine and deutetrabenazine
Use with monoamine oxidase inhibitors (MAOIs).	Avoid concomitant use with MAOIs.
Use with strong CYP3A4 inducers.	Concomitant use is not recommended.
Use with strong CYP3A4 inhibitors.	Reduce valbenazine dose to 40 mg.
Use with strong CYP2D6 inhibitors.	Consider dose reduction of valbenazine based on tolerability. Deutetrabenazine dose should not exceed 36 mg daily.

Route and Dosage
• The initial dose of valbenazine is 40 mg once daily. After 1 week, increase the dose to the recommended dose of 80 mg once daily. The initial dose of deutetrabenzine is 12 mg once a day (6 mg tablets twice daily) and may be increased by 6 mg weekly up to 48 mg daily.
• Valbenazine can be taken with or without food. Deutetrabenazine should be taken with food and should be swallowed whole (not crushed, chewed, or broken).
• The recommended dose of valbenazine for patients with moderate or severe hepatic impairment is 40 mg once daily. The use of deutetrabenazine in patients with hepatic impairment is contraindicated.
• Consider dose reduction based on tolerability in known CYP2D6 poor metabolizers.

■ NURSING DIAGNOSES RELATED TO ANTIPARKINSONIAN AGENTS

1. Risk for injury related to symptoms of Parkinson's disease or drug-induced EPS.

2. Hyperthermia related to anticholinergic effect of decreased sweating.
3. Activity intolerance related to side effects of drowsiness, dizziness, ataxia, weakness, confusion.
4. Deficient knowledge related to medication regimen.

■ NURSING IMPLICATIONS FOR ANTIPARKINSONIAN AGENTS

The plan of care should include monitoring for the following side effects from antiparkinsonian medications. Nursing implications related to each side effect are designated by an asterisk (*).

1. Anticholinergic effects. These side effects are identical to those produced by antipsychotic drugs. Taking both medications compounds these effects. For this reason, the physician may elect to prescribe an antiparkinsonian agent only at the onset of EPS rather than as routine adjunctive therapy.
   a. Dry mouth
      * Offer sugarless candy or gum, ice, frequent sips of water.
      * Ensure that the patient practices strict oral hygiene.
   b. Blurred vision
      * Explain that symptom will most likely subside after a few weeks.
      * Offer to assist with tasks requiring visual acuity.
   c. Constipation
      * Order foods high in fiber; encourage increase in physical activity and fluid intake, if not contraindicated.
   d. Paralytic ileus
      * A rare but potentially very serious side effect of anticholinergic drugs. Monitor for abdominal distension, absent bowel sounds, nausea, vomiting, epigastric pain.
      * Report any of these symptoms to physician immediately.
   e. Urinary retention
      * Instruct the patient to report any difficulty urinating; monitor intake and output.
   f. Tachycardia, decreased sweating, elevated temperature
      * Assess vital signs each shift; document and report significant changes to physician.
      * Ensure that the patient remains in cool environment, because the body is unable to cool itself naturally with this medication.
2. Nausea, gastrointestinal (GI) upset
   * May administer tablets or capsules with food to minimize GI upset.
3. Sedation, drowsiness, dizziness
   * Discuss with physician possibility of administering drug at bedtime.

* Discuss with physician possible decrease in dosage or order for less-sedating drug.
* Instruct the patient not to drive or use dangerous equipment while experiencing sedation or dizziness.

4. Exacerbation of psychoses
   * Assess for signs of loss of contact with reality.
   * Intervene during a hallucination; talk about real people and real events; reorient the patient to reality.
   * Stay with the patient during period of agitation and delirium; remain calm and reassure the patient of his or her safety.
   * Discuss with physician possible decrease in dosage or change in medication.

5. Orthostatic hypotension
   * Instruct the patient to rise slowly from a lying or sitting position; monitor blood pressure (lying and standing) each shift; document and report significant changes.

6. Risk for suicide.
   * Patients taking deutetrabenazine should be assessed regularly for evidence of worsening depression or suicidal ideation.

■ PATIENT/FAMILY EDUCATION RELATED TO ALL ANTIPARKINSONIAN AGENTS

* Take the medication with food if GI upset occurs.
* Use caution when driving or operating dangerous machinery. Drowsiness and dizziness can occur.
* Do not stop taking the drug abruptly. To do so might produce unpleasant withdrawal symptoms.
* Report occurrence of any of the following symptoms to the physician immediately: pain or tenderness in area in front of ear; extreme dryness of mouth; difficulty urinating; abdominal pain; constipation; fast, pounding heartbeat; rash; visual disturbances; mental changes.
* Rise slowly from a sitting or lying position to prevent a sudden drop in blood pressure.
* Stay inside in air-conditioned room when weather is very hot. Perspiration is decreased with antiparkinsonian agents, and the body cannot cool itself as well. There is greater susceptibility to heat stroke. Inform physician if air-conditioned housing is not available.
* Take frequent sips of water, chew sugarless gum, or suck on hard candy if dry mouth is a problem. Good oral care (frequent brushing, flossing) is very important.
* Do not drink alcohol while on antiparkinsonian therapy.

- Do not consume other medications (including over-the-counter products) without physician's approval. Many medications contain substances that interact with antiparkinsonian agents in a way that may be harmful.
- Be aware of possible risks of taking antiparkinsonian agents during pregnancy. Safe use during pregnancy and lactation has not been fully established. It is thought that antiparkinsonian agents readily cross the placental barrier; if so, fetus could experience adverse effects of the drug. Inform physician immediately if pregnancy occurs, is suspected, or is planned.
- Be aware of side effects of antiparkinsonian agents. Refer to written materials furnished by health-care providers for safe self-administration.
- Continue to take medication, even if feeling well and as though it is not needed. Symptoms may return if medication is discontinued.
- Carry card or other identification at all times describing medications being taken.

@ INTERNET REFERENCES

- www.mentalhealth.com
- https://www.nimh.nih.gov/index.shtml
- https://www.nimh.nih.gov/health/topics/mental-health-medications/index.shtml
- https://medlineplus.gov/druginformation.html
- https://www.drugguide.com/ddo (Davis's Drug Guide)
- http://centerwatch.com

CHAPTER 28

Sedative-Hypnotics

■ BENZODIAZEPINES
Examples

Generic (Trade) Name	Controlled Substance Schedule	Half-life (hr)	Indications	Available Forms (mg)
Estazolam	C-IV	8–28	• Insomnia	**TABS:** 1, 2
Flurazepam	C-IV	2–3 (active metabolite 47–100)	• Insomnia	**CAPS:** 15, 30
Temazepam (Restoril)	C-IV	9–15	• Insomnia	**CAPS:** 7.5, 15, 22.5, 30
Triazolam (Halcion)	C-IV	1.5–5.5	• Insomnia	**TABS:** 0.125, 0.25

Action
- Potentiate gamma aminobutyric acid (GABA) neuronal inhibition.
- The sedative effects involve GABA receptors in the limbic, neocortical, and mesencephalic reticular systems.

Contraindications and Precautions

Contraindicated in: • Hypersensitivity to these or other benzodiazepines • Pregnancy and lactation • Respiratory depression and sleep apnea • *(Triazolam):* concurrent use with ketoconazole, itraconazole, or nefazodone, medications that impair the metabolism of triazolam by cytochrome P450 3A (CYP3A) • *(Flurazepam):* Children younger than age 15 • *(Estazolam, temazepam, triazolam):* Children younger than age 18 • Benzodiazepines should not be combined with opiate medications. Opioids should be used with benzodiazepines only when other alternatives are indequate (**black-box warning**)

Use Cautiously in: • Elderly and debilitated patients • Hepatic or renal dysfunction • Patients with history of drug abuse and dependence • Depressed or suicidal patients • Patients with compromised respiratory function

Adverse Reactions and Side Effects

- Drowsiness
- Headache
- Confusion
- Lethargy
- Tolerance
- Physical and psychological dependence
- Potentiates the effects of other central nervous system (CNS) depressants
- May aggravate symptoms in depressed persons
- Palpitations; tachycardia; hypotension
- Paradoxical excitement
- Dry mouth
- Nausea and vomiting
- Blood dyscrasias

Interactions

- Additive CNS depression with **alcohol** and other **CNS depressants.**
- Decreased clearance and increased effects of benzodiazepines with **cimetidine, oral contraceptives, disulfiram,** and **isoniazid.**
- Increased effects of benzodiazepines with **azole antifungals** and **nefazodone** (contraindicated with **triazolam**).
- More rapid onset or more prolonged benzodiazepine effect with **probenecid.**
- Increased clearance and decreased half-life of benzodiazepines with **rifampin.**
- Increased benzodiazepine clearance with **cigarette smoking.**
- Decreased pharmacological effects of benzodiazepines with **theophylline, carbamazepine,** and **St. John's wort.**
- Increased bioavailability of triazolam with **macrolides.**
- Benzodiazepines may increase serum levels of **digoxin** and **phenytoin** and increase risk of toxicity.
- Potentiation of respiratory depression with **methadone.**

Route and Dosage

ESTAZOLAM

Insomnia: **PO** *(Adults):* 1 to 2 mg at bedtime.
    Healthy elderly: **PO:** 1 mg at bedtime. Increase with caution.
    Debilitated or small elderly patients: **PO:** 0.5 mg at bedtime.

FLURAZEPAM

Insomnia: **PO** *(Adults):* 15 to 30 mg at bedtime.
    Elderly or debilitated: **PO:** 15 mg at bedtime.

TEMAZEPAM (Restoril)

Insomnia: **PO** *(Adults):* 15 to 30 mg at bedtime; 7.5 mg may be sufficient for some patients.
    Elderly or debilitated: **PO:** 7.5 mg at bedtime.

TRIAZOLAM (Halcion)

Insomnia: **PO** *(Adults):* 0.125 to 0.5 mg at bedtime.
    Elderly or debilitated: **PO:** 0.125 to 0.25 mg at bedtime.

■ BARBITURATES
Examples

Generic (Trade) Name	Controlled Substance Schedule	Half-life (hr)	Indications	Available Forms (mg)
Amobarbital	C-II	16–40	• Sedation • Insomnia	**POWDER FOR INJECTION:** 500/vial
Butabarbital (Butisol)	C-III	66–140	• Sedation • Insomnia	**TABS:** 15, 30, 50 **ELIXIR:** 30/5 mL
Pentobarbital (Nembutal)	C-II	15–50	• Insomnia • Preanesthetic in pediatric patients • Acute convulsive episodes	**INJ:** 50/mL
Phenobarbital (Luminal)	C-IV	53–118	• Sedation • Anticonvulsant	**TABS:** 15, 16, 30, 60, 90, 100 **CAPS:** 16 **ELIXIR:** 15/5 mL; 20/5 mL **INJ (MG/ML):** 30, 60, 65, 130
Secobarbital (Seconal)	C-II	15–40	• Preoperative sedation • Insomnia	**CAPS:** 100

Action

- Depress the sensory cortex, decrease motor activity, and alter cerebellar function.
- All levels of CNS depression can occur, from mild sedation to hypnosis to coma to death.
- Can induce anesthesia in sufficiently high therapeutic doses.

Contraindications and Precautions

Contraindicated in: • Hypersensitivity to barbiturates • Severe hepatic, renal, cardiac, or respiratory disease • Individuals with history of drug abuse or dependence • Porphyria • Uncontrolled severe pain • Intra-arterial or subcutaneous administration • Lactation

Use Cautiously in: • Elderly and debilitated patients • Patients with hepatic, renal, cardiac, or respiratory impairment • Depressed or suicidal patients • Pregnancy • Children

Adverse Reactions and Side Effects

- Bradycardia
- Hypotension
- Somnolence
- Agitation
- Confusion
- Nausea, vomiting
- Constipation
- Skin rashes
- Respiratory depression
- Physical and psychological dependence

Interactions

- Additive CNS depression with **alcohol** and other **CNS depressants.**
- Decreased effects of barbiturates with **rifampin.**
- Increased effects of barbiturates with **monoamine oxidase inhibitors (MAOIs)** or **valproic acid.**
- Decreased effects of the following drugs with concurrent use of barbiturates: **anticoagulants, beta blockers, carbamazepine, clonazepam, oral contraceptives, corticosteroids, digitoxin, doxorubicin, doxycycline, felodipine, fenoprofen, griseofulvin, metronidazole, phenylbutazone, quinidine, theophylline, chloramphenicol,** and **verapamil.**
- Concomitant use with **methoxyflurane** may enhance renal toxicity.

Route and Dosage

AMOBARBITAL

Sedation: **IM** *(Adults):* 30 to 50 mg, 2 or 3 times/day.

Insomnia: **IM** *(Adults):* 65 to 200 mg at bedtime.

NOTE: Do not inject a volume >5 mL IM at any one site regardless of drug concentration. Tissue irritation can occur.

BUTABARBITAL (Butisol)

Daytime sedation: **PO** *(Adults):* 15 to 30 mg, 3 or 4 times/day.

Insomnia: **PO** *(Adults):* 50 to 100 mg at bedtime.

Preoperative sedation: **PO** *(Adults):* 50 to 100 mg, 60 to 90 minutes before surgery.
 Children: **PO:** 2 to 6 mg/kg; maximum dose: 100 mg.

PENTOBARBITAL (Nembutal)

Insomnia: **IM** *(Adults):* Usual dosage: 150 to 200 mg.

Preanesthetic sedation: **IM** *(Children):* 2 to 6 mg/kg, not to exceed 100 mg.

NOTE: Inject deeply into large muscle mass. Do not exceed a volume of 5 mL at any one site because of possible tissue irritation.

PHENOBARBITAL (Luminal)

Sedation: **PO, IM** *(Adults):* 30 to 120 mg/day in 2 to 3 divided doses not to exceed 400 mg/day.
  Children: **PO:** 2 mg/kg 3 times daily.

Preoperative sedation: **IM** *(Adults):* 100 to 200 mg, 60 to 90 minutes before the procedure.
  Children: **PO, IM, or IV:** 1 to 3 mg/kg 60 to 90 minutes before the procedure.

Insomnia: **PO, IM, or IV** *(Adults):* 100 to 320 mg at bedtime.

SECOBARBITAL (Seconal)

Preoperative sedation: **PO** *(Adults):* 200 to 300 mg 1 to 2 hours before surgery.
  Children: **PO:** 2 to 6 mg/kg, not to exceed 100 mg.

Insomnia: **PO** *(Adults):* 100 mg at bedtime.

■ MISCELLANEOUS (NONBARBITURATE)
Examples

Generic (Trade) Name	Controlled Substance Schedule	Half-life (hr)	Indications	Available Forms (mg)
Chloral hydrate	C-IV	7–10	• Insomnia • Preoperative sedation • Alcohol withdrawal	**CAPS:** 500 **SYRUP:** 250/5 mL; 500/5 mL
Eszopiclone (Lunesta)	C-IV	6	• Insomnia	**TABS:** 1, 2, 3
Ramelteon (Rozerem)	Not controlled	1–2.6	• Insomnia	**TABS:** 8
Suvorexant (Belsomra)	C-IV	12	• Insomnia	**TABS:** 5, 10, 15, 20
Zaleplon	C-IV	1	• Insomnia	**CAPS:** 5, 10
Zolpidem (Ambien)	C-IV	2–3	• Insomnia	**TABS:** 5, 10 **TABS (CR):** 6.25, 12.5 **TABS (SUBLINGUAL):** 1.75, 3.5, 5, 10 **SPRAY SOLUTION (LINGUAL):** 5 per actuation

Action

Zolpidem and Zaleplon

- Bind to GABA receptors in the central nervous system. Appear to be selective for the omega1-receptor subtype.

Eszopiclone

- Action as a hypnotic is unclear but is thought to interact with GABA-receptor complexes near benzodiazepine receptors.

Chloral hydrate

- Action unknown. Produces a calming effect through depression of the central nervous system.
- Has generally been replaced by safer and more effective agents.

Ramelteon

- Ramelteon is a melatonin receptor agonist with high affinity for melatonin MT1 and MT2 receptors.

Suvorexant

- Antagonizes the effects of orexins A and B, naturally occurring neuropeptides that promote wakefulness, by binding to their receptors.

Contraindications and Precautions

Contraindicated in: • Hypersensitivity • In combination with other CNS depressants • Pregnancy and lactation

Zolpidem, zaleplon, eszopiclone, ramelteon, suvorexant: • Children (safety not established)

Zolpidem: • May cause injury or death related to complex sleep behaviors such as sleepwalking, sleep driving, or other behaviors while not fully awake (**black-box warning**) • Contraindicated in patients with a history of complex sleep behaviors • Avoid use with opioids; may cause respiratory depression and death (**black-box warning**)

Chloral hydrate: • Severe hepatic, renal, or cardiac impairment • Esophagitis, gastritis, or peptic ulcer disease

Ramelteon: • Severe hepatic function impairment • Concomitantly with fluvoxamine

Use Cautiously in: • Elderly or debilitated patients • Depressed or suicidal patients • Patients with history of drug abuse or dependence • Patients with hepatic, renal, or respiratory dysfunction • Patients susceptible to acute intermittent porphyria (**chloral hydrate**)

Suvorexant: **Contraindicated in:** • Narcolepsy • Concurrent use of strong inhibitors of CYP3A • Severe hepatic impairment

Use Cautiously in: • History of substance abuse or drug dependence • Concurrent use of moderate inhibitors of CYP3A (dose ↓ recommended) • Obese patients (↑ levels, especially in women, dose ↓ may be warranted) • History of or concurrent psychiatric diagnoses • Underlying pulmonary disease • Use during pregnancy only if potential benefit justifies potential fetal risk • Lactation—use cautiously if breast feeding

Adverse Reactions and Side Effects

- Headache
- Drowsiness
- Dizziness
- Lethargy
- Amnesia
- Nausea
- Dry mouth
- Rash
- Paradoxical excitement
- Physical and/or psychological dependence
- Complex sleep-related behaviors, such as driving while asleep
- Abnormal thinking and behavioral changes

Chloral hydrate, eszopiclone: • Unpleasant taste

Interactions

The effects of:	Are increased by:	Are decreased by:	Concurrent use may result in:
Chloral Hydrate	**Alcohol** and other **CNS depressants,** including **antihistamines, antidepressants, opioids, sedative-hypnotics,** and **antipsychotics**		Increased effects of **oral anticoagulants;** symptoms of sweating, hot flashes, tachycardia, hypertension, weakness, and nausea with **IV furosemide;** decreased effects of **phenytoin**
Eszopiclone	Drugs that inhibit the CYP3A4 enzyme system, including **ketoconazole, itraconazole, clarithromycin, nefazodone, ritonavir,** and **nelfinavir**	**Lorazepam;** drugs that induce the CYP3A4 enzyme system, such as **rifampin;** taking eszopiclone with or immediately after a **high-fat or heavy meal**	Additive CNS depression with **alcohol** and other **CNS depressants,** including **antihistamines, antidepressants, opioids, sedative-hypnotics,** and **antipsychotics;** decreased effects of **lorazepam**

The effects of:	Are increased by:	Are decreased by:	Concurrent use may result in:
Ramelteon	**Alcohol, azole antifungals,** and **fluvoxamine**	**Rifampin;** taking ramelteon with or immediately after a **high-fat or heavy meal**	
Suvorexant	• **CNS depressants,** including **alcohol** increase risk of CNS depression, sleep-driving, and other complex behaviors while not fully awake; **strong inhibitors of CYP3A,** including **boceprevir, clarithromycin, conivaptan, indinavir, itraconazole, ketoconazole, nefazodone, nelfinavir, posaconazole, ritonavir, saquinavir,** and **telithromycin** increase risk of excessive sedation and should be avoided.	**Strong CYP3A inducers**	• Increased risk of sedation with **strong inhibitors of CYP3A,** including **boceprevir, clarithromycin, conivaptan, indinavir, itraconazole, ketoconazole, nefazodone, nelfinavir, posaconazole, ritonavir, saquinavir,** and **telithromycin** • Increased sedation with **moderate inhibitors of CYP3A,** including **aprepitant, atazanavir, ciprofloxacin, diltiazem, erythromycin, fluconazole, fosamprenavir, imatinib,** and **verapamil** (↓ dose recommended)
Zaleplon	**Cimetidine**	Drugs that induce the CYP3A4 enzyme system, including **rifampin, phenytoin, carbamazepine,** and **phenobarbital;** taking zaleplon with or immediately after a **high-fat or heavy meal**	Additive CNS depression with **alcohol** and other **CNS depressants,** including **antihistamines, antidepressants, opioids, sedative-hypnotics,** and **antipsychotics**
Zolpidem	**Ritonavir, selective serotonin reuptake inhibitors**	**Flumazenil; rifampin;** administration with **food**	Risk of life-threatening cardiac arrhythmias with **amiodarone;** additive CNS depression with **alcohol** and other **CNS depressants,** including **antihistamines, antidepressants, opioids, sedative-hypnotics,** and **antipsychotics**

Route and Dosage

CHLORAL HYDRATE

Daytime sedation: **PO** *(Adults):* 250 mg 3 times a day after meals. Maximum daily dose: 2 g.

    Children: **PO**: 25 to 50 mg/kg/day given in divided doses every 6 to 8 hours, not to exceed 500 mg per single dose.

Preoperative sedation: **PO** *(Adults):* 500 to 1000 mg 30 minutes before surgery.

Preprocedural sedation: **PO** *(Children):* 50 to 75 mg/kg 30 to 60 minutes before procedure. May repeat the dose in 30 minutes if needed. Single dose should not exceed 1 g total for infants or 2 g total for children.

Insomnia: **PO** *(Adults)*: 500 mg to 1 g 15 to 30 minutes before bedtime.

    Children: **PO**: 50 mg/kg/day, up to 1 g per single dose. May give in divided doses.

Alcohol withdrawal: **PO** *(Adults):* 500 mg to 1 g repeated at 6-hour intervals if needed. Maximum daily dose: 2 g.

ESZOPICLONE (Lunesta)

Insomnia: **PO** *(Adults):* 2 mg immediately before bedtime; may be increased to 3 mg if needed (3-mg dose is more effective for sleep maintenance).

    Elderly patients: **PO**: 1 mg immediately before bedtime for patients who have difficulty falling asleep; 2 mg immediately before bedtime for patients who have difficulty staying asleep.

RAMELTEON (Rozerem)

Insomnia: **PO** *(Adults):* 8 mg within 30 minutes of bedtime. It is recommended that ramelteon not be taken with or immediately after a high-fat meal.

SUVOREXANT (Belsomra)

    PO *(Adults):* 10 mg within 30 minutes of going to bed; if well tolerated but not optimally effective, dose may be increased next night, not to exceed 20 mg (dose may not be repeated on a single night and should be taken when at least 7 hours of sleep time is anticipated before planned awakening). *Concurrent use of moderate inhibitors of CYP3A*—5 mg initially; dose may be ↑ to 10 mg if lower dose is tolerated but not optimally effective. Lowest effective dose should be used.

ZALEPLON

Insomnia: **PO** *(Adults):* 10 mg (range 5 to 20 mg) at bedtime.

    Elderly and debilitated patients: **PO**: 5 mg at bedtime, not to exceed 10 mg.

ZOLPIDEM (Ambien)

Insomnia: **PO** *(Adults):* 10 mg at bedtime. *Extended-release tablets:* 12.5 mg at bedtime.

    Elderly or debilitated patients and patients with hepatic impairment: **PO:** 5 mg at bedtime. *Extended-release tablets:* 6.25 mg at bedtime.

■ NURSING DIAGNOSES RELATED TO ALL SEDATIVE-HYPNOTICS

1. Risk for injury related to abrupt withdrawal from long-term use or decreased mental alertness caused by residual sedation.
2. Disturbed sleep pattern/insomnia related to situational crises, physical condition, or severe level of anxiety.
3. Risk for activity intolerance related to side effects of lethargy, drowsiness, dizziness.
4. Risk for acute confusion related to action of the medication on the central nervous system.

■ NURSING IMPLICATIONS FOR SEDATIVE-HYPNOTICS

The nursing care plan should include monitoring for the following side effects from sedative-hypnotics. Nursing implications related to each side effect are designated by an asterisk (*):

1. **Drowsiness, dizziness, lethargy** (most common side effects)
   * Instruct the patient not to drive or operate dangerous machinery while taking the medication.
2. **Tolerance, physical and psychological addiction**
   * Instruct the patient to take the medication exactly as directed. Do not take more than the amount prescribed because of the habit-forming potential. Recommended for short-term use only. Abrupt withdrawal after long-term use may result in serious, even life-threatening, symptoms. *Exception:* **Ramelteon** is not considered to be a drug of abuse or dependence. It is not classified as a controlled substance. It has, however, been associated with cases of rebound insomnia after abrupt discontinuation following long-term use.
3. **Potentiates the effects of other CNS depressants**
   * Instruct the patient not to drink alcohol or take other medications that depress the CNS when taking this medication.
4. **May aggravate symptoms in depressed persons**
   * Assess mood daily.
   * Take necessary precautions for potential suicide.
5. **Orthostatic hypotension; palpitations; tachycardia**
   * Monitor lying and standing blood pressure and pulse every shift.
   * Instruct the patient to arise slowly from a lying or sitting position.

* Monitor pulse rate and rhythm and report any significant change to the physician.
6. **Paradoxical excitement**
   * Withhold drug and notify the physician.
7. **Dry mouth**
   * Have the patient take frequent sips of water, ice chips, suck on hard candy, or chew sugarless gum.
8. **Nausea and vomiting**
   * Have the patient take drug with food or milk (unless it is a drug in which taking with food is not recommended).
9. **Blood dyscrasias**
   * Symptoms of sore throat, fever, malaise, easy bruising, or unusual bleeding should be reported to the physician immediately.
10. **Abnormal thinking and behavioral changes**
    * Unusual changes in behavior, including aggressiveness, hallucinations, and suicidal ideation, have been reported. Certain complex behaviors, such as sleep-driving, preparing and eating food, and making phone calls, with amnesia for the behavior, have occurred. Although a direct correlation to the behavior with use of sedative-hypnotics cannot be made, the emergence of any new behavioral sign or symptom of concern requires careful and immediate evaluation.

■ PATIENT/FAMILY EDUCATION RELATED TO ALL SEDATIVE-HYPNOTICS

* Do not drive or operate dangerous machinery. Drowsiness and dizziness can occur.
* Do not stop taking the drug abruptly after prolonged use. Can produce serious withdrawal symptoms, such as depression, insomnia, anxiety, abdominal and muscle cramps, tremors, vomiting, sweating, convulsions, and delirium.
* Do not consume other CNS depressants (including alcohol).
* Do not take nonprescription medication without approval from physician.
* Rise slowly from the sitting or lying position to prevent a sudden drop in blood pressure.
* Report to physician immediately symptoms of sore throat, fever, malaise, easy bruising, unusual bleeding, motor restlessness, or any thinking or behavior that is outside the usual range of thinking or characterization for the individual taking the medication.

- Be aware of risks of taking these drugs during pregnancy. (Congenital malformations have been associated with use during the first trimester). If pregnancy is suspected or planned, notify the physician of the desirability to discontinue the drug.
- Be aware of possible side effects. Refer to written materials furnished by health-care providers regarding the correct method of self-administration.
- Carry card or piece of paper at all times stating names of medications being taken.
- Stop taking the drug immediately and notify the physician if an episode of complex sleeping behavior or amnesia for events occurs while taking the drug (zolpidem).

@ INTERNET REFERENCES

- www.mentalhealth.com
- https://www.nimh.nih.gov/index.shtml
- https://www.nimh.nih.gov/health/topics/mental-health-medications/index.shtml
- https://medlineplus.gov/druginformation.html
- https://www.drugguide.com/ddo (Davis's Drug Guide)
- www.centerwatch.com

CHAPTER 29

Agents Used to Treat Attention-Deficit/ Hyperactivity Disorder

■ CENTRAL NERVOUS SYSTEM (CNS) STIMULANTS (AMPHETAMINES)

Examples

Generic (Trade) Name	Controlled Substance Schedule	Half-life (hr)	Indications	Available Forms (mg)
Amphetamine (Adzenys XR ODT)	C-II	d-amphetamine: 11 (adult)/ 10 (ped) l-amphetamine: 14 (adult); 11 (ped)	• Attention-deficit/ hyperactivity disorder (ADHD)	**TABS (ER; ORALLY DISINTE-GRATING):** 3.1, 6.3, 9.4, 12.5, 15.7, 18.8
Amphetamine/ dextroamphetamine mixtures (Adderall; Adderall XR)	C-II	9–13	• ADHD • Narcolepsy	**TABS:** 5, 7.5, 10, 12.5, 15, 20, 30 **CAPS (XR):** 5, 10, 15, 20, 25, 30
Dextroamphetamine sulfate (Dexedrine; Dextrostat)	C-II	~12	• ADHD • Narcolepsy	**TABS:** 5, 10 **CAPS (ER):** 5, 10, 15 **ORAL SOLU:** 5 mg/5 mL
Methamphetamine (Desoxyn)	C-II	4–5	• ADHD • Exogenous obesity	**TABS:** 5
Lisdexamfetamine (Vyvanse)	C-II	<1	• ADHD	**CAPS:** 20, 30, 40 50, 60, 70

Action

- Central nervous system (CNS) stimulation is mediated by release of norepinephrine from central noradrenergic neurons in the cerebral cortex, reticular activating system, and brainstem.
- At higher doses, dopamine may be released in the mesolimbic system.
- Action in the treatment of attention-deficit/hyperactivity disorder (ADHD) is unclear. Recent research indicates that their effectiveness in the treatment of hyperactivity disorders is based on the activation of dopamine D_4 receptors in the basal ganglia and thalamus, which depress, rather than enhance, motor activity (Erlij et al, 2012).

Contraindications and Precautions

Contraindicated in: • Advanced arteriosclerosis • Symptomatic cardiovascular disease • Moderate to severe hypertension • Hyperthyroidism • Hypersensitivity or idiosyncrasy to the sympathomimetic amines • Glaucoma • Agitated states • History of drug abuse • During or within 14 days following administration of MAO inhibitors (hypertensive crisis may occur) • Children younger than 3 years (dextroamphetamine; amphetamine; mixtures) • Children younger than 6 years (methamphetamine; lisdexamfetamine) • Pregnancy and lactation

Use Cautiously in: • Patients with mild hypertension • Children with psychoses (may exacerbate symptoms) • Tourette's disorder (may exacerbate tics) • Anorexia • Insomnia • Elderly, debilitated, or asthenic patients • Patients with suicidal or homicidal tendencies

Adverse Reactions and Side Effects

- Overstimulation
- Restlessness
- Dizziness
- Insomnia
- Headache
- Palpitations
- Tachycardia
- Elevation of blood pressure
- Anorexia
- Weight loss
- Dry mouth
- Tolerance
- New or worsened psychiatric symptoms
- Physical and psychological addiction
- Suppression of growth in children (with long-term use)

Interactions

- Increased sensitivity to amphetamines with **furazolidone.**
- Use of amphetamines with **monoamine oxidase inhibitors (MAOIs)** can result in hypertensive crisis.
- Prolonged effects of amphetamines with **urinary alkalinizers.**
- Hastened elimination of amphetamines with **urinary acidifiers.**
- Amphetamines may reverse the hypotensive effects of **guanethidine and other antihypertensives.**
- Concomitant use of amphetamines and **tricyclic antidepressants, selective serotonin reuptake inhibitors (SSRIs), serotonin-norepinephrine reuptake inhibitor (SNRIs), or MAOIs** may result in **serotonin syndrome.**
- Patients with diabetes mellitus who take amphetamines may require **insulin** adjustment.
- **Adrenergic blockers** are inhibited by amphetamines.

Route and Dosage

ADZENYS XR ODT

ADHD: **PO:** Pediatric patients (ages 6 to 17 yr): Starting dose is 6.3 mg once daily in the morning. Maximum dose is 18.8 mg once daily for patients 6 to 12 years and 12.5 mg once daily for patients 13 to 17 years.

    Adults: 12.5 mg once daily in the morning.

AMPHETAMINE/DEXTROAMPHETAMINE MIXTURES
(Adderall; Adderall XR)

ADHD: **PO:** *(Adults and children ≥6 yr):* Initial dose: 5 mg once or twice daily. May be increased in increments of 5 mg at weekly intervals until optimal response is obtained. Maximum dose: 40 mg/day. *Extended-release caps:* Initial dosage: 10 mg once daily in the morning. May increase in increments of 10 mg at weekly intervals. Maximum dose: 30 mg/day.

    Children 3 to 5 years: **PO:** Initial dose: 2.5 mg/day. May increase in increments of 2.5 mg/day at weekly intervals until optimal response is obtained.

Narcolepsy: **PO** *(Adults and children ≥12 years):* Initial dose: 10 mg/day; may increase in increments of 10 mg/day at weekly intervals up to a maximum of 60 mg/day.

    Children 6 to 12 years: **PO:** Narcolepsy is rare in children younger than 12 years. When it does occur, initial dose is 5 mg/day. May increase in increments of 5 mg/day at weekly intervals up to a maximum of 60 mg/day.

DEXTROAMPHETAMINE SULFATE (Dexedrine; Dextrostat)

ADHD: **PO** *(Adults and children ≥6 yr):* Initial dosage: 5 mg once or twice daily. May be increased in increments of 5 mg at weekly intervals. More than 40 mg/day is seldom required. (Sustained-release capsules should not be used as initial therapy.)

> *Children 3 to 5 years:* **PO:** Initial dose: 2.5 mg/day. May increase in increments of 2.5 mg/day at weekly intervals until optimal response is achieved.

Narcolepsy: **PO** *(Adults):* 5 to 60 mg/day in single or divided doses. Sustained-release capsules should not be used as initial therapy.

> *Children ≥12 years:* **PO:** 10 mg/day. May increase by 10 mg/day at weekly intervals until response is obtained or 60 mg is reached.

> *Children 6 to 12 years:* **PO:** 5 mg/day. May increase by 5 mg/day at weekly intervals until response is obtained or 60 mg is reached.

METHAMPHETAMINE (Desoxyn)

ADHD: **PO** *(Adults and children ≥6 yr):* 5 mg once or twice daily. May increase in increments of 5 mg at weekly intervals. Usual effective dose is 20 to 25 mg/day in divided doses.

Exogenous obesity: **PO** *(Adults and children ≥12 yr):* Usual dosage: One 5 mg tablet taken 30 minutes before each meal.

LISDEXAMFETAMINE (Vyvanse)

ADHD: **PO** *(Adults and children ≥6 yr):* Initial dosage: 30 mg once daily in the morning. Dosage may be increased in increments of 10 or 20 mg/day at weekly intervals up to a maximum of 70 mg/day.

■ CNS STIMULANTS (MISCELLANEOUS AGENTS)
Examples

Generic (Trade) Name	Controlled Substance Schedule	Half-life (hr)	Indications	Available Forms (mg)
Dexmethylphenidate (Focalin; Focalin XR)	C-II	2.2	• ADHD	**TABS:** 2.5, 5, 10 **CAPS (ER):** 5, 10, 15, 20, 25, 30, 35, 40
Methylphenidate (Ritalin; Ritalin-SR; Ritalin LA; Methylin; Methylin ER; Metadate ER; Metadate CD; Concerta; Daytrana; Quillivant XR)	C-II	2–4	• ADHD • Narcolepsy (except Concerta, Metadate CD, and Ritalin LA)	**TABS (IMMEDIATE RELEASE [METHYLIN; RITALIN]):** 5, 10, 20 **CHEWABLE TABS (METHYLIN):** 2.5, 5, 10 **TABS (ER [METADATE ER; METHYLIN ER]):** 10, 20 **TABS (ER [CONCERTA]):** 18, 27, 36, 54 **TABS (SR [RITALIN-SR]):** 20

(Continued)

Generic (Trade) Name	Controlled Substance Schedule	Half-life (hr)	Indications	Available Forms (mg)
				CAPS (ER [METADATE CD; RITALIN LA]): 10, 20, 30, 40, (50, 60—*METADATE CD* ONLY)
				ORAL SOLU (METHYLIN): 5/5 mL, 10/5 mL
				TRANSDERMAL PATCH (DAYTRANA): 10, 15, 20, 30 (based on 9-hr delivery system)
				ORAL SUSPENSION (ER [QUILLIVANT XR]): 5/mL

ER, CD, LA = extended release forms; SR = sustained release.

Actions

- Dexmethylphenidate blocks the reuptake of norepinephrine and dopamine into the presynaptic neuron and increases the release of these monoamines into the extraneuronal space.
- Methylphenidate activates the brainstem arousal system and cortex to produce its stimulant effect.
- Recent research indicates that the effectiveness of CNS stimulants in the treatment of hyperactivity disorders is based on the activation of dopamine D_4 receptors in the basal ganglia and thalamus, which depress, rather than enhance, motor activity (Erlij et al., 2012).

Contraindications and Precautions

Contraindicated in: • Hypersensitivity • Pregnancy, lactation, and children younger than 6 years (safety has not been established) • Patients with marked anxiety, tension, or agitation • Glaucoma • Hyperthyroidism • Motor tics or family history or diagnosis of Tourette's syndrome • During or within 14 days of treatment with MAOIs (hypertensive crisis can occur) • Patients with structural cardiac abnormalities, cardiomyopathy, arrhythmias, recent myocardial infarction, or other serious cardiac problems • Patients with preexisting psychotic disorder

Use Cautiously in: • Patients with history of seizure disorder and/or EEG abnormalities • Hypertension • History of drug or alcohol dependence • Emotionally unstable patients • Renal or hepatic insufficiency • Diabetes mellitus

Adverse Reactions and Side Effects
- Headache
- Nausea
- Rhinitis
- Fever
- Anorexia
- Insomnia
- Tachycardia; palpitations; hypertension
- Nervousness
- Abdominal pain
- Growth suppression in children (with long-term use)
- Skin redness or itching at site of transdermal patch *(Daytrana)*

Interactions
- Decreased effectiveness of **antihypertensive agents.**
- Increased serum levels of anticonvulsants (e.g., **phenobarbital, phenytoin,** and **primidone**), **tricyclic antidepressants, SSRIs, warfarin.**
- Increased effects of **vasopressor agents** with concurrent use.
- Hypertensive crisis may occur with concurrent use (or within 2 weeks use) of **MAOIs.**
- Concurrent use with **clonidine** may result in serious adverse reactions.
- Increased sympathomimetic effects with other **adrenergics,** including **vasoconstrictors** and **decongestants.**

Route and Dosage
DEXMETHYLPHENIDATE (Focalin; Focalin XR)

ADHD: (Immediate-release tabs): **PO** *(Adults and children ≥6 yr): Patients not previously taking methylphenidate:* 2.5 mg 2 times a day. May be increased weekly as needed up to 10 mg 2 times a day. *Patients currently taking methylphenidate:* Starting dose is one-half of the methylphenidate dose, up to 10 mg 2 times a day.

(Extended-release capsules): **PO** *(Adults): Patients not previously taking methylphenidate:* 10 mg once daily. May be increased by 10 mg after 1 week to 40 mg/day. *Patients currently taking methylphenidate:* Starting dose is one-half of the methylphenidate dose, up to 40 mg/day given as a single daily dose. *Patients currently taking dexmethylphenidate:* Give same daily dose as a single dose.

PO *(Children ≥6 yr): Patients not previously taking methylphenidate:* 5 mg once daily. May be increased by 5 mg weekly up to 30 mg/day. *Patients currently taking methylphenidate:* Starting dose is one-half of the methylphenidate dose, up to 30 mg/day, given as a single daily dose. *Patients currently taking dexmethylphenidate:* Give same daily dose as a single dose.

METHYLPHENIDATE (Ritalin; Ritalin-SR; Ritalin LA; Methylin; Methylin ER; Metadate ER; Metadate CD; Concerta; Daytrana)

ADHD: (Immediate-release forms): **PO** *(Adults):* 5 to 20 mg 2 or 3 times/day preferably 30 to 45 minutes before meals. Average dose is 20 to 30 mg/day. To prevent interruption of sleep, take last dose of the day before 6 p.m.

PO *(Children ≥6 yr):* Individualize dosage. May start with low dose of 2.5 to 5 mg twice daily before breakfast and lunch. May increase dosage in 5 to 10 mg increments at weekly intervals. Maximum daily dosage: 60 mg.

(Extended-release forms):

Ritalin-SR, Methylin ER, and Metadate ER: **PO** *(Adults and children ≥6 yr):* May be used in place of the immediate release tablets when the 8-hour dosage corresponds to the titrated 8-hour dosage of the immediate release tablets. Must be swallowed whole.

Ritalin LA and Metadate CD: **PO** *(Adults and children ≥6 yr):* Initial dosage: 20 mg once daily in the morning before breakfast. May increase dosage in 10 mg increments at weekly intervals to a maximum of 60 mg taken once daily in the morning. Capsules may be swallowed whole with liquid or opened and contents sprinkled on soft food (e.g., applesauce). Ensure that entire contents of capsule are consumed when taken in this manner. **Note:** Ritalin LA may be used in place of twice-daily regimen given once daily at same total dose, or in place of sustained-release product at same dose.

Concerta: Should be taken once daily in the morning. Must be swallowed whole and not chewed, divided, or crushed.

PO *(Adults 18 to 65 yr):* Initial dosage: 18 or 36 mg/day for patients who are not currently taking methylphenidate or for patients who are on stimulants other than methylphenidate. May be increased in 18 mg increments at weekly intervals to a maximum dose of 72 mg/day.

PO *(Children 13 to 17 yr):* Initial dosage: 18 mg/day for patients who are not currently taking methylphenidate or for patients who are on stimulants other than methylphenidate. May be increased in 18-mg increments at weekly intervals to a maximum dose of 72 mg/day, not to exceed 2 mg/kg/day.

PO *(Children 6 to 12 yr):* Initial dosage: 18 mg/day for patients who are not currently taking methylphenidate or for patients who are on stimulants other than methylphenidate. May be increased in 18-mg increments at weekly intervals to a maximum dose of 54 mg/day.

QUILLIVANT XR

PO: For patients 6 years and older, recommended starting dose is 20 mg given orally once daily in the morning. Dosage may be increased weekly in increments of 10 mg to 20 mg per day. Daily dosage above 60 mg is not recommended.

Patients currently using methylphenidate: Should use following conversion table:

Previous methylphenidate dose	Recommended Concerta dose
5 mg 2 or 3 times/day or 20 mg (SR)	18 mg every morning
10 mg 2 or 3 times/day or 40 mg (SR)	36 mg every morning
15 mg 2 or 3 times/day or 60 mg (SR)	54 mg every morning

Daytrana: Transdermal Patch *(Adults and children ≥6 years):* Patch should be applied to hip area 2 hours before an effect is needed and should be removed 9 hours after application. Alternate hips with additional doses. Dosage for patients new to methylphenidate should be titrated to desired effect according to the following recommended schedule:

	Week 1	Week 2	Week 3	Week 4
Nominal delivered dose (mg/9 hours)	10 mg	15 mg	20 mg	30 mg
Delivery rate (based on 9-hr wear period)	(1.1 mg/hr)	(1.6 mg/hr)	(2.2 mg/hr)	(3.3 mg/hr)

Patients converting from another formulation of methylphenidate should follow the above titration schedule due to differences in bioavailability of Daytrana compared to other products.

***Narcolepsy:* PO** *(Adults): Ritalin, Methylin, Methylin ER, Ritalin-SR,* and *Metadate ER* indicated for this use. 10 mg 2 to 3 times a day. Maximum dose 60 mg/day.

■ ALPHA-ADRENERGIC AGONISTS
Examples

Generic (Trade) Name	Half-life (hr)	Indications	Available Forms (mg)
Clonidine (Catapres; Kapvay [ER])	12–22	• Hypertension • ADHD in children (ER only) **Unlabeled use:** • ADHD (immediate release) • Tourette's disorder	**TABS:** 0.1, 0.2, 0.3 **TABS (MODIFIED-RELEASE):** 0.1 **TABS (ER):** 0.1, 0.2 **SUSP (ER):** 0.09/mL **TRANSDERMAL PATCHES:** 0.1/24 hr, 0.2/24 hr, 0.3/24 hr
Guanfacine (Tenex; Intuniv)	16–18	• Hypertension (Tenex) • ADHD (Intuniv) **Unlabeled use:** • Tourette's disorder	**TABS (TENEX):** 1, 2 **TABS (ER) (INTUNIV):** 1, 2, 3, 4

Action

- Stimulates alpha-adrenergic receptors in the brain, thereby reducing sympathetic outflow from the CNS resulting in decreases in peripheral vascular resistance, heart rate, and blood pressure.
- Mechanism of action in the treatment of ADHD is unknown.

Contraindications and Precautions

Contraindicated in: • Hypersensitivity to the drug or any of its inactive ingredients

Use Cautiously in: • Coronary insufficiency • Recent myocardial infarction • Cerebrovascular disease • History of hypotension, bradycardia, or syncope • Chronic renal or hepatic failure • Elderly • Pregnancy and lactation

Adverse Reactions and Side Effects

- Orthostatic hypotension
- Bradycardia
- Palpitations
- Syncope
- Dry mouth
- Constipation
- Nausea
- Fatigue
- Sedation
- Erectile dysfunction
- Rebound syndrome with abrupt withdrawal

Interactions

- Increased effects of clonidine with **verapamil** and **beta blockers.**
- Decreased effects of clonidine with **prazosin** and **tricyclic antidepressants.**
- Decreased effects of **levodopa** with clonidine.
- Additive CNS effects with **CNS depressants,** including **alcohol, antihistamines, opioid analgesics,** and **sedative-hypnotics.**
- Additive hypotensive effects with other **antihypertensives** and **nitrates.**
- Decreased effects of guanfacine with **barbiturates, carbamazepine, rifampin, tricyclic antidepressants,** or **phenytoin.**
- Increased effects of guanfacine with **ketoconazole.**
- Increased effects of **valproic acid** with guanfacine.

Route and Dosage

CLONIDINE (Catapres; Kapvay)

Hypertension: **PO** *(Adults):* Initial dosage: 0.1 mg twice daily (immediate release), 0.1 mg at bedtime (modified release), or 0.17 mg once daily (suspension). May increase dosage in increments of 0.1 mg/day (0.09 mg for suspension) at weekly intervals until desired response is achieved. Maximum dose: 2.4 mg/day (immediate release) or 0.52 mg/day (suspension).

Transdermal system: Transdermal system delivering 0.1 mg to 0.3 mg/24 hours applied every 7 days. Initiate with 0.1 mg/24-hour system. Dosage increments may be made every 1 to 2 weeks when system is changed.

ADHD: **PO** *(Children ≥6 yr): Extended release:* Initial dose: 0.1 mg at bedtime. May increase in increments of 0.1 mg/day at weekly intervals to maximum dose of 0.4 mg/day.

Immediate release: Initial dose: 0.05 mg at bedtime. May increase dosage over several weeks to 0.15 to 0.3 mg/day in 3 or 4 divided doses.

Tourette's disorder: **PO** *(Children and adolescents):* 0.0025 to 0.015 mg/kg/day for 6 weeks to 3 months.

GUANFACINE (Tenex; Intuniv)

Hypertension (Immediate release): **PO** *(Adults):* 1 mg daily at bedtime. If satisfactory results are not achieved after 3 to 4 weeks, may increase to 2 mg.

ADHD (Extended release): **PO** *(Children 6 to 17 yr):* Initial dosage: 1 mg once daily. May increase dose in increments of 1 mg/day at weekly intervals until desired response is achieved. Maximum dose of 4 mg/day. Tablets should not be chewed, crushed, or broken before swallowing and should not be administered with high-fat meals.

Tourette's disorder: **PO** *(Children and adolescents):* Initial dosage: 0.5 mg at bedtime. May increase dose by 0.5 mg every 3 to 7 days to maximum dosage of 4 mg/day.

■ MISCELLANEOUS AGENTS FOR ADHD
Examples

Generic (Trade) Name	Half-life (hr)	Indications	Available Forms (mg)
Atomoxetine (Strattera)	5	• ADHD	**CAPS:** 10, 18, 25, 40, 60, 80, 100
Bupropion (Wellbutrin; Wellbutrin SR; Wellbutrin XL; Budeprion SR; Budeprion XL; Aplenzin; Zyban)	8–24	• Depression (all except Zyban) • Seasonal affective disorder (Wellbutrin XL; Aplenzin) • Smoking cessation (Zyban) **Unlabeled use:** • ADHD (Wellbutrin; Wellbutrin SR; Wellbutrin XL)	**TABS:** 75, 100 **TABS (SR):** 100, 150, 200 **TABS (XL):** 150, 300 **TABS (ER [APLENZIN]):** 174, 348, 522

SR = 12-hour tablets; XL = 24-hour tablets.

Action

- Atomoxetine selectively inhibits the reuptake of the neurotransmitter norepinephrine.
- Bupropion is a weak inhibitor of the neuronal uptake of norepinephrine, serotonin, and dopamine.
- Action in the treatment of ADHD is unclear.

Contraindications and Precautions

Contraindicated in: • Hypersensitivity • Coadministration with or within 2 weeks after discontinuing an MAOI • Lactation

Atomoxetine: • Narrow-angle glaucoma • Current or prior history of pheochromocytoma

Bupropion: • Known or suspected seizure disorder • Acute phase of myocardial infarction • Patients with current or prior diagnosis of bulimia or anorexia nervosa • Patients undergoing abrupt discontinuation of alcohol or sedatives (increased risk of seizures)

Use Cautiously in: • Patients with suicidal ideation • Patients with urinary retention • Hypertension • Hepatic, renal, or cardiovascular insufficiency • Pregnancy (use only if benefits outweigh possible risks to fetus) • Children and adolescents (may increase suicidal risk) • Elderly and debilitated patients

Atomoxetine: • Children younger than 6 years (safety not established)

Adverse Reactions and Side Effects

- Dry mouth
- Anorexia
- Nausea and vomiting
- Constipation
- Urinary retention
- Sexual dysfunction
- Headache
- Dizziness
- Insomnia or sedation
- Palpitations; tachycardia
- Weight loss
- Abdominal pain
- Increased sweating

Atomoxetine

- Fatigue
- Cough
- New or worsened psychiatric symptoms
- Severe liver damage

Bupropion

- Weight gain
- Tremor

- Seizures
- Blurred vision

Interactions

The effects of:	Are increased by:	Are decreased by:	Concurrent use may result in:
Atomoxetine	Concomitant use of **CYP2D6 inhibitors (paroxetine, fluoxetine, quinidine)**		Risk of additive hypertensive effects with pressor agents, such as **dobutamine** or **dopamine;** potentially fatal reactions with concurrent use (or use within 2 weeks of discontinuation) of **MAOIs;** increased cardiovascular effects of **albuterol** with concurrent use
Bupropion	Amantadine, levodopa, cimetidine, clopidogrel, ticlopidine, guanfacine	Carbamazepine, ritonavir	Increased risk of acute toxicity with **MAOIs;** increased risk of hypertension with **nicotine replacement agent;** adverse neuropsychiatric events with **alcohol** (alcohol tolerance is reduced); increased anticoagulant effect of **warfarin;** increased effects of drugs metabolized by CYP2D6 (e.g., **nortriptyline, imipramine, desipramine, paroxetine, fluoxetine, sertraline, haloperidol, risperidone, thioridazine metoprolol, propafenone,** and **flecainide**); increased risk of seizures with drugs that lower the seizure threshold (antidepressants, antipsychotics, theophylline, corticosteroids, stimulants/anorectics)

Route and Dosage
ATOMOXETINE (Strattera)
ADHD: PO (Adults, adolescents, and children weighing >70 kg): Initial dose: 40 mg/day. Increase after a minimum of 3 days to a target total daily dose of 80 mg, as a single dose in the morning or 2 evenly divided doses in the morning and late afternoon or early evening. After 2 to 4 weeks, total dosage may be increased to a maximum of 100 mg, if needed.

PO *(Children weighing ≤70 kg):* Initial dose: 0.5 mg/kg/day. May be increased every 3 days to a daily target dose of 1.2 mg/kg taken either as a single dose in the morning or 2 evenly divided doses in the morning and late afternoon or early evening. Maximum daily dose: 1.4 mg/kg or 100 mg daily, whichever is less.

Adjusted Dosing: Hepatic impairment: In patients with moderate hepatic impairment, reduce to 50% of usual dose. In patients with severe hepatic impairment, reduce to 25% of usual dose.

Adjusted Dosing: Coadministration with strong CYP2D6 inhibitors (e.g., quinidine, fluoxetine, paroxetine): **PO** *(Adults, adolescents, and children weighing >70 kg):* Initiate dosage at 40 mg/day and only increase to the usual target dose of 80 mg/day if symptoms fail to improve after 4 weeks and the initial dose is well tolerated. **PO** *(Children and adolescents weighing up to 70 kg):* Initiate dosage at 0.5 mg/kg/day and only increase to the usual target dose of 1.2 mg/kg/day if symptoms fail to improve after 4 weeks and the initial dose is well tolerated.

BUPROPION (Wellbutrin; Budeprion; Aplenzin; Zyban)

Depression (Wellbutrin; Budeprion): **PO** *(Adults) (immediate-release tabs):* 100 mg 2 times/day. May increase after 3 days to 100 mg given 3 times/day. For patients who do not show improvement after several weeks of dosing at 300 mg/day, an increase in dosage up to 450 mg/day may be considered. No single dose of bupropion should exceed 150 mg. To prevent the risk of seizures, administer with 4 to 6 hours between doses.

    Sustained-release tabs (Wellbutrin SR; Budeprion SR): Give as a single 150-mg dose in the morning. May increase to twice a day (total 300 mg), with at least 8 hours between doses. Maximum dose: 400 mg, administered as 200 mg twice a day, with at least 8 hours between doses.

    Extended-release tabs (Wellbutrin XL; Budeprion XL): Begin dosing at 150 mg/day, given as a single daily dose in the morning. May increase after 3 days to 300 mg/day, given as a single daily dose in the morning. Maximum dose: 450 mg administered as a single daily dose in the morning.

    Aplenzin: Initial dose: 174 mg once daily. After 4 days, may increase the dose to 348 mg once daily.

Seasonal affective disorder (Wellbutrin XL): **PO** *(Adults):* 150 mg administered each morning beginning in the autumn prior to the onset of depressive symptoms. Dose may be uptitrated to the target dose of 300 mg/day after 1 week. Therapy should continue through the winter season before being tapered to 150 mg/day for 2 weeks prior to discontinuation in early spring.

    Aplenzin: **PO** *(Adults):* 174 mg once daily beginning in the autumn prior to the onset of seasonal depressive symptoms. After 1 week, may increase the dose to 348 mg once daily. Continue treatment through the winter season.

Smoking cessation (Zyban): **PO** *(Adults):* Begin dosing at 150 mg given once a day in the morning for 3 days. If tolerated well, increase to target dose of 300 mg/day given in doses of 150 mg twice daily with an interval of 8 hours between doses. Continue treatment for 7 to 12 weeks. Some patients may need treatment for as long as 6 months.

ADHD (Wellbutrin; Wellbutrin SR; Wellbutrin XL): **PO** *(Adults):* 150 to 450 mg/day. Initiate therapy with 150 mg/day and titrate based on tolerability and efficacy. Doses can be given as divided doses or in SR or XL formulations.

   Children and adolescents (Wellbutrin; Wellbutrin SR; Wellbutrin XL): Up to 3 mg/kg/day or 150 mg/day initially, titrated to a maximum dosage of up to 6 mg/kg/day or 300 mg/day. Single dose should not exceed 150 mg. Usually given in divided doses for safety and effectiveness: twice daily for children and 3 times daily for adolescents.

■ NURSING DIAGNOSES RELATED TO AGENTS FOR ADHD

1. Risk for injury related to overstimulation and hyperactivity (CNS stimulants [or seizures] possible side effect of bupropion).
2. Risk for suicide secondary to major depression related to abrupt withdrawal after extended use (CNS stimulants).
3. Risk for suicide (children and adolescents) as a side effect of atomoxetine and bupropion (**black-box warning**).
4. Imbalanced nutrition, less than body requirements, related to side effects of anorexia and weight loss (CNS stimulants).
5. Disturbed sleep pattern related to side effects of overstimulation or insomnia.
6. Nausea related to side effects of atomoxetine or bupropion.
7. Pain related to side effect of abdominal pain (atomoxetine, bupropion) or headache (all agents).
8. Risk for activity intolerance related to side effects of sedation or dizziness (atomoxetine or bupropion).

■ NURSING IMPLICATIONS FOR ADHD AGENTS

The plan of care should include monitoring for the following side effects from agents for ADHD. Nursing implications related to each side effect are designated by an asterisk (*).

1. **Overstimulation, restlessness, insomnia** (with CNS stimulants)
   * Assess mental status for changes in mood, level of activity, degree of stimulation, and aggressiveness.
   * Ensure that the patient is protected from injury.
   * Keep stimuli low and environment as quiet as possible to discourage overstimulation.
   * To prevent insomnia, administer the last dose at least 6 hours before bedtime. Administer sustained release forms in the morning.

2. **Palpitations, tachycardia** (with CNS stimulants; atomoxetine; bupropion; clonidine) or bradycardia (clonidine, guanfacine)
   * Monitor and record vital signs at regular intervals (two or three times a day) throughout therapy. Report significant changes to the physician immediately.

NOTE: The FDA has issued warnings associated with CNS stimulants and atomoxetine of the risk for sudden death in patients who have cardiovascular disease. A careful personal and family history of heart disease, heart defects, or hypertension should be obtained before these medications are prescribed. Careful monitoring of cardiovascular function during administration must be ongoing.

3. **Anorexia, weight loss** (with CNS stimulants, atomoxetine, and bupropion)
   * To reduce anorexia, the medication may be administered immediately after meals. The patient should be weighed regularly (at least weekly) when receiving therapy with CNS stimulants, atomoxetine, or bupropion because of the potential for anorexia and weight loss, and temporary interruption of growth and development.

4. **Tolerance, physical and psychological dependence** (with CNS stimulants)
   * Tolerance develops rapidly.
   * In children with ADHD, a drug "holiday" should be attempted periodically under direction of the physician to determine the effectiveness of the medication and the need for continuation.
   * The drug should not be withdrawn abruptly. To do so could initiate the following syndrome of symptoms: nausea, vomiting, abdominal cramping, headache, fatigue, weakness, mental depression, suicidal ideation, increased dreaming, and psychotic behavior.

5. **Nausea and vomiting** (with atomoxetine and bupropion)
   * May be taken with food to minimize gastrointestinal upset.

6. **Constipation** (with atomoxetine, bupropion, clonidine, and guanfacine)
   * Increase fiber and fluid in diet if not contraindicated.

7. **Dry mouth** (with clonidine and guanfacine)
   * Offer the patient sugarless candy, ice, frequent sips of water.
   * Strict oral hygiene is very important.

8. **Sedation** (with clonidine and guanfacine)
   * Warn the patient that this effect is increased by concomitant use of alcohol and other CNS drugs.
   * Warn patients to refrain from driving or performing hazardous tasks until response has been established.

9. **Potential for seizures** (with bupropion)
   * Protect the patient from injury if seizure should occur. Instruct family and significant others of patients on bupropion therapy how to protect the patient during a seizure if one should occur. Ensure that doses of the immediate release medication are administered 4 to 6 hours apart, and doses of the sustained release medication at least 8 hours apart.
10. **Severe liver damage** (with atomoxetine)
    * Monitor for the following side effects and report to physician immediately: itching, dark urine, right upper quadrant pain, yellow skin or eyes, sore throat, fever, malaise.
11. **New or worsened psychiatric symptoms** (with CNS stimulants and atomoxetine)
    * Monitor for psychotic symptoms (e.g., hearing voices, paranoid behaviors, delusions.
    * Monitor for manic symptoms, including aggressive and hostile behaviors.
12. **Rebound syndrome** (with clonidine and guanfacine)
    * The patient should be instructed not to discontinue therapy abruptly. To do so may result in symptoms of nervousness, agitation, headache, tremor, and a rapid rise in blood pressure. Dosage should be tapered gradually under the supervision of the physician.

■ PATIENT/FAMILY EDUCATION RELATED TO AGENTS FOR ADHD

* Use caution in driving or operating dangerous machinery. Drowsiness, dizziness, and blurred vision can occur.
* Do not stop taking CNS stimulants abruptly. To do so could produce serious withdrawal symptoms.
* Avoid taking CNS stimulants late in the day to prevent insomnia. Take no later than 6 hours before bedtime.
* Do not take other medications (including over-the-counter drugs) without physician's approval. Many medications contain substances that, in combination with agents for ADHD, can be harmful.
* Diabetic patients should monitor blood sugar two or three times a day or as instructed by the physician. Be aware of need for possible alteration in insulin requirements because of changes in food intake, weight, and activity.
* Avoid consumption of large amounts of caffeinated products (coffee, tea, colas, chocolate), as they may enhance the CNS stimulant effect.
* Notify physician if symptoms of restlessness, insomnia, anorexia, or dry mouth become severe or if rapid, pounding heartbeat becomes evident. Report any of the following side effects to the physician immediately: shortness of breath, chest pain, jaw/left

arm pain, fainting, seizures, sudden vision changes, weakness on one side of the body, slurred speech, confusion, itching, dark urine, right upper quadrant pain, yellow skin or eyes, sore throat, fever, malaise, increased hyperactivity, believing things that are not true, or hearing voices.
- Be aware of possible risks of taking agents for ADHD during pregnancy. Safe use during pregnancy and lactation has not been established. Inform the physician immediately if pregnancy is suspected or planned.
- Be aware of potential side effects of agents for ADHD. Refer to written materials furnished by health-care providers for safe self-administration.
- Carry a card or other identification at all times describing medications being taken.

@ INTERNET REFERENCES

- www.mentalhealth.com
- https://www.nimh.nih.gov/index.shtml
- https://www.nimh.nih.gov/health/topics/mental-health-medications/index.shtml
- https://medlineplus.gov/druginformation.html
- www.chadd.org
- https://www.nimh.nih.gov/health/topics/attention-deficit-hyperactivity-disorder-adhd/index.shtml

Comparison of Developmental Theories

Age	Stage	Major Developmental Tasks
Freud's Stages of Psychosexual Development		
Birth–18 months	Oral	Relief from anxiety through oral gratification of needs
18 months–3 years	Anal	Learning independence and control, with focus on the excretory function
3–6 years	Phallic	Identification with parent of same gender; development of sexual identity; focus is on genital organs
6–12 years	Latency	Sexuality is repressed; focus is on relationships with same-gender peers
13–20 years	Genital	Libido is reawakened as genital organs mature; focus is on relationships with members of the opposite gender

Stages of Development in H. S. Sullivan's Interpersonal Theory		
Birth–18 months	Infancy	Relief from anxiety through oral gratification of needs
18 months–6 years	Childhood	Learning to experience a delay in personal gratification without undue anxiety
6–9 years	Juvenile	Learning to form satisfactory peer relationships
9–12 years	Preadolescence	Learning to form satisfactory relationships with persons of the same gender; the initiation of feelings of affection for another person

(Continued)

Stages of Development in H. S. Sullivan's Interpersonal Theory—cont'd		
12–14 years	Early adolescence	Learning to form satisfactory relationships with persons of the opposite gender; developing a sense of identity
14–21 years	Late adolescence	Establishing self-identity; experiencing satisfying relationships; working to develop a lasting, intimate opposite-gender relationship

Stages of Development in Eric Erikson's Psychosocial Theory		
Infancy (birth–18 months)	Trust vs. mistrust	To develop a basic trust in the mothering figure and be able to generalize it to others
Early childhood (18 months–3 years)	Autonomy vs. shame and doubt	To gain some self-control and independence within the environment
Late childhood (3–6 years)	Initiative vs. guilt	To develop a sense of purpose and the ability to initiate and direct own activities
School age (6–12 years)	Industry vs. inferiority	To achieve a sense of self-confidence by learning, competing, performing successfully, and receiving recognition from significant others, peers, and acquaintances
Adolescence (12–20 years)	Identity vs. role confusion	To integrate the tasks mastered in the previous stages into a secure sense of self
Young adulthood (20–30 years)	Intimacy vs. isolation	To form an intense, lasting relationship or a commitment to another person, a cause, an institution, or a creative effort
Adulthood (30–65 years)	Generativity vs. stagnation	To achieve the life goals established for oneself while also considering the welfare of future generations
Old age (65 years–80s)	Ego integrity vs. despair	To review one's life and derive meaning from both positive and negative events while achieving a positive sense of self-worth
80s and older	Transcendence	To face the issues related to meaning in life, well-being, life satisfaction, faith, hope, and wisdom

Stages of Development in M. Mahler's Theory of Object Relations

Birth–1 month	I. Normal autism	Fulfillment of basic needs for survival and comfort
1–5 months	II. Symbiosis	Developing awareness of external source of need fulfillment
	III. Separation–Individuation	
5–10 months	A. Differentiation	Commencement of a primary recognition of separateness from the mothering figure
10–16 months	B. Practicing	Increased independence through locomotor functioning; increased sense of separateness of self
16–24 months	C. Rapprochement	Acute awareness of separateness of self; learning to seek "emotional refueling" from mothering figure to maintain feeling of security
24–36 months	D. Consolidation	Sense of separateness established; on the way to object constancy (i.e., able to internalize a sustained image of loved object/person when it is out of sight); resolution of separation anxiety

Piaget's Stages of Cognitive Development

Birth–2 years	Sensorimotor	With increased mobility and awareness, develops a sense of self as separate from the external environment; the concept of object permanence emerges as the ability to form mental images evolves
2–6 years	Preoperational	Learning to express self with language; develops understanding of symbolic gestures; achievement of object permanence
6–12 years	Concrete operations	Learning to apply logic to thinking; development of understanding of reversibility and spatiality; learning to differentiate and classify; increased socialization and application of rules
12–15+ years	Formal operations	Learning to think and reason in abstract terms; making and testing hypotheses; capability of logical thinking and reasoning expand and are refined; cognitive maturity achieved

Kohlberg's Stages of Moral Development		
I. Preconventional (common from ages 4–10 years)	1. Punishment and obedience orientation	Behavior is motivated by fear of punishment
	2. Instrumental relativist orientation	Behavior is motivated by egocentrism and concern for self
II. Conventional (common from ages 10–13 years and into adulthood)	3. Interpersonal concordance orientation	Behavior is motivated by the expectations of others; strong desire for approval and acceptance
	4. Law and order orientation	Behavior is motivated by respect for authority
III. Postconventional (can occur from adolescence on)	5. Social contract legalistic orientation	Behavior is motivated by respect for universal laws and moral principles and guided by an internal set of values
	6. Universal ethical principle orientation	Behavior is motivated by internalized principles of honor, justice, and respect for human dignity and guided by the conscience

Stages of Development in H. Peplau's Interpersonal Theory		
Infancy	Learning to count on others	Learning to communicate in various ways with the primary caregiver to have comfort needs fulfilled
Toddlerhood	Learning to delay gratification	Learning the satisfaction of pleasing others by delaying self-gratification in small ways
Early childhood	Identifying oneself	Learning appropriate roles and behaviors by acquiring the ability to perceive the expectations of others
Late childhood	Developing skills in participation	Learning the skills of compromise, competition, and cooperation with others; establishing a more realistic view of the world and a feeling of one's place in it

Source: Adapted from Morgan, K. I. & Townsend, M. C. (2020). *Psychiatric mental health nursing: Concepts of care in evidence-based practice* (10th ed.). Philadelphia: F.A. Davis, pp. 655–656.

Ego Defense Mechanisms

Defense Mechanisms	Example	Defense Mechanisms	Example
Compensation: Covering up a real or perceived weakness by emphasizing a trait one considers more desirable	A physically handicapped boy is unable to participate in football, so he compensates by becoming a great scholar.	**Rationalization:** Attempting to make excuses or formulate logical reasons to justify unacceptable feelings or behaviors	John tells the rehab nurse, "I drink because it's the only way I can deal with my bad marriage and my worse job."
Denial: Refusing to acknowledge the existence of a real situation or the feelings associated with it	A woman who drinks alcohol every day and cannot stop fails to acknowledge that she has a problem.	**Reaction Formation:** Preventing unacceptable or undesirable thoughts or behaviors from being expressed by exaggerating opposite thoughts or types of behaviors	Jane hates nursing. She attended nursing school to please her parents. During career day, she speaks to prospective students about the excellence of nursing as a career.
Displacement: The transfer of feelings from one target to another that is	A client is angry at his physician, does not express it,	**Regression:** Responding to stress by retreating to an earlier level of	When 2-year-old Jay is hospitalized for tonsillitis, he will drink only

(Continued)

Defense Mechanisms	Example	Defense Mechanisms	Example
considered less threatening or that is neutral	but becomes verbally abusive with the nurse.	development and the comfort measures associated with that level of functioning	from a bottle, even though his mom states he has been drinking from a cup for 6 months.
Identification: An attempt to increase self-worth by acquiring certain attributes and characteristics of an individual one admires	A teenager who required lengthy rehabilitation after an accident decides to become a physical therapist as a result of his experiences.	**Repression:** Involuntarily blocking unpleasant feelings and experiences from one's awareness	An accident victim can remember nothing about the accident.
Intellectualization: An attempt to avoid expressing actual emotions associated with a stressful situation by using the intellectual processes of logic, reasoning, and analysis	S's husband is being transferred with his job to a city far away from her parents. She hides anxiety by explaining to her parents the advantages associated with the move.	**Sublimation:** Rechanneling of drives or impulses that are personally or socially unacceptable into activities that are constructive	A mother whose son was killed by a drunk driver channels her anger and energy into being the president of the local chapter of Mothers Against Drunk Driving.
Introjection: Integrating the beliefs and values of another individual into one's own ego structure	Children integrate their parents' value system into the process of conscience formation. A child says to a friend, "Don't cheat. It's wrong."	**Suppression:** The voluntary blocking of unpleasant feelings and experiences from one's awareness	Scarlett O'Hara says, "I don't want to think about that now. I'll think about that tomorrow."

Defense Mechanisms	Example	Defense Mechanisms	Example
Isolation: Separating a thought or memory from the feeling tone or emotion associated with it	A young woman describes being attacked and raped, without showing any emotion.	**Undoing:** Symbolically negating or canceling out an experience that one finds intolerable	Joe is nervous about his new job and yells at his wife. On his way home, he stops and buys her some flowers.
Projection Attributing feelings or impulses unacceptable to one's self to another person	Sue feels a strong sexual attraction to her track coach and tells her friend, "He's coming on to me!"		

Source: Morgan, K.I. & Townsend, M.C. (2020). *Psychiatric mental health nursing: Concepts of care in evidence-based practice* (10th ed.). Philadelphia: F.A. Davis, p. 19.

Levels of Anxiety

Level	Perceptual Field	Ability to Learn	Physical Characteristics	Emotional/Behavioral Characteristics
Mild	Heightened perception (e.g., noises may seem louder; details within the environment are clearer) Increased awareness Increased alertness	Learning is enhanced	Restlessness Irritability	May remain superficial with others Rarely experienced as distressful Motivation is increased
Moderate	Reduction in perceptual field Reduced alertness to environmental events (e.g., someone talking may not be heard; part of the room may not be noticed)	Learning still occurs, but not at optimal ability Decreased attention span Decreased ability to concentrate	Increased restlessness Increased heart and respiration rates Increased perspiration Gastric discomfort Increased muscular tension Increase in speech rate, volume, and pitch	A feeling of discontent May lead to a degree of impairment in interpersonal relationships as individual begins to focus on self and the need to relieve personal discomfort

(Continued)

Level	Perceptual Field	Ability to Learn	Physical Characteristics	Emotional/Behavioral Characteristics
Severe	Greatly diminished; only extraneous details are perceived, or fixation on a single detail may occur. May not take notice of an event even when attention is directed by another	Extremely limited attention span. Unable to concentrate or problem-solve. Effective learning cannot occur	Headaches Dizziness Nausea Trembling Insomnia Palpitations Tachycardia Hyperventilation Urinary frequency Diarrhea	Feelings of dread, loathing, horror. Total focus on self and intense desire to relieve the anxiety
Panic	Unable to focus on even one detail within the environment. Misperceptions of the environment are common (e.g., a perceived detail may be elaborated and out of proportion)	Learning cannot occur. Unable to concentrate. Unable to comprehend even simple directions	Dilated pupils Labored breathing Severe trembling Sleeplessness Palpitations Diaphoresis and pallor Muscular incoordination Immobility or purposeless hyperactivity Incoherence or inability to verbalize	Sense of impending doom. Terror. Bizarre behavior, including shouting, screaming, running about wildly, or clinging to anyone or anything from which a sense of safety and security is derived. Hallucinations; delusions. Extreme withdrawal into self

Source: Morgan, K.I. & Townsend, M.C. (2020). Psychiatric mental health nursing: Concepts of care in evidence-based practice (10th ed.). Philadelphia: F.A. Davis, pp. 17–18.

APPENDIX D

Stages of Grief

A Comparison of Models by Elisabeth Kübler-Ross, John Bowlby, George Engel, and William Worden

Kübler-Ross	Bowlby	Engel	Worden	Possible Time Dimension	Behaviors
		Stages/Tasks			
I. Denial	I. Numbness/ protest	I. Shock/ disbelief	I. Accepting the reality of the loss	Occurs immediately on experiencing the loss, usually lasts no more than a few weeks	Individual has difficulty believing that the loss has occurred.
II. Anger	II. Disequilibrium	II. Developing awareness		In most cases begins within hours of the loss, peaks within a few weeks	Anger is directed toward self or others. Ambivalence and guilt may be felt toward the lost object.
III. Bargaining		III. Restitution			Individual fervently seeks alternatives to improve current situation. Attends to various rituals associated with the culture in which the loss has occurred.
IV. Depression	III. Disorganization and despair	IV. Resolution of the loss	II. Processing the pain of grief	Very individual, commonly 6 to 12 months; longer for some	The actual work of grieving. Preoccupation with the lost entity. Feelings of helplessness and loneliness occur in response to realization of the loss. Feelings associated with the loss are confronted.

V. Acceptance	IV. Reorganization	V. Recovery	IV. Finding an enduring connection with the lost entity in the midst of embarking on a new life		Resolution is complete. The bereaved person experiences a reinvestment in new relationships and new goals. The lost entity is not purged or replaced but is relocated in the life of the bereaved. At this stage, terminally ill persons express a readiness to die.
		III. Adjusting to a world without the lost entity	Ongoing	How the environment changes depends on the roles the lost entity played in the life of the bereaved person. Adaptations must be made as the changes are presented in daily life. New coping skills must be developed.

(Continued)

A Comparison of Models by Elisabeth Kübler-Ross, John Bowlby, George Engel, and William Worden—cont'd

	Stages/Tasks				
Kübler-Ross	Bowlby	Engel	Worden	Possible Time Dimension	Behaviors
VI. Finding meaning. (Kessler, 2019) Kessler, expanding on the work of Kübler-Ross identified this sixth stage of the grief process.					A feeling of peace and a sense of renewed hopefulness occurs as meaning (rather than closure) is sought.

Source: Adapted from Morgan, K.I. & Townsend, M.C. (2020). *Psychiatric mental health nursing: Concepts of care in evidence-based practice* (10th ed.). Philadelphia: F.A. Davis, pp. 819–836.

Relationship Development and Therapeutic Communication

■ PHASES OF A THERAPEUTIC NURSE-PATIENT RELATIONSHIP

Psychiatric nurses use interpersonal relationship development as the primary intervention with patients in various psychiatric and mental health settings. This is congruent with Peplau's (1962) identification of counseling as the major subrole of nursing in psychiatry. If Sullivan's (1953) belief is true—that is, that all emotional problems stem from difficulties with interpersonal relationships—then this role of the nurse in psychiatry becomes especially meaningful and purposeful. It becomes an integral part of the total therapeutic regimen.

The therapeutic interpersonal relationship is the means by which the nursing process is implemented. Through the relationship, problems are identified and resolution is sought. Tasks of the relationship have been categorized into four phases: the pre-interaction phase, the orientation (introductory) phase, the working phase, and the termination phase. Although each phase is presented as specific and distinct from the others, there may be some overlapping of tasks, particularly when the interaction is limited.

The Pre-interaction Phase

The pre-interaction phase involves preparation for the first encounter with the patient. Tasks include the following:

1. Obtaining available information about the patient from the chart, significant others, or other health team members. From this information, the initial assessment is begun. During this phase the nurse also tries to become aware of his or her preconceived attitudes about the patient.

2. Examining one's feelings, fears, and anxieties about working with a particular patient. For example, the nurse may have been raised in an alcoholic family and have ambivalent feelings about caring for a patient who is alcohol dependent.

All individuals bring attitudes and feelings from prior experiences to the clinical setting. The nurse needs to be aware of how these preconceptions may affect his or her ability to care for individual patients.

The Orientation (Introductory) Phase

During the orientation phase, the nurse and patient become acquainted. Tasks include the following:

1. Creating an environment for the establishment of trust and rapport.
2. Establishing a contract for intervention that details the expectations and responsibilities of both the nurse and the patient.
3. Gathering assessment information to build a strong patient database.
4. Identifying the patient's strengths and limitations.
5. Formulating nursing diagnoses.
6. Setting goals that are mutually agreeable to the nurse and patient.
7. Developing a plan of action that is realistic for meeting the established goals.
8. Exploring feelings of both the patient and the nurse in terms of the introductory phase. Introductions are often uncomfortable, and the participants may experience some anxiety until a degree of rapport has been established. Interactions may remain on a superficial level until anxiety subsides. Several interactions may be required to fulfill the tasks associated with this phase.

The Working Phase

The therapeutic work of the relationship is accomplished during this phase. Tasks include the following:

1. Maintaining the trust and rapport that was established during the orientation phase.
2. Promoting the patient's insight and perception of reality.
3. Problem-solving in an effort to facilitate change in the patient's life.
4. Overcoming resistance behaviors on the part of the patient as the level of anxiety rises in response to discussion of painful issues.
5. Continuously evaluating progress toward goal attainment.

The Termination Phase

Termination of the relationship may occur for a variety of reasons: the mutually agreed-upon goals may have been reached, the patient may be discharged from the hospital, or in the case of a student nurse, the clinical rotation may come to an end. Termination can be a difficult phase for both the patient and nurse. Tasks include the following:

1. Bringing a therapeutic conclusion to the relationship. This occurs when:
   a. Progress has been made toward attainment of mutually set goals.
   b. A plan for continuing care or for assistance during stressful life experiences is mutually established by the nurse and the patient.
   c. Feelings about termination of the relationship are recognized and explored. Both the nurse and patient may experience feelings of sadness and loss. The nurse should share his or her feelings with the patient. Through these interactions, the patient learns that it is acceptable to undergo these feelings at a time of separation. Through this knowledge, the patient experiences growth during the process of termination.

NOTE: When the patient feels sadness and loss, behaviors to delay termination may become evident. If the nurse experiences the same feelings, he or she may allow the patient's behaviors to delay termination. For therapeutic closure, the nurse must establish the reality of the separation and resist being manipulated into repeated delays by the patient.

Therapeutic Communication Techniques

Technique	Explanation/ Rationale	Examples
Using silence	Silence encourages the patient to organize thoughts and put them into words and allows the patient time to think about the significance of events, thoughts, and feelings. Allowing the patient to break the silence often provides the nurse with important information about the patient's foremost concerns.	Pt: "My husband divorced me so I must be undesirable." Nurse: (silence) Pt: "You know, when I think about it, no matter what my husband does I always assume it's my fault or it's something wrong with me."
Accepting	Acceptance conveys an attitude of reception and regard.	"Yes, I understand what you said." Eye contact; nodding.

(Continued)

Therapeutic Communication Techniques—cont'd

Technique	Explanation/Rationale	Examples
Giving recognition	Acknowledging; indicating awareness; better than complimenting, which reflects the nurse's judgment.	"Hello, Mr. J. I notice that you made a ceramic ash tray in OT." "I see you made your bed."
Offering self	Willingness to spend time with the patient and show interest, on an unconditional basis, helps to increase the patient's feelings of self-worth.	"I'll stay with you awhile." "Let's make some time this afternoon to talk about what's been troubling you" "I'm available to talk with you, and I'd like to hear more about what kinds of things you've tried in the past for relaxation."
Giving broad openings	Broad openings allow the patient to direct the focus of the interaction and emphasizes the importance of the patient's role in the communication process.	"What would you like to talk about today?" "Is there anything you want to discuss?"
Offering general leads	General leads offer the patient encouragement to continue with minimal input from the nurse.	"Yes, I see." "Go on." "And after that?"
Placing the event in time or sequence	Encouraging the patient to identify the sequence of events and when they occurred in time facilitates organizing one's thoughts about their experiences.	"What happened first?" "What happened next?" "Was this before or after …?" "When did this happen?"
Making observations	Verbalizing observations about a patient's behavior or appearance encourages patients to develop awareness of how they	"You seem tense." "I notice you are pacing a lot." "You seem uncomfortable when you…."

Therapeutic Communication Techniques—cont'd

Technique	Explanation/ Rationale	Examples
	are perceived by others and promotes exploration of issues that may be problematic.	
Encouraging description of perceptions	Asking the patient to verbalize his or her perceptions facilitates the patient's ability to develop awareness and understanding. For the patient experiencing hallucinations, it can facilitate both nurse's and patient's clarification about what the patient's perceptual experiences are communicating.	"Tell me more about the voices you said you are hearing." "What was it that increased your agitation during the group activity?" "Are these voices you hear directing you to take some action?"
Encouraging comparison	Asking the patient to compare similarities and differences in ideas, experiences, or interpersonal relationships helps the patient recognize life experiences that tend to recur and those aspects of life that are changeable.	"Was this episode similar to …?" "How does this compare with the time when …?" "What was your response the last time this situation occurred?"
Restating	Repeating the main idea of what the patient has said. This lets the patient know that an expressed statement has been heard and gives him or her the chance to continue or to clarify if necessary.	Pt: "I can't study. My mind keeps wandering." Nurse: "Your mind keeps wandering?" Pt: "I can't take that new job. What if I can't do it?" Nurse: "You're afraid you won't be able to do it?"

(Continued)

Therapeutic Communication Techniques—cont'd

Technique	Explanation/ Rationale	Examples
Reflecting	Questions and feelings are referred back to the patient so that the patient is empowered to actively engage in problem-solving rather than simply asking the nurse for advice.	Pt: "Don't you think I should tell my boss I'm not putting up with that?" Nurse: "What do you think you should do?" Pt: "She makes me so upset!" Nurse: "So you're feeling angry at your boss?"
Focusing	Taking notice of a single idea or even a single word works especially well with a patient who is moving rapidly from one thought to another. However, focusing is very difficult for a patient with severe anxiety so, in this case, the nurse should not pursue focusing until the anxiety level decreases.	"This point seems worth looking at more closely. Perhaps you and I can discuss it together." "You say you are having pain; tell me specifically where the pain is and what it feels like."
Exploring	When the nurse hears the patient mention an issue or theme that seems relevant, the nurse asks the patient to explore this further. Exploring facilitates the patient's development of awareness and understanding about events, thoughts, and feelings. However, if the patient chooses not to disclose further information, the nurse should refrain from pushing or	"Please explain that situation in more detail." "Tell me more about that particular situation." "You mentioned feeling like no one cares about you. Tell me more about those feelings."

Therapeutic Communication Techniques—cont'd

Technique	Explanation/ Rationale	Examples
	probing in an area that obviously creates discomfort.	
Seeking clarification and validation	Striving to explain vague or incomprehensible statements and searching for mutual understanding; clarifying the meaning of what has been said facilitates and increases understanding for both patient and nurse.	"I'm not sure that I understand. Would you please explain?" "Tell me if my understanding agrees with yours." "Do I understand correctly that you said …?"
Presenting reality	When the patient has a misperception of the environment, the nurse defines reality by expressing his or her perception of the situation without challenging the patient's perceptions.	"I understand that the voices seem real to you, but I do not hear any voices." "I don't see anyone else in the room but you and me."
Voicing doubt	Expressing uncertainty as to the reality of the patient's perceptions. Often used with patients experiencing delusional thinking.	"It's difficult to believe that the President of the United States would be listening to all of your phone calls." "I find that hard to believe (or accept)." "That seems rather doubtful to me."
Verbalizing the implied	Putting into words what the patient has only implied or said indirectly is a technique that can be helpful with patients experiencing impaired verbal communication.	Pt: "I can't talk about this … you haven't been where I've been." Nurse: "Does it seem like no one could understand your thoughts and feelings unless they've had the same experiences you've had?" Pt: "I … I don't know where to begin." Nurse: "So it feels overwhelming to think about sharing the details of this experience."

(Continued)

Therapeutic Communication Techniques—cont'd

Technique	Explanation/ Rationale	Examples
Attempting to translate words into feelings	When the patient has difficulty identifying feelings or feelings are expressed indirectly, the nurse tries to "desymbolize" what has been said and to find clues to the underlying true feelings.	Pt: "I'm just an empty pit." Nurse: "It sounds like you are feeling hopeless, is that right?"
Formulating a plan of action	Encouraging the patient to identify a plan for behavior change promotes developing better coping skills.	"What could you do differently if you are faced with this situation in the future?" "What are some steps you could take to manage your anger without punching someone?" "What is one thing you might be willing to try to decrease your anxiety instead of using alcohol?"

Sources: Adapted from Hays, J.S., & Larson, K.H. (1963). *Interacting with patients.* New York: Holt, Rinehart, and Winston; Engard, B. (2019). 17 therapeutic communication techniques. Retrieved from https://online.rivier.edu/therapeutic-communication-techniques/; Sullivan, H. S. (1954). *The psychiatric interview.* New York: Norton.

Nontherapeutic Communication Techniques

Technique	Explanation/ Rationale	Examples
Giving false reassurance	False reassurance conveys that the nurse already knows the outcome of a situation and minimizes the patient's expressed concerns. It may discourage the patient from further expression of feelings if he or she believes the feelings will be downplayed or ridiculed.	Pt: "My husband doesn't love me anymore. I think he wants a divorce." Nurse: "I'm sure he must still love you. Everything will be fine." **Better alternative:** "Tell me more about what's been happening in your relationship with your husband."

Nontherapeutic Communication Techniques—cont'd

Technique	Explanation/ Rationale	Examples
Rejecting	Refusing to consider or showing contempt for the patient's ideas or behavior. This may result in the patient discontinuing interaction with the nurse for fear of further rejection.	Pt: "Since I started taking this medication I can't be intimate with my girlfriend." Nurse: "Let's not talk about that right now." **Better alternative:** "Tell me more about what you mean by not being able 'to be intimate' with your girlfriend."
Giving approval or disapproval	Sanctioning or denouncing the patient's ideas or behavior. Implies that the nurse has the right to pass judgment on whether the patient's ideas or behaviors are "good" or "bad" and that the patient is expected to please the nurse. The nurse's acceptance of the patient is then seen as conditional depending on the patient's behavior.	"It's good that you confronted your wife about her behavior." "You shouldn't yell at your wife." **Better alternative:** "What happened after you confronted your wife in a loud voice?"
Agreeing/ disagreeing	Indicating accord with or opposition to the patient's ideas or opinions implies that the nurse has the right to pass judgment on whether the patient's ideas or opinions are "right" or "wrong." Agreement discourages the patient from later modifying his or her point of view. Disagreement implies inaccuracy	Pt: "I think my doctor doesn't care about me." Nurse: "I disagree. You shouldn't think that way." Or "I can't believe that's true." **Better alternative:** "Tell me more about why you think your doctor doesn't care."

(Continued)

Nontherapeutic Communication Techniques—cont'd

Technique	Explanation/ Rationale	Examples
	and may provoke defensiveness on the part of the patient.	
Giving advice	Telling the patient what to do or how to behave implies that the nurse knows what is best and nurtures the patient in the dependent role by discouraging independent thinking and problem-solving.	"You need to do deep breathing exercises when you become anxious." "You should stop drinking alcohol and start going to Alcoholics Anonymous meetings." **Better alternative:** "What do you think you should do?" or "Let's explore some options for solving this problem."
Probing	Persistent questioning of the patient and pushing for answers to issues the patient does not wish to discuss causes the patient to feel used and valued only for what information the nurse is seeking and may place the patient on the defensive.	"Why was your family angry with you?" "How many times did you receive poor evaluations before you got fired?" "How many girlfriends were you lying to?" **Better alternative:** The nurse should actively listen to the patient's response and discontinue the interaction at the first sign of discomfort.
Defending	Defending someone or something the patient has criticized minimizes or completely ignores the patient's concerns. Defending may cause the patient to think the nurse is taking sides against him or her.	"No one here would lie to you." "You have a very capable physician. I'm sure he only has your best interests in mind." **Better to say:** "I will try to answer your questions and clarify some issues regarding your treatment." Or "Tell me more about your thoughts and feelings related to this issue."
Requesting an explanation	This nontherapeutic technique involves asking the patient why he or she has certain thoughts,	"Why do you think people are out to get you?" "Why do you feel depressed?" "Why were you taking drugs?"

Nontherapeutic Communication Techniques—cont'd

Technique	Explanation/ Rationale	Examples
	feelings, and behaviors. Asking "why" a patient did something or feels a certain way can be very intimidating and implies that the patient must defend his or her behavior or feelings.	**Better alternative:** "Describe what you were feeling just before that happened."
Indicating the existence of an external source of power	Attributing the source of thoughts, feelings, and behavior to others or to outside influences. This encourages the patient to project blame for his or her thoughts or behaviors on others rather than accepting the responsibility personally.	"What made you go on a drinking binge?" "What made you say that you are 'a worthless person'?" **Better alternative:** What was happening just before you started binge drinking?" "What do you mean when you say you are 'a worthless person'?"
Belittling or minimizing feelings	When the nurse minimizes the degree of the patient's discomfort, a lack of empathy and understanding may be conveyed. When the nurse tells the patient to "cheer up" or "everybody feels that way," the patient may feel that his or her concerns are insignificant or unimportant.	Pt: "I don't even have the energy to go to work." Nurse: "We've all felt like that at times. You've just got to 'perk up' and get moving." **Better alternative:** "Tell me more about what you are feeling right now."
Making stereotyped comments	Trite expressions are meaningless in a nurse-patient relationship. When the nurse uses meaningless expressions, it	"How are you?" "Hang in there." "It'll all work out." **Better alternative:** Choose words, sentences, and nonverbal language that convey a

(Continued)

Nontherapeutic Communication Techniques—cont'd

Technique	Explanation/ Rationale	Examples
	encourages a similar response from the patient.	sincere interest in encouraging the patient to share more about the patient's thoughts, feelings, and behaviors.
Using denial	Denying that a problem exists blocks discussion and avoids helping the patient identify and explore areas of difficulty.	Pt: "I have a problem interacting with people." Nurse: "You're doing fine." **Better alternative:** "Tell me more about that."
Interpreting	Interpreting attempts to tell the patient the meaning of his or her experience. Erroneous interpretations may leave the patient feeling that the nurse doesn't understand him or her, or that the nurse is being smug.	"What you really mean is...." "Your continued drinking is your way of avoiding discussing your anger over the divorce...." **Better technique:** "Tell me more about what you're thinking (or feeling)."
Introducing an unrelated topic	When the nurse prematurely changes the subject, it conveys to the patient that the nurse does not want to discuss the original topic any further. This may occur in order to get to something that the nurse wants to discuss with the patient or to get away from a topic that he or she would prefer not to discuss.	Pt: "I don't have anything to live for." Nurse: "How well did you sleep last night?" **Better alternative:** "Tell me more." Sometimes silence may be appropriate to convey that the nurse is willing to hear all of what the patient wants to say before moving on to a different topic.

Sources: Adapted from Hays, J.S., & Larson, K.H. (1963). *Interacting with patients.* New York: Holt, Rinehart, and Winston; Engard, B. (2019). 17 therapeutic communication techniques. Retrieved from https://online.rivier.edu/therapeutic-communication-techniques/; Sullivan, H.S. (1954). *The psychiatric interview.* New York: Norton.

Psychosocial Therapies

■ GROUP THERAPY

Group therapy is a type of psychosocial therapy with a number of patients at one time. The group is founded in a specific theoretical framework, with the goal being to encourage improvement in interpersonal functioning.

Nurses often lead *therapeutic groups*, which are based to a lesser degree in theory than is group therapy. The focus of therapeutic groups is more on group relations, interactions among group members, and the consideration of a selected issue.

Types of groups include *task groups*, in which the function is to accomplish a specific outcome or task; *teaching groups*, in which knowledge or information is conveyed to a number of individuals; *supportive-therapeutic groups*, which help prevent future upsets by teaching participants effective ways of dealing with emotional stress arising from situational or developmental crises; and *self-help groups* of individuals with similar problems who meet to help each other with emotional distress associated with those problems.

Yalom (2005) identified 11 therapeutic factors that individuals can achieve through interpersonal interactions within the group. They include the following:

1. The instillation of hope.
2. Universality (individuals come to understand that they are not alone in the problems they experience).
3. The imparting of information.
4. Altruism (mutual sharing and concern for each other).
5. The corrective recapitulation of the primary family group.
6. The development of socializing techniques.
7. Imitative behavior.
8. Interpersonal learning.
9. Group cohesiveness.
10. Catharsis (open expression of feelings).
11. Existential factors (the group is able to help individual members take direction of their own lives and to accept responsibility for the quality of their existence).

■ PSYCHODRAMA

Psychodrama is a specialized type of therapeutic group that employs a dramatic approach in which patients become "actors" in life-situation scenarios.

The group leader is called the *director*, group members are the *audience*, and the *set*, or *stage*, may be specially designed or may just be any room or part of a room selected for this purpose. Actors are members from the audience who agree to take part in the "drama" by role-playing a situation about which they have been informed by the director. Usually the situation is an issue with which one individual patient has been struggling. The patient plays the role of himself or herself and is called the *protagonist*. In this role, the patient is able to express true feelings toward individuals (represented by group members) with whom he or she has unresolved conflicts.

In some instances, the group leader may ask for a patient to volunteer to be the protagonist for that session. The patient may choose a situation he or she wishes to enact and select the audience members to portray the roles of others in the life situation. The psychodrama setting provides the patient with a safer and less threatening atmosphere than the real situation in which to express true feelings. Resolution of interpersonal conflicts is facilitated.

When the drama has been completed, group members from the audience discuss the situation they have observed, offer feedback, express their feelings, and relate their own similar experiences. In this way, all group members benefit from the session, either directly or indirectly.

Nurses often serve as actors, or role players, in psychodrama sessions. Leaders of psychodrama have graduate degrees in psychology, social work, nursing, or medicine with additional training in group therapy and specialty preparation to become a psychodramatist.

■ FAMILY THERAPY

In family therapy, the nurse-therapist works with the family as a group to improve communication and interaction patterns. Areas of assessment include communication, manner of self-concept reinforcement, family members' expectations, handling differences, family interaction patterns, and the "climate" of the family (a blend of feelings and experiences that are the result of sharing and interacting).

The Family as a System

General systems theory is a way of organizing thought according to the holistic perspective. A system is considered greater than the sum of its parts. A family can be viewed as a system composed of various subsystems. The systems approach to family therapy is composed of eight major concepts: (1) differentiation of self; (2) triangles; (3) nuclear family emotional process; (4) family projection process; (5) multigenerational transmission process; (6) sibling position profiles; (7) emotional cutoff; and (8) societal regression. The goal is to increase the level of differentiation of self while remaining in touch with the family system.

The Structural Model

In this model, the family is viewed as a social system within which the individual lives and to which the individual must adapt. The individual both contributes to and responds to stresses within the family. Major concepts include systems, subsystems, transactional patterns, and boundaries. The goal of therapy is to facilitate change in the family structure. The therapist does this by joining the family, evaluating the family system, and restructuring the family.

The Strategic Model

This model uses the interactional or communications approach. Functional families are open systems in which clear and precise messages, congruent with the situation, are sent and received. Healthy communication patterns promote nurturance and individual self-worth. In dysfunctional families, viewed as partially closed systems, communication is vague, and messages are often inconsistent and incongruent with the situation. Destructive patterns of communication tend to inhibit healthful nurturing and decrease individual feelings of self-worth. Concepts of this model include double-bind communication, pseudomutuality and pseudohostility, marital schism, and marital skew. The goal of therapy is to create change in destructive behavior and communication patterns among family members. This is accomplished by using paradoxical intervention (prescribing the symptom) and reframing (changing the setting or viewpoint in relation to which a situation is experienced and placing it in another more positive frame of reference).

■ MILIEU THERAPY

In psychiatry, milieu therapy, or a therapeutic community, constitutes a manipulation of the environment in an effort to create behavioral changes and to improve the psychological health and functioning of the individual. The goal of therapeutic community is for the patient to learn adaptive coping, interaction, and relationship skills that can be generalized to other aspects of his or her life. The community environment itself serves as the primary tool of therapy.

According to Skinner (1979), a therapeutic community is based on seven basic assumptions:

1. The health in each individual is to be realized and encouraged to grow.

2. Every interaction is an opportunity for therapeutic intervention.
3. The patient owns his or her own environment.
4. Each patient owns his or her behavior.
5. Peer pressure is a useful and a powerful tool.
6. Inappropriate behaviors are dealt with as they occur.
7. Restrictions and punishment are to be avoided.

Since the goals of milieu therapy relate to helping the patient learn to generalize that which is learned to other aspects of his or her life, the conditions that promote a therapeutic community in the hospital setting are similar to the types of conditions that exist in real-life situations. They include the following:

1. The fulfillment of basic physiological needs.
2. Physical facilities that are conducive to the achievement of the goals of therapy.
3. The existence of a democratic form of self-government.
4. The assignment of unit responsibilities according to patient capabilities.
5. A structured program of social and work-related activities.
6. The inclusion of community and family in the program of therapy in an effort to facilitate discharge from the hospital.

The program of therapy on the milieu unit is conducted by the interdisciplinary treatment (IDT) team. The team includes some, or all, of the following disciplines and may include others that are not specified here: psychiatrist, clinical psychologist, psychiatric clinical nurse specialist, psychiatric nurse, mental health technician, psychiatric social worker, occupational therapist, recreational therapist, art therapist, music therapist, psychodramatist, dietitian, and chaplain.

Nurses play a crucial role in the management of a therapeutic milieu. They are involved in the assessment, diagnosis, outcome identification, planning, implementation, and evaluation of all treatment programs. They have significant input into the IDT plans that are developed for all patients. They are responsible for ensuring that patients' basic needs are fulfilled, for continual assessment of physical and psychosocial status, for medication administration, for the development of trusting relationships, for setting limits on unacceptable behaviors, for patient education, and ultimately, for helping patients, within the limits of their capability, become productive members of society.

Milieu therapy came into its own during the 1960s through the early 1980s. During this period, psychiatric inpatient treatment provided sufficient time to implement programs of therapy that were aimed at social rehabilitation. Currently, care in inpatient psychiatric facilities is shorter and more biologically based, limiting patients' benefit from the socialization that occurs in a milieu as treatment program. Although strategies for milieu therapy are still used, they have been modified to conform to the short-term approach to care or to outpatient treatment programs.

■ CRISIS INTERVENTION

A *crisis* is "a sudden event in one's life that disturbs homeostasis, during which usual coping mechanisms cannot resolve the problem" (Lagerquist, 2012). All individuals experience crises at one time or another. This does not necessarily indicate psychopathology.

Crises are precipitated by specific, identifiable events and are determined by an individual's personal perception of the situation. They are acute, not chronic, and generally last no more than 4 to 6 weeks.

Crises occur when an individual is exposed to a stressor and previous problem-solving techniques are ineffective. This causes the level of anxiety to rise. Panic may ensue when new techniques are employed and resolution fails to occur.

Six types of crises have been identified. They include dispositional crises, crises of anticipated life transitions, crises resulting from traumatic stress, maturational or developmental crises, crises reflecting psychopathology, and psychiatric emergencies. The type of crisis determines the method of intervention selected.

Crisis intervention is designed to provide rapid assistance for individuals who have an urgent need. Aguilera (1998) suggests that the "focus is on the supportive, with the restoration of the individual to his precrisis level of functioning or possibly to a higher level of functioning" (p. 24).

Nurses regularly respond to individuals in crisis in all types of settings. Nursing process is the vehicle by which nurses assist individuals in crisis with a short-term, problem-solving approach to change. A four-phase technique is used: assessment/analysis; planning of therapeutic intervention; intervention; and evaluation of crisis resolution and anticipatory planning. Through this structured method of assistance, nurses assist individuals in crisis to develop more adaptive coping strategies for dealing with stressful situations in the future.

■ RELAXATION THERAPY

Stress is a part of our everyday lives. It can be positive or negative, but it cannot be eliminated. Keeping stress at a manageable level is a lifelong process.

Individuals under stress respond with a physiological arousal that can be dangerous over long periods. Indeed, the stress response has been shown to be a major contributor, either directly or indirectly, to coronary heart disease, cancer, lung ailments, accidental injuries, cirrhosis of the liver, and suicide—six of the leading causes of death in the United States.

Relaxation therapy is an effective means of reducing the stress response in some individuals. The degree of anxiety that an individual experiences in response to stress is related to certain predisposing factors, such as characteristics of temperament with which he or she was born, past experiences resulting in learned patterns of responding, and existing conditions, such as health status, coping strategies, and adequate support systems.

Deep relaxation can counteract the physiological and behavioral manifestations of stress. The ability to effectively use any relaxation therapies is enhanced by regular practice. Various methods of relaxation include the following:

Deep-Breathing Exercises: Tension is released when the lungs are allowed to breathe in as much oxygen as possible. Deep-breathing exercises involve inhaling slowly and deeply through the nose, holding the breath for a few seconds, and then exhaling slowly through the mouth, pursing the lips as if trying to whistle.

Progressive Relaxation: This method of deep-muscle relaxation is based on the premise that the body responds to anxiety-provoking thoughts and events with muscle tension. Each muscle group is tensed for 5 to 7 seconds and then relaxed for 20 to 30 seconds, during which time the individual concentrates on the difference in sensations between the two conditions. Soft, slow background music may facilitate relaxation. A modified version of this technique (called *passive progressive relaxation*) involves relaxation of the muscles by concentrating on the feeling of relaxation within the muscle rather than on the actual tensing and relaxing of the muscle.

Meditation: The goal of meditation is to gain mastery over attention. It brings on a special state of consciousness as attention is concentrated solely on one thought or object. During meditation, as the individual becomes totally preoccupied with the selected focus, the respiration rate, heart rate, and blood pressure decrease. The overall metabolism declines, and the need for oxygen consumption is reduced. Mindfulness meditation is a specific type of meditation in which the participant is encouraged to nonjudgmentally focus on the present moment, such as attention to one's breathing. For example, sitting in a relaxed position, focus on one's inhalation and exhalation, noting the sound, the different depths of each breath, and any other body sensations associated with breath. As the mind wanders, notice that and nonjudgmentally return focus to breathing. The benefits of practicing mindfulness meditation are both for relaxation and for developing skill in focusing on the present moment, which are both foundational to problem solving and behavior change.

Mental Imagery: Mental imagery uses the imagination in an effort to reduce the body's response to stress. The frame of reference is very personal, based on what each individual considers a relaxing environment. The relaxing scenario is most useful when taped and played back at a time when the individual wishes to achieve relaxation.

Biofeedback: Biofeedback is the use of instrumentation to become aware of processes in the body that usually go unnoticed and to help bring them under voluntary control. Biological conditions, such as muscle tension, skin surface temperature, blood pressure, and heart rate, are monitored by the biofeedback equipment. With special training, the individual learns to use relaxation and voluntary control to modify the biological condition, in turn indicating a modification of the autonomic function it represents. Biofeedback is often used together with other relaxation techniques such as deep breathing, progressive relaxation, and mental imagery.

■ ASSERTIVENESS TRAINING

Assertive behavior helps individuals feel better about themselves by encouraging them to stand up for their own basic human rights. These rights have equal representation for all individuals. But along with rights comes an equal number of responsibilities. Part of being assertive includes living up to these responsibilities.

Assertive behavior increases self-esteem and the ability to develop satisfying interpersonal relationships. This is accomplished through honesty, directness, appropriateness, and respecting one's own rights as well as the rights of others.

Individuals develop patterns of responding in various ways, such as role modeling, by receiving positive or negative reinforcement or by conscious choice. These patterns can take the form of nonassertiveness, assertiveness, aggressiveness, or passive-aggressiveness.

Nonassertive individuals seek to please others at the expense of denying their own basic human rights. *Assertive* individuals stand up for their own rights while protecting the rights of others. Those who respond *aggressively* defend their own rights by violating the basic rights of others. Individuals who respond in a *passive-aggressive* manner defend their own rights by expressing resistance to social and occupational demands.

Some important behavioral considerations of assertive behavior include eye contact, body posture, personal distance, physical contact, gestures, facial expression, voice, fluency, timing, listening, thoughts, and content. Various techniques have been developed to assist individuals in the process of becoming more assertive. Some of these include the following:

1. **Standing up for one's basic human rights.**
   Example: "I have the right to express my opinion."
2. **Assuming responsibility for one's own statements.**
   Example: "I *don't want* to go out with you tonight" instead of "I *can't* go out with you tonight." The latter implies a lack of power or ability.

3. **Responding as a "broken record."** Persistently repeating in a calm voice what is wanted.

   Example:

Telephone salesperson:	"I want to help you save money by changing long-distance services."
Assertive response:	"I don't want to change my long-distance service."
Telephone salesperson:	"I can't believe you don't want to save money!"
Assertive response:	"I don't want to change my long-distance service."

4. **Agreeing assertively.** Assertively accepting negative aspects about oneself. Admitting when an error has been made.

   Example:

Ms. Jones:	"You sure let that meeting get out of hand. What a waste of time."
Ms. Smith:	"Yes, I didn't do a very good job of conducting the meeting today."

5. **Inquiring assertively.** Seeking additional information about critical statements.

   Example:

Male board member:	"You made a real fool of yourself at the board meeting last night."
Female board member:	"Oh, really? Just what about my behavior offended you?"
Male board member:	"You were so damned pushy!"
Female board member:	"Were you offended that I spoke up for my beliefs, or was it because my beliefs are in direct opposition to yours?"

6. **Shifting from content to process.** Changing the focus of the communication from discussing the topic at hand to analyzing what is actually going on in the interaction.

   Example:

Wife:	"Would you please call me if you will be late for dinner?"
Husband:	"Why don't you just get off my back! I always have to account for every minute of my time with you!"
Wife:	"Sounds to me like we need to discuss some other things here. What are you *really* angry about?"

7. **Clouding/fogging.** Concurring with the critic's argument without becoming defensive and without agreeing to change.

   Example:

Nurse No. 1:	"You make so many mistakes. I don't know how you ever got this job!"

Nurse No. 2: "You're right. I have made some mistakes since I started this job."

8. **Defusing.** Putting off further discussion with an angry individual until he or she is calmer.

   Example: "You are very angry right now. I don't want to discuss this matter with you while you are so upset. I will discuss it with you in my office at 3 o'clock this afternoon."

9. **Delaying assertively.** Putting off further discussion with another individual until one is calmer.

   Example: "That's a very challenging position you have taken, Mr. Brown. I'll need time to give it some thought. I'll call you later this afternoon."

10. **Responding assertively with irony.**

    Example:

    Man: "I bet you're one of them so-called 'women's libbers,' aren't you?"

    Woman: "Yes, thank you for noticing."

11. **Using "I" statements.**

    "I" statements allow an individual to take ownership for his or her feelings rather than saying they are caused by another person. "I" statements are sometimes called "feeling" statements. They express directly what an individual is feeling. "You" statements are accusatory and put the receiver on the defensive. "I" statements have four parts:

    a. How I feel: *These are my feelings and I accept ownership of them.*
    b. When: *Describe in a neutral manner the behavior that is the problem.*
    c. Why: *Describe what it is about the behavior that is objectionable.*
    d. Suggest change: *Offer a preferred alternative to the behavior.*

    Example:

    John has just returned from a hunting trip and walked into the living room in his muddy boots, leaving a trail of mud on the carpet. His wife, Mary, may respond as follows:

    With a "you" statement: "You are such a jerk! Can't you see the trail of mud you are leaving on the carpet? I just cleaned this carpet. You make me so angry!"

    With an "I" statement: "I feel so angry when you walk on the carpet in your muddy boots. I just cleaned it, and now I will have to clean it again. I would appreciate it if you would remove your boots on the porch before you come in the house."

"You" statements are negative and focus on what the person has done wrong. They don't explain what is being requested of the person. "I" statements are more positive. They explain *how* one is feeling, *why* he or she is feeling that way, and *what* the individual wants instead.

■ COGNITIVE BEHAVIOR THERAPY

Cognitive behavior therapy, developed by Aaron Beck, is commonly used in the treatment of mood disorders. In cognitive behavior therapy, the individual is taught to control thought distortions that are considered to be a factor in the development and maintenance of mood disorders. In the cognitive model, depression is characterized by a triad of negative distortions related to expectations of the environment, self, and future. The environment and activities within it are viewed as unsatisfying, the self is unrealistically devalued, and the future is perceived as hopeless. In the same model, mania is characterized by a positive cognitive triad—the self is seen as highly valued and powerful, experiences within the environment are viewed as overly positive, and the future is seen as one of unlimited opportunity.

The general goals in cognitive behavior therapy are to obtain symptom relief as quickly as possible, to assist the patient in identifying dysfunctional patterns of thinking and behaving, and to guide the patient to evidence and logic that effectively test the validity of the dysfunctional thinking. Therapy focuses on changing "automatic thoughts" that occur spontaneously and contribute to the distorted affect. Examples of automatic thoughts in depression include the following:

1. **Personalizing:** "I'm the only one who failed."
2. **All or nothing:** "I'm a complete failure."
3. **Mind reading:** "He thinks I'm foolish."
4. **Discounting positives:** "The other questions were so easy. Any dummy could have gotten them right."

Examples of automatic thoughts in mania include the following:

1. **Personalizing:** "She's this happy only when she's with me."
2. **All or nothing:** "Everything I do is great."
3. **Mind reading:** "She thinks I'm wonderful."
4. **Discounting negatives:** "None of those mistakes are really important."

The patient is asked to describe evidence that both supports and disputes the automatic thought. The logic underlying the inferences is then reviewed with the patient. Another technique involves evaluating what would most likely happen if the patient's automatic thoughts were true. Implications of the consequences are then discussed.

Patients should not become discouraged if one technique seems not to be working. There is no single technique that works with all patients. He or she should be reassured that there are a number of techniques that may be used, and both therapist and patient may explore these possibilities. Cognitive behavior therapy has been shown to be an effective treatment for mood disorders, particularly in conjunction with psychopharmacological intervention.

Electroconvulsive Therapy

■ DEFINED

Electroconvulsive therapy (ECT) is a type of somatic treatment in which electric current is applied to the brain through electrodes placed on the temples. The current is sufficient to induce a grand mal seizure, from which the desired therapeutic effect is achieved.

■ INDICATIONS

ECT is primarily used in the treatment of severe depression. It is sometimes administered in conjunction with antidepressant medication, but most physicians prefer to perform this treatment only after an unsuccessful trial of drug therapy.

ECT may also be used as a fast-acting treatment for very hyperactive manic patients in danger of physical exhaustion and for individuals who are extremely suicidal.

ECT was originally attempted in the treatment of schizophrenia but with little success in most instances. There has been evidence, however, of its effectiveness in the treatment of acute schizophrenia, particularly if it is accompanied by catatonic or affective (depression or mania) symptomatology.

■ CONTRAINDICATIONS

ECT should not be used if there is increased intracranial pressure (from brain tumor, recent cardiovascular accident, or other cerebrovascular lesion). Other conditions, although not considered absolute contraindications, may render patients at high risk for complications resulting from the treatment. They are largely cardiovascular in nature and include myocardial infarction or cerebrovascular accident within the preceding 3 to 6 months, aortic or cerebral aneurysm, severe underlying hypertension, and congestive heart failure.

■ MECHANISM OF ACTION

The exact mechanism of action is unknown. However, it is thought that ECT produces biochemical changes in the brain—an increase in the levels of norepinephrine, serotonin, and dopamine—similar to the effects of antidepressant medications. A longitudinal study of imaging research shows that the therapeutic response to ECT is associated with several effects on the brain, including decreased frontal perfusion, changes in metabolism, functional connectivity, volume, and neuronal chemical metabolites, all of which support anticonvulsant and neurotrophic effects of ECT (Abbott et al, 2014). In another study, the researchers conclude that therapeutic response from ECT may be related to neuroplasticity in white matter microstructures, which are altered in major depression (Lyden et al, 2014).

Several recent studies have identified an increase in gray matter, particularly in the hippocampal and amygdala areas, following ECT (Depping et al, 2016; Pirnia et al, 2016; Sartorius et al, 2015). Because these areas of the brain show a decrease in volume in major depression, the study findings are being looked at with interest as an indication of neuroplasticity and the neurorestorative effects of ECT. The results of studies relating to the mechanism underlying the effectiveness of ECT continue to be mixed and controversial. Its effectiveness may be a complex dynamic of several effects interacting with one another.

■ SIDE EFFECTS AND NURSING IMPLICATIONS

Temporary Memory Loss and Confusion

- These are the most common side effects of ECT. It is important for the nurse to be present when the patient awakens in order to alleviate the fears that accompany this loss of memory.
- Provide reassurance that memory loss is only temporary.
- Describe to the patient what has occurred.
- Reorient the patient to time and place.
- Allow the patient to verbalize fears and anxieties related to receiving ECT.
- To minimize confusion, provide a good deal of structure for the patient's routine activities.

■ RISKS ASSOCIATED WITH ECT

1. **Mortality:** The mortality rate from ECT is about 0.002% per treatment and 0.01% for each patient (Sadock, Sadock, & Ruiz, 2015). The major cause is cardiovascular complications, such as acute myocardial infarction or cerebrovascular accident.
2. **Brain Damage:** According to Sadock and associates, "virtually all [brain imaging studies] concluded that permanent brain damage is not an adverse effect of ECT" (2015, p. 1072).
3. **Permanent Memory Loss:** Most individuals report no problems with their memory, aside from the time immediately surrounding the ECT treatments. However, some patients have reported retrograde amnesia extending back to months before treatment.

Although the potential for these effects appears to be minimal, the patient must be made aware of the risks involved before consenting to treatment.

■ POTENTIAL NURSING DIAGNOSES ASSOCIATED WITH ECT

1. Risk for injury related to risks associated with ECT.
2. Risk for aspiration related to altered level of consciousness immediately following treatment.
3. Decreased cardiac output related to vagal stimulation occurring during the ECT.
4. Impaired memory/acute confusion related to side effects of ECT.
5. Deficient knowledge related to necessity for and side effects and risks of ECT.
6. Anxiety (moderate to severe) related to impending therapy.
7. Self-care deficit related to incapacitation during postictal stage.
8. Risk for activity intolerance related to post-ECT confusion and memory loss.

■ NURSING INTERVENTIONS FOR PATIENTS RECEIVING ECT

1. Ensure that the physician has obtained informed consent and that a signed permission form is on the chart.
2. Ensure that the most recent laboratory reports (complete blood count [CBC], urinalysis) and results of electrocardiogram (ECG) and x-ray examination are available.
3. The patient should receive nothing by mouth (NPO) for 6 to 8 hours prior to the treatment.
4. Prior to the treatment, the patient should void, dress in night clothes (or other loose clothing), and remove dentures and eyeglasses or contact lenses. Bedrails should be raised.
5. Take baseline vital signs and blood pressure.
6. Administer cholinergic blocking agent (e.g., atropine sulfate, glycopyrrolate) approximately 30 minutes before treatment, as ordered by the physician, to decrease secretions (to prevent aspiration) and increase heart rate (which is suppressed in response to vagal stimulation caused by the ECT).
7. Assist physician and/or anesthesiologist as necessary in the administration of intravenous medications. A short-acting anesthetic, such as methohexital sodium (Brevital sodium), is given along with the muscle relaxant succinylcholine chloride (Anectine).
8. Administer oxygen and provide suctioning as required.
9. After the procedure, take vital signs and blood pressure every 15 minutes for the first hour. Position the patient on his or her side to prevent aspiration.

10. Stay with the patient until he or she is fully awake, oriented, and able to perform self-care activities without assistance.
11. Describe to the patient what has occurred.
12. Allow the patient to verbalize fears and anxieties associated with the treatment.
13. Reassure the patient that memory loss and confusion are only temporary.
14. Provide the patient with a highly structured schedule of routine activities in order to minimize confusion.

Medication Assessment Tool

Date ——————————— Patient's Name ——————————— Age ———————————

Marital Status ——————————— Children ———————————

Occupation ———————————

Presenting Symptoms (subjective & objective) ———————————

———————————

Diagnosis (*DSM-5*) ———————————

Current Vital Signs: Blood Pressure: Sitting ———— / ————; Standing ———— / ————; Pulse ————; Respirations ————

Height ——————————— Weight ———————————

■ **CURRENT/PAST USE OF PRESCRIPTION DRUGS (INDICATE WITH "C" OR "P" BESIDE NAME OF DRUG WHETHER CURRENT OR PAST USE):**

Name	*Dosage*	*How Long Used*	*Why Prescribed*	*By Whom*	*Side Effects/Results*

■ CURRENT/PAST USE OF OVER-THE-COUNTER DRUGS (INDICATE WITH "C" OR "P" BESIDE NAME OF DRUG WHETHER CURRENT OR PAST USE):

Name	Dosage	How Long Used	Why Prescribed	By Whom	Side Effects/Results

■ CURRENT/PAST USE OF STREET DRUGS, ALCOHOL, NICOTINE, AND/OR CAFFEINE (INDICATE WITH "C" OR "P" BESIDE NAME OF DRUG):

Name	Amount Used	How Often Used	When Last Used	Effects Produced

Any allergies to food or drugs? _____

Any special diet considerations? _____

Do you have (or have you ever had) any of the following? If yes, provide explanation on the back of this sheet.

	Yes	No		Yes	No		Yes	No
1. Difficulty swallowing	___	___	12. Chest pain	___	___	22. Shortness of breath	___	___
2. Delayed wound healing	___	___	13. Blood clots/pain in legs	___	___	23. Sexual dysfunction	___	___
3. Constipation problems	___	___	14. Fainting spells	___	___	24. Lumps in your breasts	___	___
4. Urination problems	___	___	15. Swollen ankles/legs/hands	___	___	25. Blurred or double vision	___	___
5. Recent change in elimination patterns	___	___	16. Asthma	___	___	26. Ringing in the ears	___	___
6. Weakness or tremors	___	___	17. Varicose veins	___	___	27. Insomnia	___	___
7. Seizures	___	___	18. Numbness/tingling (location?)	___	___	28. Skin rashes	___	___
8. Headaches	___	___	19. Ulcers	___	___	29. Diabetes	___	___
9. Dizziness	___	___	20. Nausea/vomiting	___	___	30. Hepatitis (or other liver disease)	___	___
10. High blood pressure	___	___	21. Problems with diarrhea	___	___	31. Kidney disease	___	___
11. Palpitations	___	___				32. Glaucoma	___	___

Are you pregnant or breast feeding? _____ Date of last menses _____ Type of contraception used _____

Describe any restrictions/limitations that might interfere with your use of medication for your current problem. _____

Prescription orders: Patient teaching related to medications prescribed:

Lab work or referrals prescribed:

_____   _____

Nurse's signature   **Patient's signature**

Cultural Assessment Tool

Patient's name _____ Ethnic origin _____

Address _____ Birthdate _____

Name of significant other _____ Relationship _____

Primary language spoken _____

Second language spoken _____

How does the patient usually communicate with people who speak a different language? _____

Is an interpreter required? _____

Available? _____

Highest level of education achieved: _____

Occupation: _____

Presenting problem: _____

_____

Has this problem ever occurred before? _____

If so, in what manner was it handled previously? _____

_____

What is the patient's usual manner of coping with stress? _____

_____

Who is (are) the patient's main support system(s)? _____

_____

Describe the family living arrangements: _____

_____

Who is the major decision maker in the family? _____

Describe the patient's/family members' roles within the family.

_____

_____

Describe religious beliefs and practices: _____

_____

Are there any religious requirements/restrictions that place limitations on the patient's care? _____
If so, describe: _____
_____

Who in the family takes responsibility for health concerns?
_____

Describe any special health beliefs and practices: _____
_____
_____

From whom does family usually seek medical assistance in time of need? _____
Describe the patient's usual emotional/behavioral response to:
_____

Anxiety: _____
Anger: _____
Loss/change/failure: _____
Pain: _____
Fear: _____
Describe any topics that are particularly sensitive or that the patient is unwilling to discuss (because of cultural taboos): _____
_____
_____

Describe any activities in which the patient is unwilling to participate (because of cultural customs or taboos): _____
_____
_____

What are the patient's personal feelings regarding touch? _____
What are the patient's personal feelings regarding eye contact?
_____

What is the patient's personal orientation to time? (past, present, future) _____
Describe any particular illnesses to which the patient may be bioculturally susceptible (e.g., hypertension and sickle cell anemia in African Americans): _____
_____

Describe any nutritional deficiencies to which the patient may be bioculturally susceptible (e.g., lactose intolerance in Native and Asian Americans)_____
_____

Describe the patient's favorite foods: _____

_____

Are there any foods the patient requests or refuses because of cultural beliefs related to this illness (e.g., "hot" and "cold" foods for Latino Americans and Asian Americans)? If so, please describe: _____

_____

Describe the patient's perception of the problem and expectations of health care: _____

_____

DSM-5 Classification: Categories and Codes*

International Classification of Diseases, 10th revision, Clinical Modification (ICD-10-CM) codes are provided.

■ NEURODEVELOPMENTAL DISORDERS

Intellectual Disabilities

Intellectual Disability (Intellectual Developmental Disorder)
Specify current severity:

70	Mild
71	Moderate
72	Severe
73	Profound
F88	Global Developmental Delay
F79	Unspecified Intellectual Disability (Intellectual Developmental Disorder)

Communication Disorders

F80.9	Language Disorder
F80.0	Speech Sound Disorder
F80.81	Childhood-Onset Fluency Disorder (Stuttering)
	NOTE: Later-onset cases are diagnosed as F98.5 adult-onset fluency disorder.
F80.89	Social (Pragmatic) Communication Disorder
(F80.9)	Unspecified Communication Disorder

Autism Spectrum Disorder

F84.0   Autism Spectrum Disorder
Specify if: Associated with a known medical or genetic condition or environmental factor; Associated with another neurodevelopmental, mental, or behavioral disorder
Specify current severity for Criterion A and Criterion B: Requiring very substantial support, Requiring substantial support, Requiring support
Specify if: With or without accompanying intellectual impairment, With or without accompanying language impairment, With catatonia (use additional code F06.1)

*Reprinted with permission from *Diagnostic and Statistical Manual of Mental Disorders, Fifth Edition.* (Copyright 2013). American Psychiatric Association.

Attention-Deficit/Hyperactivity Disorder

	Attention-Deficit/Hyperactivity Disorder
	Specify whether:
F90.2	Combined presentation
F90.0	Predominantly inattentive presentation
F90.1	Predominantly hyperactive/impulsive presentation
	Specify if: In partial remission
	Specify current severity: Mild, Moderate, Severe
F90.8	Other Specified Attention-Deficit/Hyperactivity Disorder
F90.9	Unspecified Attention-Deficit/Hyperactivity Disorder

Specific Learning Disorder

	Specific Learning Disorder
	Specify if:
F81.0	With impairment in reading (*specify* if with word reading accuracy, reading rate or fluency, reading comprehension)
F81.81	With impairment in written expression (*specify* if with spelling accuracy, grammar and punctuation accuracy, clarity or organization of written expression)
F81.2	With impairment in mathematics (*specify* if with number sense, memorization of arithmetic facts, accurate or fluent calculation, accurate math reasoning)
	Specify current severity: Mild, Moderate, Severe

Motor Disorders

F82	Developmental Coordination Disorder
F98.4	Stereotypic Movement Disorder
	Specify if: With self-injurious behavior, Without self-injurious behavior
	Specify if: Associated with a known medical or genetic condition, neurodevelopmental disorder, or environmental factor
	Specify current severity: Mild, Moderate, Severe

Tic Disorders

F95.2	Tourette's Disorder
F95.1	Persistent (Chronic) Motor or Vocal Tic Disorder
	Specify if: With motor tics only, With vocal tics only
F95.0	Provisional Tic Disorder
F95.8	Other Specified Tic Disorder
F95.9	Unspecified Tic Disorder

Other Neurodevelopmental Disorders

F88	Other Specified Neurodevelopmental Disorder
F89	Unspecified Neurodevelopmental Disorder

■ SCHIZOPHRENIA SPECTRUM AND OTHER PSYCHOTIC DISORDERS

The following specifiers apply to Schizophrenia Spectrum and Other Psychotic Disorders where indicated:

[a]*Specify* if: The following course specifiers are only to be used after a 1-year duration of the disorder: First episode, currently in acute episode; First episode, currently in partial remission; First episode, currently in full remission; Multiple episodes, currently in acute episode; Multiple episodes, currently in partial remission; Multiple episodes, currently in full remission; Continuous; Unspecified

[b]*Specify* if: With catatonia (use additional code F06.1)

[c]*Specify* current severity of delusions, hallucinations, disorganized speech, abnormal psychomotor behavior, negative symptoms, impaired cognition, depression, and mania symptoms

F21	Schizotypal (Personality) Disorder
F22	Delusional Disorder[a, c]
	Specify whether: Erotomanic type, Grandiose type, Jealous type, Persecutory type, Somatic type, Mixed type, Unspecified type
	Specify if: With bizarre content
F23	Brief Psychotic Disorder[b, c]
	Specify if: With marked stressor(s), Without marked stressor(s), With postpartum onset
F20.81	Schizophreniform Disorder[b, c]
	Specify if: With good prognostic features, Without good prognostic features
F20.9	Schizophrenia[a, b, c]
	Schizoaffective Disorder[a, b, c]
	Specify whether:
F25.0	Bipolar type
F25.1	Depressive type
	Substance/Medication-Induced Psychotic Disorder[c]
	NOTE: See the criteria set and corresponding recording procedures for substance-specific codes and ICD-10-CM coding.
	Specify if: With onset during intoxication, With onset during withdrawal
	Psychotic Disorder Due to Another Medical Condition[c]
	Specify whether:
F06.2	With delusions
F06.0	With hallucinations
F06.1	Catatonia Associated With Another Mental Disorder (Catatonia Specifier)
F06.1	Catatonic Disorder Due to Another Medical Condition
F06.1	Unspecified Catatonia
	NOTE: Code first R29.818 other symptoms involving nervous and musculoskeletal systems.
F28	Other Specified Schizophrenia Spectrum and Other Psychotic Disorder
F29	Unspecified Schizophrenia Spectrum and Other Psychotic Disorder

■ BIPOLAR AND RELATED DISORDERS

The following specifiers apply to Bipolar and Related Disorders where indicated:

[a]*Specify*: With anxious distress (*specify* current severity: mild, moderate, moderate-severe, severe); With mixed features; With rapid cycling; With melancholic features; With atypical features; With mood-congruent psychotic features; With mood incongruent psychotic features; With catatonia (use additional code F06.1); With peripartum onset; With seasonal pattern

	Bipolar I Disorder[a]
	Current or most recent episode manic
F31.11	Mild
F31.12	Moderate
F31.13	Severe
F31.2	With psychotic features
F31.73	In partial remission
F31.74	In full remission
F31.9	Unspecified
F31.0	Current or most recent episode hypomanic
F31.73	In partial remission
F31.74	In full remission
F31.9	Unspecified
	Current or most recent episode depressed
F31.31	Mild
F31.32	Moderate
F31.4	Severe
F31.5	With psychotic features
F31.75	In partial remission
F31.76	In full remission
F31.9	Unspecified
F31.9	Current or most recent episode unspecified
F31.81	Bipolar II Disorder[a]

Specify current or most recent episode: Hypomanic, Depressed

Specify course if full criteria for a mood episode are not currently met: In partial remission, In full remission

Specify severity if full criteria for a mood episode are not currently met: Mild, Moderate, Severe

F34.0	Cyclothymic Disorder

Specify if: With anxious distress

Substance/Medication-Induced Bipolar and Related Disorder

NOTE: See the criteria set and corresponding recording procedures for substance-specific codes and ICD-10-CM coding.

Specify if: With onset during intoxication, With onset during withdrawal

Bipolar and Related Disorder Due to Another Medical Condition

Specify if:

F06.33	With manic features
F06.33	With manic- or hypomanic-like episode
F06.34	With mixed features
F31.89	Other Specified Bipolar and Related Disorder
F31.9	Unspecified Bipolar and Related Disorder

■ DEPRESSIVE DISORDERS

The following specifiers apply to Depressive Disorders where indicated:

aSpecify: With anxious distress (specify current severity: mild, moderate, moderate-severe, severe); With mixed features; With melancholic features; With atypical features; With mood-congruent psychotic features; With mood-incongruent psychotic features; With catatonia (use additional code F06.1); With peripartum onset; With seasonal pattern

F34.8	Disruptive Mood Dysregulation Disorder
	Major Depressive Disordera
	Single episode
F32.0	Mild
F32.1	Moderate
F32.2	Severe
F32.3	With psychotic features
F32.4	In partial remission
F32.5	In full remission
F32.9	Unspecified
	Recurrent episode
F33.0	Mild
F33.1	Moderate
F33.2	Severe
F33.3	With psychotic features
F33.41	In partial remission
F33.42	In full remission
F33.9	Unspecified
F34.1	Persistent Depressive Disorder (Dysthymia)a
	Specify if: In partial remission, In full remission
	Specify if: Early onset, Late onset
	Specify if: With pure dysthymic syndrome; With persistent major depressive episode; With intermittent major depressive episodes, with current episode; With intermittent major depressive episodes, without current episode
	Specify current severity: Mild, Moderate, Severe
N94.3	Premenstrual Dysphoric Disorder
	Substance/Medication-Induced Depressive Disorder
	NOTE: See the criteria set and corresponding recording procedures for substance-specific codes and ICD-10-CM coding.
	Specify if: With onset during intoxication, With onset during withdrawal
	Depressive Disorder Due to Another Medical Condition
	Specify if:

F06.31	With depressive features
F06.32	With major depressive-like episode
F06.34	With mixed features
F32.8	Other Specified Depressive Disorder
F32.9	Unspecified Depressive Disorder

■ ANXIETY DISORDERS

F93.0	Separation Anxiety Disorder
F94.0	Selective Mutism
	Specific Phobia
	Specify if:
F40.218	Animal
F40.228	Natural environment
	Blood-injection-injury
F40.230	Fear of blood
F40.231	Fear of injections and transfusions
F40.232	Fear of other medical care
F40.233	Fear of injury
F40.248	Situational
F40.298	Other
F40.10	Social Anxiety Disorder (Social Phobia)
	Specify if: Performance only
F41.0	Panic Disorder
	Panic Attack Specifier
F40.00	Agoraphobia
F41.1	Generalized Anxiety Disorder
	Substance/Medication-Induced Anxiety Disorder
	NOTE: See the criteria set and corresponding recording procedures for substance-specific codes and ICD-10-CM coding.
	Specify if: With onset during intoxication, With onset during withdrawal, With onset after medication use
F06.4	Anxiety Disorder Due to Another Medical Condition
F41.9	Unspecified Anxiety Disorder

■ OBSESSIVE-COMPULSIVE AND RELATED DISORDERS

The following specifier applies to Obsessive-Compulsive and Related Disorders where indicated:

   [a]*Specify* if: With good or fair insight, With poor insight, With absent insight/delusional beliefs

F42	Obsessive-Compulsive Disorder[a]
	Specify if: Tic-related
F45.22	Body Dysmorphic Disorder[a]
	Specify if: With muscle dysmorphia
F42	Hoarding Disorder[a]
	Specify if: With excessive acquisition
F63.3	Trichotillomania (Hair-Pulling Disorder)

L98.1   Excoriation (Skin-Picking) Disorder
Substance/Medication-Induced Obsessive-Compulsive and Related Disorder
NOTE: See the criteria set and corresponding recording procedures for substance-specific codes and ICD-10-CM coding.
Specify if: With onset during intoxication, With onset during withdrawal, With onset after medication use

F06.8   Obsessive-Compulsive and Related Disorder Due to Another Medical Condition
Specify if: With obsessive-compulsive disorder–like symptoms, With appearance preoccupations, With hoarding symptoms, With hair-pulling symptoms, With skin-picking symptoms

F42   Other Specified Obsessive-Compulsive and Related Disorder

F42   Unspecified Obsessive-Compulsive and Related Disorder

■ TRAUMA- AND STRESSOR-RELATED DISORDERS

F94.1   Reactive Attachment Disorder
Specify if: Persistent
Specify current severity: Severe

F94.2   Disinhibited Social Engagement Disorder
Specify if: Persistent
Specify current severity: Severe

F43.10   Posttraumatic Stress Disorder (includes Posttraumatic Stress Disorder for Children 6 Years and Younger)
Specify whether: With dissociative symptoms
Specify if: With delayed expression

F43.0   Acute Stress Disorder
Adjustment Disorders
Specify whether:

F43.21   With depressed mood

F43.22   With anxiety

F43.23   With mixed anxiety and depressed mood

F43.24   With disturbance of conduct

F43.25   With mixed disturbance of emotions and conduct

F43.20   Unspecified

F43.8   Other Specified Trauma- and Stressor-Related Disorder

F43.9   Unspecified Trauma- and Stressor-Related Disorder

■ DISSOCIATIVE DISORDERS

F44.81   Dissociative Identity Disorder

F44.0   Dissociative Amnesia
Specify if:

F44.1   With dissociative fugue

F48.1   Depersonalization/Derealization Disorder

F44.89   Other Specified Dissociative Disorder

F44.9   Unspecified Dissociative Disorder

■ SOMATIC SYMPTOM AND RELATED DISORDERS

F45.1	Somatic Symptom Disorder
	Specify if: With predominant pain
	Specify if: Persistent
	Specify current severity: Mild, Moderate, Severe
F45.21	Illness Anxiety Disorder
	Specify whether: Care seeking type, Care avoidant type
	Conversion Disorder (Functional Neurological Symptom Disorder)
	Specify symptom type:
F44.4	With weakness or paralysis
F44.4	With abnormal movement
F44.4	With swallowing symptoms
F44.4	With speech symptom
F44.5	With attacks or seizures
F44.6	With anesthesia or sensory loss
F44.6	With special sensory symptom
F44.7	With mixed symptoms
	Specify if: Acute episode, Persistent
	Specify if: With psychological stressor (specify stressor), Without psychological stressor
F54	Psychological Factors Affecting Other Medical Conditions
	Specify current severity: Mild, Moderate, Severe, Extreme
F68.10	Factitious Disorder (includes Factitious Disorder Imposed on Self, Factitious Disorder Imposed on Another)
	Specify Single episode, Recurrent episodes
F45.8	Other Specified Somatic Symptom and Related Disorder
F45.9	Unspecified Somatic Symptom and Related Disorder

■ FEEDING AND EATING DISORDERS

The following specifiers apply to Feeding and Eating Disorders where indicated:

> a*Specify* if: In remission
> b*Specify* if: In partial remission, In full remission
> c*Specify* current severity: Mild, Moderate, Severe, Extreme

	Pica[a]
F98.3	In children
F50.8	In adults
F98.21	Rumination Disorder[a]
F50.8	Avoidant/Restrictive Food Intake Disorder[a]
	Anorexia Nervosa[b, c]
	Specify whether:
F50.01	Restricting type
F50.02	Binge-eating/purging type
F50.2	Bulimia Nervosa[b, c]
F50.8	Binge-Eating Disorder[b, c]
F50.8	Other Specified Feeding or Eating Disorder
F50.9	Unspecified Feeding or Eating Disorder

■ ELIMINATION DISORDERS

F98.0	Enuresis
	Specify whether: Nocturnal only, Diurnal only, Nocturnal and diurnal
F98.1	Encopresis
	Specify whether: With constipation and overflow incontinence, Without constipation and overflow incontinence
	Other Specified Elimination Disorder
N39.498	With urinary symptoms
R15.9	With fecal symptoms
	Unspecified Elimination Disorder
R32	With urinary symptoms
R15.9	With fecal symptoms

■ SLEEP-WAKE DISORDERS

The following specifiers apply to Sleep-Wake Disorders where indicated:

[a]*Specify* if: Episodic, Persistent, Recurrent
[b]*Specify* if: Acute, Subacute, Persistent
[c]*Specify* current severity: Mild, Moderate, Severe

G47.00	Insomnia Disorder[a]
	Specify if: With non-sleep disorder mental comorbidity, With other medical comorbidity, With other sleep disorder
G47.10	Hypersomnolence Disorder[b, c]
	Specify if: With mental disorder, With medical condition, With another sleep disorder
	Narcolepsy[c]
	Specify whether:
G47.419	Narcolepsy without cataplexy but with hypocretin deficiency
G47.411	Narcolepsy with cataplexy but without hypocretin deficiency
G47.419	Autosomal dominant cerebellar ataxia, deafness, and narcolepsy
G47.419	Autosomal dominant narcolepsy, obesity, and type 2 diabetes
G47.429	Narcolepsy secondary to another medical condition

Breathing-Related Sleep Disorders

G47.33	Obstructive Sleep Apnea Hypopnea[c]
	Central Sleep Apnea
	Specify whether:
G47.31	Idiopathic central sleep apnea
R06.3	Cheyne-Stokes breathing
G47.37	Central sleep apnea comorbid with opioid use
	NOTE: First code opioid use disorder, if present.
	Specify current severity
	Sleep-Related Hypoventilation
	Specify whether
G47.34	Idiopathic hypoventilation
G47.35	Congenital central alveolar hypoventilation

G47.36	Comorbid sleep-related hypoventilation
	Specify current severity
	Circadian Rhythm Sleep-Wake Disorders[a]
	Specify whether:
G47.21	Delayed sleep phase type
	Specify if: Familial, Overlapping with non-24-hour sleep-wake type
G47.22	Advanced sleep phase type
	Specify if: Familial
G47.23	Irregular sleep-wake type
G47.24	Non-24-hour sleep-wake type
G47.26	Shift work type
G47.20	Unspecified type

Parasomnias

	Non-Rapid Eye Movement Sleep Arousal Disorders
	Specify whether:
F51.3	Sleepwalking type
	Specify if: With sleep-related eating, With sleep-related sexual behavior (sexsomnia)
F51.4	Sleep terror type
F51.5	Nightmare Disorder[b, c]
	Specify if: During sleep onset
	Specify if: With associated non-sleep disorder, With associated other medical condition, With associated other sleep disorder
G47.52	Rapid Eye Movement Sleep Behavior Disorder
G25.81	Restless Legs Syndrome
	Substance/Medication-Induced Sleep Disorder
	NOTE: See the criteria set and corresponding recording procedures for substance-specific codes and ICD-10-CM coding.
	Specify whether: Insomnia type, Daytime sleepiness type, Parasomnia type, Mixed type
	Specify if: With onset during intoxication, With onset during discontinuation/withdrawal
G47.09	Other Specified Insomnia Disorder
G47.00	Unspecified Insomnia Disorder
G47.19	Other Specified Hypersomnolence Disorder
G47.10	Unspecified Hypersomnolence Disorder
G47.8	Other Specified Sleep-Wake Disorder
G47.9	Unspecified Sleep-Wake Disorder

■ SEXUAL DYSFUNCTIONS

The following specifiers apply to Sexual Dysfunctions where indicated:

    [a]*Specify* whether: Lifelong, Acquired
    [b]*Specify* whether: Generalized, Situational
    [c]*Specify* current severity: Mild, Moderate, Severe

F52.32	Delayed Ejaculation[a, b, c]
F52.21	Erectile Disorder[a, b, c]
F52.31	Female Orgasmic Disorder[a, b, c]
	Specify if: Never experienced an orgasm under any situation
F52.22	Female Sexual Interest/Arousal Disorder[a, b, c]
F52.6	Genito-Pelvic Pain/Penetration Disorder[a, c]
F52.0	Male Hypoactive Sexual Desire Disorder[a, b, c]
F52.4	Premature (Early) Ejaculation[a, b, c]
	Substance/Medication-Induced Sexual Dysfunction[c]
	NOTE: See the criteria set and corresponding recording procedures for substance-specific codes and ICD-10-CM coding.
	Specify if: With onset during intoxication, With onset during withdrawal, With onset after medication use
F52.8	Other Specified Sexual Dysfunction
F52.9	Unspecified Sexual Dysfunction

■ GENDER DYSPHORIA

	Gender Dysphoria
F64.2	Gender Dysphoria in Children
	Specify if: With a disorder of sex development
F64.1	Gender Dysphoria in Adolescents and Adults
	Specify if: With a disorder of sex development
	Specify if: Posttransition
	NOTE: Code the disorder of sex development if present, in addition to gender dysphoria.
F64.8	Other Specified Gender Dysphoria
64.9	Unspecified Gender Dysphoria

■ DISRUPTIVE, IMPULSE-CONTROL, AND CONDUCT DISORDERS

F91.3	Oppositional Defiant Disorder
	Specify current severity: Mild, Moderate, Severe
F63.81	Intermittent Explosive Disorder
	Conduct Disorder
	Specify whether:
F91.1	Childhood-onset type
F91.2	Adolescent-onset type
F91.9	Unspecified onset
	Specify if: With limited prosocial emotions
	Specify current severity: Mild, Moderate, Severe
F60.2	Antisocial Personality Disorder
F63.1	Pyromania

F63.2	Kleptomania
F91.8	Other Specified Disruptive, Impulse-Control, and Conduct Disorder
F91.9	Unspecified Disruptive, Impulse-Control, and Conduct Disorder

■ SUBSTANCE-RELATED AND ADDICTIVE DISORDERS

The following specifiers and note apply to Substance-Related and Addictive Disorders where indicated:

[a]*Specify* if: In early remission, In sustained remission
[b]*Specify* if: In a controlled environment
[c]*Specify* if: With perceptual disturbances
[d]The ICD-10-CM code indicates the comorbid presence of a moderate or severe substance use disorder, which must be present in order to apply the code for substance withdrawal.

Substance-Related Disorders
Alcohol-Related Disorders

	Alcohol Use Disorder[a, b]
	Specify current severity:
F10.10	Mild
F10.20	Moderate
F10.20	Severe
	Alcohol Intoxication
F10.129	With use disorder, mild
F10.229	With use disorder, moderate or severe
F10.929	Without use disorder
	Alcohol Withdrawal[c, d]
F10.239	Without perceptual disturbances
F10.232	With perceptual disturbances
	Other Alcohol-Induced Disorders
F10.99	Unspecified Alcohol-Related Disorder

Caffeine-Related Disorders

F15.929	Caffeine Intoxication
F15.93	Caffeine Withdrawal
	Other Caffeine-Induced Disorders
F15.99	Unspecified Caffeine-Related Disorder

Cannabis-Related Disorders

	Cannabis Use Disorder[a, b]
	Specify current severity
F12.10	Mild
F12.20	Moderate
F12.20	Severe
	Cannabis Intoxication[c]
	Without perceptual disturbances
F12.129	With use disorder, mild
F12.229	With use disorder, moderate or severe

F12.929	Without use disorder
	With perceptual disturbances
F12.122	With use disorder, mild
F12.222	With use disorder, moderate or severe
F12.922	Without use disorder
F12.288	Cannabis Withdrawal[d]
	Other Cannabis-Induced Disorders
F12.99	Unspecified Cannabis-Related Disorder

Hallucinogen-Related Disorders

	Phencyclidine Use Disorder[a, b]
	Specify current severity:
F16.10	Mild
F16.20	Moderate
F16.20	Severe
	Other Hallucinogen Use Disorder[a, b]
	Specify the particular hallucinogen
	Specify current severity:
F16.10	Mild
F16.20	Moderate
F16.20	Severe
	Phencyclidine Intoxication
F16.129	With use disorder, mild
F16.229	With use disorder, moderate or severe
F16.929	Without use disorder
	Other Hallucinogen Intoxication
F16.129	With use disorder, mild
F16.229	With use disorder, moderate or severe
F16.929	Without use disorder
F16.983	Hallucinogen Persisting Perception Disorder
	Other Phencyclidine-Induced Disorders
	Other Hallucinogen-Induced Disorders
F16.99	Unspecified Phencyclidine-Related Disorder
F16.99	Unspecified Hallucinogen-Related Disorder

Inhalant-Related Disorders

	Inhalant Use Disorder[a, b]
	Specify the particular inhalant
	Specify current severity:
F18.10	Mild
F18.20	Moderate
F18.20	Severe
	Inhalant Intoxication
F18.129	With use disorder, mild
F18.229	With use disorder, moderate or severe
F18.929	Without use disorder
	Other Inhalant-Induced Disorders
F18.99	Unspecified Inhalant-Related Disorder

Opioid-Related Disorders

	Opioid Use Disorder[a]
	Specify if: On maintenance therapy, In a controlled environment
	Specify current severity:
F11.10	Mild
F11.20	Moderate
F11.20	Severe
	Opioid Intoxication[c]
	Without perceptual disturbances
F11.129	With use disorder, mild
F11.229	With use disorder, moderate or severe
F11.922	Without use disorder
F11.23	Opioid Withdrawal[d]
	Other Opioid-Induced Disorders
F11.99	Unspecified Opioid-Related Disorder

Sedative-, Hypnotic-, or Anxiolytic-Related Disorders

	Sedative, Hypnotic, or Anxiolytic Use Disorder[a, b]
	Specify current severity:
F13.10	Mild
F13.20	Moderate
F13.20	Severe
	Sedative, Hypnotic, or Anxiolytic Intoxication
F13.129	With use disorder, mild
F13.229	With use disorder, moderate or severe
F13.929	Without use disorder
	Sedative, Hypnotic, or Anxiolytic Withdrawal[c, d]
F13.239	Without perceptual disturbances
F13.232	With perceptual disturbances
	Other Sedative-, Hypnotic-, or Anxiolytic-Induced Disorders
F13.99	Unspecified Sedative-, Hypnotic-, or Anxiolytic-Related Disorder

Stimulant-Related Disorders

	Stimulant Use Disorder[a, b]
	Specify current severity:
	Mild
F15.10	Amphetamine-type substance
F14.10	Cocaine
F15.10	Other or unspecified stimulant
	Moderate
F15.20	Amphetamine-type substance
F14.20	Cocaine
F15.20	Other or unspecified stimulant
	Severe
F15.20	Amphetamine-type substance
F14.20	Cocaine

F15.20	Other or unspecified stimulant
	Stimulant Intoxication[c]
	Specify the specific intoxicant
	Amphetamine or other stimulant, Without perceptual disturbances
F15.129	With use disorder, mild
F15.229	With use disorder, moderate or severe
F15.929	Without use disorder
	Cocaine, Without perceptual disturbances
F14.129	With use disorder, mild
F14.229	With use disorder, moderate or severe
F14.929	Without use disorder
	Amphetamine or other stimulant, With perceptual disturbances
F15.122	With use disorder, mild
F15.222	With use disorder, moderate or severe
F15.922	Without use disorder
	Cocaine, With perceptual disturbances
F14.122	With use disorder, mild
F14.222	With use disorder, moderate or severe
F14.922	Without use disorder
	Stimulant Withdrawal[d]
	Specify the specific substance causing the withdrawal syndrome
F15.23	Amphetamine or other stimulant
F14.23	Cocaine
	Other Stimulant-Induced Disorders
	Unspecified Stimulant-Related Disorder
F15.99	Amphetamine or other stimulant
F14.99	Cocaine

Tobacco-Related Disorders

	Tobacco Use Disorder[a]
	Specify if: On maintenance therapy, In a controlled environment
	Specify current severity:
Z72.0	Mild
F17.200	Moderate
F17.200	Severe
F17.203	Tobacco Withdrawal[d]
	Other Tobacco-Induced Disorders
F17.209	Unspecified Tobacco-Related Disorder

Other (or Unknown) Substance-Related Disorders

	Other (or Unknown) Substance Use Disorder[a, b]
	Specify current severity:
F19.10	Mild
F19.20	Moderate
F19.20	Severe
	Other (or Unknown) Substance Intoxication
F19.129	With use disorder, mild
F19.229	With use disorder, moderate or severe
F19.929	Without use disorder
F19.239	Other (or Unknown) Substance Withdrawal[d]
	Other (or Unknown) Substance-Induced Disorders
F19.99	Unspecified Other (or Unknown) Substance-Related Disorder

Non-Substance-Related Disorders

F63.0	Gambling Disorder[a]
	Specify if: Episodic, Persistent
	Specify current severity: Mild, Moderate, Severe

■ NEUROCOGNITIVE DISORDERS

	Delirium[a]
	NOTE: See the criteria set and corresponding recording procedures for substance-specific codes and ICD-10-CM coding.
	Specify whether:
	Substance intoxication delirium[a]
	Substance withdrawal delirium[a]
	Medication-induced delirium[a]
F05	Delirium due to another medical condition
F05	Delirium due to multiple etiologies
	Specify if: Acute, Persistent
	Specify if: Hyperactive, Hypoactive, Mixed level of activity
R41.0	Other Specified Delirium
R41.0	Unspecified Delirium

Major and Mild Neurocognitive Disorders

Specify whether due to: Alzheimer's disease, Frontotemporal lobar degeneration, Lewy body disease, Vascular disease, Traumatic brain injury, Substance/medication use, HIV infection, Prion disease, Parkinson's disease, Huntington's disease, Another medical condition, Multiple etiologies, Unspecified

> [a]Specify Without behavioral disturbance, With behavioral disturbance. For possible major neurocognitive disorder and for mild neurocognitive disorder, behavioral disturbance cannot be coded but should still be indicated in writing.
> [b]Specify current severity: Mild, Moderate, Severe. This specifier applies only to major neurocognitive disorders (including probable and possible).

NOTE: As indicated for each subtype, an additional medical code is needed for probable major neurocognitive disorder or major neurocognitive disorder. An additional medical code should *not* be used for possible major neurocognitive disorder or mild neurocognitive disorder.

Major or Mild Neurocognitive Disorder Due to Alzheimer's Disease

	Probable Major Neurocognitive Disorder Due to Alzheimer's Disease[b]
	NOTE: Code first G30.9 Alzheimer's disease.
F02.81	With behavioral disturbance
F02.80	Without behavioral disturbance
G31.9	Possible Major Neurocognitive Disorder Due to Alzheimer's Disease[a, b]
G31.84	Mild Neurocognitive Disorder Due to Alzheimer's Disease[a]

Major or Mild Frontotemporal Neurocognitive Disorder

Probable Major Neurocognitive Disorder Due to Frontotemporal Lobar Degeneration[b]
NOTE: Code first G31.09 frontotemporal disease.

F02.81	With behavioral disturbance
F02.80	Without behavioral disturbance
G31.9	Possible Major Neurocognitive Disorder Due to Frontotemporal Lobar Degeneration[a, b]
G31.84	Mild Neurocognitive Disorder Due to Frontotemporal Lobar Degeneration[a]

Major or Mild Neurocognitive Disorder With Lewy Bodies

Probable Major Neurocognitive Disorder With Lewy Bodies[b]
NOTE: Code first G31.83 Lewy body disease.

F02.81	With behavioral disturbance
F02.80	Without behavioral disturbance
G31.9	Possible Major Neurocognitive Disorder With Lewy Bodies[a, b]
G31.84	Mild Neurocognitive Disorder With Lewy Bodies[a]

Major or Mild Vascular Neurocognitive Disorder

Probable Major Vascular Neurocognitive Disorder[b]
NOTE: No additional medical code for vascular disease.

F01.51	With behavioral disturbance
F01.50	Without behavioral disturbance
G31.9	Possible Major Vascular Neurocognitive Disorder[a, b]
G31.84	Mild Vascular Neurocognitive Disorder[a]

Major or Mild Neurocognitive Disorder Due to Traumatic Brain Injury

Major Neurocognitive Disorder Due to Traumatic Brain Injury[b]
NOTE: For ICD-10-CM, code first S06.2X9S diffuse traumatic brain injury with loss of consciousness of unspecified duration, sequela.

F02.81	With behavioral disturbance
F02.80	Without behavioral disturbance
G31.84	Mild Neurocognitive Disorder Due to Traumatic Brain Injury[a]

Substance/Medication-Induced Major or Mild Neurocognitive Disorder[a]

NOTE: No additional medical code. See the criteria set and corresponding recording procedures for substance-specific codes and ICD-10-CM coding.

Specify if: Persistent

Major or Mild Neurocognitive Disorder Due to HIV Infection

Major Neurocognitive Disorder Due to HIV Infection[b]
NOTE: Code first B20 HIV infection.

F02.81	With behavioral disturbance
F02.80	Without behavioral disturbance
G31.84	Mild Neurocognitive Disorder Due to HIV Infection[a]

Major or Mild Neurocognitive Disorder Due to Prion Disease

Major Neurocognitive Disorder Due to Prion Disease[b]
NOTE: Code first A81.9 prion disease.

F02.81	With behavioral disturbance
F02.80	Without behavioral disturbance
G31.84	Mild Neurocognitive Disorder Due to Prion Disease[a]

Major or Mild Neurocognitive Disorder Due to Parkinson's Disease

Major Neurocognitive Disorder Probably Due to Parkinson's Disease[b]
NOTE: Code first G20 Parkinson's disease.

F02.81	With behavioral disturbance
F02.80	Without behavioral disturbance
G31.9	Major Neurocognitive Disorder Possibly Due to Parkinson's Disease[a, b]
G31.84	Mild Neurocognitive Disorder Due to Parkinson's Disease[a]

Major or Mild Neurocognitive Disorder Due to Huntington's Disease

Major Neurocognitive Disorder Due to Huntington's Disease[b]
NOTE: Code first G10 Huntington's disease.

F02.81	With behavioral disturbance
F02.80	Without behavioral disturbance
G31.84	Mild Neurocognitive Disorder Due to Huntington's Disease[a]

Major or Mild Neurocognitive Disorder Due to Another Medical Condition

Major Neurocognitive Disorder Due to Another Medical Condition[b]
NOTE: Code first the other medical condition.

F02.81	With behavioral disturbance
F02.80	Without behavioral disturbance
G31.84	Mild Neurocognitive Disorder Due to Another Medical Condition[a]

Major or Mild Neurocognitive Disorder Due to Multiple Etiologies

Major Neurocognitive Disorder Due to Multiple Etiologies[b]
NOTE: Code first all the etiological medical conditions (with the exception of vascular disease).

F02.81	With behavioral disturbance
F02.80	Without behavioral disturbance
G31.84	Mild Neurocognitive Disorder Due to Multiple Etiologies[a]

Unspecified Neurocognitive Disorder

R41.9	Unspecified Neurocognitive Disorder[a]

■ PERSONALITY DISORDERS

Cluster A Personality Disorders

F60.0	Paranoid Personality Disorder
F60.1	Schizoid Personality Disorder
F21	Schizotypal Personality Disorder

Cluster B Personality Disorders

F60.2	Antisocial Personality Disorder
F60.3	Borderline Personality Disorder
F60.4	Histrionic Personality Disorder
F60.81	Narcissistic Personality Disorder

Cluster C Personality Disorders

F60.6	Avoidant Personality Disorder
F60.7	Dependent Personality Disorder
F60.5	Obsessive-Compulsive Personality Disorder

Other Personality Disorders

F07.0	Personality Change Due to Another Medical Condition
	Specify whether: Labile type, Disinhibited type, Aggressive type, Apathetic type, Paranoid type, Other type, Combined type, Unspecified type
F60.89	Other Specified Personality Disorder
F60.9	Unspecified Personality Disorder

■ PARAPHILIC DISORDERS

The following specifier applies to Paraphilic Disorders where indicated:

[a]*Specify* if: In a controlled environment, In full remission

F65.3	Voyeuristic Disorder[a]
F65.2	Exhibitionistic Disorder[a]
	Specify whether: Sexually aroused by exposing genitals to prepubertal children, Sexually aroused by exposing genitals to physically mature individuals, Sexually aroused by exposing genitals to prepubertal children and to physically mature individuals.

F65.81	Frotteuristic Disorder[a]
F65.51	Sexual Masochism Disorder[a]
	Specify if: With asphyxiophilia
F65.52	Sexual Sadism Disorder[a]
F65.4	Pedophilic Disorder
	Specify whether: Exclusive type, Nonexclusive type
	Specify if: Sexually attracted to males, Sexually attracted to females, Sexually attracted to both
	Specify if: Limited to incest
F65.0	Fetishistic Disorder[a]
	Specify: Body part(s), Nonliving object(s), Other
F65.1	Transvestic Disorder[a]
	Specify if: With fetishism, With autogynephilia
F65.89	Other Specified Paraphilic Disorder
F65.9	Unspecified Paraphilic Disorder

■ OTHER MENTAL DISORDERS

F06.8	Other Specified Mental Disorder Due to Another Medical Condition
F09	Unspecified Mental Disorder Due to Another Medical Condition
F99	Other Specified Mental Disorder
F99	Unspecified Mental Disorder

■ MEDICATION-INDUCED MOVEMENT DISORDERS AND OTHER ADVERSE EFFECTS OF MEDICATION

G21.11	Neuroleptic-Induced Parkinsonism
G21.19	Other Medication-Induced Parkinsonism
G21.0	Neuroleptic Malignant Syndrome
G24.02	Medication-Induced Acute Dystonia
G25.71	Medication-Induced Acute Akathisia
G24.01	Tardive Dyskinesia
G24.09	Tardive Dystonia
G25.71	Tardive Akathisia
G25.1	Medication-Induced Postural Tremor
G25.79	Other Medication-Induced Movement Disorder
	Antidepressant Discontinuation Syndrome
T43.205A	Initial encounter
T43.205D	Subsequent encounter
T43.205S	Sequelae
	Other Adverse Effect of Medication
T50.905A	Initial encounter
T50.905D	Subsequent encounter
T50.905S	Sequelae

■ OTHER CONDITIONS THAT MAY BE A FOCUS OF CLINICAL ATTENTION

Relational Problems

Problems Related to Family Upbringing

Z62.820	Parent-Child Relational Problem
Z62.891	Sibling Relational Problem
Z62.29	Upbringing Away From Parents
Z62.898	Child Affected by Parental Relationship Distress

Other Problems Related to Primary Support Group

Z63.0	Relationship Distress With Spouse or Intimate Partner
Z63.5	Disruption of Family by Separation or Divorce
Z63.8	High Expressed Emotion Level Within Family
Z63.4	Uncomplicated Bereavement

Abuse and Neglect

Child Maltreatment and Neglect Problems

CHILD PHYSICAL ABUSE, CONFIRMED

T74.12XA	Initial encounter
T74.12XD	Subsequent encounter

CHILD PHYSICAL ABUSE, SUSPECTED

T76.12XA	Initial encounter
T76.12XD	Subsequent encounter

OTHER CIRCUMSTANCES RELATED TO CHILD PHYSICAL ABUSE

Z69.010	Encounter for mental health services for victim of child abuse by parent
Z69.020	Encounter for mental health services for victim of nonparental child abuse
Z62.810	Personal history (past history) of physical abuse in childhood
Z69.011	Encounter for mental health services for perpetrator of parental child abuse
Z69.021	Encounter for mental health services for perpetrator of nonparental child abuse

CHILD SEXUAL ABUSE, CONFIRMED

T74.22XA	Initial encounter
T74.22XD	Subsequent encounter

CHILD SEXUAL ABUSE, SUSPECTED

T76.22XA	Initial encounter
T76.22XD	Subsequent encounter

OTHER CIRCUMSTANCES RELATED TO CHILD SEXUAL ABUSE

Z69.010	Encounter for mental health services for victim of child sexual abuse by parent
Z69.020	Encounter for mental health services for victim of nonparental child sexual abuse

Z62.810	Personal history (past history) of sexual abuse in childhood
Z69.011	Encounter for mental health services for perpetrator of parental child sexual abuse
Z69.021	Encounter for mental health services for perpetrator of nonparental child sexual abuse

CHILD NEGLECT, CONFIRMED
| T74.02XA | Initial encounter |
| T74.02XD | Subsequent encounter |

CHILD NEGLECT, SUSPECTED
| T76.02XA | Initial encounter |
| T76.02XD | Subsequent encounter |

OTHER CIRCUMSTANCES RELATED TO CHILD NEGLECT
Z69.010	Encounter for mental health services for victim of child neglect by parent
Z69.020	Encounter for mental health services for victim of nonparental child neglect
Z62.812	Personal history (past history) of neglect in childhood
Z69.011	Encounter for mental health services for perpetrator of parental child neglect
Z69.021	Encounter for mental health services for perpetrator of nonparental child neglect

CHILD PSYCHOLOGICAL ABUSE, CONFIRMED
| T74.32XA | Initial encounter |
| T74.32XD | Subsequent encounter |

CHILD PSYCHOLOGICAL ABUSE, SUSPECTED
| T76.32XA | Initial encounter |
| T76.32XD | Subsequent encounter |

OTHER CIRCUMSTANCES RELATED TO CHILD PSYCHOLOGICAL ABUSE
Z69.010	Encounter for mental health services for victim of child psychological abuse by parent
Z69.020	Encounter for mental health services for victim of nonparental child psychological abuse
Z62.811	Personal history (past history) of psychological abuse in childhood
Z69.011	Encounter for mental health services for perpetrator of parental child psychological abuse
Z69.021	Encounter for mental health services for perpetrator of nonparental child psychological abuse

Adult Maltreatment and Neglect Problems

SPOUSE OR PARTNER VIOLENCE, PHYSICAL, CONFIRMED
| T74.11XA | Initial encounter |
| T74.11XD | Subsequent encounter |

SPOUSE OR PARTNER VIOLENCE, PHYSICAL, SUSPECTED
T76.11XA	Initial encounter
T76.11XD	Subsequent encounter

OTHER CIRCUMSTANCES RELATED TO SPOUSE OR PARTNER VIOLENCE, PHYSICAL
Z69.11	Encounter for mental health services for victim of spouse or partner violence, physical
Z91.410	Personal history (past history) of spouse or partner violence, physical
Z69.12	Encounter for mental health services for perpetrator of spouse or partner violence, physical

SPOUSE OR PARTNER VIOLENCE, SEXUAL, CONFIRMED
T74.21XA	Initial encounter
T74.21XD	Subsequent encounter

SPOUSE OR PARTNER VIOLENCE, SEXUAL, SUSPECTED
T76.21XA	Initial encounter
T76.21XD	Subsequent encounter

OTHER CIRCUMSTANCES RELATED TO SPOUSE OR PARTNER VIOLENCE, SEXUAL
Z69.81	Encounter for mental health services for victim of spouse or partner violence, sexual
Z91.410	Personal history (past history) of spouse or partner violence, sexual
Z69.12	Encounter for mental health services for perpetrator of spouse or partner violence, sexual

SPOUSE OR PARTNER NEGLECT, CONFIRMED
T74.01XA	Initial encounter
T74.01XD	Subsequent encounter

SPOUSE OR PARTNER NEGLECT, SUSPECTED
T76.01XA	Initial encounter
T76.01XD	Subsequent encounter

OTHER CIRCUMSTANCES RELATED TO SPOUSE OR PARTNER NEGLECT
Z69.11	Encounter for mental health services for victim of spouse or partner neglect
Z91.412	Personal history (past history) of spouse or partner neglect
Z69.12	Encounter for mental health services for perpetrator of spouse or partner neglect

SPOUSE OR PARTNER ABUSE, PSYCHOLOGICAL, CONFIRMED
T74.31XA	Initial encounter
T74.31XD	Subsequent encounter

SPOUSE OR PARTNER ABUSE, PSYCHOLOGICAL, SUSPECTED
T76.31XA	Initial encounter
T76.31XD	Subsequent encounter

OTHER CIRCUMSTANCES RELATED TO SPOUSE OR PARTNER ABUSE, PSYCHOLOGICAL

Z69.11	Encounter for mental health services for victim of spouse or partner psychological abuse
Z91.411	Personal history (past history) of spouse or partner psychological abuse
Z69.12	Encounter for mental health services for perpetrator of spouse or partner psychological abuse

ADULT PHYSICAL ABUSE BY NONSPOUSE OR NONPARTNER, CONFIRMED

T74.11XA	Initial encounter
T74.11XD	Subsequent encounter

ADULT PHYSICAL ABUSE BY NONSPOUSE OR NONPARTNER, SUSPECTED

T76.11XA	Initial encounter
T76.11XD	Subsequent encounter

ADULT SEXUAL ABUSE BY NONSPOUSE OR NONPARTNER, CONFIRMED

T74.21XA	Initial encounter
T74.21XD	Subsequent encounter

ADULT SEXUAL ABUSE BY NONSPOUSE OR NONPARTNER, SUSPECTED

T76.21XA	Initial encounter
T76.21XD	Subsequent encounter

ADULT PSYCHOLOGICAL ABUSE BY NONSPOUSE OR NONPARTNER, CONFIRMED

T74.31XA	Initial encounter
T74.31XD	Subsequent encounter

ADULT PSYCHOLOGICAL ABUSE BY NONSPOUSE OR NONPARTNER, SUSPECTED

T76.31XA	Initial encounter
T76.31XD	Subsequent encounter

OTHER CIRCUMSTANCES RELATED TO ADULT ABUSE BY NONSPOUSE OR NONPARTNER

Z69.81	Encounter for mental health services for victim of nonspousal adult abuse
Z69.82	Encounter for mental health services for perpetrator of nonspousal adult abuse

Educational and Occupational Problems
Educational Problems

Z55.9	Academic or Educational Problem

Occupational Problems

Z56.82	Problem Related to Current Military Deployment Status
Z56.9	Other Problem Related to Employment

Housing and Economic Problems

Housing Problems

Z59.0	Homelessness
Z59.1	Inadequate Housing
Z59.2	Discord With Neighbor, Lodger, or Landlord
Z59.3	Problem Related to Living in a Residential Institution

Economic Problems

Z59.4	Lack of Adequate Food or Safe Drinking Water
Z59.5	Extreme Poverty
Z59.6	Low Income
Z59.7	Insufficient Social Insurance or Welfare Support
Z59.9	Unspecified Housing or Economic Problem

Other Problems Related to the Social Environment

Z60.0	Phase of Life Problem
Z60.2	Problem Related to Living Alone
Z60.3	Acculturation Difficulty
Z60.4	Social Exclusion or Rejection
Z60.5	Target of (Perceived) Adverse Discrimination or Persecution
Z60.9	Unspecified Problem Related to Social Environment

Problems Related to Crime or Interaction With the Legal System

Z65.4	Victim of Crime
Z65.0	Conviction in Civil or Criminal Proceedings Without Imprisonment
Z65.1	Imprisonment or Other Incarceration
Z65.2	Problems Related to Release From Prison
Z65.3	Problems Related to Other Legal Circumstances

Other Health Service Encounters for Counseling and Medical Advice

Z70.9	Sex Counseling
Z71.9	Other Counseling or Consultation

Problems Related to Other Psychosocial, Personal, and Environmental Circumstances

Z65.8	Religious or Spiritual Problem
Z64.0	Problems Related to Unwanted Pregnancy
Z64.1	Problems Related to Multiparity
Z64.4	Discord With Social Service Provider, Including Probation Officer, Case Manager, or Social Services Worker
Z65.4	Victim of Terrorism or Torture
Z65.5	Exposure to Disaster, War, or Other Hostilities
Z65.8	Other Problem Related to Psychosocial Circumstances
Z65.9	Unspecified Problem Related to Unspecified Psychosocial Circumstances

Other Circumstances of Personal History

Z91.49	Other Personal History of Psychological Trauma
Z91.5	Personal History of Self-Harm
Z91.82	Personal History of Military Deployment
Z91.89	Other Personal Risk Factors
Z72.9	Problem Related to Lifestyle
Z72.811	Adult Antisocial Behavior
Z72.810	Child or Adolescent Antisocial Behavior

Problems Related to Access to Medical and Other Health Care

Z75.3	Unavailability or Inaccessibility of Health Care Facilities
Z75.4	Unavailability or Inaccessibility of Other Helping Agencies

Nonadherence to Medical Treatment

Z91.19	Nonadherence to Medical Treatment
E66.9	Overweight or Obesity
Z76.5	Malingering
Z91.83	Wandering Associated With a Mental Disorder
R41.83	Borderline Intellectual Functioning

Mental Status Assessment

Gathering the correct information about the patient's mental status is essential to the development of an appropriate plan of care. The mental status examination is a description of all the areas of the patient's mental functioning. The following are the components that are considered critical in the assessment of a patient's mental status. Examples of interview questions and criteria for assessment are included.

■ IDENTIFYING DATA

1. Name
2. Gender
3. Age
   a. How old are you?
   b. When were you born?
4. Race/culture
   a. What country did you (your ancestors) come from?
   b. Are there cultural practices that are important to you?
5. Occupational/financial status
   a. How do you make your living?
   b. How do you obtain money for your needs?
6. Educational level
   a. What was the highest grade level you completed in school?
7. Significant other
   a. Are you married?
   b. Do you have a significant relationship with another person?
8. Living arrangements
   a. Do you live alone?
   b. With whom do you share your home?
9. Religious preference
   a. Do you have a religious preference?
   b. Is religion something that is important to you?
10. Allergies
    a. Are you allergic to anything?
    b. Foods? Medications?

11. Special diet considerations
    a. Do you have any special diet requirements?
    b. Diabetic? Low sodium?
12. Chief complaint
    a. For what reason did you come for help today?
    b. What seems to be the problem?
13. Medical diagnosis

■ GENERAL DESCRIPTION

Appearance

1. Grooming and dress
    a. Note unusual modes of dress.
    b. Evidence of soiled clothing?
    c. Use of makeup?
    d. Neat; unkempt?
2. Hygiene
    a. Note evidence of body or breath odor.
    b. Condition of skin, fingernails.
3. Posture
    a. Note if standing upright, rigid, slumped over.
4. Height and weight
    a. Perform accurate measurements.
5. Level of eye contact
    a. Intermittent?
    b. Occasional and fleeting?
    c. Sustained and intense?
    d. No eye contact?
6. Hair color and texture
    a. Is hair clean and healthy-looking?
    b. Greasy, matted, tangled?
7. Evidence of scars, tattoos, or other distinguishing skin marks
    a. Note any evidence of swelling or bruises.
    b. Birth marks?
    c. Rashes?
8. Evaluation of patient's appearance compared with chronological age.

Motor Activity

1. Tremors
    a. Do hands or legs tremble?
       • Continuously?
       • At specific times?
2. Tics or other stereotypical movements
    a. Any evidence of facial tics?
    b. Jerking or spastic movements?

3. Mannerisms and gestures
   a. Specific facial or body movements during conversation?
   b. Nail biting?
   c. Covering face with hands?
   d. Grimacing?
4. Hyperactivity
   a. Gets up and down out of chair.
   b. Paces.
   c. Unable to sit still.
5. Restlessness or agitation
   a. Lots of fidgeting.
   b. Clenching hands.
6. Aggressiveness
   a. Overtly angry and hostile.
   b. Threatening.
   c. Uses sarcasm.
7. Rigidity
   a. Sits or stands in a rigid position.
   b. Arms and legs appear stiff and unyielding.
8. Gait patterns
   a. Any evidence of limping?
   b. Limitation of range of motion?
   c. Ataxia?
   d. Shuffling?
9. Echopraxia
   a. Evidence of mimicking the actions of others?
10. Psychomotor retardation
    a. Movements are very slow.
    b. Thinking and speech are very slow.
    c. Posture is slumped.
11. Freedom of movement (range of motion)
    a. Note any limitation in ability to move.
12. Apraxia
    a. Evidence of difficulty performing tasks or movements when asked, even though the request is understood.

Speech Patterns

1. Slowness or rapidity of speech
   a. Note whether speech seems very rapid or slower than normal.
2. Pressure of speech
   a. Note whether speech seems frenzied.
   b. Unable to be interrupted?
3. Intonation
   a. Are words spoken with appropriate emphasis?
   b. Are words spoken in monotone, without emphasis?

4. Volume
   a. Is speech very loud? Soft?
   b. Is speech low-pitched? High-pitched?
5. Stuttering or other speech impairments
   a. Hoarseness?
   b. Slurred speech?
6. Aphasia
   a. Difficulty forming words.
   b. Use of incorrect words.
   c. Difficulty thinking of specific words.
   d. Making up words (neologisms).

General Attitude

1. Cooperative/uncooperative
   a. Answers questions willingly.
   b. Refuses to answer questions.
2. Friendly/hostile/defensive
   a. Is sociable and responsive.
   b. Is sarcastic and irritable.
3. Uninterested/apathetic
   a. Refuses to participate in interview process.
4. Attentive/interested
   b. Actively participates in interview process.
5. Guarded/suspicious
   a. Continuously scans the environment.
   b. Questions motives of interviewer.
   c. Refuses to answer questions.

■ EMOTIONS

Mood

1. Depressed; despairing
   a. Do you have overwhelming feelings of sadness?
   b. Have you experienced a loss of interest in regular activities?
2. Irritable
   a. Are you easily annoyed and provoked to anger?
3. Anxious
   a. Are you feeling anxious, apprehensive, or worried?
   b. Does the patient appear anxious?
4. Elated
   a. Expresses feelings of joy and intense pleasure.
   b. Is intensely optimistic.
5. Euphoric
   a. Demonstrates a heightened sense of elation.
   b. Expresses feelings of heightened elation ("Everything is wonderful!").

6. Fearful
   a. Demonstrates or verbalizes feeling of apprehension associated with real or perceived danger.
7. Guilty
   a. Expresses a feeling of discomfort associated with real or perceived wrongdoing.
   b. May be associated with feelings of sadness and despair.
8. Labile
   a. Exhibits mood swings that range from euphoria to depression or anxiety.

Affect

1. Congruence with mood
   a. Outward emotional expression is consistent with mood (e.g., if depressed, emotional expression is sadness, eyes downcast, may be crying).
2. Constricted or blunted
   a. Minimal outward emotional expression is observed.
3. Flat
   a. There is an absence of outward emotional expression.
4. Appropriate
   a. The outward emotional expression is what would be expected in a certain situation (e.g., crying upon hearing of a death).
5. Inappropriate
   a. The outward emotional expression is incompatible with the situation (e.g., laughing upon hearing of a death).

■ THOUGHT PROCESSES
Form of Thought

1. Flight of ideas
   a. Verbalizations are continuous and rapid, and flow from one to another.
2. Loose associations
   a. Verbalizations shift from one unrelated topic to another.
3. Circumstantiality
   a. Verbalizations are lengthy and tedious, and because of numerous details, are delayed reaching the intended point.
4. Tangentiality
   a. Verbalizations that are lengthy and tedious, and never reach an intended point.
5. Neologisms
   a. The individual is making up nonsensical-sounding words, which have meaning only to him or her.

6. Concrete thinking
   a. Thinking is literal; elemental.
   b. Absence of ability to think abstractly.
   c. Unable to translate simple proverbs.
7. Clang associations
   a. Speaking in puns or rhymes; using words that sound alike but have different meanings.
8. Word salad
   a. Using a mixture of words that have no meaning together; sounding incoherent.
9. Perseveration
   a. Repetition of words or phrases in the absence or cessation of socially appropriate context.
10. Echolalia
    a. Persistently repeating what another person says.
11. Mutism
    a. Does not speak (either cannot or will not).
12. Poverty of speech
    a. Speaks very little; may respond in monosyllables.
13. Ability to concentrate and disturbance of attention
    a. Does the person hold attention to the topic at hand?
    b. Is the person easily distractible?
    c. Is there selective attention (e.g., blocks out topics that create anxiety)?

Content of Thought

1. Delusions (Does the person have unrealistic ideas or beliefs?)
   a. Persecutory: A belief that someone is out to get him or her is some way (e.g., "The FBI will be here at any time to take me away").
   b. Grandiose: An idea that he or she is all-powerful or of great importance (e.g., "I am the king … and this is my kingdom! I can do anything!").
   c. Reference: An idea that whatever is happening in the environment is about him or her (e.g., "Just watch the movie on TV tonight. It is about my life").
   d. Control or influence: A belief that his or her behavior and thoughts are being controlled by external forces (e.g., "I get my orders from Channel 27. I do only what the forces dictate").
   e. Somatic: A belief that he or she has a dysfunctional body part (e.g., "My heart is at a standstill. It is no longer beating").
   f. Nihilistic: A belief that he or she, or a part of the body, or even the world does not exist or has been destroyed (e.g., "I am no longer alive").

2. Suicidal or homicidal ideas
   a. Is the individual expressing ideas of harming self or others?
   b. Does the individual have a plan?
   c. Does the individual have access to the identified means for his or her plan?
   d. How strong is his or her intent to die?
3. Obsessions
   a. Is the person verbalizing about a persistent thought or feeling that he or she is unable to eliminate from their consciousness?
4. Paranoia/suspiciousness
   a. Continuously scans the environment.
   b. Questions motives of interviewer.
   c. Refuses to answer questions.
5. Magical thinking
   a. Is the person speaking in a way that indicates his or her words or actions have power (e.g., "If you step on a crack, you break your mother's back!")?
6. Impaired religiosity
   a. Is the individual demonstrating obsession with religious ideas and behavior that is causing marked distress and impairing ability to function?
7. Phobias
   a. Is there evidence of irrational fears (of a specific object, or a social situation)?
8. Poverty of content
   a. Is little information conveyed by the patient because of vagueness or stereotypical statements or clichés?

■ PERCEPTUAL DISTURBANCES

1. Hallucinations. (Is the person experiencing unrealistic sensory perceptions?)
   a. Auditory. (Is the individual hearing voices or other sounds that do not exist?)
   b. Visual. (Is the individual seeing images that do not exist?)
   c. Tactile. (Does the individual feel unrealistic sensations on the skin?)
   d. Olfactory. (Does the individual smell odors that do not exist?)
   e. Gustatory. (Does the individual have a false perception of an unpleasant taste?)
2. Illusions
   a. Does the individual misperceive or misinterpret real stimuli within the environment? (Sees something and thinks it is something else?)

3. Depersonalization (altered perception of the self)
   a. Does the individual verbalize feeling "outside the body," visualizing himself or herself from afar?
4. Derealization (altered perception of the environment)
   a. Does the individual verbalize that the environment feels "strange or unreal?" A feeling that the surroundings have changed?

■ SENSORIUM AND COGNITIVE ABILITY

1. Level of alertness/consciousness
   a. Is the individual clear-minded and attentive to the environment?
   b. Or is there disturbance in perception and awareness of the surroundings?
2. Orientation. Is the person oriented to the following?
   a. Time.
   b. Place.
   c. Person.
   d. Circumstances.
3. Memory
   a. Recent. (Is the individual able to remember occurrences of the past few days?)
   b. Remote. (Is the individual able to remember occurrences of the distant past?)
   c. Confabulation. (Does the individual fill in memory gaps with experiences that have no basis in fact?)
4. Capacity for abstract thought
   a. Can the individual interpret proverbs correctly?
      • "What does 'no use crying over spilled milk' mean?"

■ IMPULSE CONTROL

1. Ability to control impulses. (Does psychosocial history reveal problems with any of the following?)
   a. Aggression.
   b. Hostility.
   c. Fear.
   d. Guilt.
   e. Affection.
   f. Sexual feelings.

■ JUDGMENT

1. Ability to solve problems and make decisions
   a. What are your plans for the future?
   b. What do you plan to do to reach your goals?
2. Does the patient demonstrate adaptive or maladaptive coping strategies?

■ INSIGHT

1. Knowledge about self
   a. Awareness of limitations.
   b. Awareness of consequences of actions.
   c. Awareness of illness.
      - "Do you think you have a problem?"
      - "Do you think you need treatment?"
2. Does the patient demonstrate awareness or lack of awareness of adaptive/maladaptive use of coping strategies and ego defense mechanisms (e.g., rationalizing maladaptive behaviors, projection of blame, displacement of anger)?

Assigning Nursing Diagnoses to Patient Behaviors

Following is a list of patient behaviors and the NANDA International nursing diagnoses (NANDA-I, 2018) that correspond to the behaviors and that may be used in planning care for the patient exhibiting the specific behavioral symptoms.

Behaviors	NANDA Nursing Diagnoses
Aggression; hostility	Risk for injury; Risk for other-directed violence
Anorexia or refusal to eat	Imbalanced nutrition: Less than body requirements; Ineffective adolescent eating dynamics
Anxious behavior	Anxiety (specify level); Acute substance withdrawal syndrome; Complicated grieving; Imbalanced energy field
Confusion; memory loss	Confusion, acute/chronic; Impaired memory; Disturbed thought processes*
Delusions	Disturbed thought processes*
Denial of problems	Ineffective denial
Depressed mood or anger turned inward	Complicated grieving
Detoxification; withdrawal from substances	Risk for injury; Acute substance withdrawal syndrome
Difficulty accepting new diagnosis or recent change in health status	Risk-prone health behavior; Ineffective denial
Difficulty making important life decision	Decisional conflict
Difficulty sleeping	Insomnia; Disturbed sleep pattern
Difficulty with interpersonal relationships	Impaired social interaction; ineffective relationship

Behaviors	NANDA Nursing Diagnoses
Disruption in capability to perform usual responsibilities	Ineffective role performance; fatigue
Dissociative behaviors (depersonalization; derealization)	Disturbed sensory perception (kinesthetic)*
Expresses feelings of disgust about body or body part	Disturbed body image
Expresses anger at God	Spiritual distress
Expresses lack of control over personal situation	Powerlessness
Fails to follow prescribed therapy	Ineffective health management;
Flashbacks, nightmares, obsession with traumatic experience	Posttrauma syndrome; Rape-trauma syndrome
Hallucinations	Disturbed sensory perception (auditory; visual)*
Highly critical of self or others	Low self-esteem (chronic; situational)
Inability to meet basic needs	Self-care deficit (feeding; bathing; dressing; toileting)
Loose associations or flight of ideas	Impaired verbal communication
Loss of a valued entity, recently experienced	Risk for complicated grieving
Manic hyperactivity	Risk for injury; Labile emotional control
Manipulative behavior	Ineffective coping
Multiple personalities; gender dysphoria	Disturbed personal identity
Orgasm, problems with; lack of sexual desire; erectile dysfunction	Sexual dysfunction
Overeating, compulsive Overweight; Obesity	Risk for imbalanced nutrition: More than body requirements; Risk for metabolic imbalance syndrome
Phobias	Fear
Physical symptoms as coping behavior	Ineffective coping
Potential or anticipated loss of significant entity	Grieving
Projection of blame; rationalization of failures; denial of personal responsibility	Defensive coping
Ritualistic behaviors	Anxiety (severe); ineffective coping
Seductive remarks; inappropriate sexual behaviors	Impaired social interaction
Self-inflicted injuries (non-life-threatening)	Self-mutilation; Risk for self-mutilation
Sexual behaviors (difficulty, limitations, or changes in; reported dissatisfaction)	Ineffective sexuality pattern

(Continued)

Behaviors	NANDA Nursing Diagnoses
Stress from caring for chronically ill person	Caregiver role strain
Stress from locating to new environment	Relocation stress syndrome
Substance use as a coping behavior	Ineffective coping
Substance use (denies use is a problem)	Ineffective denial
Suicidal gestures/threats; suicidal ideation	Risk for suicide; Risk for self-directed violence
Suspiciousness	Ineffective coping; Disturbed thought processes*
Vomiting, excessive, self-induced	Risk for deficient fluid volume
Withdrawn behavior	Social isolation

*These diagnoses have been retired from the NANDA-I list of approved nursing diagnoses.

Brief Mental Status Evaluation

Area of Mental Function Evaluated	Evaluation Activity
Orientation to time	"What year is it? What month is it? What day is it?" (3 points)
Orientation to place	"Where are you now?" (1 point)
Attention and immediate recall	"Repeat these words now: bell, book, & candle." (3 points) "Remember these words and I will ask you to repeat them in a few minutes."
Abstract thinking	"What does this mean: No use crying over spilled milk." (3 points)
Recent memory	"Say the three words I asked you to remember earlier." (3 points)
Naming objects	Point to eyeglasses and ask, "What is this?" Repeat with one other item (e.g., calendar, watch, pencil). (2 points possible)
Ability to follow simple verbal command	"Tear this piece of paper in half and put it in the trash container." (2 points)
Ability to follow simple written command	Write a command on a piece of paper (e.g., TOUCH YOUR NOSE), give the paper to the patient and say, "Do what it says on this paper." (1 point for correct action)
Ability to use language correctly	Ask the patient to write a sentence. (3 points if sentence has a subject, a verb, and has valid meaning)
Ability to concentrate	"Say the months of the year in reverse, starting with December." (1 point each for correct answers from November through August; 4 points possible)

(Continued)

Area of Mental Function Evaluated	Evaluation Activity
Understanding spatial relationships	Instruct the patient to draw a clock; put in all the numbers; and set the hands on 3 o'clock. (clock circle = 1 point; numbers in correct sequence = 1 point; numbers placed on clock correctly = 1 point; two hands on the clock = 1 point; hands set at correct time = 1 point. (5 points possible)

Scoring: 21–30 = normal; 11–20 = mild cognitive impairment; 0–10 = severe cognitive impairment (scores are not absolute and must be considered within the comprehensive diagnostic assessment).

Sources: Folstein, M.F., Folstein, S.E., & McHugh, P.R. (1975). Mini-mental state: A practical method for grading the cognitive state of patients for the clinician. *Journal of Psychiatric Research, 12*(3), 189–198; Kaufman, D.M., & Zun, L. (1995). A quantifiable, brief mental status examination for emergency patients. *Journal of Emergency Medicine, 13*(4), 440–456; Kokman, E., Smith, G.E., Petersen, R.C., Tangalos, E., & Ivnik, R.C. (1991). The short test of mental status: Correlations with standardized psychometric testing. *Archives of Neurology, 48*(7), 725–728; *Merck manual of health & aging.* (2005). New York: Random House; Pfeiffer, E. (1975). A short portable mental status questionnaire for the assessment of organic brain deficit in elderly patients. *Journal of the American Geriatric Society, 23*(10), 433–441.

Trauma-Informed Care

History of trauma is associated with many physical, psychological, and mental symptoms. Trauma-informed care recognizes the importance of screening all patients for history of trauma and providing care that is sensitive to the impact of trauma in provision of health care. The following are selected interventions essential to this approach.

Screening and Assessment:

1. Ask patients if they have had any history of traumatic events.
2. For patients with history of exposure to traumatic events, screen for physical, psychological, and mental symptoms associated with trauma. Many validated screening tools are available at (http://www.ptsd.va.gov/professional/pages/assessments/assessment.asp).
   Key aspects to include in the assessment process are:
   a. Trauma-related symptoms.
   b. Depressive or dissociative symptoms, sleep disturbances, and intrusive experiences.
   c. Past and present mental disorders, including typically trauma-related disorders (e.g., mood disorders).
   d. Specific trauma type (e.g., forms of interpersonal violence, adverse childhood events, combat experiences).
   e. Substance abuse.
   f. Social support and coping styles.
   g. Availability of resources.
   h. Risks for self-harm, suicide, and violence.
   i. Health screenings.
3. Be aware of the patient's emotional response to discussing traumatic events. Don't require patient to describe in detail any traumatic experiences that are emotionally overwhelming to discuss.
4. Focus assessment on how trauma symptoms are affecting the patient's current functioning. Note that not all patients make the connection between their trauma history and current maladaptive behaviors (such as substance use or avoidant behaviors).

5. Recognize symptoms that are often associated with trauma history, including:
   a. Emotional dysregulation – difficulty managing emotional reactions such as anger, fear, and anxiety.
   b. Numbing – feelings are detached from thoughts and behaviors.
   c. Somatization – focusing on physical symptoms.
   d. Misinterpretation of current events as dangerous.
   e. Trauma-induced hallucinations and delusions.
   f. Intrusive thoughts or memories.
   g. Guilt.
   h. Hyperarousal.
   i. Sleep disturbances.
   j. Flashbacks.

Education:

1. Educate the patient about how this historical information is important in guiding current treatment.
2. Educate the patient that symptoms such as flashbacks of a traumatic event, sleep disturbances, hyperarousal or hypervigilance, as well as many physical symptoms, are reactions to extreme psychological distress.
3. Communicate that treatment and other wellness activities can improve both psychological and physiological symptoms (e.g., therapy, meditation, exercise, yoga).
4. Explain that trauma symptoms are not a character flaw, weakness, or even unexpected responses. In other words, normalize the trauma symptoms.

Support:

1. Communicate a message of hope, that the patient is not alone, not at fault, and recovery is very possible.
2. Approach the patient with a matter-of-fact, supportive attitude.
3. Communicate with honesty and transparency.
4. Respect the patient's personal space and boundaries. Request permission before touching the patient.
5. Allow the patient time to reduce anxiety and become oriented to the present if needed.
6. Avoid any communication that implies judgment about the trauma.
7. Empower the patient to make decisions and collaborate in care and treatment.

Interventions for Acute Trauma Symptoms (Such as Flashbacks):

1. Create a safe environment.
2. Assist the patient to focus on the here and now.
3. Reassure the patient that he or she is safe.
4. When the patient is calm and present-oriented, assist the patient to identify triggers that might place the patient at greater risk for retraumatization.

Referral

1. Discuss with the patient options for longer-term therapy to address and resolve trauma symptoms.
2. Facilitate referral in collaboration with the patient and other members of the health care team.

Source: Adapted from Substance Abuse and Mental Health Services Administration (SAMHSA). (2014). *Trauma-informed care in behavioral health services: Treatment improvement protocol 57*. Retrieved from https://www.ncbi.nlm.nih.gov/books/NBK207191/

APPENDIX O

DEA Controlled Substances Schedules

Classes or schedules are determined by the Drug Enforcement Agency (DEA), an arm of the U.S. Justice Department, and are based on the potential for abuse and dependence liability (physical and psychological) of the medication. Some states may have stricter prescription regulations. Physicians, dentists, podiatrists, and veterinarians may prescribe controlled substances. Nurse practitioners and physician's assistants may prescribe controlled substances with limitations that vary from state to state.

Schedule I (C-I)

Potential for abuse is so high as to be unacceptable. May be used for research with appropriate limitations. Examples are LSD and heroin.

Schedule II (C-II)

High potential for abuse and extreme liability for physical and psychological dependence (amphetamines, opioid analgesics, dronabinol, certain barbiturates). Outpatient prescriptions must be in writing. In emergencies, telephone orders may be acceptable if a written prescription is provided within 72 hours. No refills are allowed.

Schedule III (C-III)

Intermediate potential for abuse (less than C-II) and intermediate liability for physical and psychological dependence (certain nonbarbiturate sedatives, certain nonamphetamine CNS stimulants, and certain opioid analgesics). Outpatient prescriptions can be refilled five times within 6 months from date of issue if authorized by prescriber. Telephone orders are acceptable.

Schedule IV (C-IV)

Less abuse potential than Schedule III with minimal liability for physical or psychological dependence (certain sedative-hypnotics, certain antianxiety agents, some barbiturates, benzodiazepines, chloral hydrate, pentazocine, and propoxyphene).

Outpatient prescriptions can be refilled six times within 6 months from date of issue if authorized by prescriber. Telephone orders are acceptable.

Schedule V (C-V)

Minimal abuse potential. Number of outpatient refills determined by prescriber. Some products (cough suppressants with small amounts of codeine, antidiarrheals containing paregoric) may be available without prescription to patients older than 18 years of age.

Source: Vallerand, A.H., & Sanoski, C.A. (2019). *Davis's drug guide for nurses* (16th ed.). Philadelphia: F.A. Davis. With permission.

APPENDIX **P**

Abnormal Involuntary Movement Scale (AIMS)

Name _____ Rater Name _____
Date _____

Instructions: Complete the examination procedure before making ratings. For movement ratings, circle the highest severity observed. Rate movements that occur upon activation one *less* than those observed spontaneously. Circle movement as well as code number that applies.

Code: 0 = None
1 = Minimal, may be normal
2 = Mild
3 = Moderate
4 = Severe

Facial and Oral Movements		
	1. **Muscles of facial expression** (e.g., movements of forehead, eyebrows, periorbital area, cheeks, including frowning, blinking, smiling, grimacing)	0 1 2 3 4
	2. **Lips and perioral area** (e.g., puckering, pouting, smacking)	0 1 2 3 4
	3. **Jaw** (e.g., biting, clenching, chewing, mouth opening, lateral movement)	0 1 2 3 4
	4. **Tongue** (Rate only increases in movement both in and out of mouth. NOT inability to sustain movement. Darting in and out of mouth)	0 1 2 3 4

Extremity Movements	5. **Upper (arms, wrists, hands, fingers)** (Include choreic movements [i.e., rapid, objectively purposeless, irregular, spontaneous] and athetoid movements [i.e., slow, irregular, complex serpentine]. *Do not include tremor* [i.e., repetitive, regular, rhythmic])	0 1 2 3 4
	6. **Lower (legs, knees, ankles, toes)** (e.g., lateral knee movement, foot tapping, heel dropping, foot squirming, inversion and eversion of foot)	0 1 2 3 4
Trunk Movements	7. **Neck, shoulders, hips** (e.g., rocking, twisting, squirming, pelvic gyrations)	0 1 2 3 4
Global Judgments	8. **Severity of abnormal movements overall**	0 1 2 3 4
	9. **Incapacitation due to abnormal movements**	0 1 2 3 4
Dental Status	10. **Patient's awareness of abnormal movements** (Rate only the patient's report)	0 No awareness 1 Aware, no distress 2 Aware, mild distress 3 Aware, moderate distress 4 Aware, severe distress
	11. **Current problems with teeth and/or dentures?**	No Yes
	12. **Are dentures usually worn?**	No Yes
	13. **Edentia?**	No Yes
	14. **Do movements disappear in sleep?**	No Yes

Either before or after completing the Examination Procedure, observe the patient unobtrusively, at rest (e.g., in waiting room). The chair to be used in this examination should be a hard, firm one without arms.

1. Ask patient to remove shoes and socks.
2. Ask patient whether there is anything in his/her mouth (i.e., gum, candy, etc.) and, if there is, to remove it.
3. Ask patient about the current condition of his/her teeth. Ask the patient if he/she wears dentures. Do teeth or dentures bother the patient now?
4. Ask patient whether he/she notices any movements in mouth, face, hands, or feet. If yes, ask to describe and to what extent they currently bother the patient or interfere with his/her activities.
5. Have patient sit in chair with both hands on knees, legs slightly apart, and feet flat on floor. (Look at entire body for movements while in this position.)
6. Ask patient to sit with hands hanging unsupported. If male, between legs, if female and wearing a dress, hanging over knees. (Observe hands and other body areas.)
7. Ask patient to open mouth. (Observe tongue at rest within mouth.) Do this twice.
8. Ask patient to protrude tongue. (Observe abnormalities of tongue movement.) Do this twice.
9. Ask patient to tap thumb with each finger as rapidly as possible for 10 to 15 seconds; separately with right hand, then with left hand. (Observe facial and leg movements.)
10. Flex and extend patient's left and right arms (one at a time). (Note any rigidity.)
11. Ask patient to stand up. (Observe in profile. Observe all body areas again, hips included.)
12. Ask patient to extend both arms outstretched in front with palms down. (Observe trunk, legs, and mouth.)
13. Have patient walk a few paces, turn, and walk back to chair. (Observe hands and gait.) Do this twice.

Interpretation of AIMS Score

Add patient scores and note areas of difficulty.
   Score of:
   • 0 to 1 = Low risk
   • 2 in only ONE of the areas assessed = borderline/observe closely
   • 2 in TWO or more of the areas assessed **or** 3 to 4 in ONLY ONE area = indicative of TD

Source: From U.S. Department of Health and Human Services. Available for use in the public domain.

Hamilton Depression Rating Scale (HDRS)

Instructions: For each item, circle the number to select the one "cue" that best characterizes the patient.

1. **Depressed Mood** (sadness, hopeless, helpless, worthless)
   0 = Absent
   1 = These feeling states indicated only on questioning
   2 = These feeling states spontaneously reported verbally
   3 = Communicates feeling states nonverbally (i.e., through facial expression, posture, voice, tendency to weep)
   4 = Patient reports virtually only these feeling states in spontaneous verbal and nonverbal communication

2. **Feelings of Guilt**
   0 = Absent
   1 = Self-reproach; feels he/she has let people down
   2 = Ideas of guilt or rumination over past errors or sinful deeds
   3 = Present illness is a punishment. Delusions of guilt
   4 = Hears accusatory or denunciatory voices and/or experiences threatening visual hallucinations

3. **Suicide**
   0 = Absent
   1 = Feels life is not worth living
   2 = Wishes he/she were dead or any thoughts of possible death to self
   3 = Suicidal ideas or gesture
   4 = Attempts at suicide (any serious attempt rates 4)

4. **Insomnia: Early in the Night**
   0 = No difficulty falling asleep
   1 = Complains of occasional difficulty falling asleep (i.e., more than one-half hour)
   2 = Complains of nightly difficulty falling asleep

5. **Insomnia: Middle of the Night**
   0 = No difficulty
   1 = Complains of being restless and disturbed during the night
   2 = Waking during the night—any getting out of bed rates as 2 (except for purposes of voiding)

6. **Insomnia: Early Hours of the Morning**
   0 = No difficulty
   1 = Waking in early hours of the morning but goes back to sleep
   2 = Unable to fall asleep again if he/she gets out of bed

7. **Work and Activities**
   0 = No difficulty
   1 = Thoughts and feelings of incapacity, fatigue, or weakness related to activities, work, or hobbies
   2 = Loss of interest in activity, hobbies, or work—either directly reported by patient or indirectly in listlessness, indecision, and vacillation (feels he/she has to push self to work or activities)
   3 = Decrease in actual time spent in activities or decrease in productivity. Rate 3 if patient does not spend at least 3 hours a day in activities (job or hobbies), excluding routine chores
   4 = Stopped working because of present illness. Rate 4 if patient engages in no activities except routine chores, or if does not perform routine chores unassisted

8. **Psychomotor Retardation** (slowness of thought and speech, impaired ability to concentrate, decreased motor activity)
   0 = Normal speech and thought
   1 = Slight retardation during the interview
   2 = Obvious retardation during the interview
   3 = Interview difficult
   4 = Complete stupor

9. **Agitation**
   0 = None
   1 = Fidgetiness
   2 = Playing with hands, hair, etc.
   3 = Moving about, can't sit still
   4 = Hand wringing, nail biting, hair pulling, biting of lips

10. **Anxiety (Psychic)**
    0 = No difficulty
    1 = Subjective tension and irritability
    2 = Worrying about minor matters
    3 = Apprehensive attitude apparent in face or speech
    4 = Fears expressed without questioning

11. **Anxiety (Somatic):** Physiological concomitants of anxiety (e.g., dry mouth, indigestion, diarrhea, cramps, belching, palpitations, headache, tremor, hyperventilation, sighing, urinary frequency, sweating, flushing)
    0 = Absent
    1 = Mild
    2 = Moderate
    3 = Severe
    4 = Incapacitating

12. **Somatic Symptoms (Gastrointestinal)**
    0 = None
    1 = Loss of appetite, but eating without encouragement. Heavy feelings in abdomen
    2 = Difficulty eating without urging from others. Requests or requires medication for constipation or gastrointestinal symptoms

13. **Somatic Symptoms (General)**
    0 = None
    1 = Heaviness in limbs, back, or head. Backaches, headache, muscle aches. Loss of energy and fatigability
    2 = Any clear-cut symptom rates 2.

14. **Genital Symptoms** (e.g., loss of libido, impaired sexual performance, menstrual disturbances)
    0 = Absent
    1 = Mild
    2 = Severe

15. **Hypochondriasis**
    0 = Not present
    1 = Self-absorption (bodily)
    2 = Preoccupation with health
    3 = Frequent complaints, requests for help, etc.
    4 = Hypochondriacal delusions

16. **Loss of Weight (Rate *either* A *or* B)**
    A. According to subjective patient history:
    0 = No weight loss
    1 = Probably weight loss associated with present illness
    2 = Definite weight loss associated with present illness
    B. According to objective weekly measurements:
    0 = Less than 1 lb. weight loss in week
    1 = Greater than 1 lb. weight loss in week
    2 = Greater than 2 lb. weight loss in week

17. **Insight**
    0 = Acknowledges being depressed and ill
    1 = Acknowledges illness but attributes cause to bad food, climate, overwork, virus, need for rest, etc.
    2 = Denies being ill at all

SCORING:

    0–6 = No evidence of depressive illness
    7–17 = Mild depression
    18–24 = Moderate depression
    >24 = Severe depression
    TOTAL SCORE _____

Source: Hamilton, M. (1960). A rating scale for depression. *Journal of Neurology, Neurosurgery, & Psychiatry, 23,* 56–62. The HDRS is in the public domain.

Hamilton Anxiety Rating Scale (HAM-A)

Below are descriptions of symptoms commonly associated with anxiety. Assign the patient the rating between 0 and 4 (for each of the 14 items) that best describes the extent to which he/she has these symptoms.

0 = Not present
1 = Mild
2 = Moderate
3 = Severe
4 = Very severe

	Rating		Rating
1. **Anxious mood** Worries, anticipation of the worst, fearful anticipation, irritability	_____	5. **Intellectual** Difficulty in concentration, poor memory	_____
2. **Tension** Feelings of tension, fatigability, startle response, moved to tears easily, trembling, feelings of restlessness, inability to relax	_____	6. **Depressed mood** Loss of interest, lack of pleasure in hobbies, depression, early waking, diurnal swing	_____
3. **Fears** Of dark, of strangers, of being left alone, of animals, of traffic, of crowds	_____	7. **Somatic (muscular)** Pains and aches, twitching, stiffness, myoclonic jerks, grinding of teeth, unsteady voice, increased muscular tone	_____
4. **Insomnia** Difficulty in falling asleep, broken sleep, unsatisfying sleep and fatigue on waking, dreams, nightmares, night terrors	_____	8. **Somatic (sensory)** Tinnitus, blurred vision, hot/cold flushes, feelings of weakness, tingling sensation	_____

	Rating		Rating
9. **Cardiovascular symptoms** Tachycardia, palpitations, pain in chest, throbbing of vessels, feeling faint	_____	13. **Autonomic symptoms** Dry mouth, flushing, pallor, tendency to sweat, giddiness, tension headache	_____
10. **Respiratory symptoms** Pressure or constriction in chest, choking feelings, sighing, dyspnea	_____	14. **Behavior at interview** Fidgeting, restlessness or pacing, tremor of hands, furrowed brow, strained face, sighing or rapid respiration, facial pallor, swallowing, clearing throat	_____
11. **Gastrointestinal symptoms** Difficulty swallowing, flatulence, abdominal pain and fullness, burning sensations, nausea/vomiting, borborygmi, diarrhea, constipation, weight loss	_____		
12. **Genitourinary symptoms** Urinary frequency, urinary urgency, amenorrhea, menorrhagia, loss of libido, premature ejaculation, impotence	_____		

Patient's Total Score _____

SCORING:

    14–17 = Mild Anxiety
    18–24 = Moderate Anxiety
    25–30 = Severe Anxiety

Source: Hamilton, M. (1959). The assessment of anxiety states by rating. *British Journal of Medical Psychology, 32,* 50–55. The HAM-A is in the public domain.

APPENDIX S

Columbia-Suicide Severity Rating Scale

Columbia-Suicide Severity Rating Scale
Screen Version - Recent

Ask questions that are bolded and <u>underlined</u>.	Past Month		Lifetime (Worst Point)	
	Yes	No	Yes	No
Ask Questions 1 and 2				
1) *Have you wished you were dead or wished you could go to sleep and not wake up?*				
2) *Have you actually had any thought of killing yourself?*				
If YES to 2, ask questions 3, 4, 5, and 6. If NO to 2, go directly to question 6.				
3) *Have you been thinking about how you might do this?* E.g., *"I thought about taking an overdose but I never made a specific plan as to when, where, or how I would actually do it...and I would never go through with it."*				
4) *Have you had these thoughts and had some intention of acting on them?* As opposed to *"I have the thought but I definitely will not do anything about them."*				
5) *Have you started to work out or worked out the details of how to kill yourself? Do you intend to carry out this plan?*				

How long ago did the Worst Point Ideation occur? _____

	Yes	No
6) *Have you ever done anything, started to do anything, or prepared to do anything to end your life?* Examples: Collected pills, obtained a gun, gave away valuables, wrote a will or suicide note, took out pills but didn't swallow any, held a gun but changed your mind or it was grabbed from your hand, went to the roof but didn't jump; or actually took pills, tried to shoot yourself, cut yourself, tried to hang yourself, etc... If YES, ask: *Was this within the past three months?*		

☐ Low risk ☐ Moderate risk ☐ High risk

Reprinted with Permission from The Columbia Lighthouse Project.

Bibliography

Academy for Eating Disorders. (2009). Position statement: The role of the family in eating disorders. Retrieved from http://www.aedweb.org/index.php/23-get-involved/position-statements/88-the-role-of-the-family-in-eating-disorders

Acosta, M.T., Swanson, J., Stehli, A., Molina, B., Martinez, A.F., Arcos-Burgos, ... MTA Team. (2016). ADGRL3 (LPHN3) variants are associated with a refined phenotype of ADHD in the MTA study. *Molecular Genetics and Genomic Medicine, 4*(5), 540–547. doi:10.1002/mgg3.230

Adelson, S. (2012). Practice parameter on gay, lesbian, or bisexual sexual orientation, gender nonconformity, and gender discordance in children and adolescents. *Journal of the American Academy of Child and Adolescent Psychiatry, 51*(9), 957–974. doi:http://dx.doi.org/10.1016/j.jaac.2012.07.004

ADHD Institute. (2016). *Environmental risk factors.* Retrieved from www.adhd-institute.com/burden-of-adhd/aetiology/environmental-risk-factors

Aguilera, D.C. (1998). *Crisis intervention: Theory and methodology* (8th ed.). St. Louis, MO: C.V. Mosby.

Alzheimer's Australia. (2017). *Dementia care research.* Retrieved from https://nsw.fightdementia.org.au/research-publications/research/areas-of-dementia-research/dementia-care-research

American Academy of Child and Adolescent Psychiatry. (2019). *Children of alcoholics.* Retrieved from https://www.aacap.org/AACAP/Families_and_Youth/Facts_for_Families/FFF-Guide/Children-Of-Alcoholics-017.aspx

American Academy of Child and Adolescent Psychiatry. (2016). *Military families resource center.* Retrieved from www.aacap.org/AACAP/Families_and_Youth/Resource_Centers/Military_Families_Resource_Center/FAQ.aspx

American Addiction Centers. (2017). *Using desipramine (Norpramin) for drug withdrawal & cocaine addiction.* Retrieved from http://americanaddictioncenters.org/addiction-medications/desipramine

American Chiropractic Association (ACA). (2019). Key facts about the chiropractic profession. Retrieved from www.acatoday.org/Patients/Why-Choose-Chiropractic/Key-Facts

American Medical Association (AMA). (2010). *Unconventional medical care in the United States.* Policy #H-480-973. Advocacy Resource Center. Chicago: AMA.

American Nurses Association (no date). *What is nursing?* Retrieved from https://www.nursingworld.org/practice-policy/workforce/what-is-nursing/

American Nurses Association (ANA). (2010a). *Nursing's social policy statement: The essence of the profession.* Silver Spring, MD: ANA.

American Nurses Association (2015). *Scope and standards of practice* (3rd ed.) Silver Spring, MD: ANA.

American Nurses Association (ANA) and International Association of Forensic Nurses (IAFN). (2015). *Forensic nursing: Scope and standards of practice.* Retrieved from http://c.ymcdn.com/sites/www.forensicnurses. org/resource/resmgr/Docs/SS_Public_Comment_Draft_1505.pdf? hhSearchTerms=%222015protect%20$elax%20pm%20$andprotect %20$elax%20pm%20$draft%22

American Psychiatric Association. (2013). *Diagnostic and statistical manual of mental disorders* (5th ed.). Washington, DC: American Psychiatric Publishing.

American Psychological Association. (2015). Guidelines for psychological practice with transgender and gender nonconforming people. *American Psychologist 70*(9), 832–864.

American Psychological Association. (2019). *Trauma.* Retrieved from www.apa.org/topics/trauma

American Society of Addiction Medicine. (2019). Definition of addiction. Available at https://www.asam.org/resources/definition-of-addiction

Anxiety and Depression Association of America. (2018). Facts and statistics. Retrieved from https://www.adaa.org/about-adaa/press-room/ facts-statistics

Avants, S.K., Margolin, A., Holford, T.R., & Kosten, T.R. (2000). A randomized controlled trial of auricular acupuncture for cocaine dependence. *Archives of Internal Medicine, 160*(15), 2305–2312.

Balodis, I.M., Grilo, C.M., & Potenza, M.N. (2015). Neurobiological underpinnings of obesity and addiction: A focus on binge eating disorder and implications for treatment. *Psychiatric Times.* Retrieved from www. psychiatrictimes.com/cme/neurobiological-underpinnings-obesity-and-addiction-focus-binge-eating-disorder-and-implications/page/0/2

Banks, M.R., & Banks, W.A. (2002). The effects of animal-assisted therapy on loneliness in an elderly population in long-term care facilities. *Journals of Gerontology Series A: Biological Sciences and Medical Sciences, 57*(7), M428–M432.

Beck, A., Rush, A.J., Shaw, B.F., & Emery, G. (1979). *Cognitive theory of depression.* New York, NY: Guilford Press.

Benson, P.J., Beedie, S.A., Shephard, E., Giegling, I., Rujescu, D., & St. Clair, D. (2012). Simple viewing tests can detect eye movement abnormalities that distinguish schizophrenia cases from controls with exceptional accuracy. *Biological Psychiatry, 72*(9): 716. doi:10.1016/ j.biopsych.2012.04.019

Bergeron, S., Rosen, N.O., & Corsini-Munt, S. (2016). Painful sex. In S. Levine, C. Risen, & S. Althof (Eds.), *Handbook of clinical sexuality for mental health professionals* (3rd ed., pp. 71–85). New York, NY: Routledge.

Bernstein, B.E. (2018). *Conduct disorder.* Retrieved from http://emedicine. medscape.com/article/918213-overview#a3

Blumenthal, M. (Ed.). (1998). *The complete German Commission E monographs: Therapeutic guide to herbal medicines.* Austin, TX: American Botanical Garden.

Bornstein, R.F., Bianucci, V., Fishman, D.P., & Biars, J.W. (2104). Toward a firmer foundation for *DSM-5.1:* Domains of impairment in *DSM IV/DSM-5* personality disorders. *Journal of Personality Disorders, 28*(2), 212–224.

Bowlby, J. (1961). Processes of mourning. *International Journal of Psychoanalysis, 42,* 317–322.

Brancu, M., Straits-Troster, K., & Kudler, H. (2011). Behavioral health conditions among military personnel and veterans: Prevalence and best practices for treatment. *North Carolina Medical Journal*, 72(1), 54–60.

Brasic, J.R. (2016). *Catatonia*. Retrieved from http://emedicine.medscape.com/article/1154851-differential

Breslau, N. (2009, July). The epidemiology of trauma, PTSD, and other posttrauma disorders. *Trauma, Violence, & Abuse*, 10(3), 198–210.

Burgess, A. (2010). *Rape violence*. Gannett Education Course #60025. Retrieved from http://ce.nurse.com/60025/Rape-Violence

Burgess, A.W., Slattery, D.M., & Herlihy, P.A. (2013). Military sexual trauma: A silent syndrome. *Journal of Psychosocial Nursing*, 51(2), 20–26.

Byne, W., Bradley, S., Coleman, E., Eyler, A.E., Green, R., Menvielle, E., … Tompkins, D.A. (2012). Report of the APA task force on treatment of gender identity disorder. *American Journal of Psychiatry*, 169(8), 1–35.

Call, C.C., Attia, E., & Walsh, B.T. (2017). Feeding and eating disorders. In B.J. Sadock, V.A. Sadock, & P. Ruiz (Eds.), *Comprehensive textbook of psychiatry* (10th ed., pp. 2065–2082). Philadelphia, PA: Wolters Kluwer.

Catalano, J.T. (2020). *Nursing now! Today's issues, tomorrow's trends* (8th ed.). Philadelphia, PA: F.A. Davis.

Centers for Disease Control and Prevention (CDC). (2013). *Burden of mental illness*. Retrieved from https://www.cdc.gov/mentalhealth/basics/burden.htm

Centers for Disease Control and Prevention. (CDC). (2019a). *Autism Spectrum Autism and Developmental Disabilities Monitoring Network*. Retrieved from www.cdc.gov/ncbddd/autism/addm.html

Centers for Disease Control and Prevention. (CDC). (2019b). *FastStats: Attention deficit hyperactivity disorder*. Retrieved from www.cdc.gov/nchs/fastats/adhd.htm

Centers for Disease Control and Prevention (CDC). (2019c). *About Adverse Childhood Experiences*. Retrieved from https://www.cdc.gov/violenceprevention/childabuseandneglect/acestudy/aboutace.html

Chess, S., Thomas, A., & Birch, H. (1970). The origins of personality. *Scientific American 223*,102.

Child Welfare Information Gateway (CWIG). (2013). *What is child abuse and neglect? Recognizing the signs and symptoms*. Retrieved from www.childwelfare.gov/pubs/factsheets/whatiscan.pdf

Clarke, T.C., Black, L.I., Stussman, B.J., Barnes, P.M., & Nahin, R.L. (2015). Trends in the use of complementary health approaches among adults: United States, 2002–2012. National Health Statistics Reports; no 79. Hyattsville, MD: National Center for Health Statistics.

CNN (2013). By the numbers: Women in the U.S. military. (2013, January). Retrieved from https://www.cnn.com/2013/01/24/us/military-women-glance/index.html

Cohen, M.A. (2018). *American Medical Association supports alternative medicine*. Retrieved from www.camlawblog.com/articles/health-trends/american-medical-association-supports-alternative-medicine

Connor, D. (2017). Disruptive behavior disorders in children and adolescents. In B.J. Sadock, V.A. Sadock, & P. Ruiz (Eds.), *Comprehensive textbook of psychiatry* (10th ed., pp. 3605–3621). Philadelphia, PA: Wolters Kluwer.

Constantino, R.E., Crane, P.A., & Young, S.E. (2013). *Forensic nursing: Evidence-based principles and practice*. Philadelphia, PA: F.A. Davis.

Cooper, B.E., & Sejnowski, C.A. (2013). Serotonin syndrome: Recognition and treatment. *AACN Advanced Critical Care*, *24*(1), 15–20.

Corr, C.A., & Corr, D.M. (2013). *Death & dying: Life & living* (7th ed.). Belmont, CA: Wadsworth.

Council of Acupuncture and Oriental Medicine Associations (CAOMA). (2013). *Conditions treated by acupuncture and oriental medicine*. Retrieved from www.acucouncil.org/conditions_treated.htm

Crosby, K. (2015). FDA and the Department of Defense: A Joint Force to Reduce Tobacco Use in the Military (FDA blog, September 2015). Retrieved from http://blogs.fda.gov/fdavoice/index.php/2015/09/fda-and-the-department-of-defense-a-joint-force-to-reduce-tobacco-use-in-the-military-2/?utm_source=CTPtwitter&utm_medium=socialmedia&utm_campaign=HealthyBase

Crystal, H.A. (2018). Dementia with Lewy bodies: Treatment and management. *Medscape*. Retrieved from emedicine.medscape.com/article/1135041-treatment

Delgado, J., Traub, S.J., & Grayzel, J. (2017). *Intoxication from LSD and other common hallucinogens*. Retrieved from www.uptodate.com/contents/intoxication-from-lsd-and-other-common-hallucinogens

Department of Defense (DoD). (2015). *About the Department of Defense*. Retrieved from www.defense.gov/About-DoD

Department of Veterans Affairs. (2018). How common is PTSD? Retrieved from www.ptsd.va.gov/understand/common/common_adults.asp

Department of Veterans Affairs & Department of Defense (DVA/DoD). (2016). *Clinical practice guideline for management of concussion/mild traumatic brain injury*. Retrieved from https://www.healthquality.va.gov/guidelines/Rehab/mtbi/mTBICPGFullCPG50821816.pdf

Devries, M.R., Hughes, H.K., Watson, H., & Moore, B.A. (2012). Understanding the military culture. In B.A. Moore (Ed.), *Handbook of counseling military couples* (pp. 7–18). New York, NY: Routledge.

Doenges, M.E., Moorhouse, M.F., & Murr, A.C. (2013). *Nurse's pocket guide: Diagnoses, prioritized interventions, and rationales* (13th ed.). Philadelphia, PA: F.A. Davis.

Doenges, M.E., Moorhouse, M.F., & Murr, A.C. (2016). *Nursing diagnosis manual: Planning, individualizing, and documenting client care* (5th ed.). Philadelphia, PA: F.A. Davis.

Donahey, K. (2016). Problems with orgasm. In S. Levine, C. Risen, & S. Althof (Eds.), *Handbook of clinical sexuality for mental health professionals* (3rd ed., pp. 60–70). New York, NY: Routledge.

Drug Facts and Comparisons. (2014). St. Louis, MO: Wolters Kluwer.

Eisendrath, S.J., & Lichtmacher, J.E. (2012). Psychiatric disorders. In S.J. McPhee, M.A. Papadakis, & M.W. Rabow (Eds.), *Current medical diagnosis and treatment 2012* (pp. 1010–1064). New York, NY: McGraw-Hill.

Endocrine Society. (2017). *Full Guideline: Endocrine Treatment of Gender-Dysphoric/Gender-incongruent persons: An Endocrine Society clinical practice guideline*. Retrieved from https://www.endocrine.org/guidelines-and-clinical-practice/clinical-practice-guidelines/gender-dysphoria-gender-incongruence

Engel, G. (1964). Grief and grieving. *American Journal of Nursing*, *64*, 93.

Epstein, S. (1991). Beliefs and symptoms in maladaptive resolutions of the traumatic neurosis. In D. Ozer, J.M. Healy, Jr., & A.J. Stewart (Eds.), *Perspectives on personality* (Vol. 3). London, UK: Jessica Kingsley.

Erikson, E.H. (1963). *Childhood and society*. New York, NY: W.W. Norton.

Erlij, D., Acosta-Garcia, J., Rojas-Marquez, M., Gonzalez-Hernandez, B., Escartin-Perez, E., Aceves, J., & Floran, B. (2012). Dopamine D4 receptor stimulation in GABAergic projections of the globus pallidus to the reticular thalamic nucleus and the substantia nigra reticulate of the rat decreases locomotor activity. *Neuropharmacology, 62*(2), 1111–1118.

Ernst, L.S. (2012). Animal-assisted therapy: Using animals to promote healing. *Nursing 2012, 42*(10), 54–58.

Escobar, J.I., & Dimsdale, J.E. (2017). Somatic symptom and related disorders. In B.J. Sadock, V.A. Sadock, & P. Ruiz (Eds.), *Comprehensive textbook of psychiatry* (10th ed., pp. 1827–1845). Philadelphia, PA: Wolters Kluwer.

Fabian, T J., & Solai, L.K. (2017). Neurocognitive disorders. In B.J. Sadock, V.A. Sadock, & P. Ruiz (Eds.), *Comprehensive textbook of psychiatry* (10th ed., pp. 1178–1191). Philadelphia, PA: Wolters Kluwer

Family and Youth Services Bureau. (2016). Domestic violence and homelessness: Statistics (2016). Retrieved from https://www.acf.hhs.gov/fysb/resource/dv-homelessness-stats-2016

Folstein, M.F., Folstein, S.E., & McHugh, P.R. (1975). Mini-mental state: A practical method for grading the cognitive state of patients for the clinician. *Journal of Psychiatric Research, 12*(3), 189–198.

Ford, J.D., & Courtois, C.A. (2014). Complex PTSD, affect dysregulation, and borderline personality disorder. *Borderline Personality Disorder and Emotion Dysregulation, 1*(9). doi:10.1186/2051-6673-1-9

Froehlich, T.E., Lanphear, B.P., Auinger, P., Hornung, R., Epstein, J.N., Braun, J., & Kahn, R.S. (2009). Association of tobacco and lead exposures with attention-deficit/hyperactivity disorder. *Pediatrics* 124, 1054–1063. Retrieved from www.ncbi.nlm.nih.gov/pmc/articles/PMC2853804

Freud, S. (1962). The neuro-psychoses of defense. In J. Strachey (Ed.), *Standard edition of the complete psychological works of Sigmund Freud* (Vol. 3). London, NY: Hogarth Press (original work published 1894).

Freudenreich, O. (2010). Differential diagnosis of psychotic symptoms: Medical "mimics." *Psychiatric Times, 27*(12), 52–61.

Friedmann, E., & Thomas, S.A. (1995). Pet ownership, social support, and one-year survival after acute myocardial infarction in the cardiac arrhythmia suppression trial. *American Journal of Cardiology, 76*(17), 1213.

Gabany, E., & Shellenbarger, T. (2010). Caring for families with deployment stress: How nurses can make a difference in the lives of military families. *American Journal of Nursing, 110*(11), 36–41.

Galéra, C., Côté, S.M., Bouvard, M.P., Pingault, J.B., Melchior, M., Michel, G.M., … Tremblay, R.E. (2011). Early risk factors for hyperactivity-impulsivity and inattention trajectories from age 17 months to 8 years. *Archives of General Psychiatry, 68*(12), 1267–1275. doi:10.1001/archgenpsychiatry.2011.138

Gibbons, R.D., Hur, K., Brown, C.H., & Mann, J.J. (2009). Relationship between antiepileptic drugs and suicide attempts in patients with bipolar disorder. *Archives of General Psychiatry, 66*(12), 1354–1360.

Glaze, L.E., & Parks, E. (2012). *Correctional populations in the United States, 2011*. Bureau of Justice Statistics. Retrieved from http://bjs.ojp.usdoj.gov/content/pub/pdf/cpus11.pdf

Godenne, G. (2001). The role of pets in nursing homes …and psychotherapy. *The Maryland Psychiatrist, 27*(3), 5–6.

, & Harari, E. (2019). Research sheds light on two types of treatment for ADHD. *Psychiatric Times*, *36*(7). Retrieved from https://www.psychiatrictimes.com/adhd/research-sheds-light-two-types-treatment-adhd

Gunderson, J.G. (2011). An introduction to borderline personality disorder: Diagnosis, origins, course, and treatment. *National Education Alliance—Borderline Personality Disorder*. Retrieved from www.borderlinepersonalitydisorder.com/understanding-bpd/a-bpd-brief

Haberman, C. (2014). Debate persists over diagnosing mental disorders, long after 'Sybil.' *New York Times*. Retrieved from www.nytimes.com/2014/11/24/us/debate-persists-over-diagnosing-mental-health-disorders-long-after-sybil.html?_r=0

Haddad, P.M. (2001). Antidepressant discontinuation syndromes: Clinical relevance, prevention, and management. *Drug Safety*, *24*(3), 183–197.

Hall, L.K. (2012). The military lifestyle and the relationship. In B.A. Moore (Ed.), *Handbook of counseling military couples* (pp. 137–156). New York, NY: Routledge.

Hamilton, M. (1959). The assessment of anxiety states by rating. *British Journal of Medical Psychology*, *32*, 50–55.

Harrisberger, F., Smieskova1, R., Vogler, C., Egli, T., Schmidt, A., Lenz, C.S., ... Borgwardt, S. (2016). Impact of polygenic schizophrenia-related risk and hippocampal volumes on the onset of psychosis. *Translational Psychiatry*, *6*, e868. doi:10.1038/tp.2016.143

Harvard Medical School. (2001, April). Bipolar disorder—Part I. *The Harvard Mental Health Letter*. Boston, MA: Harvard Medical School Publications Group.

Harvard Medical School. (2005). The homeless mentally ill. *Harvard Mental Health Letter*, *21*(11), 4–7.

Hatchett, G. (2015). Treatment guidelines for clients with antisocial personality disorder. *Journal of Mental Health Counseling*, *37*(1), 15–27.

Hays, J.S., & Larson, K.H. (1963). *Interacting with patients*. New York, NY: Holt, Rinehart, & Winston.

Hensley, P.L., & Clayton, P.J. (2013). Why the bereavement exclusion was introduced in DSM-III. *Psychiatric Annals*, *43*(6), 256–260.

Hill, J. (2003). Early identification of individuals at risk for antisocial personality disorder. *British Journal of Psychiatry*, *182*(suppl. 44), s11–s14.

Holt, G.A., & Kouzi, S. (2002). Herbs through the ages. In M.A. Bright (Ed.), *Holistic health and healing* (pp. 135–160). Philadelphia, PA: F.A. Davis.

Hopper, E.K., Bassuk, E.L., & Olivet, J. (2010). Shelter from the storm: Trauma-informed care in homelessness services settings. *Open Health Services and Policy Journal*, *3*, 80–100.

Htay, T.T. (2016). *Premenstrual dysphoric disorder treatment and management*. Retrieved from http://emedicine.medscape.com/article/293257-treatment#d8

Huntington's Disease Society of America (HDSA). (2019). *What is Huntington's disease?* Retrieved from http://hdsa.org/what-is-hd

Institute of Medicine (IOM). (2013). *Returning home from Iraq and Afghanistan: Preliminary assessment of readjustment needs of veterans, service members, and their families*. Washington, DC: National Academies Press. Retrieved from http://iom.nationalacademies.org/~/media/Files/Report%20Files/2013/Returning-Home-Iraq-Afghanistan/Returning-Home-Iraq-Afghanistan-RB.pdf

International Association of Forensic Nurses. (2019). *Areas of forensic nursing practice.* Retrieved from https://iafn.site-ym.com/?page=FNFAQs

International Association of Forensic Nurses (IAFN) & American Nurses Association (ANA). (2015). *Forensic nursing: Scope and standards of practice.* Silver Spring: MD: American Nurses Association

International Association for the Study of Pain. (2012). IASP taxonomy. Retrieved from https://www.iasp-pain.org/Taxonomy

International Society for the Study of Trauma and Dissociation. (2011). Guidelines for treating dissociative identity disorder in adults, third revision, *Journal of Trauma & Dissociation, 12*(2), 115–187. http://dx.doi.org/10.1080/15299732.2011.537247

Jakupcak, M., Vannoy, S., Imel., Z., Cook, J.W., Fontana, A., Rosenheck, R., & McFall, M. (2010). Does PTSD moderate the relationship between social support and suicide risk in Iraq and Afghanistan war veterans seeking mental health treatment? *Depression and Anxiety, 27*(11), 1001–1005.

Jaret, P. (2010). *Eating disorders and depression.* Retrieved from www.webmd.com/depression/features/eating-disorders

Jensen, J.E., & Miller, B. (2004). *Home health psychiatric care: A guide to understanding home health psychiatric care as covered under Medicare Part A.* Seattle, WA: The Washington Institute for Mental Illness Research & Training.

Kabat-Zinn, J. (2012). *Mindfulness for beginners: Reclaiming the present moment and your life.* Boulder, CO: Sounds True, Inc.

Kahn, D. (2018). Illness anxiety disorder (formerly hypochondriasis). Retrieved from https://emedicine.medscape.com/article/290955-overview#a6

Kaplan, K. (2012). Update on trichotillomania. *Psychiatric Times.* Retrieved from www.psychiatrictimes.com/apa2012/update-trichotillomania

Kaufman, D.M., & Zun, L. (1995). A quantifiable, brief mental status examination for emergency patients. *Journal of Emergency Medicine, 13*(4), 440–456.

Kearns, C. (2014). *PTSD and the bereaved parent.* Retrieved from http://carolkearns.com/columns/col_ptsd-bereaved.html

Kelsoe, J.R. & Greenwood, T.A. (2017). Mood disorders: Genetics. In B.J. Sadock, V.A. Sadock, & P. Ruiz (Eds.), *Comprehensive textbook of psychiatry* (10th ed., pp.1619–1630). Philadelphia, PA: Wolters Kluwer.

Kessler, D. (2019). *Finding meaning: The sixth stage of grief.* New York, NY: Scribner.

Khazan, O. (2015). Most prisoners are mentally ill: Can mental health courts, in which people are sentenced to therapy, help? Retrieved from www.theatlantic.com/health/archive/2015/04/more-than-half-of-prisoners-are-mentally-ill/389682

Killgore, W.D., Cotting, D.I., Thomas, J.L., Cox, A.L., McGurk, D., Vo, A.H., Castro, C.A., & Hoge, C.W. (2008). Post-combat invincibility: Violent combat experiences are associated with increased risk-taking propensity following deployment. *Journal of Psychiatric Research, 42*(13), 1112–1121.

Kime, P. (2015). DoD military suicide rate declining. *Military Times.* Retrieved from www.militarytimes.com/story/military/pentagon/2015/01/16/defense-department-suicides-2013-report/21865977

King, B.M., & Regan, P. (2014). *Human sexuality today* (8th ed.). Upper Saddle River, NJ: Prentice Hall.

anthan, M., Petersen, I., Jones, L. Marston, L., & Nazareth, I. (2013). Mortality and medical care after bereavement: A practical cohort study. *PloS ONE, 8*(1), 1–7. doi:10.1371/journal.pone.0052561

Kokman, E., Smith, G.E., Petersen, R.C., Tangalos, E., & Ivnik, R.C. (1991). The short test of mental status: Correlations with standardized psychometric testing. *Archives of Neurology, 48*(7), 725–728.

Kolla, N.J., Malcolm, C., Attard, S., Arenovich, T., Blackwood, N., & Hodgins, S. (2013). Childhood maltreatment and aggressive behavior in violent offenders with psychopathy. *Canadian Journal of Psychiatry, 58*(8), 487–494.

Kranjac, D. (2016). *In vitro modeling of early brain overgrowth in autism.* Retrieved from www.psychiatryadvisor.com/neurodevelopmental-disorder/modeling-early-brain-overgrowth-in-autism/article/508852

Krastins, A., Francis, A.J., Field, A.M., & Carr, S.N. (2014). Childhood predictors of adult antisocial personality disorder symptomatology. *Australian Psychologist, 49*, 142–150.

Kübler-Ross, E. (1969). *On death and dying.* New York, NY: Macmillan.

Ladd, G.W. (1999). Peer relationships and social competence during early and middle childhood. *Annual Review of Psychology, 50*, 333–359.

Lagerquist, S.L. (2012). *Davis's NCLEX-RN Success* (3rd ed.). Philadelphia, PA: F.A. Davis.

Lanius, U. (2013). *Neurobiology and treatment of traumatic dissociation.* Retrieved from www.isst-d.org/downloads/AnnualConference/2013/Baltimore2013handout.pdf

Lawn, S., Diped, B.A., & McMahon, J. (2015). Experience of family carers of people diagnosed with borderline personality disorder. *Journal of Psychiatric and Mental Health Nursing, 22*, 234–243.

Ledray, L.E. (2009). Evidence collection and care of the sexual assault survivor: The SANE-SART response. *Minnesota Center Against Violence and Abuse.* Retrieved from www.mincava.umn.edu/documents/commissioned/2forensicevidence/2forensicevidence.html

Leiblum, S.R. (1999). Sexual problems and dysfunction: Epidemiology, classification, and risk factors. *The Journal of Gender-Specific Medicine, 2*(5), 41–45.

Levine, G.N., Allen, K., Braun, L.T., Christian, H.E., Friedmann, E., Taubert, K.A., … Lange, R.A. (2013). Pet ownership and cardiovascular risk: A scientific statement from the American Heart Association. *Circulation Journal of the American Heart Association, 127*(23), 2353–2363. doi:10.1161/CIR.0b013e31829201e1

Lubit, R.H. (2016). Borderline personality disorder. *eMedicine Psychiatry.* Retrieved from http://emedicine.medscape.com/article/913575-overview

Lyden, H., Espinoza, R.T., Pirnia, T., Clark, K., Joshi, S.H., Leaver, A.M., … Narr, K.L. (2014). Electroconvulsive therapy mediates neuroplasticity of white matter microstructure in major depression. *Translational Psychiatry 4*, e380; doi:10.1038/tp.2014.21

Lynch, V.A. (2011). *Forensic nursing science* (2nd ed.). St. Louis, MO: Mosby.

Lynch, V.A., & Koehler, S.A. (2011). Forensic investigation of death. In V.A. Lynch (Ed.), *Forensic nursing science* (2nd ed., pp. 179–194). St. Louis, MO: Mosby.

MacIntosh, H.B., Godbout, N., & Dubash, N. (2015). Borderline personality disorder: Disorder of trauma or personality, a review of the empirical literature. *Canadian Psychology, 56*(2), 227–241.

Mahler, M., Pine, F., & Bergman, A. (1975). *The psychological birth of the human infant*. New York, NY: Basic Books.

Marashly, E.T., & Bohlega, S.A. (2017). Riboflavin has neuroprotective potential: Focus on Parkinson's disease and migraine. *Frontiers in Neurology*. https://doi.org/10.3389/fneur.2017.00333

Marx, M.S., Cohen-Mansfield, J., Regier, N.G., Dakheel-Ali M., Srihari, A., & Thein, K. (2010). The impact of different dog-related stimuli on engagement of persons with dementia. *American Journal of Alzheimer's Disease and Other Dementia*, 25(1), 37–45. doi:10.1177/1533317508326976

Massachusetts General Hospital Center for Women's Mental Health. (2015). *PMS and PMDD*. Retrieved from https://womensmentalhealth.org/specialty-clinics/pms-and-pmdd/?doing_wp_cron=1489094332.2227799892425537109375

Matheson, S.L., Shepherd, A.M., & Carr, V.J. (2014). How much do we know about schizophrenia and how well do we know it? Evidence from the Schizophrenia Library. *Psychological Medicine*, 44, 3387–3405. doi:10.1017/S0033291714000166

Mathewson, J. (2011). In support of military women and families. In R.B. Everson & C.R. Figley (Eds.), *Families under fire* (pp. 215–235). New York, NY: Routledge.

Mayo Clinic. (2019a). *Hoarding*. Retrieved from www.mayoclinic.com/health/hoarding/DS00966

Mayo Clinic. (2019b). *Oppositional defiant disorder*. Retrieved from www.mayoclinic.org/diseases-conditions/oppositional-defiant-disorder/basics/risk-factors/con-20024559

Mayo Clinic (2019c). *Alcohol poisoning*. Retrieved from http://www.mayoclinic.org/diseases-conditions/alcohol-poisoning/diagnosis-treatment/treatment/txc-20227934

Mayo Clinic. (2017a). *Drugs and supplements*. Retrieved from https://www.mayoclinic.org/drugs-supplements/

Mayo Clinic. (2017b). *Tourette syndrome*. Retrieved from www.mayoclinic.org/diseases-conditions/tourette-syndrome/diagnosis-treatment/treatment/txc-20163628

Mazur, E.E., & Litch, N.A. (2019). *Nutrition and diet therapy: Evidence-based applications* (7th ed.). Philadelphia, PA: F.A. Davis.

McClintock, S.M., & Husain, M.M. (2011). Electroconvulsive therapy does not damage the brain. *Journal of the American Psychiatric Nurses Association*, 17(3), 212–213.

McGough, J.J., Sturm, A., Cowen, J., Tung, K., Salgari, G.C., Leuchter, A. F., ... Loo, S.K. (2019). Double-blind, sham-controlled, pilot study of trigeminal nerve stimulation for attention-deficit/hyperactivity disorder. *Journal of the American Academy of Child and Adolescent Psychiatry*, 58(4), 403–411. DOI: https://doi.org/10.1016/j.jaac.2018.11.013

Medicare.gov. (no date). *What's home health care?* Retrieved from https://www.medicare.gov/what-medicare-covers/home-health-care/home-health-care-what-is-it-what-to-expect.html

Merck manual of health & aging. (2005). New York, NY: Random House.

Minzenberg, M.J., Poole, J.H., & Vinogradov, S. (2008). A neurocognitive model of borderline personality disorder: Effects of childhood sexual abuse and relationship to adult social attachment disturbance. *Development and Psychopathology*, 20(1), 341–368. doi:10.1017/S0954579408000163

Moore, T.J., Glenmullen, J., & Mattison, J.R. (2014). Reports of pathological gambling, hypersexuality, and compulsive shopping associated mine receptor agonist drugs. *JAMA Internal Medicine*, 30–1933. doi:10.1001/jamainternmed.2014.5262

Moretti, F., De Ronchi, D., Bernabei, V., Marchetti, L., Ferrari, B., Forlani, C., & Atti, A.R. (2011). Pet therapy in elderly patients with mental illness. *Psychogeriatrics, 11*(2), 125–129. doi:10.1111/j.1479-8301. 2010.00329.x

Morgan, K. I. & Townsend, M.C. (2020). *Essentials of psychiatric mental health nursing* (8th ed.). Philadelphia, PA: F.A. Davis.

Morrow, A. (2016). *Grief and mourning: What's normal and what's not?* Retrieved from https://www.verywell.com/grief-and-mourning-process-1132545

National Alliance on Mental Illness (NAMI). (2015). President Obama signs Veterans Suicide Prevention Act [blog]. Retrieved from https://www.nami.org/Search?searchtext=Clayton+Hunt+Act&searchmode=anyword

National Alliance to End Homelessness. (2019). *The state of homelessness.* Retrieved from https://endhomelessness.org/homelessness-in-america/homelessness-statistics/state-of-homelessness-report/

NANDA International. (2018). *Nursing diagnoses: Definitions & classification 2018–2020* (11th ed.). New York, NY: Thieme.

National Center for Complementary and Alternative Medicine (NCCAM). (2008). *The use of complementary and alternative medicine in the United States.* NCCAM Publication No. D424. Bethesda, MD: National Institutes of Health.

National Center for Complementary and Alternative Medicine (NCCAM). (2012a). *Acupuncture: An introduction.* NCCAM Publication No. D404. Bethesda, MD: National Institutes of Health.

National Center for Complementary and Alternative Medicine (NCCAM). (2012c). *What is complementary and alternative medicine?* NCCAM Publication No. D347. Bethesda, MD: National Institutes of Health.

National Center for Complementary and Integrative Health (NCCIH). (2017a). *NCCIH facts-at-a-glance and mission.* Retrieved from https://nccih.nih.gov/about/ataglance

National Center for Complementary and Integrative Health (NCCIH). (2017b). *Acupuncture: In depth.* Retrieved from https://nccih.nih.gov/health/acupuncture/introduction

National Center on Elder Abuse. (no date). *Statistics and data: Challenges in elder abuse research.* Retrieved from https://ncea.acl.gov/What-We-Do/Research/Statistics-and-Data.aspx#challenges

National Coalition for the Homeless (NCH). (2017). Mental illness and homelessness. Retrieved from http://nationalhomeless.org/wp-content/uploads/2017/06/Mental-Illness-and-Homelessness.pdf

National Council of State Boards of Nursing (NCSBN). (2016). *Test plan for the National Council Licensure Examination for Registered Nurses.* Retrieved from www.ncsbn.org

National Institutes of Health (NIH). (2019). *Tourette's syndrome fact sheet.* Retrieved from www.ninds.nih.gov/disorders/tourette/detail_tourette. htm#3231_1

National Institute on Drug Abuse (NIDA). (2013). *Drug facts: Substance abuse among the military.* Retrieved from https://www.drugabuse.gov/publications/drugfacts/substance-abuse-in-military.

National Institute on Drug Abuse (NIDA). (2018). *Synthetic cannabinoids.* Retrieved from www.drugabuse.gov/publications/drugfacts/synthetic-cannabinoids

National Institute of Mental Health. (2017). *Bipolar disorder.* Retrieved https://www.nimh.nih.gov/health/statistics//bipolar-disorder.shtml

Os, J.V., & Reininghaus, U. (2017). The clinical epidemiology of schizophrenia. In B.J. Sadock, V.A. Sadock., & P. Ruiz (Eds.), *Comprehensive textbook of psychiatry* (10th ed., pp. 1445–1457). Philadelphia, PA: Wolters Kluwer.

Ouellet-Morin, I., Côté, S.M., Vitaro, F., Hébert, M., Carbonneau, R., Lacourse, E., &Tremblay, R.E. (2016). Effects of the MAOA gene and levels of exposure to violence on antisocial outcomes. *British Journal of Psychiatry, 208*(1), 42–48. doi:10.1192/bjp.bp.114.162081

Parcell, S. (2008). Biochemical and nutritional influences on pain. In J.F. Audette & A. Bailey (Eds.), *Integrative pain medicine* (pp. 133–172). New York: Springer-Verlag.

Parris, R.J. (2011). Initial management of bereaved relatives following trauma. *Trauma, 14*(2), 139–155.

PDR for herbal medicines (4th ed.). (2007). Montvale, NJ: Thomson Healthcare Inc.

Peacock, S.C., Hammond-Collins, K., & Ford, D.A. (2014). The journey with dementia from the perspective of bereaved caregivers: A qualitative descriptive study. *BioMed Central Nursing, 13*(42), 1–10.

Pedersen, E.R., Marshall, G.N., & Kurz, J. (2016). Behavioral health treatment receipt among a community sample of young adult veterans. *Journal of Behavioral Health Services & Research,* 1–15.

Peplau, H.E. (1962). Interpersonal techniques: The crux of psychiatric nursing. *American Journal of Nursing, 62*(6), 50–54.

Peplau, H.E. (1991). *Interpersonal relations in nursing.* New York, NY: Springer.

Pfeiffer, E. (1975). A short portable mental status questionnaire for the assessment of organic brain deficit in elderly patients. *Journal of the American Geriatric Society, 23*(10), 433–441.

Phillips, N.A. (2000, July). Female sexual dysfunction: Evaluation and treatment. *American Family Physician, 62*(1), 127–136, 141–142.

Piaget, J., & Inhelder, B. (1969). *The psychology of the child.* New York, NY: Basic Books.

Pier, K., Marin, L.K., Wilsnack, J., & Goodman, M. (2016). The neurobiology of borderline personality disorder. *Psychiatric Times.* Retrieved from www.psychiatrictimes.com/special-reports/neurobiology-borderline-personality-disorder/page/0/1

Pies, R.W. (2013, April 29). Grief and depression: The sages knew the difference. *Psychiatric Times.* Retrieved from www.psychiatrictimes.com/display/article/10168/2140230

Pranthikanti, S. (2007). Ayurvedic treatments. In J.H. Lake & D. Spiegel (Eds.), *Complementary and alternative treatments in mental health care* (pp. 225–272). Washington, DC: American Psychiatric Publishing.

Prator, B.C. (2006). Serotonin syndrome. *Journal of Neuroscience Nursing, 38*(2), 102–105.

Presser, A.M. (2000). *Pharmacist's guide to medicinal herbs.* Petaluma, CA: Smart Publications.

t, T.J., McLean, R.M., Forciea, M.A., for the Clinical Guide-
ittee of the American College of Physicians. (2017). Nonin-
vasive treatments for acute, subacute, and chronic low back pain: A clinical
practice guideline from the American College of Physicians. *Annals of
Internal Medicine, 166*(7), 514. https://doi.org/10.7326/M16-2367

Radhakrishnan, R., Wilkinson, S.T., & D'Souza, D.C. (2014). Gone to
pot—A review of the association between cannabis and psychosis. *Frontiers in Psychiatry, 5*(54). doi:10.3389/fpsyt.2014.00054

Registered Nurses Association of British Columbia (RNABC). (2003).
Nurse-client relationships. Vancouver, BC: RNABC.

Research Center for Human-Animal Interaction (ReCHAI). (2008).
Veterans and shelter dogs initiative. Retrieved from http://vabenefitblog.
com/rechai-veterans-and-shelter-dogs-initiative

Rodriguez, T. (2017). Bipolar disorder, borderline personality disorder
may represent the same disorder. Retrieved from http://www.
psychiatryadvisor.com/bipolar-disorder/bipolar-disordersame-as-
borderline-personality-disorder/article/712397

Rossignol, D.A., & Frye, R.E. (2016). Environmental toxicants and autism
spectrum disorder. Retrieved from http://www.psychiatrictimes.com/
special- reports/environmental-toxicants-and-autism-spectrum-disorder

Sadock, B.J., Sadock, V.A., & Ruiz, P. (2015). *Synopsis of psychiatry: Behavioral sciences/clinical psychiatry* (11th ed.). Philadelphia, PA: Lippincott
Williams & Wilkins.

Saraswat, A., Weinand, J. D., & Sasfer, J.D. (2015). Evidence supporting
the biologic nature of gender identity. *Endocrine Practice, 21*(2),
199–204.

Schatzberg, A.F., Cole, J.O., & DeBattista, C. (2010). *Manual of clinical
psychopharmacology* (7th ed.). Washington, DC: American Psychiatric
Publishing.

Schoenen, J., Jacquy, J., & Lenaerts, M. (1998). Effectiveness of high-dose
riboflavin in migraine prophylaxis: A randomized controlled trial. *Neurology, 50,* 466–469.

Schroeder, B. (2013). Getting started in home care. *Nurse.com Nursing
CE Courses.* Retrieved from http://ce.nurse.com/course/60085/getting-
started-in-home-care

Schuster, P.M. (2012). *Concept mapping: A critical-thinking approach to care
planning* (3rd ed.). Philadelphia, PA: F.A. Davis.

Seligman, M. (1974). Depression and learned helplessness. In R. Friedman
& M. Katz (Eds.), *The psychology of depression: Contemporary theory and
research.* Washington, DC: V.H. Winston & Sons.

Selye, H. (1956). *The stress of life.* New York, NY: McGraw-Hill.

Shah, S.M., Carey, I.M., Harris, T., DeWilde, S., Victor, C.R., & Cook, D.G.
(2013). The effect of unexpected bereavement on mortality in older
couples. *American Journal of Public Health, 103*(6), 1140–1145.

Siegel, J.M., Angulo, F.J., Detels, R., Wesch, J., & Mullen, A. (1999). AIDS
diagnosis and depression in the Multicenter AIDS Cohort Study: The
ameliorating impact of pet ownership. *AIDS Care, 11*(2), 157–170.

Skinner, K. (1979, August). The therapeutic milieu: Making it work.
Journal of Psychiatric Nursing and Mental Health Services, 17, 38–44.

Souter, M.A., & Miller, M.D. (2007). Do animal-assisted activities effectively treat depression? A meta-analysis. *Anthrozoos, 20*(2), 167–180.
doi:10.2752/175303707X207954

Stein, T. (2015). *Natural remedies for PMS and premenstrual dysphoric disorder*. Retrieved from www.goodtherapy.org/blog/natural-remedies-pms-pmdd-0419124

Substance Abuse and Mental Health Services Administration (SAMHSA). (2012). Behavioral health issues among Afghanistan and Iraq U.S. war veterans. *SAMHSA In Brief*, 7(1).

Substance Abuse and Mental Health Services Administration (SAMHSA). (2015). *Trauma informed care and alternatives to seclusion and restraint*. Retrieved from https://www.samhsa.gov/nctic/trauma-interventions

Substance Abuse and Mental Health Services Administration (SAMHSA). (2017). *Critical issues facing veterans and military families*. Retrieved from https://www.samhsa.gov/veterans-military-families/critical-issues

Substance Abuse and Mental Health Services Administration (SAMHSA). (2019). *Homelessness programs and resources*. Retrieved from https://www.samhsa.gov/homelessness-programs-resources

Sullivan, H.S. (1953). *The interpersonal theory of psychiatry*. New York, NY: W.W. Norton.

Sullivan, H.S. (1956). *Clinical studies in psychiatry*. New York, NY: W.W. Norton.

Sullivan, H.S. (1962). *Schizophrenia as a human process*. New York, NY: W.W. Norton.

Sullivan, M., Bisaga, A., Pavlicova, M., Choi, C.J., Mishlen, K. Carpenter, K.M., ... Nunes, E.V. (2017). Long-acting injectable naltrexone induction: A randomized trial of outpatient opiate detoxification with naltrexone versus buprenorphine. *American Journal of Psychiatry*. doi:http://dx.doi.org/10.1176/appi.ajp.2016.16050548

Thompson, D.F., Ramos, C.L., & Willett, J.K. (2014). Psychopathy: Clinical features, developmental basis, and therapeutic challenges. *Journal of Clinical Pharmacology and Therapeutics, 39*, 485–495.

Toulany, A. & Katzman, D.K. (2019). Restrictive anorexia nervosa. *Psychiatric Advisor*. Retrieved from https://www.psychiatryadvisor.com/home/decision-support-in-medicine/pediatrics/restrictive-anorexia-nervosa/

Townsend, M.C., & Morgan, K.I. (2018). *Psychiatric mental health nursing: Concepts of care in evidence-based practice* (9th ed.). Philadelphia, PA: F.A. Davis.

Tucker, J., Fischer, T., Upjohn, L., Mazzera, D., & Kumar, M. (2018). Unapproved pharmaceutical ingredients included in dietary supplements associated with U.S Food and Drug Administration warnings. *JAMA Network Open, 1*(6), e183337. doi:10.1001/jamanetworkopen.2018.3337

Ulbricht, C. (2011). *Davis's pocket guide to herbs and supplements*. Philadelphia, PA: F.A. Davis.

Urvakhsh, M.M., Thirthalli, J., Aneelraj, D., Jadhav, P., Gangadhar, B.N., & Keshavan, M.S. (2014). Mirror neuron dysfunction in schizophrenia and its functional implications: A systematic review. *Schizophrenia Research, 160*(1-3), 9–19. doi:http://dx.doi.org/10.1016/j.schres.2014.10.040

USA.gov. (2013). *Military personnel records and statistics*. Retrieved from www.usa.gov/Federal-Employees/Active-Military-Records.shtml

U.S. Census Bureau. (2016). *Quick facts United States*. Retrieved from www.census.gov/quickfacts/table/PST045215/00

of Mayors (USCM). (2014). *A status report on hunger and America's cities: 2014.* Washington, DC: U.S. Conference of Mayors.

U.S. Department of Agriculture & U.S. Department of Health and Human Services. (2015). *Dietary guidelines for Americans 2015–2020* (8th ed.). Washington, DC: U.S. Government Printing Office.

U.S. Food and Drug Administration (FDA). (2016). *FDA requires strong warnings for opioid analgesics, prescription opioid cough products, and benzodiazepine labeling related to serious risks and death from combined use.* Retrieved from https://www.fda.gov/NewsEvents/Newsroom/Press Announcements/ucm518697.htm

U.S. Department of Justice. (2013). *A national protocol for sexual assault medical forensic examination: Adults/adolescents* (2nd ed.). Retrieved from https://www.ncjrs.gov/pdffiles1/ovw/241903.pdf

Valentino, R.J., & Van Bockstaele, E. (2015). Endogenous opioids: The downside to opposing stress. *Neurobiology of Stress, 1,* 23–32. doi:http://dx.doi.org/10.1016/j.ynstr.2014.09.006

Vallerand, A.H., Sanoski, C.A., & Deglin, J.H. (2017). *Davis's drug guide for nurses* (15th ed.). Philadelphia, PA: F.A. Davis.

Verona, E., & Patrick, C.J. (2015). Psychobiological aspects of antisocial personality disorder, psychopathy, and violence. *Psychiatric Times,* 1–7. Retrieved from wwwpsychiatrictimes.com

Victoroff, J. The neuropsychiatry of human aggression. In B.J. Sadock, V.A. Sadock, & P. Ruiz (Eds.). *Comprehensive textbook of psychiatry* (10th ed., pp. 2471–2504). Philadelphia, PA: Wolters Kluwer.

Viher, P.V., Stegmayer, K., Giezendanner, S, Federspiel, A., Bohlhalter, S., Vanbellingen, T., … Walthera, S. (2016). Cerebral white matter structure is associated with DSM-5 schizophrenia symptom dimensions. *Neuroimage: Clinical, 12,* 93–99.

Vlahos, K.B. (2012). The rape of our military women. *Anti-War.Com.* Retrieved from http://original.antiwar.com/vlahos/2012/05/14/the-rape-of-our-military-women

Volkmar, F.R., Klin, A., Schultz, R.T., & State, M.W. (2017). Autism spectrum and social communication disorder. In B.J. Sadock, V.A. Sadock, & P. Ruiz (Eds.), *Comprehensive textbook of psychiatry* (10th ed., pp. 3571–3586). Philadelphia, PA: Wolters Kluwer.

Wakefield, M. (2007). Guarding the military home front. *Counseling Today.* Retrieved from http://ct.counseling.org/2007/01/from-the-president-guarding-the-military-home-front

Wang, S., Hongling, Y., Zhang, J., Zhang, B., Liu, T., Gan, L., & Zheng, J. (2016). Efficacy and safety assessment of acupuncture and nimodipine to treat mild cognitive impairment after cerebral infarction: A randomized controlled trial. *BioMedCentral Complementary and Alternative Medicine, 16,* 361. doi:10.1186/s12906-016-1337-0

Weiss, H.D., & Pontone, G.M. (2014). Dopamine receptor agonist drugs and impulse control disorders. *JAMA Internal Medicine, 174*(12), 1935-1937. doi:10.1001/jamainternmed.2014.4097

Wertsch, M.E. (1996). *Military brats: Legacies of childhood inside the fortress.* St. Louis, MO: Brightwell.

Whitaker, J. (2000). Pet owners are a healthy breed. *Health & Healing 10*(10), 1–8.

Wisse, B. (2015). *Prolactinoma.* Retrieved from https://www.nlm.nih.gov/medlineplus/ency/article/000336.htm

Wolfe, J., Sharkansky, E.J., Read, J.P., Dawson, R., Martin, J.A., & Oimette, P.C. (1998). Sexual harassment and assault as predictors of PTSD symptomatology among U.S. female Persian Gulf military personnel. *Journal of Interpersonal Violence, 13*(1), 40–57.

Woolridge, T., & Lemberg, R. (2016). Macho, bravado, and eating disorders in men: Special issues in diagnosis and treatment. *Psychiatric Times, 33*(5). Retrieved from http://www.psychiatrictimes.com/special-reports/macho-bravado-and-eating-disorders-men-special-issues-diagnosis-and-treatment

Wootton, J. (2008). Meditation and chronic pain. In J.F. Audette & A. Bailey (Eds.), *Integrative pain medicine* (pp. 195–210). New York, NY: Springer-Verlag.

Worden, J.W. (2009). *Grief counseling and grief therapy: A handbook for the mental health practitioner* (4th ed.). New York, NY: Springer.

Yalom, I. (2005). *The theory and practice of group psychotherapy* (5th ed.). New York, NY: Basic Books.

Yates, W. (2019). Somatic symptom disorders. *Medscape.* Retrieved from http://emedicine.medscape.com/article/294908-overview

Yurkovich, E., & Smyer, T. (2000). Health maintenance behaviors of individuals with severe mental illness in a state prison. *Journal of Psychosocial Nursing and Mental Health Services, 38*(6), 20–31.

Subject Index

Drug Index

Nursing Diagnoses Index